WARM PATHOGEN DISEASES
A CLINICAL GUIDE

REVISED EDITION

WARM PATHOGEN DISEASES

A CLINICAL GUIDE

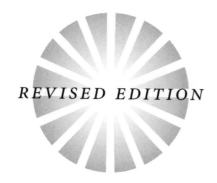

REVISED EDITION

Guohui Liu

EASTLAND PRESS • SEATTLE

©2001, 2005 by Eastland Press, Incorporated
P.O. Box 99749, Seattle, WA 98139 USA
www.eastlandpress.com

Library of Congress Control Number: 2005923285
International Standard Book Number: 0-939616-45-9
Printed in the United States of America

2   4   6   8   10   9   7   5   3   1

Edited by Dan Bensky, Jeff Gould, Louis Poncz, and John O'Connor
Indexed by Cynthia Landeen

Book design by Gary Niemeier

Table of Contents

Foreword

WHAT IS THE difference between Western and Chinese medicine? If one asks this question of a Chinese person today they will most likely point to differences in speed and application of treatment. Western medicine, they say, works fast and is best for acute disorders. Chinese medicine, by comparison, is slow and suited more for treating chronic illness. This response accords well with the use of Chinese medicine in the West where patients use it for those conditions that biomedicine finds difficult to treat. Infectious diseases are not widely perceived to fall within that category.

Not that long ago Chinese people provided very different answers to the same question. As late as the 1930s the general view, expressed most notably in an essay by the nationalist revolutionary and intellectual Zhang Tai-Yan (1869–1936), was that Western medicine excelled in treating organic illness while Chinese medicine was superior in treating seasonal disorders (時病 *shí bìng)*. Seasonal disorders are those diseases thought to have discernible external causes and thus include all kinds of infectious diseases, from colds and flu to meningitis and cholera. In line with Zhang's statement is the observation that in the twentieth century, as throughout its long history, the development of Chinese medicine remained inextricably linked to the treatment of seasonal disorders.

Shanghai-based physicians like Ding Gan-Ren (1865–1926), Xia Ying-Tang (1871–1936), Cao Ying-Fu (1868–1937), Yun Tie-Qiao (1878–1935), or Lu Yuan-Lei (1894–1955) who set Chinese medicine on its course of modernization in the early years of the last century, all became well-known by treating and discoursing about seasonal disorders. The money they earned in doing so and the viiiprestige they accumulated gave them the power and influence to establish the schools, societies, and journals that made Chinese medicine what it is today. Half a century later, it was the medical acumen shown by Pu Fu-Zhou (1888–1975), a physician from Sichuan, in getting on top of two meningitis epidemics in northern China, that vindicated the use of pattern differentiation (辯證 *biàn zhèng*) in the eyes of skeptical politicians and helped to safeguard a space for tradition within a process of rapid modernization.

Changes in morbidity and cheaply available antibiotic therapy have radically transformed contexts of practice in contemporary China. As a consequence, urban hospital based Chinese medicine has come to focus on the chronic disorders of modern living, while acute and life-threatening illness is treated in biomedical wards. And yet, many of Chinese medicine's most famous representatives continue to define themselves, and thereby the medicine they practice, through an affinity to seasonal disorders. All textbooks of internal medicine still start with chapters on such diseases. Formularies and materia medica begin with sections devoted to treating invasion of pathogens from the outside. And the collected writings and case records of venerated senior physicians all include prominent chapters on these problems.

Practitioners of Chinese medicine in the West usually begin their studies with a different set of priorities. During my own education in the early 1980s, for instance, the lecture on seasonal disorders lasted about as long as that on Four-Gentleman Decoction (*sì jūn zǐ tāng*). Constitution, spirit, and emotion rather than summerheat, dampness, or autumn dryness are the buzzwords that most easily catch the attention of modern students. While this situation is slowly changing, the scarcity of Western language literature on seasonal disorders still is striking to anyone who has ever browsed a Chinese bookshop or library.

This is unfortunate for two reasons. First, it effectively denies the average practitioner access to one of the most important disciplines in the history of Chinese medicine. Throughout the ages texts on seasonal disorders have been crucial in shaping Chinese medicine, not merely by providing therapeutic strategies. They defined how Chinese physicians thought about illness and demarcated fields of study. Affiliation to different streams of thought regarding the nature and treatment of seasonal disorders was expressed in the formation of schools, factions, and lineages whose genealogies make up the history of Chinese medicine. The combining of drugs for the treatment of seasonal disorders created aesthetics of prescribing that filtered into the treatment of other illnesses and thereby made Chinese medicine.

Second, if the availability of cheap antibiotic treatment marked a distinctive change in how Chinese medicine came to be practiced and perceived, then so will the post-antibiotic period that may be just around the corner. The spread of new strains of tuberculosis, super-bugs resistant to even the most potent antibiotics, and the emergence of new viral disorders conjoined to the effects of an ever accelerating process of globalization will, in all likelihood, radically transform the epidemiological landscapes of the twenty-first century. Chinese medicine may have an important role to play here, but only if we, as its practitioners, are ready.

Thus, publication of the present volume could not have come at a more opportune moment. It is the first English language text that provides more than a superficial introduction to the doctrines and practices of the warm pathogen disease stream (溫病學派 *wēn bìng xué pài*) in Chinese medicine. Starting in the Jin and Yuan dynasties, but accelerating from the late Ming onwards, the ideas of physicians belonging to this stream transformed traditional cold damage (傷寒 *shāng hán*) based approaches to the treatment of seasonal disorders. If previously wind and cold invasion or inopportune climatic conditions had been seen as the sole causes of such disorders, an entire universe of new pathogens and pathologies was gradually identified. These included not merely climatic factors such as warmth, heat, damp warmth, and dryness, but a wide array of pestilential (癘 *lì*) or heterogeneous (雜 *zá*) qi whose existence radically altered Chinese possibilities of thinking about illness in general.

These new ideas were diverse, and their proponents disagreed amongst themselves on many crucial issues. As a consequence, texts that sought to provide a coherent form to what had been invented emerged in the course of the nineteenth century. They defined the new medicine against, though not necessarily in opposition to, older cold damage therapeutics, centering it on the notion of warm pathogens. Most of these authors lived in the Yangzi River area of southern China, and before long issues of cultural and political identity infiltrated therapeutics. Hence, by the end of the nineteenth century, warm pathogen disease therapeutics had been defined as a medicine of the south, and placed in opposition to the cold damage medicine of the north.

While in practice physicians continued to build individual treatment strategies from a core of shared ideas, the revolution in Chinese medical education in the 1920s and 30s led to the compilation of the first textbooks devoted to the systematic study of warm pathogen diseases. This disciplining of an extremely heterogeneous and still developing tradition was accelerated in the 1950s and 60s, and again in the 1980s, through the formation of warm pathogen disease studies (溫病學 *wēn bìng xué*) as a core subject of Chinese medical education. A creative tension between mature systematization and innovative challenges to prevailing orthodoxies, however, prevails also in the present. While national textbooks present the discipline in systematic terms as a coherent whole, individual university departments and professors teach it based on personal experience, sometimes providing alternative teaching material. Individual physicians continue to produce new commentaries on older texts, try out new treatments, and advance innovative analysis. In doing so, they make the field of warm pathogen diseases one of the most lively and exciting in contemporary Chinese medicine.

What I admire most, therefore, about Dr. Liu's book—and there is much to admire—is his ability to condense all of this into a single text. Dr. Liu presents the field of warm pathogen disease studies in a clear and systematic manner without ever reducing its immanent vitality to principles set in stone. He has written a highly original textbook that is, at the same time, an important contribution to the development of warm pathogen disease studies as a medical discipline. As such, he addresses himself to three diverse groups of readers. He meets the demands of students for an introductory textbook that is sufficiently general to allow for an overall understanding of the discipline, yet specific enough to guide them toward clinically useful application. He considerably deepens the understanding of readers already familiar with basic principles of warm pathogen disease studies, helping them to develop a more sure-footed practice. And he expands the knowledge of anyone already regularly using warm pathogen disease treatment strategies in clinical practice through his keen insights and considerable experience. Dr. Liu's learning consistently opens up new horizons, yet never constrains readers from developing their own insights.

I warmly recommend this book to anyone interested in warm pathogen diseases. For the foreseeable future it will be the definitive English language textbook on the topic, but it is more than that—a guide into a field of medicine that no serious practitioner of Chinese medicine should be without.

—Volker Scheid, Ph.D.
London

Note to Revised Edition

The changes in this revised edition were primarily made to make it fit better with the new 3rd edition of *Chinese Herbal Medicine: Materia Medica*. Changes include updating both the pharmaceutical and pinyin names of the herbs, updating the formula names, addition of tone marks to herb and formula pinyin names, and new translations of book titles. There are also a few changes in terminology, most notably, *warm disease* is now *warm pathogen disease*, and *warm-febrile disease* is now *warm-heat pathogen disease*. We also took this opportunity to correct some minor errors in the text.

Preface

Background

THIS BOOK WAS written to describe the most important aspects and concepts of the warm pathogen disease school (溫病學說 *wēn bìng xúe shuō*) of Chinese medicine, and to convey how these can be used in understanding and treating disease. In this preface I would like to explain why I wrote the book, and to provide more background to help the reader understand the importance of this information.

Chinese medicine has developed rapidly over the past twenty-five years in the West. For example, today in the United States there are more than ten-thousand licensed acupuncturists and three thousand students enrolled in over forty schools of acupuncture. However, even today many people in the West have the mistaken idea that Chinese medicine is simply acupuncture. This is far from the truth. There are two general types of treatment in Chinese medicine: internal treatment, which is performed through the ingestion of oral medications; and external treatment, which includes such modalities as acupuncture, massage, and the topical application of herbs. While acupuncture is just a small part of Chinese medicine, it has some advantages that made it easier to introduce and be accepted by people in the West. It is safe, has very few side effects, and is relatively easy to learn and apply. In addition, its utility in treating pain syndromes and musculoskeletal disorders (due to its ability to promote the flow of qi and blood) without the side effects of biomedical pharmaceuticals has made it attractive. Still, acupuncture, like all modalities, has its shortcomings. It is particularly difficult to use acupuncture successfully in the treatment of diseases that are due to processes such as blood or yin deficiency, toxin, or damp-heat (which are the usual reasons for such biomedical conditions as hepatitis C, ulcerative colitis, viral myocarditis, and diabetes). I believe that this is due to the fact that acupuncture does not really add anything to the body that it might need to deal with these problems. It is also difficult to use acupuncture to treat pathogenic factors that have form, especially interior dampness. These types of conditions demand a medicine that can directly work on the yin and yang organs, can tonify qi, blood, yin, and essence, and can eliminate dampness, clear heat, and resolve toxicity. In Chinese medicine, this means the use of herbs.

I agree with the common sentiment that using herbs requires a deeper understanding of Chinese medical theories, and greater clarity of differentiation and treatment methods, than is necessary in the practice of acupuncture. In the West, most practitioners differentiate on the basis of the yin and yang organs for internal diseases. This is of great value, but still insufficient in many respects for treating a wide variety of illness, especially those that are externally contracted (外感 *wài gǎn*). To treat these diseases effectively, one must understand in a systematic and detailed manner how to predict and measure their progression, and then how to appropriately treat them. Organ differentiation alone is often insufficient for these purposes.

Traditionally, there have been three approaches in Chinese medicine to the differentiation and treatment of diseases caused by externally-contracted pathogens. The first is six-stage differentiation theory, first described in *Discussion of Cold Damage (Shāng hán lùn)* written by Zhang Ji (also known by his honorific name, Zhang Zhong-Jing) around the beginning of the third century. The second and third approaches are four-level and three-burner differentiation, developed by several physicians during the Qing dynasty (1644–1911). It is the latter approaches that comprise the main focus of this book. However, because these concepts have been used by a multitude of practitioners for hundreds of years, their use has been expanded beyond diseases caused by externally-contracted pathogens (e.g., wind-cold, wind-heat), and they are now also applied to internal disharmonies that may not be the direct result of such pathogens (e.g., internal dampness, blood stasis, blood, yin, and essence deficiency). In China for at least the last hundred years, it would be inconceivable for any medical practitioner to attempt to treat a highly difficult disease of any type without a full understanding of these three types of differentiation. As Chinese medicine continues to develop in the West, more and more acupuncturists are realizing that they need to learn more about these ideas if they are going to treat more difficult and serious diseases.

Over the past two decades, several Western language textbooks have introduced and discussed these three theories, thereby providing Chinese medicine students with a useful overview. However, such coverage has been simple and basic, such that many Western readers have not been exposed to the full sophistication and utility of these theories, particularly four-level and three-burner differentiation.

Both of these systems were developed and used by the warm pathogen disease school, which identified a group of diseases caused by warm-heat pathogens and developed concepts to address such diseases. As explained in Chapter 1 of this book, this school emerged in response to several epidemics that occurred in China two to four hundred years ago. In a world that values cutting-edge up to the minute ideas, these concepts may seem archaic, and some acupuncturists may view them as poor substitutes for modern biomedicine in the treatment of contemporary diseases. They present many questions. Are warm-heat pathogens equivalent to viruses, bacteria, and parasites? Are diseases caused by warm-heat pathogens the same as infectious diseases? Can these ancient theories still be used to treat current diseases in modern society, especially those caused by viruses, bacteria, and parasites, or allergies and cancers that may result from environmental pollution? Can herbs used by practitioners of the warm pathogen disease school be as effective as antibiotics? These are the questions that I am asked by students and practitioners alike during my classes and workshops.

These questions are easily answered, for the most part. From a Chinese perspective, the scope of externally-contracted diseases is not limited to infectious diseases, but also includes conditions due to allergies, environmental pollution, as well as some of those related to immune system dysfunction. In addition, while many of these problems can be approached with the theories related to diseases caused by cold and six-stage differentiation, the general opinion in China is that the majority of infectious diseases are best treated using the concepts of the warm pathogen disease school.

It is true that the effects of warm pathogen disease treatment are generally not as fast as those of antibiotics for bacterial diseases. However, antibiotics have many significant side effects, and their overusage has led to the development of resistant strains of bacteria. In addition, from a Chinese medical perspective, antibiotics are considered bitter and cold. This means that, if used indiscriminately, they can trap pathogenic factors inside the body. Moreover, while most viral diseases (e.g., influenza, mumps, hepatitis) cannot be treated by pharmaceuticals at the present time, there are effective treatments based on warm pathogen disease concepts. For example, during encephalitis B epidemics in China in the 1950s, and the influenza epidemic in the winter of 1999, warm pathogen disease treatments played an important role. Theories on diagnosis and the progression of disease derived from the warm pathogen disease school may even be helpful in treating some relatively new diseases, such as the opportunistic infections experienced by those living with AIDS.

Nor should we limit warm pathogen disease treatments to viral conditions, as they can also be effective for bacterial infections. The biomedical approach to bacterial infections is rather straightforward—find out what bacteria are responsible for the disease and choose an appropriate antibiotic to eradicate them. However, even from a biomedical perspective, this approach may be too simplistic. For example, should one not worry about the possible consequences of the residue of the killed bacteria that remain in the patient's body? This residue is made up of alien proteins that may stimulate the patient's immune system to produce corresponding antibodies, leading to an overactive or imbalanced immune system which may, in turn, lead to such common and irritating problems as sinusitis or allergies. In severe cases, autoimmune diseases or even cancer may be related to this breakdown of the immune system. Clinically, it is very common to see in patients with sinusitis or allergies a history of multiple antibiotic usage. From the viewpoint of Chinese medicine, when treating externally-contracted disease, one must spare no effort to *rid the body* of the exogenous factors, instead of simply killing them and then letting them stay in some form within the body. There are many ways in Chinese medicine to rid the body of exogenous pathogenic factors, including sweating, vomiting, purging, promoting urination, and bleeding, as well as friction modalities such a *gua sha*. To be sure, there is a wide variety of Chinese medicinals that can suppress or kill bacteria. However, according to the warm pathogen disease school, the overarching strategy must be to guide the pathogen out of the body. We never use antimicrobial herbs in isolation, but combine them with other herbs to remove the exogenous pathogens from the body.

Another concern with antibiotics, once considered to be the answer to many infectious diseases, is that they are losing their effectiveness against a number of illnesses because the bacteria are mutating and developing resistance. In general, bacterial resistance does not seem to develop in response to Chinese medicine. In part this is because we are treating the person's response to the disease instead of the disease itself, and in part it is because it is rare that we use a fixed combination of herbs. That is, we change the ingredients and dosage in an herbal prescription based on a patient's particular condition and constellation of symptoms. Even though a patient may seem to have the same common cold, sore throat, or cough at different times when he or she catches a cold, their physical constitution and the attacking pathogens may have changed, and the treatment is changed accordingly. Both Chinese medical theory and the experience of modern doctors of traditional Chinese medicine agree that antibiotics are more likely to keep a warm-heat pathogen (e.g., bacteria, viruses, and parasites) trapped and "lurking" inside the body, even though, from a Western biomedical point of view, they have been killed. This is because antibiotics are cold in nature and bitter in flavor, and cold and bitter substances readily suppress and block the qi, constrict the pores of the skin, and thereby trap warm-heat pathogens in the body. Thus, the advantage of warm pathogen disease treatment is that warm-heat pathogens will not remain in the body in any form, and they will build no resistance to the next treatment, even if the patient "caught" them again. What is more, there is a unique theory—called lurking pathogenic factors (伏氣學說 *fú qì xué shuō*), detailed in Chapter 3—which explains why warm-heat pathogens can stay hidden in the body and only present with signs and symptoms at a later time.

This theory provides a useful way to think of the side effects of the left over remnants of bacteria, viruses, and parasites, and offers an approach to treatment.

Living in the modern age, our bodies are affected by environmental factors like polluted air and water and chemicals in food, as well as natural changes such as abrupt changes in the weather. Also, our mental and physical condition is influenced by our lifestyle, including spending the majority of our time in air conditioned and centrally-heated environments, which can put us out of touch with the seasons. Concepts from the warm pathogen disease school can be used to treat the effects of these phenomena.

How to Use this Book

This book is divided into two parts. Part one discusses the history and theory of warm pathogen diseases, while part two discusses seven different types of warm pathogen disease. Traditionally, diseases caused by warm-heat pathogens have been classified and discussed according to the order of the seasons: wind-warmth in spring, spring-warmth in spring, summerheat-warmth in summer, damp-warmth in late summer or early autumn, autumn-dryness in autumn, and lurking summerheat in autumn or winter. This method of classification has been the dominant paradigm for teaching warm pathogen diseases in China for over forty years. While it does have the advantage of helping students identify certain types of warm pathogen disease, it gives a false impression that can affect diagnosis in the clinic. Many warm pathogen diseases can appear in two or three seasons, not just one particular season. Moreover, this approach ignores differences among the various warm-heat pathogens as to how they combine, especially between those with a significant aspect of dampness and those without. In this book, warm pathogen diseases are classified into two groups, those caused by heat and those caused by both heat and dampness. This was done because the presence or absence of dampness has a great impact on the resulting disease and treatment. My experience leads me to believe that readers will find it much easier to grasp differentiation and treatment of warm pathogen diseases by simply checking to see if dampness is involved.

In part two of the book, in addition to a discussion of etiology, factors used in identifying the disease, and treatment principles, the clinical manifestations have been grouped into several concurrent presentations which I believe will help the reader identify the patterns more easily. In addition, in order to help gain a deeper understanding of both the patterns and their treatment, comparisons are often made between similar patterns and formulas. One of the strengths of Chinese medicine is that a given problem can be understood and treated from a variety of perspectives. In this book I have tried to provide examples of some of the many approaches that can be used in the clinic.

The standard dosage for herbs can be found in *Chinese Herbal Medicine: Materia Medica* by Dan Bensky, Steven Clavey, and Erich Stöger.[1] Of course, in the clinic the dosage must be adjusted based on the condition of the patient. For example, for a heavy patient the dosage should be increased, while for a child it should be decreased. The dosage for herbs used in this book are *recommended ones* based on the source text in which a particular formula is found. Readers should choose the actual dosage according to the clinical situation. In general, I take the measurement of 1 *liáng* from the Han (206 BCE–280 CE) and Jin (280–420) dynasty texts as equal to 1 *qián* (3g). For formulas that are found in books written after that time, I consider 1 *liáng* equal 1 *liáng* (30g) today.[2]

Over the course of this book, citations to over one hundred and fifty ancient and modern Chinese medical texts can be found. This was done to deepen the reader's understanding of the development of the warm pathogen disease concept. Among these references are famous adages, short and to the point, that have become part of the fundamental way in which warm pathogen diseases are understood in Chinese medicine. In fact, these adages have become important to understanding many aspects of Chinese medicine, not just those of warm pathogen disease theory. I very much hope that the reader will enjoy reading these adages, and will apply them in their clinical practice. All of the books cited in the text are listed in the bibliography.

Chinese medicine has developed over a period of thousands of years. Throughout this book, as in this preface, are references to the various dynasties by which the Chinese measure their history. For the convenience of readers who are unfamiliar with Chinese history, we have included a table of Chinese dynasties in the back of the book (Appendix A).

In ancient China, people were born with both a family name (always placed first) and a given or personal name. However, men, when they became adults, often took another personal name, known as a style name (字 *zì*). Because the style name is more honorific, it is the one often referred to in the Chinese literature. For example Ye Gui had the style name Tian-Shi, and is often referred to as Ye Tian-Shi. To avoid confusion, both the given and style names for each of the cited authors is provided in Appendix B, together with the dates that they lived.

In order to help the reader understand the application of warm pathogen disease theory, especially the clinical usage of the formulas, a number of case studies are presented. Most of them are selected from famous practitioners in contemporary China, while some are from my own practice. Even if the manifestations described in these case studies are not exactly like those described in the main text, the basic pathology is the same. These cases are included to show the flexibility of warm pathogen disease theory and formulas in the clinic. Most of the cases that clearly mirror the description of a topic discussed in the text are placed right after the discussion of the pattern. Those which describe a somewhat different condition from that in the text, or a clinical extension of the concept and theory of warm pathogen disease, are placed in Appendix C. In some cases, the writers of the case studies have not specifically noted the name of the formula used, and in those cases I have added the name of the formula in parenthesis.

While many of the formulas discussed in this book have been described before in English, others have not. To facilitate access, a cross reference to the names of the formulas from pinyin to English is provided in Appendix D. In addition, a full index to every herb and formula mentioned in the text is provided at the back of the book.

Technical Considerations

Clinical results will almost always be better if the patient cooks the dried herbs and drinks the strained decoction. However, this can be time consuming (generally at least an hour), and the taste of a decoction is often not pleasant, to say the least. Both of these factors limit patient cooperation, especially for children, and herbs in granular form are an alternative. However, at the present time there are not many prepared or patent medicines on the market for warm pathogen disease formulas, except for those used in the early stages. In addition, if one uses prepared medicines, the practitioner cannot adjust the prescription to optimally fit the patient's condition. In my experience, while there is not much difference between the prepared medicines and herbal decoctions used for enriching the yin, the herbs in granular form are not as strong as the decoction in terms of eliminating warm-heat pathogens.

It is a general practice to tell the patient to take a packet of herbs each day. However, you might consider spreading this out over two days, as many people in the West appear to be more sensitive to Chinese herbs than is the average Chinese. This may be due to the fact that they seldom take Chinese herbs. Another possible reason is that, in general, the quality of exported herbs is better than for herbs used internally in China (although there are many exceptions). On the other hand, for severe and urgent cases, the patient may need to use two packets of herbs a day.

The following are my recommendations for making decoctions:

1. *Cooking pot:* In general, herbs should be prepared using ceramic pots and utensils. If this is not possible, enamel or stainless steel pots can be used. Do not use other metals.

2. *Cooking procedures:*
   - Normally, only one packet of herbs is cooked at a time. If there are herbs that need to be cooked for shorter or longer periods, they are put into separate bags.
   - Place the contents of one packet of loose herbs into the pot. Any herbs in separate bags are placed in other containers and soaked in a small amount of water.
   - Add water, usually until the level is one inch above the loose herbs. If most of the herbs are grassy, the water level should be higher, as dried grasses absorb more water than do other herbs. If most of the substances are minerals or

shells, the water level can be lower, as they absorb less water than grass. Soak for about 30 minutes.

- Bring the soaked herbs to a boil, cover the pot and let it simmer for 20 minutes. There are exceptions, of course. If the herbs are to be used for treating protective level patterns, they are cooked at medium-high for just 7 to 10 minutes. If they are to be used to enrich the yin, they should be cooked for 40 minutes. If there are any herbs that need to be cooked for a longer period of time, soak them in a separate pot for half an hour and cook for half an hour. Then add the herbs and liquid to the pot that contains the remaining herbs, and cook as described above. If there is a separate bag for herbs that should be added near the end, do so about five minutes from the end.

- After cooking, strain the liquid into a small glass or ceramic container. Save the cooked herbs to cook a second time. Herbs used to enrich the yin should be cooked three times.

- For the second or third cooking, cover the herbs with water to a level that is half an inch above the herbs, bring to a boil, and then simmer for an additional 15 minutes. Strain the liquid and mix with the liquid from the previous cooking. When done, discard the dregs. At this point the strained decoction is ready to drink.

3. *Administration:* In general, herbs should be taken half an hour after meals, as there is less chance of the herbs (whatever the form) irritating the stomach if there is some food in it. If the herbs are too bitter, patients without diabetes may add honey to the strained decoction, or mix the granules with applesauce. Alternatively, the granules can be put into capsules and taken with water.

We should be aware of the possibility of interactions between Chinese herbs and biomedical pharmaceuticals. According to John Chen, a pharmacologist and president of an herb company, there are a few steps that should be taken to avoid these interactions. First, allow 3-4 hours between the time that herbs are taken and the time when pharmaceuticals are taken. This is particularly important when the patient is taking drugs for gastrointestinal problems or antipsychotics. In addition, for patients taking pharmaceuticals, the herbs should be initiated at a low dosage and gradually increased. If a patient is taking a pharmaceutical that requires monitoring of its blood level (e.g., dilantin or warfarin) the blood levels should be monitored very carefully and more frequently than normal when taking herbs[3]

The liquid made from cooking herbs should usually be taken three times a day. For acute or critical conditions, the patient can take it every 4 to 6 hours, or even every hour. If a patient has lost consciousness, a nasogastric tube can be used.

The herbal liquid can be stored in a refrigerator for up to two days. It should be warmed up before being ingested. As there is some concern that microwaves could conceivably alter the effectiveness of the decoctions, I recommend that patients remove the saved decoctions from the refrigerator and either warm them up over a stove, or simply wait ten minutes or so until the liquid returns to room temperature.

This book includes a few topical herbal formulas. In order to avoid or minimize possible allergic skin reactions, I recommend that the topical paste or powder first be applied under the arms as a test. If there is no skin rash, itching or blistering, then you can apply it to the diseased area.

The reader should be alerted that some formula or patent remedies discussed in this book may contain substances that are illegal in certain countries, either because they contain endangered plant or animal species, or because they include toxic substances. While we have endeavored to give reasonable substitutions when possible, the reader should check with local laws before using them.

For the most part, the terminology used in this book follows the relatively literal gloss developed by Eastland Press. However, I have chosen to translate a few terms less literally when in my opinion a literal translation would be overly obscure. For example, the term 逆傳 *nì chuán* literally means rebellious or reversed progression. This is somewhat misleading, as it is a progression which has a worse prognosis than its counterpart 順傳 *shùn chuán*, which means smooth or normal progression. Therefore in this book *nì chuán* is translated as 'abnormal progression.' Another example is 'antipathogenic qi' instead of 'normal qi' for 正氣 *zhèng qì*, as I believe this more readily conveys the meaning of the term in Chinese medicine.

Acknowledgements

First, I would like to acknowledge my teacher Zhang Zhi-Wen, a professor at the Chengdu University of Traditional Chinese Medicine. He is the one who first taught me about warm pathogen disease theory during my college years. Ever since that time he has strongly supported my endeavors.

Because English is my second language, writing this book has been a big challenge. Also, because I presently live outside of China, it has been quite difficult for me to find the necessary references for this book. For these and other reasons, without help from the following people, this book could not have been written.

I owe Heiner Fruehauf, who brought me to United States, a debt of gratitude that is difficult to repay. Not only has he been a continuous support and inspiration for me here, he also provided many texts from his wonderful library, which were of great help in writing this book. The medical editor at Eastland Press, Dan Bensky, worked with great care and much patience on this project. During the editorial process, not only did he help me with the English itself, he also provided useful guidelines and valuable input on many technical issues. I am very grateful to Elizabeth Goldblatt for introducing me to Eastland Press, and supporting me in this writing for six years. I am indebted to Jeff Gould and Louis Poncz for editing the early versions of the manuscript and providing many useful suggestions, and to John O'Connor for his meticulous editing of the final version. I would also like to thank Volker Scheid and Charles Chace for their helpful criticism of the manuscript. I especially appreciate the excellent foreword for this book written by Dr. Scheid. I am very grateful to Meng-Ke Kou for supplying many useful books, and to Zheng Zeng for providing useful information about some rare herbs.

I deeply appreciate the patience, enthusiasm, and encouragement of my students at the Oregon College of Oriental Medicine, particularly Andrew Sutherland and Peter Borten, who respectively performed some of the initial editing and helped me with the botanical names for certain rare herbs.

Finally, I would especially like to thank Junlan Cai and Ruolan Liu for their boundless love, support, and forgiveness in keeping me in line throughout this long project. Also, I would like to thank my father Luyan Liu, my mother Yixin Liu, and my brother Lianghui Liu, for their continuous support, and for inspiring my medical career.

Endnotes

1. Dan Bensky, Steven Clavey, and Erich Stöger, with Andrew Gamble. *Chinese Herbal Medicine: Materia Medica, 3rd edition.* Seattle: Eastland Press, 2004.

2. These equivalencies are the standard in modern China. See Hubei College of Traditional Chinese Medicine, *Selected Readings from the Discussion of Cold Damage (Shāng hán lùn xuǎn dú).* Shanghai: Shanghai Science and Technology Publishing House, 1979: 162; Guangzhou College of Traditional Chinese Medicine, *Formulas (Fāng jì xué).* Shanghai: Shanghai Science and Technology Publishing House, 1983: 13.

3. John Chen, "Recognition and Prevention of Herb-Drug Interactions." Seminar in Portland, Oregon, 2001.

List of Tables

PART ONE

Introductory Materials

Historical Development of Warm Pathogen Disease Theory

1

Early Concepts in Warm Pathogen Disease Theory

WARM PATHOGEN DISEASE theory is now an integral part of Chinese medicine, although it took over a thousand years to mature. In the earliest Chinese medical texts, warm pathogen diseases were not regarded as a distinct group of disorders deserving their own theories and treatment. Instead they were subsumed under the general category of cold damage, as the accepted concept was that warm pathogen diseases were due to invasion of cold. It was not until the fourteenth century that the writer Wang Lü (Wang An-Dao, 1332-1391) first pointed out that warm pathogen diseases should not be confused with cold damage.[1] Then, in the fifteenth century, the physician Wang Ji (Wang Shi-Shan, 1463–1539) proposed that warm pathogen diseases could be contracted directly.[2] Thereafter, the development of warm pathogen disease theory accelerated as it came out from under the umbrella of cold damage theory, ultimately leading to a real revolution in the development of warm pathogen disease theory and treatment during the Qing dynasty (1644–1911). It was during this period that a number of important figures made major contributions to the development and maturation of warm pathogen disease theory and treatment protocols.

One important aspect of warm pathogen disease theory, that of lurking warm pathogen disease (伏氣溫病 *fú qì wēn bìng*), took even longer to gain acceptance. Its concepts were not generally adopted until the late nineteenth century. Unfortunately, even today this category of warm pathogen diseases is largely ignored or is regarded as only "a supplementary explanatory tool."[3] Recently, however, as practitioners of

3

Chinese medicine have been forced to deal with such problems as allergies that might develop subsequent to antibiotic treatment, they have realized the potential utility of the concepts of lurking warm pathogen disease. While these theories are not yet fully mature, they probably represent the next direction in the development of warm pathogen disease theory.

Clearly, warm pathogen disease theory is an important subject in traditional Chinese medicine because it includes unique systems of differentiation and has a long, venerable history of effective treatments. Moreover, the four level and three burner theories—hallmarks of the warm pathogen disease approach—are so effective that they cannot be replaced by other theories. It is said that knowing the theories described in the *Discussion of Cold Damage* is like fighting with only one arm, but with the theories and treatment methods of the warm pathogen disease school, you have another arm that enables you to fight disease more effectively.

In this chapter we will review the history and development of warm pathogen disease theory. Since this occurred over such a long period of time, it is easy to get lost. In order to help the reader review and grasp the key points, tables are provided that will summarize the following areas:

- Development of the concept of warm pathogen diseases
- Development of ideas concerning toxins within warm pathogen diseases
- Development of the theory and treatment of lurking warm pathogen diseases
- Development of the three burner differentiation of warm pathogen diseases
- Development of the theory of epidemic diseases within warm pathogen diseases
- Development of the concept of treating warm pathogen diseases by enriching the yin
- Development of the concept of treating warm pathogen diseases based on their type: damp-heat versus heat

YELLOW EMPEROR'S INNER CLASSIC *(Huáng dì nèi jīng)*

The first coherent attempt to explain the etiology of diseases was presented in the *Yellow Emperor's Inner Classic,* which was probably compiled in the second century.[4] In this book, the major factors in the generation of disease are said to be the individual's constitution, environmental factors, improper dietary habits, overwork, and emotional imbalance. Chinese medicine accordingly groups diseases into two principal categories:

1. Miscellaneous diseases from internal damage (內傷雜病 *nèi shāng zá bìng*) due to internal disharmony from problems relating to constitution, diet, work, or emotions
2. Externally-contracted seasonal diseases (外感時病 *wài gǎn shí bìng*) caused by environmental factors or external pathogenic factors such as wind, cold, summerheat, dampness, dryness, or fire.

Externally-contracted diseases were further subdivided into those caused by pathogenic factors that are primarily cold in nature and have a yin quality, and those that are hot in nature and have a yang quality. Those caused by cold pathogenic factors were called cold damage (傷寒 *shāng hán*) while those due to warm or hot pathogens were called warm pathogen diseases (溫病 *wēn bìng*).

Chapter 4 of *Basic Questions (Sù wēn)*, one component of the *Inner Classic*, contains the earliest reference to the term warm pathogen diseases[5] (see Table 1.1) as well as the observation that a body attacked by cold in the winter can suffer from warm pathogen disease in the spring, if that person's essence is inadequate.[6] In Chapter 33, "Discussion of Febrile Diseases" *(Rè bìng lùn)*, various symptoms of warm pathogen diseases are mentioned, including an initial fever that may return following an episode of sweating, rapid pulse, poor appetite, and delirium.[7] The treatment of warm pathogen diseases is addressed in Chapter 74, where it is advised to cool what is hot and to moisten what is dry.[8] In Chapter 72 it is recommended that a dispersing method be used to treat fire (heat) from constraint (鬱火 *yù huǒ*).[9] This idea had an immense influence on the treatment strategies devised by scholars and practitioners in the Qing dynasty.

Table 1.1	Development of the Concept of Warm Pathogen Diseases
Content	**Source**
First mention of warm pathogen diseases; only refers to warm pathogen diseases from lurking cold transforming into heat	Anonymous, *Yellow Emperor's Inner Classic*, c. 2nd century, Chapter 3
Proposed that warm pathogen diseases are specifically heat-related, and distinct from cold damage diseases	Zhang Ji, *Discussion of Cold Damage*, c. 200–210, Paragraph 6
Proposed that warm pathogen diseases should not be put into the same category as cold damage diseases	Wang An-Dao, *Discourse on Tracing Back to the Medical Classics*, 1368
First mention of the difference between newly-contracted warm pathogen diseases and lurking warm pathogen disease	Wang Ji, *Case Studies from Wang Shi-Shan*, 1519
Suggested that epidemic diseases are caused by specific pestilential qi	Wu You-Xing, *Discussion of Warm Epidemics*, 1642
Differentiated warm pathogen diseases into various types	Wu Tang, *Systematic Differentiation of Warm Pathogen Diseases*, 1798
Defined warm pathogen diseases as a group of acute, externally contracted, epidemic, febrile diseases that are caused by warm-heat pathogens at any time of year	Meng Shu-Jiang and Wang Le-Tao, *Warm Pathogen Diseases*, 1985

5

The first use of the term epidemic disease (疫 *yì*) was in Chapter 72 of *Basic Questions* where it was regarded as a form of toxin. Methods of prevention were also described.[10] In addition, five types of epidemic disease were said to be contagious, and their clinical manifestations similar, regardless of the age of the patient. It was also noted that "If the antipathogenic qi (正氣 *zhèng qì*) is strong enough, toxin cannot attack the body."[11] In Chapter 23 of the *Divine Pivot (Líng shū)*, the other component of the *Inner Classic*, it was suggested that one could clear the heat caused by warm-heat pathogens by inducing sweating and enriching the yin with acupuncture.[12]

Interestingly enough, the *Inner Classic* does not clearly distinguish between the concept of warm pathogen disease and that of cold damage, both of which can manifest with exterior signs and symptoms including chills, aversion to cold, and fever. This conceptual confusion is also reflected in the *Classic of Difficulties (Nán jīng)*, which was written slightly later than the *Inner Classic*.[13] There, cold damage is said to include five different diseases: wind-attack, cold damage, damp-warmth, hot disease, and warm pathogen disease. The relationship between heat and cold in externally-contracted diseases is unclear in these works.

DISCUSSION OF COLD DAMAGE *(SHANG HAN LUN)*

In his book *Discussion of Cold Damage and Miscellaneous Disorders (Shāng hán zá bìng lùn)*, Zhang Ji (Zhang Zhong-Jing, early third century), one of the most important figures in Chinese medical history, systematically discussed the differentiation and treatment of diseases caused by external pathogenic factors as well as those due to internal disharmony. He wrote in response to epidemics that occurred throughout China at the end of the Eastern Han dynasty (25–220). Unfortunately, the original version of this book is no longer extant, and was apparently lost during the wars and ensuing social disruption at the end of that era. However, portions of the book were found, reconstructed, and revised by Wang Xi (Wang Shu-He, dates unknown) at the end of the third century. That part which focused on diseases caused by cold was called *Discussion of Cold Damage*. In the sixth paragraph of this book, the term warm pathogen disease is applied to specific diseases marked by fever and thirst without aversion to cold.[14]

During the period 1023–1063 in the Song dynasty, Wang Zhu (dates unknown) discovered another portion of Zhang Ji's writings, which Li Yi (eleventh century) reconstructed and revised as *Essentials from the Golden Cabinet (Jin gui yao lue fang lun)*.[15] This was the first text to use the concept of the three burners to differentiate and treat internal disharmonies, which was a prelude to the three burner differentiation of warm pathogen diseases. For example, a passage in Chapter 11 of *Essentials from the Golden Cabinet* observes:

> If heat is in the upper burner, it can lead to cough and then develop into atrophy of the Lung; if heat is in the middle burner, it can lead to dry hard stools; and

if heat is in the lower burner, it can lead to bloody urine and disturbance and retention of urine.[16]

Zhang Ji also described two types of toxin patterns, yin toxin and yang toxin, with the following properties:

The manifestations of a yang toxin are a red area on the face like brocade, a sore throat, cough with pus, and blood. The manifestations of a yin toxin are a purple and blue color on the face and around the eyes, severe body aches like being beaten, and a sore throat.[17]

Zhang's approach to diagnosis and treatment was found to be very effective and was highly valued by both contemporary and later practitioners. Hua Tuo (Hua Yuan-Hua, died c. 208), a famous contemporary of Zhang Ji's, said that Zhang's book was one that could save lives.[18] About four-hundred years later, the renowned early-Tang physician and author Sun Si-Miao reported excellent results from using formulas listed in *Discussion of Cold Damage*.[19] For over a thousand years, the theories and treatments described by Zhang Ji were the chief means of differentiating and treating diseases caused by external pathogenic factors. As a result, his books became classics and gained him the appellation of "a secondary sage [of medicine]" (亞聖 *yà shèng*) relative to the Yellow Emperor.[20]

Although *Discussion of Cold Damage* focuses on diseases caused by cold, several of the treatment approaches described by Zhang had a tremendous influence on the later development of treatment protocols of the warm pathogen disease school, and are discussed elsewhere in this book. Examples include the heat-clearing formula White Tiger Decoction *(bái hǔ tāng)*, the formula to disperse heat from constraint, Gardenia and Prepared Soybean Decoction *(zhì zǐ chǐ tāng)*, and the yin-enriching and heat-clearing formula Coptis and Ass-Hide Gelatin Decoction *(huáng lián ē jiā tāng)*.

Early Developments in the Theory and Treatment of Warm Pathogen Diseases

While the theories in *Discussion of Cold Damage* were very successful, they could not explain every case of externally-contracted disease. The tantalizingly brief description of warm pathogen diseases in *Discussion of Cold Damage* piqued the interest of many and became a focal point for discussions about externally-contracted diseases that did not appear to be related to cold. These discussions were considered important even to those writers who held Zhang in high regard. For example, Wang Xi, who reconstructed and revised the *Discussion of Cold Damage*, stated in his preface to the book:

If a disease occurs immediately after exposure to cold, the disease is caused by cold. However, the cold does not bring out the disease [immediately]; rather, it can lurk in the skin and muscles. A warm pathogen disease will occur if the cold emerges in the spring, and summerheat disease will occur if the cold emerges during the summer.[21]

Wang distinguished cold damage from warm pathogen disease based on whether the cold was latent for a period of time, a concept not originally discussed by Zhang, but which further extends the idea first formulated in the *Inner Classic* concerning lurking pathogens.

The precise location of lurking cold in the body was addressed by Chao Yuan-Fang (c. 610) in *Discussion of the Origins of Symptoms of Disease (Zhū bìng yuán hòu lùn)*: the cold lurks in both the muscles and the bones.[22] This book also described various types of toxins (see Table 1.2), including cold damage toxin, febrile disease toxin, and warm pathogen disease toxin. Nevertheless, warm pathogen diseases were still regarded as a subcategory of cold damage in this book.

Table 1.2	Development of Ideas Concerning Toxins within Warm Pathogen Diseases	
Content		**Source**
First used the term 'toxin' as a cause of epidemic disease		Anonymous, *Yellow Emperor's Inner Classic: Basic Questions*, c. 2nd century
Described two types of toxin patterns: yin toxin and yang toxin		Zhang Ji, *Essentials from the Golden Cabinet*, c. 200
Described the signs and symptoms of several types of toxin-based disease		Chao Yuan-Fang, *Discussion of the Origins of Symptoms of Disease*, 610
Proposed that the common cause of all externally-contracted diseases is toxin, and that toxin can be divided into yin, yang, cold, and heat types		Pang An-Shi, *General Discussion for the Discussion of Cold Damage*, c. 1100
Regarded epidemic qi in the body as toxin; recommended using purgatives to eliminate the toxin		Wu You-Xing, *Discussion of Warm Epidemics*, 1642
Proposed that hot epidemic qi is a kind of formless toxin that will likely invade the Lung and Stomach; used many herbs with large dosages to clear heat and resolve toxicity for epidemic diseases caused by hot epidemic qi		Yu Lin, *Achievements Regarding Epidemic Rashes*, 1794

Table 1.2, cont.	
Advocated bitter and cold herbs that clear heat and clean toxin to stop and reverse the progression of warm pathogen diseases as early as possible, and at every level	Jiang Chun-Hua, "Ye Tian-Shi's Theory and Treatment for Warm Pathogen Disease and Internal Disease," 1978
Pointed out that pathogenic factors contain toxins which attack the body and give rise to heat patterns and progression; recommended focusing on clearing heat and resolving toxicity	Huang Xing-Yuan and Tian Ling-Qun, "General Description on Research and Study of Protective Qi, Ying, and Blood Theory in Warm Pathogen Diseases," 1986

By the Tang dynasty (618–896) there were some indications that treatments could be aimed at externally-contracted diseases not due to cold. Thus, although prior to this time the *Discussion of Cold Damage* was regarded as the "progenitor of all formulas" (眾方之祖 *zhòng fāng zhī zǔ*),[23] by the Tang dynasty formulas based on other principles were noted. For example, *Important Formulas Worth a Thousand Gold Pieces for any Emergency (Bèi jí qiān jīn yào fāng)* by the famous Taoist and physician Sun Si-Miao (581–682) included the formulas Solomon's seal Decoction *(wēi ruí tāng)*[24] to treat wind-warmth occurring in the spring; Rhinoceros Horn and Rehmannia Decoction *(xī jiāo dì huáng tāng)*[25] to treat heat-related bleeding trouble; and Purple Snow Special Pill *(zǐ xuě dān)*[26] to treat changes in consciousness due to intense heat. Another important book from this era, *Arcane Essentials from the Imperial Library (Wài tái mì yào)* by Wang Tao (c. 752), included Black Paste Formula *(hēi gāo fāng)*[27] for treating maculopapular rashes that appear as a result of warm toxin. This formula was based on a dispersing method for the treatment of what would later be regarded as warm pathogen diseases in the nutritive and blood levels. All of these formulas served as the bases for later approaches.

Nevertheless, during the Song dynasty (960–1279), the position of Zhang Ji's *Discussion of Cold Damage* became even stronger and dominated medical practice. It was, for example, required reading for all who hoped to enter the medical service of the emperor and his family.[28] An important event at this time was the first known annotation of *Discussion of Cold Damage* by Chen Wu-Ji (Chen Liao-She, c. 1115-1235).[29] These events helped to entrench the theory set forth by Zhang Ji in the minds of all physicians. However, while warm pathogen diseases were still regarded as being under the umbrella of cold damage, there were no treatments for them in *Discussion of Cold Damage* itself, forcing many physicians to face a contradiction. On the one hand, they were reluctant to question Zhang Ji, who by now was a medical icon; but on the other hand, they had to find a solution to deal with clinical cases that did not respond to the treatments described in his book. Their solution was to modify and adjust the approaches set forth in *Discussion of Cold Damage* to their own particular circumstances.

One such approach was to adapt the formulas to different climates. Pang An-Shi (Pang An-Shang, 1042–1099) noted:

> You will always be successful for patients who live in the north or west of China in any season when you use Cinnamon Twig Decoction *(guì zhī tāng)*.[30] But it can only be used in the winter and spring for patients who live between the Yangzi River and Huai River [in south-central China] where the climate is warmer than in the north and west of China. Scutellariae Radix *(huáng qín)* should be added for patients [in these areas] to Cinnamon Twig Decoction, Ephedra Decoction *(má huáng tāng)*[31] and Minor Bluegreen Dragon Decoction *(xiǎo qīng lóng tāng)*[32] from the end of spring to summer solstice. After the summer solstice, Anemarrhenae Rhizoma *(zhī mǔ)*, Gypsum fibrosum *(shí gāo)*, Isatidis Folium *(dà qīng yè)*, and Cimicifugae Rhizoma *(shēng má)* should be added when Cinnamon Twig Decoction is used to induce sweating.[33]

He also stressed that a common cause for all externally-contracted disease was toxin, which could be divided into yin, yang, cold, and heat types.[34]

Another approach was to broaden the understanding of externally-contracted diseases. Zhu Gong (Zhu Yi-Zhong, c. 1108) devised a system of classification that included cold damage, wind attack, summerheat attack, warm pathogen disease, wind-warmth, warm malarial disorders,[35] damp-warmth, epidemic disease, and warm toxin.[36] Zhu noted that a new attack from the outside was required to provoke the manifestation of lurking cold. This idea became important later (see Table 1.3).[37]

Table 1.3	Development of the Theory and Treatment of Lurking Warm Pathogen Diseases
Content	**Source**
Discussed warm pathogen diseases caused by an attack of cold in winter that remains in the body as a result of essence deficiency, and manifests in the spring; the term 'lurking' is not used	Anonymous, *Yellow Emperor's Inner Classic*, Chapter 3, c. 2nd century
Proposed the concept of a lurking pathogenic factor	Wang Xi, preface to *Discussion of Cold Damage*, c. 3rd century
Proposed that lurking cold manifests later after an attack by seasonal pathogenic factors	Zhu Gong, *Book to Safeguard Life Arranged According to Pattern*, 1108

Table 1.3, cont.	
Proposed the term 'lurking warm pathogen disease'	Case Studies from Wang Shi-Shang, 1519
Proposed the term 'lurking summerheat' and briefly discussed its causes	Wang Ken-Tang, *Indispensable Tools for Pattern Treatment*, 1602
Proposed that epidemic qi attacks the body through the mouth and nose and lurks in the membrane source	Wu You-Xing, *Discussion of Warm Epidemics*, 1642
Outlined a treatment protocol for newly-contracted warm pathogen diseases and lurking warm pathogen diseases, and divided lurking warm pathogen diseases into two types:spring warmth caused by an attack of cold in the winter, and lurking summerheat disease	Ye Gui, *Case Studies as a Guide to Clinical Practice*, 1746
Refuted the idea that cold damage transforms into warm pathogen disease	Yang Xuan, *Systematic Differentiation of Cold Damage and Warm Epidemics*, 1784
Proposed that damage to the essence, which allows cold to lurk in the body, is caused not only by excessive sexual activity, but by other activities as well	Wu Tang, *Systematic Differentiation of Warm Pathogen Diseases*, 1798
Summarized the different pathological changes and treatment protocols for newly-contracted warm pathogen diseases and lurking warm pathogen diseases	Wang Shi-Xiong, *Warp and Woof of Warm- Febrile Diseases*, 1852
Proposed the treatment method for eliminating the lurking warm-heat pathogen by enriching the Kidney yin	Shao Deng-Yin, *Mechanisms for Diseases of the Four Seasons*, 1879
Divided warm pathogen diseases into two types: newly-contracted diseases and seasonal lurking warm pathogen diseases	Lei Feng, *Discussion of Seasonal Diseases*, 1882
Proposed that wind-heat and the seven abnormal emotions can induce a lurking pathogen to manifest	Ye Lin, *Explanation of Lurking Qi*, c. 1897
Proposed that pathogens can lurk in the body due to improper treatment; discussed six lurking warm pathogen diseases	Liu Ji-Ren, *New Treatise on Lurking Pathogens*, c. 1898

Table 1.3, cont.	
Proposed the treatment method of both enriching the Kidney yin and clearing and venting lurking warm-heat pathogens	Liu Bao-Yi, *Encountering the Sources of Warm-Heat Pathogen Diseases*, c. 1900
Divided lurking disease into two types:that caused by cold and that caused by summer- heat; compared newly-contracted warm pathogen diseases and lurking warm pathogen diseases, and set forth a general treatment principle for lurking warm pathogen diseases	He Lian-Chen, *Revised and Expanded Discussion of Warm-Heat Pathogen Diseases*, 1907
Proposed that warm-heat pathogens lurk in the Triple Burner and that the progression of the lurking warm pathogen disease depends on constitutional factors	Zhang Xi-Chun, *Essays on Medicine Esteeming the Chinese and Respecting the Western*, 1918

Zhang Yuan-Su (Zhang Jie-Gu, c. 1186) was the first person to be openly skeptical about the applicability of the concepts and treatments of Zhang Ji. He noted that the patterns of climate and other cosmic forces were not unchanging, and that the "past and present are on different tracks. Ancient formulas are not efficacious for new diseases."[38]

Liu Wan-Su (Liu Shou-Zhen, 1120–1200), known as the founder of the cold and cooling school of medicine, modified many formulas from *Discussion of Cold Damage.* He used more bitter, acrid, and cold herbs because he observed that many practitioners used acrid and warm herbs to treat febrile diseases without success. He pointed out that all the patterns of progression in the six stages are heat patterns, even if they derive from external cold.[39] He also discussed the pathology of febrile diseases, and was the first to point out that such diseases could be due to cold constraining the yang qi, which thereupon produces heat.[40] Based on these observations, he recommended the use of acrid and cooling herbs such as Allii fistulosi Bulbus *(cōng bái)* and Sojae Semen preparatum *(dàn dòu chǐ)* to disperse the constrained yang qi and eliminate the pathogen.[41] One of his formulas, Double Resolving Powder *(shuāng jiě sǎn),* also known as Relieve Exterior and Treat Interior Powder *(jiě biǎo zhì lǐ sǎn),* contains Gardeniae Fructus *(zhī zǐ)* and Sojae Semen preparatum *(dàn dòu chǐ)* for both an exterior pattern and interior heat.[42] This was a radical departure from the use of acrid and warm herbs in treating exterior patterns. It marked an important step in the differentiation of warm pathogen diseases from cold damage, and greatly affected later practitioners.

Liu Wan-Su also made important contributions to the use of the three burners in diagnosis and treatment (see Table 1.4). In *Collection of Writings on the Mechanism of Disease, Suitability of Qi, and the Safeguarding of Life as Discussed in Basic Questions (Sù wèn bìng jī qì yí bǎo míng jí),* he used the three burners to differentiate the stages of warm pathogen diseases. For example, "Maculas and papules cannot be purged when they appear at the onset of a disease that is located in the upper burner, nor at the end when they are located in the lower burner."[43] The clinician should therefore devise a treatment based on which burner was affected.

In light of his many contributions, it is clear why practitioners began to follow Liu Wan-Su's ideas when treating diseases caused by heat,[44] and why he has been regarded as one of the founders of warm pathogen disease theory.[45] Even so, most practitioners at this time were still too constrained by the concepts in *Discussion of Cold Damage,* and confused about the differences between cold damage and warm pathogen diseases. Looking back from the vantage point of the late eighteenth century, Wu Tang (Wu Ju-Tong, 1758–1836), who features prominently in the balance of this chapter, thought a milestone had been reached when Wang Lü (Wang An-Dao, 1332–1391) proposed that warm pathogen diseases should not be put in the same category with cold damage.[46] In *Discourse on Tracing Back to the Medical Classics (Yī jīng sù huí jí),* Wang observed:

> After being attacked by cold, should a patient become immediately ill, this immediate illness is called cold damage. If the illness appears later, especially in the spring and summer, it is called warm pathogen disease or summerheat disease.

Table 1.4	Development of Three-Burner Differentiation of Warm Pathogen Diseases	
Content	**Source**	
First used three burners to differentiate and treat internal disharmonies	Zhang Ji, *Essentials from the Golden Cabinet,* c. 200	
First used three burners to categorize the various stages of warm pathogen diseases	Liu Wan-Su, *Collection of Writings on the Mechanism of Disease, Suitability of Qi, and the Safeguarding of Life as Discussed in Basic Questions,* 1186	
Proposed the concept of treating epidemic diseases according to their location in the three burners	Yu Chang, *Writing on the Esteemed Discussion,* 1658	
Developed the three-burner method of differentiation, promoted the idea of using qi circulation, and transformed and drained dampness for three-burner patterns	Ye Gui, *Case Records as a Guide to Clinical Practice,* 1746; Ye Gui, *Discussion of Warm-Heat Pathogen Disorders,* 1792	
Located diseases caused by epidemic qi according to three-burner theory	Yang Xuan, *Systematic Differentiation of Cold Damage and Warm Epidemics,* 1784	
Used the concept of three burners to differentiate the onset and progression of various stages of warm pathogen diseases	Wu Tang, *Systematic Differentiation of Warm Pathogen Diseases,* 1798	

Because all of these diseases have been caused by an attack of cold, they could be called cold damage, but the treatments should vary. If practitioners do not realize the difference between them, it is not fair for those practitioners to attribute their mistakes to Zhang Ji. This is just like blaming Su Ren [credited with finding a method to drill wood and make fire] for all the disasters due to improper management of fire because he devised a method for making fire.[47]

Although he provided neither detailed explanations nor methods of treatment, Wang Lü's new idea about differentiating warm pathogen diseases from cold damage strongly influenced later scholars and practitioners.

Further Developments in the Theory and Treatment of Warm Pathogen Diseases

Following the Song dynasty there were many outbreaks of epidemic disease in China. There were approximately sixty-four major epidemics during the Ming dynasty (1368–1644) and seventy-four during the Qing era.[48] These were very important events to the physicians of those times, just as the epidemics at the end of the Han dynasty had influenced Zhang Ji. The epidemics also left practitioners demoralized since they could not treat them successfully using the methods described in *Discussion of Cold Damage*. Thus, they were motivated to find new theories to explain the etiology of these epidemics, as well as new methods for treating them. For example, in a neighborhood that had once housed several hundred people near the home of Wu You-Xing (Wu You-Ke, c. 1582–1652), the epidemic of 1642 was so severe that no one survived.[49] These outbreaks inspired Wu to write *Discussion of Warm Epidemics (Wēn yì lùn)*, which describes epidemic and warm pathogen diseases in some depth; this had not been previously done. Wu stated that epidemic diseases are caused pestilential qi (癘氣 *lì qì*), a special contagious pathogenic factor that:

- Can be transmitted from one person to another, unlike wind, cold, or dampness (see Table 1.5)
- Acts as a toxin once it invades the body[50]
- Attacks through the mouth and nose, rather than through the skin and muscles, as cold damage is said to do[51]
- Does not manifest symptoms soon after the exposure to the pathogen.

All of this implied that special treatment would be needed to treat pestilential qi.

Wu distinguished epidemic diseases from cold damage based on differences in onset, transmission, treatment, and prognosis. He said that these two types of disease were as different as heaven and earth, and that confusing them would be like mistaking a deer for a horse.[52] According to Wu, epidemic qi resides and lurks in the membrane source (膜原 *mó yuán*).[53] He developed a formula for treating this known as Reach the Source Drink (*dá yuán yǐn*).[54]

14

Table 1.5	Development of the Theory of Epidemic Diseases within Warm Pathogen Diseases
Content	**Source**
First to discuss epidemic diseases and prevention method; thought that all five types of epidemic disease are contagious	Anonymous, *Yellow Emperor's Inner Classic: Basic Questions*, c. 2nd century
Explored the real cause and natural history of epidemic diseases	Wu You-Xing, *Discussion of Warm Epidemics*, 1642
Distinguished epidemic diseases from cold damage based on observation, odor, and pulse; also divided epidemic diseases into exterior and interior patterns	Dai Tian-Zhang, *Expanded Discussion of Warm Epidemics*, 1778
Located the diseases caused by epidemic qi based on three-burner theory	Yang Xuan, *Systematic Differentiation of Cold Damage and Warm Epidemics*, 1784
Identified the cause of epidemic diseases as toxic qi	Liu Kui, *Song-Feng Explains Epidemics*, c. 1789
Pointed out that hot epidemic qi is a type of formless toxin that will likely invade the Lung and Stomach	Yu Lin, *Achievements Regarding Epidemic Rashes*, 1794

Wu also strongly recommended the use of Rhei Radix et Rhizoma *(dà huáng)* and other purgatives to lead toxins out of the body. He realized that both the epidemic qi and purging method itself would injure the yin. In order to protect it, he combined purging with herbs that enrich the yin in formulas like Order Qi and Nourish the Nutritive Decoction *(chéng qì yǎng yíng tāng)*. [55] He also recommended that sweet and warm herbs, such as Ginseng Radix *(rén shēn)*, Astragali Radix *(huáng qí)*, and Atractylodis macrocephalae Rhizoma *(bái zhú)*, be avoided after purging since they could lead to an increase in heat and thereby further damage the yin. Instead, he suggested that these patients drink pear juice, fresh lotus node juice, and sugar cane juice, and eat watermelon.[56] These ideas influenced later writers such as Wu Tang, who developed formulas like Increase the Fluids and Order the Qi Decoction *(zēng yè chéng qì tāng)*[57] and Five Juice Drink *(wǔ zhī yǐn)*[58] along the same lines (see Table 1.6).

These concepts had a huge influence on the development of the theories and treatment of warm pathogen diseases. Wu was particularly influential as his was the first book to discuss any type of externally-contracted disease, in this case epidemic disease, as something different from cold damage. Later writers, however, did take him to task for confusing epidemic diseases, which are but one type of warm pathogen disease, with the category of warm pathogen diseases in general.

Table 1.6	Development of Concept of Treating Warm Pathogen Diseases by Enriching the Yin	
Content	**Source**	
Suggested reducing the heat caused by a warm-heat pathogen by inducing sweating and enriching the yin with acupuncture	Anonymous, *Yellow Emperor's Inner Classic: Divine Pivot*, Chapter 23, c. 2nd century	
Recorded several formulas for enriching the yin that are widely used for treating warm pathogen diseases	Zhang Ji, *Discussion of Cold Damage*, c. 200	
Suggested using sweet, moist, and slightly cold herbs to nourish Lung yin	Yu Chang, *Precepts for Physicians*, 1658	
Proposed protecting the Kidney, which was not yet affected by a disease, by using salty and cold herbs	Ye Gui, *Discussion of Warm-Heat Pathogen Disorders*, 1792	
Discussed treating the upper and middle burners with sweet and cold herbs to enrich the yin, and treating the lower burner with sweet, salty, and cloying herbs to enrich the yin and support the essence	Wu Tang, *Systematic Differentiation of Warm Pathogen Diseases*, 1798	

Many people were influenced by Wu. One of the most important was Dai Tian-Zhang (Dai Lin-Jiao, 1644–1722), author of *Expanded Discussion of Warm Epidemics (Guǎng wēn yì lùn).*[59] Dai distinguished epidemic diseases from cold damage based on differences in the patient's complexion, smell, and pulse, and was the first to enumerate the different methodologies for treating warm pathogen diseases: sweating, purging, clearing, harmonizing, and tonifying. He also suggested that purgatives could eliminate heat from constraint and should be used as early as possible. To him, purgatives removed the fuel that allowed the fire to burn and therefore could not be used too early in the course of a disease. Based on my own experience, this approach can indeed shorten the course of treatment, and sometimes even improve the outcome.

Yang Xuan (Yang Li-Shan, c. 1700–1784) wrote *Systematic Differentiation of Cold Damage and Warm Epidemics (Shāng hán wēn yì tiáo biàn).*[60] Unlike Wu You-Xing, who suggested that epidemic qi resides in the membrane source, Yang Xuan located the epidemic qi within the Triple Burner. In Yang's opinion, heat from constraint was an important aspect of epidemic diseases, and he recommended that treatment combine clearing heat as well as dispersing the stagnation within the Triple Burner.[61] Yet irrespective of the treatment method, his formulas always included the combination of Bombyx batryticatus *(bái jiāng cán)* and Cicadae Periostracum *(chán tuì)*, which are the main ingredients in Ascending and Descending Powder *(shēng jiàng sǎn)*,[62] his flagship formula for dispersing heat from constraint. In addition, Yang described fifteen modifications for specific problems. Many highly-regarded contemporary practitioners in China follow this approach. One, Pu Fu-Zhou, who counted the leaders of the Chinese Communist Party among his patients, stated that "[Our] clinical results with warm pathogen diseases will be very good if we use the fifteen formulas of Yang Xuan."[63]

Because of the recurrent and devastating epidemics and related social upheaval that occurred during the Qing dynasty, old ways of thinking were challenged and many new ideas appeared. The importance and location of hot epidemic qi (熱疫 *rè yì*) was emphasized by Yu Lin (Yu Shi-Yu, 1736–1795) in *Achievements Regarding Epidemic Rashes (Yì zhěn yī dé)*. [64] For Yu, hot epidemic qi was a type of formless toxin that was more likely to invade the Stomach than the membrane source.[65] The work of Yu Lin, Wu, and Yang established the epidemic disease school, which is one important component of warm pathogen disease. Their strategy of aggressively attacking epidemic qi or toxin by clearing and purging with bitter, cold herbs is still useful in the clinic today.

The terms newly-contracted warm pathogen disease (新感溫病 *xīn gǎn wēn bìng)* and lurking warm pathogen disease (伏氣溫病 *fú qì wēn bìng)* were coined by Wang Ji, who also argued that lurking pathogens may not be the only cause of warm pathogen diseases, and that they may be contracted directly. Wang observed:

> If a patient is attacked by cold in the winter and manifests a disease in the spring without being attacked by a secondary external pathogenic factor, it is called warm pathogen disease and its condition is mild. If the patient is attacked by warm-heat pathogen in the spring and the pathogenic factor has transformed into warm toxin, this is still called warm pathogen disease and its condition is serious. These two types of warm pathogen disease belong to [the categor y of] lurking warm pathogen disease. However, there is a type of warm pathogen disease in the spring that is not caused by an attack of cold in the winter, and this type of warm pathogen disease is called spring-warmth. It is similar to an attack of cold in the winter, of dampness in the autumn, and of summerheat in the summer. All of these are called newly-con-tracted warm pathogen disease.[66]

These ideas had a receptive audience, as evidenced by Wang Ken-Tang (Wang Yu-Tai, c. 1549–1613), who wrote in *Indispensable Tools for Pattern Treatment (Zhèng zhì zhǔn shéng)* that "Warm pathogen diseases that manifests with no aversion to cold and thirst can occur in [any of] the four seasons, rather than just in the spring."[67] This idea of newly-contracted warm pathogen disease was a breakthrough concept. Not only did it add another type of warm pathogen disease, but more importantly, it was a clear and open acknowledgement that there were pathogens that lead directly to warm pathogen disease. This idea allowed the concept of warm pathogen disease to become something distinct from cold damage, as it was no longer thought of as simply lurking cold transforming into heat.

Another important contribution of Wang's was the idea of lurking summer-heat, which he only briefly discussed. Because of its prevalence, summerheat came to the forefront during the latter days of the Ming dynasty. The first book to systematically discuss the differentiation and treatment of summerheat disease was *Revised and Expanded Complete Treatise on Summerheat Damage (Zēng dìng shāng shǔ quán shū)*,[68] written by Zhang He-Teng (Zhang Fen-Kui, c. 1623). Zhang stated that summerheat disease was derived from an attack of summerheat during the summer season, and not from lurking cold that had transformed into summerheat. This idea influenced Ye Gui (see below) who wrote approvingly in *Differentiating Lurking Pathogens and Externally Contracted Diseases during Three Seasons (Sān shí fú xié wài gǎn piàn)*[69] of Zhang's idea of forgoing the use of purgatives, and instead treating summerheat from the start with acrid and cool herbs, then with sweet and cold herbs, and finally (in a later stage) with sour and sweet or sour and bitter herbs. At around the same time, the famous late-Ming-dynasty physician Zhang Jie-Bin (Zhang Jing-Yue, 1563-1640) also wrote about summerheat, suggesting that it be divided into yin and yang types.[70] Summerheat diseases with relatively more dampness were considered relatively yin, while those with less dampness were considered yang.

The Flourishing of Warm Pathogen Disease Theory and Practice

As we have seen, by the early sixteenth century, which was well over a thousand years since the initial appearance of *Discussion of Cold Damage*, new ways of analyzing and treating warm pathogen diseases had begun to emerge. This process accelerated during the next few centuries. For example, Yu Chang (Yu Jia-Yan, c. 1585–1664) in *Writing on the Esteemed Discussion (Shàng lùn piān)*, advanced the idea of differentiating and treating epidemic diseases according to their location in the three burners: "[Warm-heat pathogens] attack the body through the mouth and nose, first invading the middle burner, and then progressing to the upper burner or lower burner. … This is how the three burners are used to identify the location of a warm-heat pathogen."[71] He also said that warm-heat pathogens should be eliminated with aromatic herbs, and that treatment should vary depending on which of the three burners was affected:

> The upper burner is like mist, so lift up and drive out [warm pathogens in it] while also resolving toxicity. The middle burner is like foam, so disperse and drive out [warm pathogens in it] while also resolving toxicity. The lower burner

is like a drainage ditch, so dredge and drive out [warm pathogens in it] while also resolving toxicity.[72]

These ideas, based on concepts that can be traced to the *Inner Classic*[73] and the works of early practitioners like Yang Xuan and Liu Wan-Su, greatly influenced Wu Tang (see below), who is credited with devising the system of three-burner differentiation.[74]

However, the most important developments in warm pathogen disease theory did not occur until a series of physicians fully developed its ideas during the Qing dynasty. Ye Gui (Ye Tian-Shi, c. 1666–1745), Xue Xue (Xue Sheng-Bai, 1681–1770), Wu Tang (Wu Ju-Tong, 1758–1836), and Wang Shi-Xiong (Wang Meng-Ying, c. 1808–1867) developed and elaborated upon the theories of differentiation of warm pathogen diseases according to the four levels (protective, qi, nutritive, blood) and three burners (upper, middle, lower). These works form the core of the warm pathogen disease school's approach to medicine.

The period from 1663 to 1795 is referred to as the Kang-Qian era after the titles of the emperors who ruled China during this time. It was an extremely prosperous period for the Chinese economy during which many aspects of Chinese culture flourished, including Chinese medicine. For example, the great compendium known as the *Golden Mirror of the Medical Tradition (Yī zōng jīn jiàn)*[75] was compiled and edited by Wu Qian (Wu Liu-Jie, 1736-1795) at the behest of the Qianglong emperor. In the relatively short span of one-hundred fifty years, dramatic advances were made in warm pathogen disease theory and practice, including methods for differentiating and treating a wide variety of warm pathogen diseases. The center for this work was the Wu area of southern China, which includes the present provinces of Jiangsu, Anhui, and Zhejiang, as well as the city of Shanghai. These advances were the product of a struggle between those who stuck solely to the concepts found in *Discussion of Cold Damage* and those who were developing new ideas for treating and understanding warm pathogen diseases.

YE GUI (1666–1745)

Ye Gui is regarded as the most brilliant of the physicians who developed the concept of warm pathogen diseases. He came from a family of physicians that included his father and grandfather. His father, a specialist in skin disorders and pediatrics, taught him the medical classics, including the *Inner Classic* and *Discussion of Cold Damage*. In addition, Ye Gui actively sought out other teachers. It is said that by the time he was eighteen, Ye had studied with seventeen different teachers.[76]

In *Discussion of Warm-Heat Pathogen Disorders (Wēn rè lùn)*,[77] Ye set forth the protocols for differentiating the various disease stages according to the four levels, and discussed the etiology, pathology, location, transmission, and treatment of warm pathogen diseases in detail. He was the first person to systematically describe a four-

19

level theory to differentiate and treat warm pathogen diseases. Moreover, his book *Case Records as a Guide to Clinical Practice (Lìn zhèng zhǐ nán yī àn)*[78] contains more than two thousand case histories which demonstrate how to treat warm pathogen diseases using these concepts.

Ye made many other contributions to the understanding and treatment of warm pathogen diseases:

- He identified two types of warm pathogen disease: those associated with dampness and those that lack dampness (see Table 1.7).[79]
- Ye outlined the treatments for both newly-contracted warm pathogen diseases and lurking warm pathogen diseases.[80] He divided lurking warm pathogen diseases into two types: spring-warmth (春溫 *chūn wēn),* which is caused by an attack of cold in the winter but manifests in the spring;[81] and lurking summerheat (伏暑 *fú shǔ),* which is caused by lurking summerheat during the summer season, but is induced by cold in late autumn.[82]
- Ye believed that the lurking cold of winter resides in the Kidney.[83]
- Ye further developed the three-burner method of differentiation first mentioned by Liu Wan-Su, and recommended the use of promoting qi circulation, transforming dampness, and draining dampness for three-burner patterns.
- Ye was the first to treat various levels of warm pathogen disease with acrid, aromatic, cool, and light herbs to dissipate and vent heat from constraint from the body.[84]
- Influenced by the classical idea that it was better to treat a disease *before* it manifests,[85] Ye suggested that one should protect the Kidney, which was not yet affected by disease but had a preexisting deficiency, by adding salty and cold herbs to the more commonly prescribed sweet and cold herbs. An example would be the use of herbs that enrich Kidney yin, in patients with underlying Kidney yin deficiency, when treating these patients for recalcitrant fever after an eruption of maculas.

Among Ye's many contributions was his expansion of the tools of diagnosis. While tongue diagnosis had been used in China since at least the time of the *Inner Classic,* Ye described some unique qualities on the tongue. He also wrote in detail about the diagnostic value of differentiating various types of skin eruptions in patients with warm pathogen diseases, as well as differences in their teeth. (These subjects will be further explored in Chapter 5.) All of these contributions distinguish Ye Gui as the foremost physician in the development of the theory and treatment of warm pathogen diseases.

Xue Xue (1681-1770)

Xue Xue was a contemporary of Ye Gui. In *Systematic Differentiation of Damp-Heat (Shī rè tiáo biàn)* Xue discussed the etiology, pathology, differentiation, and treat-

Table 1.7	Development of Concept of Treating Warm Pathogen Diseases Based on Their Type: Heat vs. Damp-Heat
Content	**Source**
Identified diseases due to damp-heat; treated them with sweet and bland herbs, promoting qi circulation, and transforming dampness	Ye Gui, *Discussion of Warm-Heat Pathogen Disorders*, 1792
Recognized that damp-heat diseases are different not only from cold damage, but also from warm pathogen diseases caused only by heat; chose herbs according to which burner is affected	Xue Xue, *Systematic Differentiation of Damp- Heat*, 1770
Identified two types of warm pathogen disease: those with dampness and those without	Wu Tang, *Systematic Differentiation of Warm Pathogen Diseases*, 1798
Formally divided warm pathogen diseases into two types based on whether or not dampness is involved	Lou Jie, *Guide for Warm Pathogen Diseases*, c.1903
Used four-level differentiation for diagnosing warm-heat diseases and three-burner differentiation for diagnosing damp-heat diseases	Zhao Shao-Qin, *Length and Breadth of Warm Pathogen Disease [Differentiation]*, 1979
Adamant about classifying warm pathogen diseases into heat and damp-heat types; discussed the pathology and treatment methods for these two types of warm pathogen disease	Song Lu-Bing, *Brief Discussion of Two Types of Warm Pathogen Disease and Their Pathology and Treatment Principles*, 1980

ment of warm pathogen diseases caused by damp-heat.[86] His basic idea is that damp-heat disorders are different not only from those caused by cold, but also from warm pathogen diseases caused only by heat.[87] Xue emphasized:

- Treating these diseases via the Spleen and Stomach, while adding herbs according to the location of the affected burner(s). He believed that diseases caused by damp-heat were more likely to attack the Spleen and Stomach. The Stomach would be mainly involved if the qi in the middle burner was strong, and the Spleen if the qi in the middle burner was weak. The disease will then progress either to the exterior (Gallbladder and Triple Burner) or the interior (Liver).[88]
- Paying attention to the relative predominance of dampness or heat when treating damp-heat diseases.[89]

Both of these principles were important contributions to the understanding and treatment of damp-warmth.

WU TANG (1758–1836)

Wu Tang was a late eighteenth-century practitioner and author who built upon the works of many of the writers discussed above, especially Ye Gui.[90] While strongly influenced by Ye, Wu traveled quite a different path in coming to medicine. He did not come from a medical family, and didn't begin the study of medicine until he was nineteen when the death of his father pushed him in that direction. Furthermore, he studied medicine without a teacher, relying instead on extensive readings from the medical literature, both ancient and contemporary. He applied this knowledge in the clinic, analyzed his patients' responses to his treatments, and in this way built up his clinical experience.[91] He associated each of the yin and yang organs with one of the burners—Heart and Lung with the upper burner, Spleen and Stomach with the middle burner, and Liver and Kidney with the lower burner. He then used the three burners as an elaborate tool for differentiating the onset and progression of warm pathogen diseases, and for devising treatment protocols.[92] For example, when treating diseases located in the different burners, the practitioner should:

> Use herbs that are as light as the feathers of a bird for disease in the upper burner; use herbs to lift the Spleen qi and cause the Stomach qi to descend in the middle burner, just like calibrating a scale that should always be in balance; and use heavy and cloying herbs to treat yin deficiency for the Liver and Kidney in the lower burner, like adding a heavy weight to a scale to tip the balance.[93]

In the treatment of warm pathogen diseases, Wu stressed that "from beginning to end, one must focus on saving yin and essence."[94] He used the three burners as a tool to differentiate the onset, progression, and treatment of warm pathogen diseases. He noted that:

> The warm-heat pathogen attacks the body through the nose and mouth. The Lung opens to the nose and the Stomach to the mouth. Disease in the Lung can progress to the Pericardium. If untreated or treated improperly in the upper burner, the disease will progress to the middle burner. If untreated or treated improperly in the middle burner, the disease will progress to the lower burner. The progression of the disease is to begin in the upper burner and end in the lower burner.[95]

In *Systematic Differentiation of Warm Pathogen Diseases (Wēn bìng tiáo biàn)*, published in 1798, Wu discussed how to treat warm pathogen diseases caused by warm-heat pathogens in each of the four seasons based on his three-burner differentiation scheme. Following the initial classification made by the early twelfth-century writer Zhu Gong (discussed above), he differentiated warm pathogen diseases as wind-warmth, warm-heat, epidemic disease, warm toxin, winter-warmth, summer-heat-warmth, lurking summer-heat, damp-warmth, warm malaria, and autumn dryness. Each type of disease was further analyzed based on the three-burner differentiation scheme. This system of classification is still basically used in Chinese medical textbooks today. In addition to stressing three-burner differentiation, Wu also realized that there were two types of warm pathogen disease: those that involved dampness and those that did not.[96]

The publication of *Systematic Differentiation of Warm Pathogen Diseases* was very important in popularizing the theory and treatment of warm pathogen diseases. In this book, enriching the yin of the organs is achieved through various means. To generate fluids for the Lung and Stomach, use sweet and cold herbs; for the Large Intestine, use salty and cold herbs. Sweet and sour herbs are used to enrich the Liver yin, while heavy, cloying products, sometimes animal derived, are used for the Kidney. Wu developed many formulas that are widely used today, including Honeysuckle and Forsythia Powder *(yín qiào sǎn)*, Three Nut Decoction *(sān rén tāng)*, and Increase the Fluids Decoction *(zēng yè tāng)*.[97] Many others appear in the pages of this book.

Another of Wu's contributions was to expand the concept of the loss of storage of essence. Up to his time, it was thought that the only way to lose essence was through overindulgence in sexual activity. In turn, this loss of essence was an underlying cause for the development of warm pathogen diseases in the spring. Wu pointed out that "the words 'loss of storage of essence' should be looked at flexibly, and not explained exclusively as too much sex. Rather, it is the case that all human activity can agitate and disturb the essence."[98] This has since become an important concept in understanding and treating disease.

However, it is not the case that later writers were slavishly devoted to Wu's theories. For example, his notion that all warm pathogen diseases begin in the Lungs is no longer believed to be true. Lurking summerheat can begin in either the qi or nutritive level, summerheat-warmth can attack the *yang ming* or Pericardium (Heart) directly, and damp-warmth can begin in the Spleen and Stomach.

Wang Shi-Xiong (1808–1867)

In *Warp and Woof of Warm-Heat Pathogen Diseases (Wēn rè jīng wěi)*,[99] Wang Shi-Xiong systematized the theories set forth in the *Inner Classic, Discussion of Cold Damage*, and the writings of Ye Gui and Xue Xue, and included many other important titles on warm pathogen disease by earlier writers, some of which would otherwise have been lost. His commentaries on these books are regarded by many as definitive. The publication of this book marked the fully mature phase of warm pathogen disease theory. It is regarded as a classic in this aspect of Chinese medicine, and has played a major role in the development of warm pathogen disease theory. In addition, Wang

- Clarified the concept of summerheat and pointed out that as a pathogenic factor, summerheat is independent of dampness[100]
- Summarized the pathological changes and differences in treatment between newly-contracted warm pathogen diseases and lurking warm pathogen diseases[101]
- Warned that using herbs that were too cold in the early stage of a warm pathogen disease can cause the warm-heat pathogen to congeal.[102]

INFLUENCE OF COLD DAMAGE THEORY ON THE DEVELOPMENT OF WARM PATHOGEN DISEASE CONCEPTS

The annotation and explanation of *Discussion of Cold Damage* also reached a peak during the Kang-Qian period (1663–1795) of the Qing dynasty, in part because of the emphasis placed at that time on scholarly revisitation of ancient texts. Many important commentaries on the book were written during this era, among them *Collected Writings on Renewal of the Discussion of Cold Damage (Shāng hán lái sū jí)* by Ke Qin (Ke Yun-Bo, c. 1674), *Direct Explanations of the Discussion of Cold Damage (Shang han lun zhi jie)* by Zhang Xi-Ju (Zhang Ling-Shao, c. 1712), and *String of Pearls from the [Discussion] of Cold Damage (Shāng hán guàn zhū jí)* by You Yi (You Zai-Jing, c. 1729). Unquestionably, there was significant interaction between practitioners who relied on six-stage differentiation, as set forth in *Discussion of Cold Damage,* and proponents of the relatively new theories of warm pathogen disease. Respect for Zhang Ji was still expected of any serious practitioner of medicine during this time. To demonstrate this respect, and to make their ideas easier for other people to accept, the proponents of warm pathogen disease sometimes used terminology from *Discussion of Cold Damage* but gave it different meaning. Wu Tang himself said that his book was a supplement to that classic.[103] He even went so far as to recommend that Cinnamon Twig Decoction, the crown jewel of formulas in *Discussion of Cold Damage,* be used for treating warm pathogen diseases,[104] which to us is obviously wrong.

Immersion in the world of *Discussion of Cold Damage* not only affected practitioners' ideas about the diagnosis and progression of disease, but also the treatment of disease. Ye Gui begins his *Discussion of Warm-Heat Pathogen Disorders,* the title of which is clearly related to that of the older classic, with the admission that he thought about dividing up the progression of warm pathogen diseases to match Zhang Ji's conceptualization of the progression of cold damage.[105] As we will see later in the present volume, many of the formulas from *Discussion of Cold Damage* were adopted, and sometimes adapted, by those practicing in the warm pathogen disease school.

Then again, the main reason that these practitioners studied *Discussion of Cold Damage* was to compare and contrast its approaches with their own. For example, Ye Gui noted that

> Cold damage is more likely to linger in the exterior, gradually transform into heat, and then progress to the interior. Warm pathogen disease [which is caused by a warm-heat pathogen], can progress very quickly to the interior … When warm pathogen disease progresses to the qi level and resides in the Triple Burner, it can present with clinical symptoms and signs that are similar to the *shao yang* pattern described in *Discussion of Cold Damage.* However, the treatment is quite different, that is, one harmonizes and resolves the *shao yang* for *shao yang* patterns, while the other promotes qi circulation and transforms dampness for warm pathogen disease in the three burners.[106]

Wu Tang also noted some differences between his approach and the one found in *Discussion of Cold Damage* in that the latter emphasized a transverse transmission, from outside to inside, while he emphasized a vertical transmission, from above to below.[107]

However, some writers during this period still thought that six-stage theory was the universal method of differentiation for all externally-contracted diseases. Yu Gen-Chu (Yu Zhao-Yuan, 1734–1799) was among the first to state definitively that the six stages from *Discussion of Cold Damage* could encompass all diseases caused by external pathogenic factors.[108] His book *Revised Popular Guide to the Discussion of Cold Damage (Chóng dìng tōng sú shāng hán lùn)* discussed etiology, pathology, patterns, and treatment in detail, and included many formulas that are still widely used today, such as Sweet Wormwood and Scutellaria Decoction to Clear the Gallbladder *(hāo qín qīng dǎn tāng)*.[109] Yu was also the first person to clearly differentiate the two types of dryness, warm-dryness and cold-dryness, each with its own treatment methods. Interestingly, he utilized the three-burner approach when discussing dryness: "Autumn-dryness first damages the Lung fluids, then the Stomach fluids, and finally Liver blood and Kidney yin. … It manifests with cough when it attacks the upper burner, thirst when it attacks the middle burner, and constipation when it attacks the lower burner."[110]

In conclusion, from their deep immersion in *Discussion of Cold Damage,* physicians who relied primarily on warm pathogen disease theory have applied what they learned from that text to further expand the theory and treatment of warm pathogen disease.

DEVELOPMENTS IN LURKING WARM PATHOGEN DISEASE THEORY

There were also new developments in the realm of lurking warm pathogen diseases during the Qing dynasty. In general, these developments tied the concepts in this area closer to everyday clinical practice. One of the first was made by Shao Deng-Yin (Shao Bu-Qing, c. 1749) in *Mechanisms for Diseases of the Four Seasons (Sì shí bìng jī).* Shao discussed an approach that was slightly different from that espoused by Ye Gui for lurking warm pathogen disease in the Kidney. While Ye had focused on the excess aspects by using Scutellaria Decoction *(huáng qín tāng)*,[111] Shao Deng-Yin emphasized the deficiency aspects with his formula, Modified Restore the Pulse Decoction *(Jiā jiǎn fù mài tāng)*.[112]

In *Discussion of Seasonal Diseases (Shí bìng lùn)*, Lei Feng (Lei Shao-Yi, 1833–1888) discussed the different types of lurking warm pathogen disease found in each season, a novel approach at the time.[113] In addition, he managed to tie together differentiation based on the six stages, the yin and yang organs, four levels, and the three burners.[114] This was a valiant effort to unify the different ideas about externally-contracted disease.

Other writers had slightly different ideas. Liu Bao-Yi (Liu Gu-Sun, 1842-1900) believed that the warm-heat pathogen lurked in the *shao yin* (Kidney) and that the severity of Kidney yin deficiency correlated with the severity of the disease.[115] One of his contributions was to treat lurking heat by simultaneously clearing heat, venting the lurking pathogens, and enriching the Kidney yin. One way to do this, he suggested, was to add Sojae Semen preparatum *(dàn dòu chǐ)* and Scrophulariae Radix *(xuán shēn)* to Scutellaria Decoction *(huáng qín tāng).*[116]

The idea that an attack by a lurking pathogen could be triggered by many factors, including emotional upset, was proposed by the late nineteenth-century writer Ye Lin (Ye Zi-Yu, c. 1895).[117] This concept was further expanded upon by Liu Ji-Ren (Liu Bing-Sheng, late nineteenth century) in his book *New Treatise on Lurking Pathogens (Fú xié xīn shū),* published in 1898, where he pointed out that external pathogens can lurk in the body due to improper treatment. Liu discussed six types of lurking disease: lurking dryness, lurking cold, lurking wind, lurking dampness, lurking summerheat, and lurking heat.[118] These ideas are very important today, especially in the context of patients who have been treated with drugs such as antibiotics and antidepressants.

Modern Developments in Warm Pathogen Disease Theory and Practice

In the early twentieth century, most developments relating to warm pathogen disease revolved around the issue of classification. For example, while Wu Tang noted that some warm pathogen diseases were associated with dampness, he did not make a formal differentiation. This was left to the early twentieth-century physician Lou Jie (Lou Shou-Zhi). Assisted by his student Xiao Hui (dates unknown), Lou wrote a book called *Guide to Warm Pathogen Diseases (Wēn bìng zhǐ nán)*[119] which formally divides warm pathogen disease into two types depending on the presence of dampness. Following in the footsteps of Wu Tang, Lou organized the contents of *Systematic Differentiation of Warm Pathogen Diseases* into two parts: wind-warmth and damp-warmth. Regarding the treatment of warm pathogen diseases, he said that "We have to identify whether dampness is involved and then the ratio of dampness to heat when there is damp-heat. Then we can decide how to use the herbs."[120] For the first time, Wu clearly divided warm pathogen diseases into wind-warmth (without any associated dampness) and damp-warmth, and then subdivided these categories in accordance with three-burner differentiation. This has become the standard approach in China.

Work on understanding and applying warm pathogen disease theory continued during the Republican period (1911-1949). Among the more important writers, He Lian-Chen (He Bing-Yuan, 1860–1929) continued the work on lurking warm pathogen diseases, dividing them into two types: those caused by cold and those caused by summer-heat. In *Revised and Expanded Discussion of Warm-Heat Pathogen Diseases*

(*Chóng dìng guǎng wēn rè lùn*) he compared lurking warm pathogen disease with newly-contracted warm pathogen disease in terms of severity and transmission, and proposed treating lurking diseases by promoting qi circulation and clearing heat from the blood.[121] Another influential physician of this period, Zhang Xi-Chun (Zhang Shou-Fu, 1860–1933), believed that warm-heat pathogens lurk in the Triple Burner and that the transmission of lurking warm pathogen disease is dependent on the body's constitution, that is, the illness will likely progress to the organ where the antipathogenic qi is weakest.[122]

In the People's Republic of China (1949–) one of the core courses at colleges of traditional Chinese medicine has been warm pathogen disease theory. The various editions of the national textbooks on this subject reflect an attempt to systematize the concepts found in the etiology, pathology, differentiation, and treatment of warm pathogen diseases. This is not to say, however, that there has been no diversity of views. For example, in 1979, Zhao Shao-Qin (1916-) published *Length and Breadth of Warm Pathogen Disease [Differentiation] (Wēn bìng zòng héng)*[123] in which he divided warm pathogen disease into warm-heat pathogen disease and damp-heat disease. In this book, Zhao used four-level differentiation for warm-heat pathogen diseases and three-burner differentiation for damp-heat disorders. This book has enormous clinical value and has influenced many contemporary teachers and practitioners.

Another example is that of Song Lu-Bing (1905–1985), who taught at the Chengdu College of Traditional Chinese Medicine. Song devised a classification system for warm pathogen diseases that divides them into two major categories: heat and damp-heat. In this scheme, the heat-type of warm pathogen disease includes wind-warmth, winter-warmth, spring-warmth, autumn dryness, warm toxin, warm-heat, summerheat, and epidemic disease caused by summerheat and dryness. This heat-type of warm pathogen disease first attacks the Lung and protective level, focusing on the Lung and Stomach, and should be treated by draining heat to save the yin. The damp-heat type of warm pathogen disease includes damp-warmth, summerheat-damp, damp-heat epidemic disease, summerheat-warmth, and lurking summerheat in which dampness is involved. This kind of warm pathogen disease accumulates in the *tai yin* (Spleen) and *yang ming* (Stomach), and causes stagnation of the qi circulation in the Triple Burner. It should be treated by separately dealing with heat from dampness and promoting qi circulation.[124] While there is some debate about the details of this classification system, I believe that this framework simplifies the differentiation of warm pathogen diseases and is practical in the clinic; I have basically followed Song's framework in this book.

There has been an abundance of writing, discussion, and debate regarding the various aspects of warm pathogen diseases in recent years. One hotly debated topic is the role of toxin in the onset and progression of these diseases. Two contemporary authors, Huang Xing-Yuan and Tian Ling-Qun, currently senior researchers at the Chongqing Institute of Traditional Chinese Medicine, have made the following hypothesis. Toxin follows the pathogenic factors into the body, and it is the toxin that causes both the generation of heat as well as the subsequent transmission of the disease. Therefore, the treatment of warm pathogen diseases should focus on both clearing heat and resolving toxicity at all levels.[125] This idea has been accepted by many practitioners as a good approach for treating those contagious diseases that fall under the warm pathogen disease rubric, especially when the infection is acute.

Another approach to warm pathogen diseases is typified by Jiang Chun-Hua (1908-). Jiang advocates the use of bitter and cold herbs to clear heat and resolve toxicity as early as possible in the treatment, regardless of the level of the illness.[126] While this idea has been accepted by some practitioners as a good approach for contagious disease, I believe that this approach can lead to severe side effects, especially if the patient's constitution is ignored or the diagnosis is inaccurate. For example, the use of bitter and cold herbs to treat a sore throat can lead to the congealing of the warm-toxin, which should be dispersed. In addition, we have noticed that patients with underlying Spleen and Stomach qi deficiency can develop severe abdominal cramps, vomiting, and/or diarrhea when treated in this manner.

In China, traditional Chinese medical practitioners regularly utilize warm pathogen disease differentiation, treatment strategies, and formulas for simple and common illnesses as well as for difficult and severe infectious diseases, including influenza, various types of hepatitis, scarlet fever, bacterial dysentery, measles, pneumonia, acute bile tract infection, acute urethra infection, encephalitis, meningitis, and hemorrhagic fever. In addition, treating acutely ill, hospitalized patients requires a willingness to experiment with new forms of herbal preparations beyond the traditional decoctions, such as granules, pills, and injections.

Endnotes

1. Wang Lü, *Discourse on Tracing Back to the Medical Classics (Yī jīng sù huí jí)*. Nanjing: Jiangsu Science and Technology Publishing House, 1984: 15-24.

2. Discussions of the ideas of Wang Ji can be found in Song Nai-Guang et al., *Warm Pathogen Diseases (Wēn bìng xué)*. Beijing: Learning Garden Publishing House, 1995: 4. See also He Lian-Chen (He Bing-Yuan, 1860–1929), *Revised and Expanded Discussion of Warm-Heat Pathogen Diseases (Chóng dìng guǎng wēn rè lùn*. Beijing: People's Health Publishing House, 1960: 30.

3. Meng Shu-Jiang,"Discussion of several issues relating to warm pathogen diseases *(Duì wēn bìng xué zhōng yǒu guān wèn tí de tǎo lùn),"* in Fang Yao-Zhong and Xu Jia-Song (eds.), *Collection of Lectures on Warm Pathogen Diseases (Wēn bìng huì jiǎng)*. Beijing: People's Health Publishing House, 1986: 145.

4. Anonymous, *Yellow Emperor's Inner Classic: Basic Questions (Huáng Dì nèi jīng sù wèn)*. Beijing: People's Health Publishing House, 1963: 21.

5. *Yellow Emperor's Inner Classic: Basic Questions* is also the first Chinese medical text to refer to the idea of lurking pathogens. See Anonymous, *Yellow Emperor's Inner Classic: Basic Questions*, 24.

6. Anonymous, *Yellow Emperor's Inner Classic: Basic Questions,* 21. Stated another way, the belief was that a person with sufficient essence would not suffer from a heat-related disease in the spring even if the individual was attacked by cold in the winter.

7. Ibid., 194–197.

8. Ibid., 523.

9. Ibid., 501.

10. This is one of the lost chapters of the *Inner Classic* that has recently been reconstituted from other sources. While there is some controversy about the authenticity of these chapters, they are accepted by most contemporary medical scholars in China.

11. Wang Qi et al., *Modern Translation and Explanation of Basic Questions (Sù wèn jīn shì).* Guiyang: Guizhou People's Publishing House, 1981: 417.

12. Anonymous, *Yellow Emperor's Inner Classic: Divine Pivot (Huáng Dì nèi jīng líng shū).* Beijing: People's Health Publishing House, 1963: 60.

13. Anonymous, *Classic of Difficulties (Nán jīng).* Beijing: People's Health Publishing House, 1979:128. While this book was traditionally attributed to the fourth century BCE physician Qin Yue-Ren, it is now thought to have been written during the Eastern Han dynasty after the *Inner Classic,* but before the *Discussion of Cold Damage.*

14. Hubei College of Traditional Chinese Medicine, *Selected Readings from the Discussion of Cold Damage (Shāng hán lùn xuǎn dú),* 4th ed. Shanghai: Shanghai Science and Technology Publishing House, 1980: 8.

15. Zhang Ji, *Essentials from the Golden Cabinet (Jīn guì yào luè fāng lùn).* Beijing: People's Publishing House, Beijing: 1963.

16. Ibid., 110.

17. Ibid., 39.

18. Ren Ying-Qiu, *Doctrines of the Various Schools of Chinese Medicine (Zhōng yī gè jiā xué shuō),* 4th ed. Shanghai: Shanghai Science and Technology Publishing House, 1980: 91.

19. Ibid.

20. Xie Zhong-Mo, *Key Points for Warm Pathogen Diseases (Wēn bìng yào yì).* Beijing: People's Health Publishing House, 1983: 4.

21. Teaching and Research Section on Discussion of Cold Damage of the Nanjing College of Traditional Chinese Medicine, *Translation and Explanation of the Discussion of Cold Damage (Shāng hán lùn yì shì).* Shanghai: Shanghai Science and Technology Publishing House, 1980: 268. Essentially, over a thousand years before the terms were coined, Wang discussed what would later be referred to as spring-warmth (春溫 *chūn wēn*) and lurking summerheat (伏暑 *fú shǔ*).

22. Chao Yuan-Fang, *Discussion of the Origins of Symptoms of Disease (Zhū bìng yuán hòu lùn).* Beijing: People's Health Publishing House, 1992: 218.

23. Tao Hong-Jing, *Collection of Commentaries on the Classic of Materia Medica (Běn cǎo jīng jí zhù).* Beijing: People's Health Publishing House, 1994: 24.

24. Sun Si-Miao, *Important Formulas Worth a Thousand Gold Pieces for any Emergency (Bèi jí qiān jīn yào fāng).* Beijing: People's Health Publishing House, 1982: 178.

25. See Chapter 8 for further details.

26. See Chapter 7 for further details.

27. Wang Tao, *Arcane Essentials From the Imperial Library (Wài tái mì yào).* Shanghai: Shanghai Ancient Literature Publishing House, 1991: 143.

28. Warm Pathogen Disease Research and Teaching Section of the Chengdu College of Traditional Chinese Medicine, *Self-Study Book for Chinese Medicine: Warm Pathogen Diseases (Zhōng yī zì xué jiào cái: Wēn bìng xué).* Chengdu: Chengdu College of Traditional Chinese Medicine, 1985: 2.

29. Ren Ying-Qiu, *Doctrines of the Various Schools of Chinese Medicine*, 91.

30. This popular formula is the first one listed in *Discussion of Cold Damage.* It can be found in Dan Bensky and Randall Barolet, *Chinese Herbal Medicine: Formulas and Strategies.* Seattle: Eastland Press, 1990: 35.

31. This formula was first discussed in *Discussion of Cold Damage* and can be found in Bensky and Barolet, *Chinese Herbal Medicine: Formulas and Strategies*, 33.

32. This formula was first discussed in *Discussion of Cold Damage* and can be found in Bensky and Barolet, *Chinese Herbal Medicine: Formulas and Strategies*, 39.

33. Pang An-Shi, *General Discussion for the Discussion of Cold Damage (Shāng hán zǒng bìng lùn)* can be found in Institute of Chinese Medical Literature of Shanghai College of Traditional Chinese Medicine (ed.), *Historical Collection of Rare Chinese Medical Books (Lì dài zhōng yī zhēn běn jí chéng).* Shanghai: Joint Publishing Company, 1990: 3.

34. Guo Zi-Guang, "Informal discussion on the concept of toxin *(Màn tán dú de gài nián)." Zhejiang Journal of Traditional Chinese Medicine* 1985(5): 227.

35. The term malarial disorder (瘧 *nuè*) in Chinese medicine refers to diseases that manifest with regularly alternating chills and fever, as well as sweating. There is some overlap with the biomedical concept of malaria. See Chapter 35 of *Basic Questions* for further details.

36. Meng Shu-Jiang et al., *Teaching Reference Books for Traditional Chinese Medical Colleges: Warm Pathogen Diseases (Gāo děng zhōng yī yuàn xiào jiào xué cān kǎo shū: wēn bìng xué).* Beijing: People's Health Publishing House, 1989: 7.

37. Zhu Gong, *Book to Safeguard Life Arranged According to Pattern (Lèi zhèng huó rén shū).* Shanghai: Commercial Press, 1957: 15.

38. Marta Hanson, "Inventing a Tradition in Chinese Medicine." Ph.D. dissertation, University of Pennsylvania: History and Sociology of Science Department, Philadelphia, Pennsylvania, 1997: 9–10.

39. Liu Wan-Su, *Direct Investigation of Cold Damage (Shāng hán zhí gé).* Shanghai: Shanghai Ancient Literature Publishing House, 1991: 863.

40. Liu Wan-Su, *Formulas from the Discussion Illuminating the Yellow Emperor's Basic Questions (Huáng Dì sù wèn xuán míng lùn fāng).* Shanghai: Shanghai Ancient Literature Publishing House, 1991: 780.

41. Liu Wan-Su, *Collection of Writings on the Mechanism of Disease, Suitability of Qi, and the Safeguarding of Life as Discussed in Basic Questions (Sù wèn bìng jī qì yí bǎo míng jí).* Shanghai: Shanghai Ancient Literature Publishing House, 1991: 11.

42. Double Resolving Powder was first recorded in Liu Wan-Su, *Formulas from the Discussion Illuminating the Yellow Emperor's Basic Questions,* 780.

43. Liu Wan-Su, *Collection of Writings on the Mechanism of Disease, Suitability of Qi, and the Safeguarding of Life as Discussed in Basic Questions,* 94.

44. Ren Ying-Qiu, *Doctrines of the Various Schools of Chinese Medicine,* 57.

45. Meng Shu-Jiang et al., *Teaching Reference Books for Traditional Chinese Medical Colleges: Warm Pathogen Diseases,* 8.

46. Ibid.

47. Wang Lü, *Discourse on Tracing Back to the Medical Classics,* 15–24.

48. Beijing College of Traditional Chinese Medicine, *A Series of National Textbooks for Medical College: Chinese Medical History (Zhōng guó yī xué shǐ),* 4th ed. Shanghai: Shanghai Science and Technology Publishing House, 1978: 4.

49. Meng Shu-Jiang et al., *Teaching Reference Books for Traditional Chinese Medical Colleges: Warm Pathogen Diseases,* 682.

49. Meng Shu-Jiang et al., *Teaching Reference Books for Traditional Chinese Medical Colleges: Warm Pathogen Diseases,* 682.

50. Wu You-Xing, *Discussion of Warm Epidemics (Wēn yì lùn).* Shenyang: Liaoning Science and Technology Publishing House, 1997: 3–5, 7, 9, 18–20.

51. This difference in the manner of attack by epidemic qi, that is, through the mouth and nose, rather than through the skin and muscles, is largely theoretical. Clinically, the difference may not exist, and epidemic qi may have the capacity to attack the body through the nose and mouth as well as the skin and muscles. It is important to note that many practitioners mistakenly assume that the site where symptoms first manifest in the body is always associated with the place where the pathogen first attacks. This is not necessarily the case.

52. Wu You-Xing, *Discussion of Warm Epidemics,* 1–2.

53. See Chapter 6 for further information on the membrane source.

54. Wu You-Xing, *Discussion of Warm Epidemics,* 2. See Chapter 12 for further details.

55. Ibid., 12.

56. Ibid., 25.

57. See Chapter 8 for further details.

58. See Chapter 7 for further details.

59. Dai Tian-Zhang, *Discussion of Widespread Warm Epidemics (Guǎng wēn yì lùn)* can be found in Cao Bing-Zhang (ed.), *Compendium of Medicine in China (Zhōng guó yī xué dà chéng).* Shanghai: Shanghai Science and Technology Publishing House, 1990. Note that *Discussion of Widespread Warm Epidemics* is also called *Clear Differentiation of Epidemic Diseases (Wēn yì míng biàn).*

60. Yang Xuan, *Systematic Differentiation of Cold Damage and Warm Epidemics (Shāng*

hán wēn yì tiáo biàn) can be found in Yu Bo-Hai et al. (ed.), *Collection of Famous Books on Discussion of Cold Damage, Essentials from the Golden Cabinet and Warm Pathogen Disease (Shāng hán jīn guì wēn bìng míng zhù jí chéng)*. Beijing: China Publishing House, 1997: 699-815.

61. Lin Zhi-Nan, "Looking at the application of the method of dispersing and draining heat from constraint in treating warm pathogen diseases from [analyzing] ascending and descending powder *(Cóng shēng jiàng sǎn kàn xuān xiè yù rè fǎ zài wēn bìng zhōng de yùn yòng),"* in *Beijing College of Traditional Medicine Collection of First Class Graduate Papers (Běijīng zhōng yī xué yuàn shōu jiè yán jiū shēng lùn wén huì biān)*. Beijing: Beijing College of Traditional Chinese Medicine, 1981: 169.

62. The formula was first recorded in Yang Xuan, *Systematic Differentiation of Cold Damage and Warm Epidemics*, 758.

63. Chinese Academy of Traditional Chinese Medicine, *Collected Medical Experience of Pu Fu-Zhou (Pú Fǔ-Zhōu yī liǎo jīng yàn jí)*. Beijing: People's Health Publishing House, 1976: 39.

64. Yu Lin, *Achievements Regarding Epidemic Rashes (Yì zhěn yī dé)* only survives as a part of the book by Wang Shi-Xiong (Wang Meng-Ying) entitled *Warp and Woof of Warm-Heat Pathogen Diseases (Wēn rè jīng wěi)*. This title is contained in Lu Zhen, *Collected Rare Recent Books on Chinese Medicine: Warm Pathogen Disease Section (Jīn dài zhōng yī zhēn běn jí: wēn bìng fēn cè)*. Hangzhou: Zhejiang Science and Technology Publishing House, 1987: 134.

65. Ibid.

66. Song Nai-Guang et al., *Warm Pathogen Diseases (Wēn bìng xué)*. Beijing: Learning Garden Publishing House, 1995: 4. See also He Lian-Chen (He Bing-Yuan, 1860–1929), *Revised and Expanded Discussion of Warm-Heat Pathogen Diseases (Chóng dìng guǎng wēn rè lùn.)*. Beijing: People's Health Publishing House, 1960: 30.

67. Wang Ken-Tang, *Indispensable Tools for Pattern Treatment (Zhèng zhì zhǔn shéng)*. Shanghai: Shanghai Science and Technology Publishing House, 1959: 318.

68. Zhang He-Teng, *Revised and Expanded Complete Treatise on Summerheat Damage (Zēng dìng shāng shǔ quán shū)*, can be found in Cao Bing-Zhang (ed.), *Compendium of Medicine in China (Zhōng guó yī xué dà chéng)*.

69. Ye Gui, *Differentiating Lurking Pathogens and Externally Contracted Diseases during Three Seasons (Sān shí fú xié wài gǎn piàn)*. This book is not available as a separate work but can be found in Ye Gui, *Case Records as a Guide to Clinical Practice (Lín zhèng zhǐ nán yī àn)*. Shanghai: Shanghai Science and Technology Publishing House, 1959: 734-744.

70. Zhang Jie-Bin, *Collected Treatises of [Zhang] Jing-Yue (Jǐng-Yuè quán shū)*. Beijing: People's Health Publishing House, 1991: 327-328. This book was first published in 1636.

71. Yu Chang, *Writings on the Esteemed Discussion (Shàng lùn piān)* found in *Collection of Famous Books on Discussion of Cold Damage, Essentials from the Golden Cabinet and Warm Pathogen Disease*, 217.

72. Ibid.

73. Anonymous, *Yellow Emperor's Inner Classic: Divine Pivot*, 52.

74. Meng Shu-Jiang et al., *Teaching Reference Books for Traditional Chinese Medical Colleges: Warm Pathogen Diseases*, 10.

75. Wu Qian, *Golden Mirror of the Medical Tradition (Yī zōng jīn jiàn)*. Beijing: People's Health Publishing House, 1973.

76. Meng Shu-Jiang et al., *Teaching Reference Books for Traditional Chinese Medical Colleges: Warm Pathogen Diseases*, 694.

77. *Discussion of Warm-Heat Pathogen Disorders* was first recorded as *Patterns and Treatment for Warm Pathogen Diseases (Wēn zhèng lùn zhì)* in Tang Da-Lie (Tang Li-San), *Collection of Papers of Physicians from Wu (Wú yī huì jiǎng)*. Shanghai: Shanghai Science and Technology Publishing House, 1983. According to Tang, *Discussion of Warm-Heat Pathogen Disorders* was not actually written by Ye Gui, but was transcribed from notes made of Ye's lectures by his student Gu Jin-Wen. It was also included in (a) Wang Shi-Xiong, *Warp and Woof of Warm-Heat Pathogen Diseases (Wēn rè jīng wěi)*, 1852, where it was called *Discourses on Externally Contracted Diseases Caused by Warm-Heat [Pathogens] (Wài gǎn wēn rè piàn)*; and (b) Zhang Nan (Zhang Xu-Gu), *A Stick to Awaken Physicians (Yī mén bàng hè)*, 1825, where it was called *Discussion of Warm-Heat Pathogen Disorders (Wēn rè lùn)*.

78. Ye Gui, *Case Records as a Guide to Clinical Practice (Lín zhèng zhǐ nán yī àn)*. Shanghai: Shanghai Science and Technology Publishing House, 1959. This book, which was edited by Ye's students, including Hua Xiu-Yun and Zou Ci-Jiu, was first published in about 1746, and is based on Ye's clinical cases.

79. Tang Da-Lie, *Collection of Papers of Physicians from Wu*, 4.

80. Ye Gui, *Differentiating Lurking Pathogens and Externally Contracted Diseases during Three Seasons*, 734. See Chapter 3 for further details.

81. Ye Gui, *Case Records as a Guide to Clinical Practice*, 734.

82. Ibid., 335-36.

83. Ibid., 734.

84. Tang Da-Lie, *Collection of Papers of Physicians from Wu*, 4–7, 9. See also Sheng Qin-Fa, "On venting method in treating warm pathogen disease *(Lùn wēn bìng de tòu fǎ)*," in *Selected Essays from Traditional Chinese Medicine Teachers' Training Seminar (Zhōng yī shī xùn bān lùn wén xuǎn)*. Shanghai: Shanghai College of Traditional Chinese Medicine, 1980: 75.

85. Zhang Ji, *Essentials from the Golden Cabinet (Jīn guì yào luè fāng lùn)*. Beijing: People's Publishing House, 1963: 1.

86. Xue Xue, *Systematic Differentiation of Damp-Heat (Shī rè tiáo biàn)*, can be found in Song Zhao-Qi (Song You-Fu), *Distinguishing [Aspects] of Southern Diseases (Nán bìng bié jiàn)*. Shanghai: Shanghai Health Publishing House, 1958: 1-22.

87. Ibid., 3.

88. Ibid., 1.

89. Ibid., 10–11.

90. Wu Tang, *Systematic Differentiation of Warm Pathogen Diseases (Wēn bìng tiáo biàn)*. Beijing: People's Health Publishing House, 1963: 7, 9.

91. Ibid., 6. See also Meng Shu-Jiang et al., *Warm Pathogen Diseases*, 694.

92. Ibid., 60.

93. Ibid., 176.

94. Ibid., 167.

95. Ibid., 60.

96. Ibid., 11.

97. These formulas can be found in Chapters 7, 12, and 7 respectively.

98. Wu Tang, *Systematic Differentiation of Warm Pathogen Diseases*, 3.

99. Wang Shi-Xiong, *Warp and Woof of Warm-Heat Pathogen Diseases (Wēn rè jīng wěi)*. This title is contained in Lu Zhen, *Collected Rare Recent Books on Chinese Medicine: Warm Pathogen Disease Section*, 4-150.

100. Wang Shi-Xiong, *Warp and Woof of Warm-Heat Pathogen Diseases*, 63.

101. Ibid., 61.

102. Ibid., 54.

103. Ibid., 9.

104. Ibid., 15.

105. Tang Da-Lie, *Collection of Papers of Physicians from Wu*, 4.

106. Tang Da-Lie, *Collection of Papers of Physicians from Wu*, 3, 4. See also Meng Shu-Jiang et al., *Teaching Reference Books for Medical Colleges: Warm Pathogen Diseases*, 307.

107. Wu Tang, *Systematic Differentiation of Warm Pathogen Diseases*, 10. See Chapter 4 for further details.

108. Yu Gen-Chu, *Revised Popular Guide to the Discussion of Cold Damage (Chóng dìng tōng sú shāng hán lùn)*. Hangzhou: New Medicine Press, 1956: 35.

109. Ibid., 55. See Chapter 13 for further details.

110. Ibid., 32.

111. It was first recorded in *Discussion of Cold Damage*, and contains Scutellariae Radix *(huáng qín)* (9g), Paeoniae Radix alba *(bái sháo)* (6g), Glycyrrhizae Radix preparata *(zhì gān cǎo)* (6g), and Jujubae Fructus *(dà zǎo)* (12 pieces).

112. Meng Shu-Jiang et al., *Teaching Reference Books for Medical Colleges: Warm Pathogen Diseases*, 722.

113. Lei Feng, *Discussion of Seasonal Diseases (Shí bìng lùn)*. Beijing: People's Health Publishing House, 1956: 5-10, 37-48, 83-93, 125-26.

114. Lei Feng, *Discussion of Seasonal Diseases*. See also Meng Shu-Jiang et al., *Teaching Reference Books for Medical Colleges: Warm Pathogen Diseases*, 12.

115. Liu Bao-Yi, *Encountering the Sources of Warm-Heat Pathogen Diseases (Wēn rè féng yuán)*. Beijing: People's Health Publishing House, 1959: 65.

116. Ibid., 64-65.

117. Ye Lin, *Explanation of Lurking Qi (Fú qì jiě)*, in Cao Bing-Zhang (ed.), *Compendium of Medicine in China (Zhōng guó yī xué dà chéng)*, 8.

118. Liu Ji-Ren, *New Treatise on Lurking Pathogens (Fú xié xīn shū)*, which can be found in Cao Bing-Zhang (ed.), *Compendium of Medicine in China (Zhōng guó yī xué dà chéng)*, 1.

119. This book was edited by Li An-Qing who changed its name to *Outline of Warm-Heat Pathogen Diseases (Wēn rè bìng gāng yào)*. Zhengzhou: Henan People's Publishing House, 1956.

120. Xie Zhong-Mo, *Key Points of Warm Pathogen Diseases (Wēn bìng yào yì)*. Beijing: People's Health Publishing House, 1956: 41.

121. He Lian-Chen, *Revised and Expanded Discussion of Warm-Heat Pathogen Diseases*, 6.

122. Zhang Xi-Chun, *Essays on Medicine Esteeming the Chinese and Respecting the Western (Yī xúe zhōng zhōng cān xī lù)*. Shijiazhuang: Hebei People's Publishing House, 1957: 506.

123. Zhao Shao-Qin, Hu Ding-Bang, and Liu Jing-Yuan, *Length and Breadth of Warm Pathogen Diseases [Differentiation] (Wēn bìng zòng héng)*. Beijing: Beijing College of Traditional Chinese Medicine, 1979: 25, 157.

124. Song Lu-Bing, "Brief discussion of two types of warm pathogen diseases and their pathologies and treatment principles *(Wēn bìng de liǎng dà lèi bié jí qí bìng jī zhì zé jiǎn lùn)*," can be found in *Collection of Literature About Research and Study on Protective, Qi, Ying, and Blood Theory in Warm Pathogen Diseases (Zhōng yī wēn bìng wèi qì yíng xuè lǐ lùn yán jiù zī liào huì biān)*. Chongqing: Sichuan Cooperative Panel on Research and Study of Protective, Qi, Nutritive, and Blood [Levels] in Warm Pathogen Diseases, 1980: 1–4.

125. Huang Xing-Yuan and Tian Ling-Qun, "General description of research and study on protective, qi, ying and blood theory in warm pathogen diseases *(Wēn bìng wèi qì yíng xuè yán jiù gài kuàng)*," in Fang Yao-Zhong and Xu Jia-Song (eds.), *Collection of Lectures on Warm Pathogen Diseases (Wēn bìng huì jiǎng)*. Beijing: People's Health Publishing House, 1986: 80.

126. Jiang Chun-Hua, "Ye tian-shi's theory and treatment for warm pathogen diseases and miscellaneous [internal] diseases *(Yè Tiān-Shì de wēn bìng hé zá bìng de lǐ lùn yǔ zhì liáo)*." *New Medicine Journal*, 1978: 8.

2 General Description of Warm Pathogen Diseases

Concept of Warm Pathogen Diseases

THE TERM WARM pathogen diseases (溫病 *wēn bìng*) refers to a group of acute, externally-contracted febrile diseases that are caused by warm-heat pathogens. Depending on the pathogen, they can occur at any time of year. They are diagnosed and treated by the application of four-level or three-burner differentiation, and are marked primarily by signs and symptoms of heat. In addition, warm pathogen diseases can readily injure the yin. While most of the time a warm pathogen disease results from the acute attack of one or another type of warm-heat pathogen, there is an exception, namely, lurking warm pathogen disease. This is caused by a warm-heat pathogen that has become trapped in the body where it 'lurks' until provoked by an attack of an external pathogenic factor like wind-heat, summerheat, or even wind-cold.

In general, fever is the main manifestation of warm pathogen diseases at the early stage. In addition, there are three other key clinical features:

- Symptoms appear very quickly.
- Heat signs and symptoms often predominate.
- The hot nature of the pathogens means that they readily injure the fluids and yin.

The majority of warm pathogen diseases are contagious, seasonal, endemic, and epidemic. *Contagious* means that the disease can be transmitted to others; contagious diseases were described in Chapter 72 of *Basic Questions* where they were said to be "easily passed (染易 *rǎn yì*) [between people]."[1] In the same chapter it is noted that "All five kinds of epidemic disease can be transmitted from one person to another person, regardless of the person's age, whether they be an elder or a child."[2] There were special terms for the different ways in which a contagion was received in ancient China. For example, if a person contracts a disease by inhaling contaminated air, it was called 'received from heaven' (天受 *tiān shòu*);[3] if it was contracted by directly touching another person or her belongings, it was called 'contagion' (傳染 *chuán rǎn*).[4]

Seasonal means that most warm pathogen diseases appear in certain seasons. For example, wind is predominant in the spring, and thus wind-warmth caused by the wind-heat pathogen is most common in spring.

Endemic means that a disease is relatively more common in a particular area. For example, the coastal regions of southeast China are warm and humid, which makes damp-heat-induced disease more common there than in the cold and dry northeastern areas of China.

Epidemics affect many people in the same area within a relatively short span of time. The related terms used in ancient times were 'prevailing throughout the world' (天行 *tiān xíng*)[5] and 'prevailing in a particular time period' (時行 *shí xíng*).[6]

Characteristics of Warm Pathogen Diseases

Warm pathogen diseases are mostly caused by the warm-heat type of external pathogens. These include wind-heat, summerheat, damp-heat, dryness, and warm-toxin. As will be shown below, there are five warm-heat pathogens that can lead to seven warm pathogen diseases. While their names are quite similar, it is crucial that the practitioner be able to distinguish among each of the pathogens and the diseases they cause. Each will be discussed in greater detail in Chapter 3.

UNIQUE CLINICAL ATTRIBUTES OF WARM PATHOGEN DISEASES

Warm-heat pathogens affect the body in specific ways, giving rise to distinctive clinical attributes:

The onset of the disease is acute. Clinically, unlike the patient who suffers from a disease caused by internal disharmony, most people who are attacked by a warm-heat pathogen and develop a warm pathogen disease can tell precisely when they began to feel sick. Even the onset of an illness due to externally-contracted wind-cold generally occurs over a longer period of time—hours versus minutes—than do most diseases caused by warm-heat pathogens.

There are often remarkable heat symptoms at the very beginning of the disease such as **high fever, thirst, irritability, restlessness, concentrated dark urine, red** tongue, and rapid pulse. Fever is the principal manifestation. Here, fever does not simply mean the subjective feeling of warmth or feverishness that often accompanies an internal disharmony, and which cannot be measured by a thermometer. Rather, in addition to the subjective sensation, there is almost always a measurable increase in temperature. Generally speaking, this type of fever is acute, shows a temperature over 37°C, and is accompanied by other signs and symptoms of heat from excess like thirst, scanty and yellow urine, irritability, restlessness, red tongue, and rapid pulse. However, in the later stage of a warm pathogen disease when only remnants of the pathogen remain, accompanied by a deficiency of qi and yin, or in a disease due to damp-heat, there might only be the subjective feeling of fever, or a low-grade fever.

Heat readily injures the yin and fluids and can sink inside and attack different organs. Therefore, the manifestations of the disease frequently change. For example, the heat of a warm pathogen disease can force blood out of the vessels, leading to bleeding and eruptions. It can attack and block the Pericardium, congealing fluids into phlegm and misting the spirit of the Heart, which in a few days can lead to muddled consciousness or even coma. Extreme heat can stir up internal wind in the Liver, giving rise to convulsions. As the illness progresses, heat can also injure the yin leading to thirst, dry tongue coating, dry lips, throat, and nose, dry skin, dry and hard stools, scanty urine, and spasms and rigidity of the muscles. Compared with externally-contracted cold disorders, warm pathogen diseases progress much more rapidly.

PROGRESSION OF WARM PATHOGEN DISEASES

If left untreated, or if treated improperly, warm pathogen diseases progress from the exterior to the interior, from mild to severe, and from excess to deficiency. Conversely, if they are properly treated, the progress of warm pathogen diseases will reverse, that is, regressing from the interior to the exterior, from internal organs to the surface, and becoming milder as the disease becomes more superficial.

Classification of Warm Pathogen Diseases

Historically, warm pathogen diseases have been classified three ways:

According to the seasons. One classification of warm pathogen diseases follows the five-phase correspondences of the seasons. In this scheme, a warm pathogen disease that occurs in the spring is called wind-warmth; in the summer it is called summer-heat-warmth; in late summer, damp-warmth; and if in autumn, autumn-dryness. While this scheme can help identify the seasonal nature of the diseases, it has certain limitations:

- It fails to identify exactly which of the many warm-heat pathogens are involved. Most importantly, it does not help determine if dampness is involved, since damp-warmth is not the only disease that includes dampness. These are very important issues in predicting the progression and providing treatment for a warm pathogen disease.
- Some types of warm pathogen disease do not occur in just one season. For example, wind-warmth may occur during either the spring or winter.
- Some warm-heat pathogens can attack and lurk within the body, without any clinical manifestations, until induced to emerge at a later point by a secondary pathogen. This type of disease is not included under this scheme.

According to the nature of the pathogen. Is the warm-heat pathogen solely one of heat without dampness, or is there also a damp component? These two categories, the warm-heat type and the damp-heat type, which are summarized in Table 2.1, are commonly used in the clinic. Warm-heat pathogen diseases include:

- Wind-warmth (風溫 *fēng wēn*)
- Spring-warmth (春溫 *chūn wēn*)
- Autumn-dryness (秋燥 *qiū zào*)
- Warm-toxin (溫毒 *wēn dú*)

Table 2.1	Classification of Warm Pathogen Diseases According to Pathogen
Without dampness	**With dampness**
Wind-warmth	Summerheat-warmth
Spring-warmth	Damp-warmth
Autumn-dryness	Lurking summerheat
Warm-toxin	

Signs and symptoms of heat from excess and yin damage comprise the principal clinical presentation of these four types of warm-heat pathogen disease. Clearing heat and enriching the yin are the main treatment principles (see Table 2.2).

Dampness, on the other hand, has a sticky and tenacious nature, making it very difficult to eliminate. Therefore, diseases in which dampness is a factor take a long time to resolve, and are more difficult to treat. In order to correctly diagnose and treat this type of warm pathogen disease, the practitioner must determine whether dampness is involved. Damp-heat diseases include:

- Summerheat-warmth (暑溫 *shǔ wēn*)
- Damp-warmth (濕溫 *shī wēn*)
- Lurking summerheat (伏暑 *fú shǔ*)

Table 2.2	Characteristics of Warm-Heat Diseases
Subclassification	**Characteristics**
Wind-warmth	Fever, aversion to cold, cough floating pulse; occurs in spring and winter
Spring-warmth	High fever, restlessness, strong thirst, and possibly convulsions and coma; occurs in spring
Autumn-dryness	Dry cough, dryness of mouth, nose, and throat; occurs in autumn
Warm-toxin	Local redness, swelling, heat, and pain, and possibly ulcerations; may occur in any season; some, like mumps and scarlet fever, are highly contagious

These three types of warm pathogen disease will present with signs and symptoms of qi stagnation and qi or yang damage, attributable to the dampness, in addition to some degree of heat and yin damage. Therefore, not only must treatment address clearing heat and enriching yin, but also promoting qi circulation and preventing dampness from damaging the qi or yang. This classification scheme is very practical because it identifies the specific warm-heat pathogen that is involved, thereby allowing treatment to be more precise. Table 2.3 sets out the differences between these two types of warm pathogen disease.[7]

Table 2.3	Differences Between Warm-Heat and Damp-Heat Types of Warm Pathogen Disease	
Different Aspects	**Warm-Heat Type**	**Damp-Heat Type**
Location in early stages	Primarily Lung and protective level	Primarily Spleen and Stomach
Onset	Acute with clear heat signs and symptoms	Slower, without clear heat signs and symptoms
Progression	Rapid	Usually slow, but can quicken if damp-heat transforms into dryness or fire
Course of disease	Short	Lingering
Prognosis	Readily damages yin	Damages yang, but can also damage yin

41

Note that, while in this scheme summerheat-warmth is always classified as a damp-heat disease, this is not always the case. The reader is referred to Chapter 11 for further discussion. See Table 2.4 for more detail about the damp-heat type of warm pathogen diseases, and Table 2.5 for the seasons in which warm-heat and damp-heat diseases occur.

Table 2.4	Characteristics of Damp-Heat Diseases
Subclassification	**Characteristics**
Summerheat-warmth	*Non-damp-related manifestations:* high fever, strong thirst, profuse sweating, flooding pulse; occurs in summer *Damp-related manifestations:* chills, no sweating, fever, epigastric distention, greasy tongue coating; occurs in summer
Damp-warmth	Aversion to cold, low-grade fever, heaviness of the head and body, stifling sensation in the chest and distention in the epigastric region, greasy tongue coating, soggy and moderate pulse; occurs in late summer
Lurking summerheat	Fever, restlessness, thirst, epigastric distention, greasy tongue coating; *or* fever, restlessness, dry mouth, deep-red tongue with little coating; occurs in autumn or winter

Table 2.5	Seasonal Associations of Warm Pathogen Disease (Theoretical)			
	Spring	**Summer**	**Autumn**	**Winter**
Wind-warmth	X			X
Spring-warmth	X			
Autumn-dryness			X	
Warm-toxin	X	X	X	X
Summerheat-warmth		X		
Damp-warmth		X		
Lurking summerheat	X		X	X

According to when the disease occurs. Does the disease occur immediately following an initial attack of the warm-heat pathogen (newly-contracted warm pathogen disease, 新感溫病 *xīn gǎn wēn bìng*) or after a period of incubation (lurking warm pathogen disease, 伏氣溫病 *fú qì wēn bìng*)? These two categories of warm pathogen disease are discussed more fully in Chapter 3.

Most warm pathogen diseases progress from the exterior to the interior, as would be expected of an externally-contracted disease. However, spring-warmth and lurking summerheat, which belong to the category of lurking warm pathogen disease, have a different progression: they can progress from either the exterior to the interior or from the interior to the exterior. The former progression indicates that the disease is getting worse, and the latter progression indicates that the disease will soon be cured. Thus, the treatment strategy for these types of warm pathogen disease is to vent the pathogens to the surface, rather than suppressing them.

Warm Pathogen Disease and Cold Damage

DISPUTES BETWEEN ADHERENTS OF WARM PATHOGEN DISEASE AND COLD DAMAGE

As mentioned in the first chapter, diseases caused by external pathogens can be divided into those related to cold and those related to heat. Yet all externally-con-tracted diseases may present with similar signs and symptoms in the clinic such as fever, aversion to cold, slight chills, nasal congestion, cough, and floating pulse. But since the treatment regimen is quite different for each type of externally-contracted disease, they must be carefully differentiated. In addition, different diagnostic schemes are utilized when diagnosing these diseases: six-stage differentiation for externally-contracted diseases due to cold, and four-level and three-burner differentiation for those related to heat.

How and when to use each of these two methods of differentiation has been a major issue for scholars and practitioners for hundreds of years. Since the theory and treatment of warm pathogen diseases was first devised, there have been intense discussions about whether such diseases are merely a subset of cold damage. The related question is whether the six-stage method of differentiation and treatment, first described in *Discussion of Cold Damage*, is appropriate for treating warm pathogen diseases. To answer these two questions, we must explore the three meanings of the term cold damage (傷寒 *shāng hán*) in the Chinese medical literature. One meaning is very broad, and includes all types of externally-contracted disease that manifest with fever and chills. This usage can be traced to Chapter 58 of the *Classic of Difficulties (Nán jīng)*.[8] The second meaning is narrower and is restricted to only those diseases caused by external cold. The third meaning of the term, which is the most narrow, refers to just one type of externally-contracted cold disease marked by an exterior, cold, excess presentation.

Before the establishment of warm pathogen disease theory, conventional wisdom held that warm pathogen diseases were a type of cold damage, and that the six-stage approach should therefore serve as the guideline for the differentiation and treatment of warm pathogen diseases. For example, the seventh-century annotator of the *Inner Classic,* Wang Bing, argued that cold was the main pathogen underlying externally-contracted diseases, and that a cold damage disease was marked by the appearance of symptoms immediately after contracting the disease. If, however, the cold lurked in the skin and muscles and emerged in the spring, there would be a warm pathogen disease, and if in the summer, a summerheat disease. For this reason, all types of febrile disease could be regarded as cold damage.[9]

However, as explained in Chapter 1, by the seventeenth century the idea had formed that there were externally-contracted diseases caused by heat that should be differentiated from those caused by cold. Ye Gui, one of the leaders of this movement, expressed it this way:

> Liu Wan-Su put forward a new idea that [we] should use the three burners as a tool to differentiate warm pathogen disease, and that bitter and acrid herbs should be selected. This is an excellent idea that is much better than [those ideas of] other practitioners and scholars. If we limit ourselves to six-stage differentiation, we will still be treating cold damage which often makes for incorrect treatment.[10]

In the very first paragraph of *Discussion of Warm-Heat Pathogen Disorders (Wēn rè lùn),* Ye Gui directly states that "The differentiation and treatment of warm pathogen disease is quite different from cold damage."[11] In addition, practitioners who focused on warm pathogen diseases felt that many important aspects of externally-contracted disease, such as patterns of heat or yin deficiency, were not adequately dealt with in *Discussion of Cold Damage.* They therefore set themselves the task of addressing these issues.

Even after the theory of warm pathogen diseases had been firmly established with the publication of works by such authors as Ye Gui, Xue Xue, and Wu Tang, discussed in Chapter 1, this issue was not resolved. Many writers continued to vigorously argue that not only are warm pathogen diseases included in the scheme of cold damage, their treatment can properly be guided by six-stage differentiation. This view was quite prevalent in the late nineteenth and early twentieth centuries, represented by such figures as Lu Mao-Xiu (Lu Jiu-Zhi, active c. 1866), Lu Yuan-Lei (Lu Peng-Nian, 1894-1955), and Yun Tie-Qiao (Yun Shu-Jue, active c. 1922).[12] Part of the problem was that they could not understand that different types of disease required different approaches. With this mindset, not only did they continue to use a six-stage approach to treat warm pathogen diseases, they also accused proponents of the warm pathogen disease school of abandoning six-stage differentiation.[13] This charge was, however, without foundation. For example, in *Systematic Differentiation of Warm Pathogen Diseases,* Wu Tang clearly stated that it was intended to supplement the *Discussion of Cold Damage*.[14] In terms of treatment, the proponents of cold damage argued that some of the innovations introduced by the warm pathogen disease school were baseless and could be dispensed with. For example, they believed that all states of muddled consciousness or coma were related to *yang ming* heat. Accordingly, clearing and purging heat from the *yang ming* was, in their view, all that was needed, and other ideas, such as Ye Gui's notion that such states could be due to heat attacking the Pericardium, were baseless and dangerous.[15]

This was clearly a conservative overreaction, and was probably related to the deep-rooted conservatism which affected much of the literati during this period as imperial China limped to its end.[16] This was even acknowledged by many scholars and practitioners who were dedicated to six-stage differentiation. One of the leading early twentieth-century specialists in the works of Zhang Ji was Cao Jia-Da (Cao Ying-Fu, 1866-1937). In *Records of Experiences with Classic Formulas (Jīng fāng shì yàn lù)*, edited by his student Jiang Zuo-Jin, Cao noted that classic formulas such as Major Order the Qi Decoction *(dà chéng qì tāng)* were ineffective for treating severe diseases of the central nervous system with such manifestations as talking to oneself, hallucinations, and convulsions. These problems were due to the stirring up of Liver wind and required the use of formulas devised much later, which included such substances as Saigae tataricae Cornu *(líng yáng jiǎo)*.[17] Cao observed that this demonstrates that "There are critical presentations that cannot be treated by classic formulas, and for which formulas made by excellent scholars and practitioners after Zhang Ji are needed."[18]

In conclusion, this dispute stimulated scholars and practitioners to explore both the similarities and differences between cold damage and warm pathogen disease. It also gave added impetus to the development of warm pathogen disease theory. This dispute, which began several hundred years ago, still continues today. In my own view, it is clear that each of these methods of diagnosis and treatment has its place in the toolbox of every practitioner of Chinese medicine. It is not a question of which is correct, but rather when each is appropriate to use.

RELATIONSHIP BETWEEN WARM PATHOGEN DISEASE AND COLD DAMAGE

The relationship between the theories of warm pathogen disease and cold damage has been somewhat complex. On the one hand, warm pathogen disease theory is deeply rooted in concepts from Discussion of Cold Damage. On the other hand, it articulates new ideas and utilizes new approaches to treatment that are far different from those of the cold damage school. It is based both on the realization that warm-heat pathogens can directly cause disease, and an understanding of the peculiarities of the presentation and progress of these diseases.

This is not to say, however, that the treatment methods of the warm pathogen disease school are completely different from those based on cold damage. Certainly the originators of the warm pathogen disease school were profoundly influenced by Zhang Ji. This is reflected in the fact that in *Systematic Differentiation of Warm Pathogen*

Diseases, Wu Tang uses no less than twenty-eight formulas from *Discussion of Cold Damage*. However, the warm pathogen disease school developed some concepts which were incomplete in the *Discussion of Cold Damage*. One example is that, while purging is recommended in the *Discussion of Cold Damage* to treat intense interior heat that clumps with the stool, other important aspects of such conditions, for example, injury to the qi, fluids, and yin, were not addressed adequately until the development of warm pathogen disease theory.

Differences between Warm Pathogen Diseases and Cold Damage

Etiology. As mentioned above, a warm pathogen disease is caused by a warm-heat pathogen and presents at onset with an exterior heat pattern. By contrast, a cold damage disease is caused by an attack of wind-cold and presents at onset with a corresponding exterior cold pattern.

Pathogenesis of warm pathogen diseases versus cold damage. The warm-heat pathogens associated with warm pathogen diseases enter the body through the mouth and nose and first attack the Lung. Cold damage diseases attack the body through the skin and muscles, beginning with the greater yang, including the greater yang channel *(tai yang)* and its associated organ, the Bladder. However, as previously noted, this theoretical distinction is not always helpful in the clinic.

Pathology and development of the diseases. Warm-heat pathogens in warm pathogen disease, like all yang pathogens, open the pores of the skin and readily injure the yin and fluids. If not properly treated, the disease can progress to exhaustion of the yin and fluids along with collapse of the yang qi, which can be terminal. Conversely, diseases caused by cold, like all yin pathogens, readily injures the yang qi. However, they can gradually transform into heat due to the closing of the pores of the skin and stagnation of the yang qi. A cold pathogenic factor sometimes attacks yin organs (Spleen, Heart, Kidney, Liver) directly through their channel connections, because the yang qi in these organs is often relatively weak prior to catching cold. If not treated properly, the yang qi can collapse and the patient will die.

Clinical manifestations in the early stage. In the early stage, warm pathogen diseases, with the exception of spring-warmth and lurking summerheat, present with exterior heat signs as their main manifestation. The predominant symptoms are relatively severe fever and slight aversion to cold, chills, sore throat, cough with yellow and sticky sputum, slightly increased thirst, red tip and edge of the tongue, and floating and rapid pulse. In general, warm pathogen diseases first attack the Lung through the nose, mouth, and throat, and affect the protective qi.

The struggle between protective qi and the warm-heat pathogen leads to a relatively high fever. Diverted by its struggle with the warm-heat pathogen, the protective qi fails to do its job of warming the body. This leads to slight aversion to cold and slight chills, which are mild because the warm-heat pathogen is yang in nature, and thus does not significantly constrict the protective qi. The warm-heat pathogen injures the Lung fluids, leading to a slight thirst. The Lung fails to disseminate and cause its qi to descend, and its fluids are congealed by heat into phlegm, leading to cough with yellow and sticky sputum. A red tip and edge of the tongue reflects the involvement of the warm-heat pathogen. A floating and rapid pulse indicates that a warm-heat pathogen is in the exterior.

During their early stages, cold damage diseases often present with patterns of exterior cold from excess as their main manifestation. The predominant symptoms include severe chills and aversion to cold, slight fever, stiffness in the neck, body aches (especially affecting the back), no special thirst, and a floating and tight pulse. This presentation is due to cold attacking the *tai yang* Bladder channel. Cold obstructs qi and blood in the *tai yang* channel, resulting in stiffness in the neck and body aches, especially in the back. Cold contracts the protective qi and prevents it from warming the exterior, resulting in chills as well as severe aversion to cold. Since the fluids are undamaged by cold, there is no special thirst, and since the struggle between the protective qi and cold is not as severe as in warm pathogen diseases, the individual usually experiences only slight fever. The floating pulse indicates an attack by cold on the exterior, and the tight pulse reflects contraction of the channel by cold.

Patients who suffer from warm pathogen diseases may or may not sweat. This depends on the extent to which dampness is involved, and whether there are sufficient fluids or yin to produce sweat. Generally speaking, if dampness is a predominant factor in the disease, the patient will not sweat; otherwise, sweating will occur. Lack of sweating due to dampness is also accompanied by stiffness and a sensation of heaviness on the surface. In addition, as expected, if there are enough fluids or yin, sweating may occur. Otherwise, there will be no sweat. Therefore, in the clinic, it is crucial to observe or ask about perspiration in order to ascertain the presence or absence of dampness, fluids, or yin. These decisions will play an important role in determining the choice of treatment.

It should be noted that, in the clinic, a disease caused by cold may present with no sweating, which ostensibly looks similar to the lack of sweating caused by dampness or yin deficiency in a warm pathogen disease. The difference is that, with cold damage, there are no signs or symptoms of heat, such as increased thirst, red tip and edge of the tongue, and rapid pulse. A warm pathogen disease *must* present with heat signs and symptoms.

Treatment approaches. In general, the early stages of a warm pathogen disease are treated by eliminating the exterior signs and symptoms with acrid, cool herbs. Cold damage diseases are treated by eliminating exterior signs and symptoms with acrid, warm herbs.

ATTEMPTS TO RECONCILE THE THEORIES OF WARM PATHOGEN DISEASE AND COLD DAMAGE

Because yin and yang are the bedrock of Chinese thought, there is a tendency in Chinese culture to view seemingly contradictory concepts as complementary, and to understand them in a larger framework. This is the case with the theories of warm pathogen disease and cold damage. One way is to have the six-stage differentiation from *Discussion of Cold Damage* encompass the four-level and three-burner differentiations of warm pathogen disease. This was first espoused by the late eighteenth-century scholar Yu Gen-Chu in *Revised Popular Guide to the Discussion of Cold Damage (Chóng dìng tōng sú shāng hán lùn)*. It is still given credence in contemporary times, as noted in *Cold Damage and Warm Pathogen Diseases in Chinese Medicine (Zhōng yī shāng hán yǔ wēn bìng)* by Shi Yi-Ren (Shi Yi-Xing, 1896-1966).[19] From this perspective, the six-stage differentiation can be used in different ways. Not only may it be used to describe the progression of externally-contracted diseases, but also the state of the body through the parameters of yin and yang, deficiency and excess, heat and cold, and exterior and interior.[20]

Another way to reconcile the theories of warm pathogen disease and cold damage is to rely on the eight parameters to unite all three types of differentiation: the six stages, four levels, and three burners. This is a modern idea that was first advanced by Wan You-Sheng, currently at the Jiangxi College of Traditional Chinese Medicine.[21] It is based on the premise that the eight parameters can be seen as a general methodology for any disease, and can be easily adapted for describing the onset and progression of externally-contracted diseases.

As in every other facet of Chinese medicine, the yin or yang aspects of a pathogen are not immutable. In terms of the effects of external pathogens, the patient's constitution can determine the course of the disease. For example, in a patient with underlying yin deficiency, any externally-contracted disease, even one due to cold, will tend to become hot once it has entered the body. When this occurs, treatment must be aimed directly at how the pathogen is manifesting at that time, regardless of its origin. Similarly, in a patient with underlying yang deficiency, any externally-contracted disease, even one due to heat, will tend to become cold once it has entered the body. Again, treatment must be aimed directly at the how the pathogen is manifesting at that time. If a cold damage disorder enters the interior and, for any reason, produces heat, the treatment of that condition is no different than the same presentation due to a warm pathogen disease. Similarly, if profuse sweating or excessive purging during the course of a warm pathogen disease leads to a cold pattern, it should be treated as such. Clinically, it is not uncommon for a patient to present with cold and heat patterns at different times in the course of the same illness.

With this degree of overlap, it would appear that one could use six-stage differentiation as an overarching framework, and include four-level or three-burner differentiation under it. However, I think this would be a mistake, for two reasons.

First, given its place in the history of Chinese medicine, using six-stage differentiation to discuss warm pathogen diseases would be confusing, as those terms are associated with cold damage. Second, this arrangement would unnecessarily narrow the options available to practitioners, as cold damage and warm pathogen diseases take quite different trajectories. They usually affect the body in different ways, which is why the warm pathogen disease school developed new schemes of diagnosis and treatment in the first place. For example, both the *tai yang* stage of cold damage diagnosis and the protective level and upper burner of warm pathogen disease diagnosis have something to do with dysfunction of the protective qi. However, the *tai yang* stage focuses more on the relationship between the protective qi and nutritive qi, while the protective level and upper burner deal primarily with dysfunction of both the protective qi and the Lung. If one way of looking at disease is subsumed in the other, important information will be lost.

While the eight parameters work as a methodology for general differentiation, they are much too broad to be used effectively for diagnosing externally-contracted diseases. And while they can be used as a tool for beginners to help them learn about the location and quality of a disease, the information filtered in this way is neither specific nor precise enough to be effective in the clinic. In addition, looking at disease in this manner provides no indication about the exact location of the disease or its progress.

As we have seen, attempts to unify the approaches to warm pathogen disease and cold damage have focused more on the terminology and formal structures of diagnosis than on the reality in the clinic. This effort involves more than simply choosing one term to encompass another. Rather, we must figure out the relationships, connections, and especially the transformations between these two types of disease. Only in this way can we establish overarching principles of differentiation and treatment for both types of disease. Otherwise, the reconciliation of warm pathogen disease and cold damage will be nothing more than a formality, with no clinical significance.

Summary

This chapter has provided a brief introduction to the concept of warm pathogen diseases, their general characteristics, the types of diseases caused by warm-heat pathogens, disputes regarding the relationship between warm pathogen disease and cold damage, and the reconciliation of the two. The following chapter will address the etiology, onset, and pathogenesis of warm pathogen diseases, and subsequent chapters will provide more specific information regarding their diagnosis and treatment.

Endnotes

1. Anonymous, *Yellow Emperor's Inner Classic: Basic Questions (Huáng Dì nèi jīng sù wèn).* Beijing: People's Health Publishing House, 1963: 581.

2. Wang Qi et al., *Modern Translation and Explanation of Basic Questions (Sù wèn jīn shì).* Guiyang: Guizhou People's Publishing House, 1981: 417.

3. Wu You-Xing, *Discussion of Warm Epidemics (Wēn yì lùn).* Changchun: Liaoning Science and Technology Publishing House, 1997: 1.

4. ibid.

5. Pang An-Shi, *General Discussion for the Discussion of Cold Damage (Shāng hán zǒng bìng lùn),* reproduced in *Historical Collection of Rare Chinese Medical Books (Lì dài zhōng yī zhēn běn jí chéng).* Shanghai: Joint Publishing Company, 1990: 100.

6. Cold Damage Teaching and Research Section of the Nanjing College of Traditional Medicine, *Translation and Explanation of the Discussion of Cold Damage (Shāng hán lùn yì shì).* Shanghai: Shanghai Science and Technology Publishing House, 1980: 270.

7. For the sake of simplicity, in this text we use the term 'warm-heat disease' to represent those warm pathogen diseases that have no significant dampness, and 'damp-heat disease' to represent those that do. It is important to remember, however, that both warm-heat and damp-heat diseases are included under the rubric of warm pathogen diseases.

8. Anonymous, *Classic of Difficulties (Nán jīng).* Beijing: People's Health Publishing House, 1979: 128.

9. Anonymous, *Yellow Emperor's Inner Classic: Basic Questions,* 183.

10. Ye Gui, *Case Records as a Guide to Clinical Practice (Lín zhèng zhǐ nán yī àn).* Shanghai: Shanghai Science and Technology Publishing House, 1959: 736.

11. Tang Da-Lie, *Collection of Papers of Physicians from Wu (Wú yī huì jiǎng).* Shanghai: Shanghai Science and Technology Publishing House, 1983: 4

12. Meng Shu-Jiang et al., *Teaching Reference Books for Traditional Chinese Medical Colleges: Warm Pathogen Diseases (Gāo děng zhōng yī yuàn xiào jiào xué cān kǎo shū: wēn bìng xué).* Beijing: People's Health Publishing House, 1989: 13.

13. Ibid.

14. Wu Tang, *Systematic Differentiation of Warm Pathogen Diseases (Wēn bìng tiáo biàn).* Beijing: People's Health Publishing House, 1963: 2.

15. Warm Pathogen Disease Teaching and Research Section of the Chengdu College of Traditional Chinese Medicine, *Self-Study Book for Chinese Medicine: Warm Pathogen Diseases (Zhōng yī zì xué jiào cái: Wēn bìng xué).* Chengdu: Chengdu College of Traditional Chinese Medicine, 1985:

16. Meng Shu-Jiang et al., *Teaching Reference Books for Traditional Chinese Medical Colleges: Warm Pathogen Diseases,* 13.

17. Cao Jia-Da, *Records of Experiences with Classic Formulas (Jīng fāng shì yàn lù).* Shanghai: Shanghai Science and Technology Publishing House, 1979: 35-36.

18. Ibid., 36.

19. Shi Yi-Ren, *Cold Damage and Warm Pathogen Diseases in Chinese Medicine (Zhōng yī shāng hán yǔ wēn bìng)*. Shanghai: Shanghai Qian Qin Tang Press, 1956.

20. Xiao De-Xin, "My views on uniting the differentiation systems of cold [damage] and warm [diseases] *(Tǒng yī hán wēn biàn zhèng tǐ xì zhī wǒ jiàn),*" in Fang Yao-Zhong and Xu Jia-Song (eds.), *Collection of Lectures on Warm Pathogen Diseases (Wēn bìng huì jiǎng)*. Beijing: People's Health Publishing House, 1986: 380-81.

21. Wan You-Sheng, "Establish differentiation system for febrile disease by uniting the theory of warm pathogen disease and the theory of cold damage under the eight parameters *(Bā gāng tǒng yī hán wēn zhèng zhì, jiàn lì rè bìng xué kē tǐ xì).*" *Journal of Beijing College of Traditional Chinese Medicine,* 1983(3): 2-5.

3 Etiology, Onset, and Pathogenesis of Warm Pathogen Diseases

Etiology

CLASSICAL AND MODERN textbooks of Chinese medicine describe six external pathogenic factors or evils (邪氣 *xié qì*): wind, cold, summerheat, dampness, dryness, and fire. While not listed among the original six, toxin and pestilential qi must also be taken into account *as* external pathogens. Although there are exceptions, warm pathogen diseases generally result from an attack on the body by some combination of these factors, where at least one aspect is hot (or yang) in nature. The warm-heat pathogens that often combine to cause warm pathogen diseases include wind-heat, summerheat, damp-heat, dry-heat, and warm-toxin.

The principal features of these external warm-heat pathogens are that they quickly attack different areas of the body and give rise to diseases that are hot in nature. Dryness has two aspects: dry-heat and cool-dryness (Table 3.1). Each of the warm-heat pathogens has an affinity for a particular part of the body. That is to say, those involving wind or dryness are more likely to attack the upper and superficial aspects of the body (Lung and protective qi), while those involving dampness are more apt to attack the Spleen and Stomach.

WIND-HEAT CAUSES WIND-WARMTH

Wind-heat (風熱 *fēng rè*) is the pathogen that causes wind-warmth (風溫 *fēng wēn*). Wind-heat prevails in the spring or winter, which accordingly are the two seasons

53

Table 3.1	Warm-Heat Pathogens
• Wind-heat	
• Summerheat	
• Damp-heat	
• Dryness (warm-dryness and cool-dryness)	
•Warm-toxin	

when wind-warmth usually appears. Wind-heat has three characteristic features:

1. *Wind-heat attacks the Lung and protective level first.* Both heat and wind are yang pathogens characterized by upward and outward dispersion. Therefore, wind-heat always attacks the exterior and upper part of the body first. As noted in Chapter 46 of *Basic Questions,* the Lung serves as a lid over the other organs and is located at the highest place in the body.[1] The Lung distributes protective qi, circulating it over the exterior to provide protection. Thus, the Lung and protective qi serve as the first line of defense against an attack by wind-heat. When it is attacked, the Lung cannot properly disseminate its qi and make it descend, and the protective qi is thus unable to circulate smoothly. This impairs Lung function and leads to stagnation of protective qi, resulting in high fever, chills, aversion to wind and cold, slight sweating, cough, slightly increased thirst, red tipped tongue with a thin and white coating, and a floating and rapid pulse. Among these signs and symptoms, chills and aversion to wind and cold reflect stagnation of protective qi, and the fever indicates that there is a fierce struggle between the protective qi and wind-heat. The cough reflects the failure of the Lung to disseminate its qi and cause it to descend. Slight sweating is attributable to the stagnation of protective qi, impairing its ability to control the pores. The slight increase in thirst shows that the wind-heat pathogen has slightly injured the fluids.

2. *Wind-heat transforms into fire and readily injures the yin.* Compared with other combinations of external pathogenic factors, wind and heat—two yang pathogens—have a tendency to progress rapidly, transform into fire, and injure the yin. Wind-heat first injures the yin of the Lung and Stomach when it invades the interior of the body, causing dry cough, dry throat and nose, strong thirst for cold beverages, red tongue with little coating, and a thin pulse.

3. *Wind-heat quickly advances to the Pericardium.* One of the characteristics of wind is its **rapid movement**. When this occurs in conjunction with weakness in the body's resistance due to injury of the Lung and Stomach yin, wind-heat can

readily attack the Pericardium directly. Lu Ting-Zhen (Lu Zi-Xian) discussed this phenomenon in *Systematic Differentiation of the Six Etiologies (Liù yīn tiáo biàn)*, published in 1868. Lu noted that "Wind-heat progresses very quickly and the patterns that arise from such progression are the most critical when compared to patterns of other warm-heat pathogens."[2] Wind-heat can progress from the Lung and the protective level to the Pericardium at the nutritive level in a very short time, leading to blockage of the Heart spirit. This in turn can lead to mental disorders, such as muddled consciousness and delirium, or even coma. Clinically, this can be seen in a child suffering from high fever, cough, and difficult breathing, such as occurs in pneumonia. The child can slip into muddled consciousness or coma, or experience convulsions and delirium, within twenty-four hours of the initial attack. This occurs because both the Lung and Pericardium are located in the upper burner, and as the Pericardium is the protector of the Heart, it can be readily attacked.

Summerheat Causes Summerheat-Warmth

According to five-phase theory, fire prevails in the early summer and corresponds to the Heart. When fire becomes too strong, it causes the water in the ground to steam upward, producing dampness. During summer people like to drink cold beverages, and many go camping in the mountains, where it is damp in the evening. The yang qi floats on the exterior at this time because of its strong attraction to the hot climate. As a result, the yang qi is relatively weak inside the body, increasing the individual's susceptibility to cold, especially cold from food. Thus, drinking cold beverages at this time can actually injure the Spleen yang more severely than drinking cold beverages in the winter, when the yang sinks more deeply into the body's core.

Accordingly, summerheat is often associated with dampness and is related to the Spleen and Stomach, as well as the Heart. The summerheat pathogen (暑熱 *shǔ rè*) causes summerheat-warmth (暑溫 *shǔ wēn*). This pathogen strikes only in the summer, except when it lurks within the body and gives rise to lurking summerheat (伏暑 *fú shǔ*) at a later time as a result of an attack by a secondary pathogen.

The summerheat pathogen has four characteristic features:

1. *Summerheat attacks the Stomach and qi level first.* Summerheat, a yang pathogen, is characterized by fierce heat and rapid movement; it often attacks the body in combination with dampness. In accordance with five-phase theory, dampness, and the Spleen (yin) and Stomach (yang), correspond to earth. Thus, if there is more yang (heat), summerheat will attack the Stomach; if there is more yin (dampness), summerheat will attack the Spleen. In the absence of dampness, or if heat is the predominant factor, summerheat will first attack the Stomach, entering the qi level directly, without first manifesting protective level signs

and symptoms. In this case, summerheat presents with vigorous fever, profuse sweating, severe thirst, and a flooding pulse. On the other hand, if dampness is the predominant factor, summerheat can readily attack the Spleen as well as the Stomach. Since dampness moves more slowly than heat, and thus penetrates the body slowly, summerheat with a strong dampness component is more likely to appear first in the protective level. Associated signs and symptoms include aversion to cold, chills, fever, heavy sensation in the body, chest distention, absence of sweating, and a white and yellow tongue coating.

2. *Summerheat can attack the Pericardium directly and block the spirit of the Heart.* When the pathogen is strong, and especially in the absence of dampness, summerheat can attack the Pericardium directly and suddenly, blocking the spirit of the Heart and leading to sunstroke. This occurs most frequently in people who are exposed to direct sunlight during summer, or who work in front of furnaces in factories.

3. *Summerheat readily injures the fluids and source qi.* According to Chapter 5 of *Basic Questions*, extreme fire (heat) will injure the qi.[3] Summerheat injures both the source qi and the fluids, resulting in severe shortness of breath, fatigue, strong thirst, a large pulse at the superficial level, and a very frail pulse at the deep level. This is unique among external pathogens such as wind-heat, damp-heat, or dry-heat, which injure yin or qi, but not both simultaneously.

4. *External dampness often accompanies summerheat when attacking the body.* As previously mentioned, during the summer season, summerheat descends and dampness steams upward. Therefore, external dampness often joins with summerheat in attacking the body. It focuses on the Stomach and Spleen, giving rise to such signs and symptoms as poor appetite, distention in the epigastrium, loose stools, and a greasy tongue coating. Clinically, these signs and symptoms are often found in individuals who drink lots of iced beverages during the daytime, eat lots of ice cream, or get cold in the evening while camping outdoors. In such cases, not only will summerheat be accompanied by dampness, but also by cold. The cold can attack the exterior as well as the Spleen and Stomach. Patients will present with severe cramping in the epigastric region or abdomen, severe body aches, chills, aversion to cold, and the absence of sweating. When treating summerheat with dampness, it is important to remember that this is a combination of yin (dampness) and yang (summerheat) pathogens, and to weigh their relative strength.

DAMP-HEAT CAUSES DAMP-WARMTH

Damp-heat generally prevails in the late summer, although it can be seen in other seasons. The damp-heat pathogen (濕熱 *shī rè*) which causes damp-warmth (濕溫 *shī wēn*) has four characteristic features:

1. *Damp-heat develops slowly and has a prolonged course.* Dampness is character-ized by turbidity and stagnation, gradual onset, and gradual conversion into heat. According to Yang Shi-Yin, author of the 13th century work *Straight Directions from [Yang] Ren-Zhai (Rén-Zhāi zhí zhǐ),* "Dampness can attack without notice a person when walking, sitting, or sleeping."[4] Unlike what is ob-served in summerheat-warmth, in the early stages of damp-warmth there are no remarkable heat symptoms, such as high fever with no aversion to cold, or strong thirst. When dampness predominates over heat, damp-warmth presents with slight fever or contained fever,[5] no increase in thirst, a white and greasy tongue coating, and a soggy and moderate pulse. The disease will likely remain in a particular level of the body, especially the qi level, for a long time. It can also progress slowly, taking anywhere from a few days to weeks for the disease to progress from one place in the body to another. Finally, the course of the disease can be weeks, months, or even years.

2. *Damp-heat mainly affects the Spleen and Stomach.* According to five-phase the-ory, dampness is associated with earth, which corresponds to the Spleen and Stomach. Therefore, while manifesting symptoms of exterior dampness, such as a heavy head and body and aversion to cold, damp-heat always attacks and tenaciously adheres to the Spleen and Stomach. It manifests with such signs and symptoms as distention in the epigastrium and the abdomen, nausea, loose stools, either normal thirst or absence of thirst, and a greasy tongue coating.

3. *Damp-heat stagnates the circulation of qi and blocks the clear yang from reaching the head.* Since dampness is a yin pathogenic factor characterized by heaviness, it is apt to stagnate the circulation of qi, especially in the middle burner and Liver. This will present with chest and epigastric distention, abdominal bloat-ing, and depression.[6] When it blocks clear yang from reaching the head, there will be a sensation of heaviness in the head as if it were wrapped in a bandage, nasal congestion, plugged ears, diminished hearing, and a dull expression. If the dampness is particularly extreme, it will descend to the lower burner and injure the Kidney yang, leading to retention of water and dampness, and presenting with intolerance to cold, edema, loose stools, cold extremities, and a white and moist tongue coating.

4. *The combination of dampness and heat is difficult to treat.* Traditional Chinese medicine likens the combination of heat which is without form, and damp-ness which has form, to a mixture of wheat flour and oil. Once mixed, they are very difficult to treat separately. Any disease caused by a combination of heat and dampness is more difficult to treat than a disease caused by heat alone. According to Xue Xue, author of *Systematic Differentiation of Damp-Heat (Shī rè tiáo biàn):*

Heat will be intense if it mixes with dampness [which can block the qi, and qi stagnation may then transform into heat]. And dampness will become severe when it mixes with heat [because it congeals dampness, making it more tenacious]. Therefore, damp-warmth will become worse when dampness and heat mix, and improve when dampness and heat are separated.7

This is because dampness blocks the qi, causing it to stagnate. Stagnation of qi can transform into heat or exacerbate existing heat. In addition, heat can cause the dampness to steam upward in the body, while dampness itself usually attacks the lower part of the body.

DRYNESS CAUSES AUTUMN-DRYNESS

In theory, the dry pathogen (燥 *zào*) only prevails in the autumn. This belief was formed because herbal theory developed in a part of the world with a particular climate and particular living conditions. In fact, however, dryness can be seen in the clinic at any time of year. For example, people living in high altitudes where the air is dry can contract the dry pathogen any time of the year. Air-conditioning can also dry the air, and people living or working in air-conditioned buildings can develop diseases associated with dryness. It is called autumn-dryness (秋燥 *qiū zào*) because historically, it almost always occurred during the autumn.

The effect of dryness, both as an aspect of normal weather change and as a pathogenic factor, was first discussed in Chapter 5 of *Basic Questions*, where it is noted that excessively dry weather will injure the fluids.[8] To classical theorists it seemed that dryness was more yang and warm in nature because it could injure the fluids. External dryness was not systematically discussed until the Qing dynasty (1644-1911). Based on an idea in *Basic Questions*, Yu Chang (Yu Jia-Yan, 1585-1664) offered the first systematic discussion of autumn-dryness in his book *Precepts for Physicians (Yī mén fǎ lù)*. Yu pointed out that dryness attacks the body like something being baked by fire and is therefore heat-oriented.[9] However, in *Discussion of Warm-Heat Diseases (Wēn rè bìng lùn)*, Shen Ming-Zong (Shen Mu-Nan, c. 1693) countered that dryness is cold.[10] Other scholars like Yu Gen-Chu (Yu Zhao-Yuan, c. 1776), Wang Meng-Ying (Wang Shi-Xiong, 1808-1867), and Fei Bo-Xiong (Fei Jin-Qing, c. 1883) thought that dryness, as an external pathogenic factor, could cause two distinct diseases: warm-dryness (溫燥 *wēn zào*) and cool-dryness (涼燥 *liáng zào*).[11] These are caused by two different aspects of the dry pathogen. Warm-dry-ness is caused by dry-heat and cool-dryness by the cool-dry pathogen. The former occurs during early autumn, when the weather first turns from summer, and is associated with the remnants of heat left over from summer. The latter occurs in late autumn, when the weather approaches winter-like conditions; it is associated with cold.

Clinically, the warm-dryness type of autumn-dryness presents with distinct signs and symptoms of heat, while cool-dryness does not. Rather, it may present with signs and symptoms of cold in addition to its dry characteristics. For this reason, the authors of the fifth edition of *Warm Pathogen Diseases (Wēn bìng xué)* in the People's Republic of China are divided as to whether cool-dryness is a warm pathogen disease.[12]

Dryness has two principal features:

1. *Dryness mainly attacks the Lung.* In accordance with five-phase theory, dryness is associated with metal and corresponds to the Lung. Therefore, dryness is apt to attack the Lung through the mouth and nose, giving rise to signs and symptoms of dryness in the Lung system such as dry cough with little sputum, dryness of the nose, sore and dry throat, and a hoarse voice in the early stage of the disease.

2. *Dryness is apt to injure the fluids of the Lung.* Because dryness affects the fluids in the yin and yang organs, it manifests in signs and symptoms of injury to the fluids, particularly those of the Lung. When dryness first attacks the Lung, it presents with dry lips, nose, throat, and mouth, thirst, dry cough with little or no sputum, and a dry, red tongue. This is quite different from wind-heat, which injures the fluids at a more advanced stage, although it also slightly injures the fluids at the onset of the disease.

PESTILENTIAL QI AND WARM-TOXIN CAUSE WARM PATHOGEN DISEASES

In addition to the four pathogens discussed above, there are two other pathogens mentioned in some of the classics that can give rise to warm pathogen diseases: pestilential qi (癘氣 *lì qì*) and warm-toxin (溫毒 *wēn dú*). The existence of pestilential qi was first mentioned in Chapter 71 of *Basic Questions*: "When pestilential qi comes strongly, populations will tend to die suddenly."[13] Pestilential qi refers to a pathogenic factor that is infectious in nature; the diseases it causes occur suddenly and progress quickly. These diseases are commonly known as epidemics and the pathogen sometimes described as epidemic qi (疫氣 *yì qì*). However, there is no systematic description in classical texts about the characteristics of pestilential qi, such as its identification, diagnosis, and treatment. The practitioner should vigorously eliminate pestilential qi using cool and acrid herbs, or bitter and cold herbs, that clear heat and resolve toxicity from the qi and nutritive levels. This is regarded as the main treatment approach for pestilential qi. Currently, many scholars argue that pestilential qi is related to infectious diseases that have a warm-toxin nature. However, pestilential qi is not exactly equivalent to warm-toxin because the latter is not necessarily infectious, while epidemic qi is always infectious. Regardless, many clinicians use treatments that address heat and toxins to treat pestilential qi and epidemics.

The term toxin (毒 *dú*) was first introduced in *Basic Questions*. In Chapter 72 it is noted that toxin is a cause of five types of infectious disease.[14] Currently, the term has three meanings. The first refers to the toxic nature of herbs, for example, Pinelliae Rhizoma preparatum *(zhì bàn xià)* or Scorpio *(quán xiē)*. The second refers to particular patterns in dermatology, for example, herpes zoster. The third refers to pathogens that can injure the body, which are called pathogenic toxin (毒邪 *dú xié*).

According to Zhao Xu-Chu in his recent book *Compendium of Modern Chinese Medicine Applications and Research: Warm Pathogen Diseases (Xiàn dài zhōng yī yào yìng yòng yǔ yán jiù dà xì: wēn bìng)*, pathogenic toxins can be divided into externally-con-tracted and internally-generated types. The externally-contracted toxins can result from an extreme buildup of other pathogenic factors such as wind-heat, summer-heat, damp-heat, dry-heat, cold, and dampness. Zhao also thinks that externally-contracted toxins include toxin from animals and insects, pharmaceutical drugs that are toxic from the perspective of Western biomedicine, and from food.[15]

Internally-generated toxin can result from other internal pathogenic factors such as heat, fire, blood stasis, and phlegm-heat. Generally speaking, externally-con-tracted toxins act as primary pathogenic factors when attacking the body. By contrast, internal pathogenic toxins, because they are usually the by-product of the other pathogenic factors listed above, are regarded as secondary pathogenic factors. Once the pathogenic factor attacks the body or is produced within the body, it can give rise to heat by blocking the circulation of qi, leading to stagnation of qi. This in turn gives rise to additional heat, as well as fire, phlegm, and blood stasis, which can injure the tissues, muscles, and organs. When pathogenic toxin and heat mix, they readily injure the source qi and yin, and force blood out of the vessels.

The term warm-toxin first appeared in *Emergency Formulas to Keep Up One's Sleeve (Zhǒu hòu bèi jí fāng)* by Ge Hong (Ge Ya-Chuan, 281-341). It is now a term used for mostly externally-contracted pathogenic toxins. Warm-toxin is the result of a warm-toxin pathogen, which manifests with acute and severe heat, develops faster than other types of warm pathogen disease, and can give rise to localized red, painful, and swollen throat or tonsils with pus. Theoretically, all pathogenic factors can transform into toxin. According to Wu Tang, author of *Systematic Differentiation of Warm Pathogen Diseases (Wēn bìng tiáo biàn)*, "Warm-toxin actually [represents] all warm-heat pathogens associated with toxin"[16] such as wind-heat with toxin, summerheat with toxin, or dryness with toxin. In *A Series of Self-Study Textbooks, Warm Pathogen Disease Section (Zhōng yī zì xué jiào cái: Wēn bìng xué)*, Zhang Zhi-Wen[17] points out that, unlike heat or wind, warm-toxin is not an independent pathogen. Rather, it results from extreme heat or accumulation of a warm-heat pathogen.

To treat diseases caused by warm-toxin pathogens, herbs that clear heat, drain fire, and purge toxins should be used. If the warm-toxin pathogen is in the blood, the practitioner should use herbs that cool the blood and resolve toxicity. In *Systematic Differentiation of Cold Damage and Warm Epidemics (Shāng hán wēn yì tiáo biàn)*, Yang Xuan (Yang Yu-Heng, 1705-1784) pointed out that one can treat warm-toxin pathogens utilizing three-burner differentiation:

> The physical function of the upper burner is to disperse qi and distribute blood that has been transformed from digested food in the form of vapors; one can disperse and dissipate the pattern caused by warm-toxin in the upper burner.

The physical function of the middle burner is to grind, transform, and transport food in the form of foam; one can purge warm-toxin through bowel movements when warm-toxin is in the middle burner. The physical function of the lower burner is to separate the clear from the turbid, and to discharge the turbid like a sluice; one can purge warm-toxin through bowel movements and urination when warm-toxin is in the lower burner.[18]

According to Yu Lin (Yu Shi-Yu, 1736-1795), author of *Achievements Regarding Epidemic Rashes (Yì zhěn yī dé)*, the combination of a warm-heat pathogen and toxin can have the following two different presentations:[19]

1. *It is confined to a certain area of the body, leading to local swelling, redness, pain, and ulceration.* The diseases caused by this type of warm-toxin are massive head febrile disorder (大頭溫 *dà tóu wēn*) and putrefying throat granular disorder (爛喉痧 *làn hóu shā*). Massive head febrile disorder was first mentioned in *Collected Treatises of [Zhang] Jing-Yue (Jǐng-Yuè quán shū)* by Zhang Jie-Bin (Zhang Jing-Yue, c. 1636). Zhang observed that:

   > Massive head febrile disorder is an attack on the three yang channels by infectious toxin, leading to fever, chills, swelling in the neck, eye, head, or throat, or even a red and swollen face, cheeks, shoulders, and back. The swelling looks like the bulging cheeks of a toad.[20]

   Putrefying throat granular disorder was first described in *Case Records as a Guide to Clinical Practice(Lín zhèng zhǐ nán yī àn)*. This book was written by Ye Gui's students, although Ye's name appears on the book as author. Here it is observed that:

   > There was a disease called putrefying throat granular disorder that occurred at the end of winter and the beginning of spring in 1733. Regardless of whether one was elderly, young, female or male, the disease could spread from one person to another. The patient who suffered from this disease presented with high fever, strong thirst, irritability, restlessness, red skin eruptions, and a painful and swollen throat.[21]

2. *It spreads over the entire body, including the exterior and interior, and affects the qi and blood.* It presents with a high fever, eruptions over the entire body, vomiting with blood, and epistaxis.

Onset and Pathogenesis of Warm Pathogen Diseases

FACTORS AFFECTING THE ONSET OF A WARM PATHOGEN DISEASE

Whether or not an individual develops a warm pathogen disease depends upon four factors:

1. *The strength of the individual's antipathogenic qi.* If the antipathogenic qi is strong relative to the strength of a warm-heat pathogen, it will defend the body and overcome an attack. No warm pathogen disease will occur. However, if the antipathogenic qi is weak relative to the strength of an assaulting warm-heat pathogen, a warm pathogen disease will appear. Many factors play important roles in one's vulnerability to warm-heat pathogens. These include one's constitution and lifestyle. A poor lifestyle, including overwork, irregular eating, excessive alcohol intake, drug use, and cigarette smoking, compromises the antipathogenic qi. It can also generate internal problems, including dampness and heat, which resonate with externally-contracted pathogens and make the situation worse.

2. *The severity of the warm-heat pathogen.* If the warm-heat pathogen is so strong that it can overcome the resistance of the body's antipathogenic qi, regardless of its strength, a warm pathogen disease will definitely appear.

3. *A change in the weather.* If the weather changes too drastically, or if one kind of weather persists for an unnatural length of time and the individual cannot adapt, the resistance of the antipathogenic qi will diminish. Under these circumstances, the attack of a warm-heat pathogen on the body will be successful.

4. *Sociological factors.* These include the individual's living standards, level of health, and approaches used to prevent diseases from attacking. If the living standards and level of health are high, and if there are numerous practical approaches for preventing the attack by disease, then it is less likely that a warm-heat pathogen will successfully attack the body.

Mechanism of Attack by Warm-Heat Pathogens

We cannot say that each pathogen always attacks a particular area of the body or always enters the body through a particular pathway. We can only say that certain pathogens are more likely to attack certain organs, and more likely to enter the body through certain pathways (Table 3.2). For example, the preferred mode of attack by wind-warmth and autumn-dryness is via the Lungs during respiration. Damp-warmth will more likely attack the Stomach and Spleen through the intake of food. Pestilential qi is not included here since it is unclear, based on ancient writings, which organs are affected by an initial attack of pestilential qi. They can also enter through the skin or muscles, especially if the person has any preexisting internal dampness, a condition that attracts external dampness to the body. These are tendencies, but only tendencies.

Attack through the skin. The skin is the first layer of defense against pathogenic factors. It is therefore the first target of attack by externally-contracted wind and cold, as well as warm-heat pathogens.

Attack through the nose and mouth. Since the latter part of the Ming dynasty (1368-1644), scholars and practitioners have attached great importance to the nose and mouth as the main route of attack for warm-heat pathogens. In his book *Systematic Differentiation of Damp-Heat (Shī rè tiáo biàn)*, Xue Xue (1681–1770) noted that "The chances of damp-heat attacking the body through the exterior are 10-20 percent, and the chances of damp-heat attacking the body through mouth and nose are 80-90 percent."[22] Since the nose is the organ through which we communicate with heavenly qi, a warm-heat pathogen is apt to attack the body through the nose when we inhale qi from the atmosphere. The Lung opens onto the nose, and thus a warm-heat pathogen can readily attack the Lung in the upper burner. Wind-warmth and autumn-dryness mostly enter the Lung via respiration. The Stomach opens onto the mouth, which takes in food. Warm-heat pathogens, if accompanied by the ingestion of improper foods, readily attack the body through the mouth. Damp-warmth, often caused by damp-heat pathogens that accompany the ingestion of improper foods, initially attacks the Spleen and Stomach in the middle burner.

Table 3.2	Organs Affected by an Initial Attack of a Warm-Heat Pathogen	
Lung	**Spleen and Stomach**	**Lung and Stomach**
Wind-heat	Summerheat	Warm-toxin
Dryness	Damp-heat	

Onset of Warm Pathogen Diseases

Warm-heat pathogens evolve into warm pathogen diseases by one of two pathways. The first is newly-contracted warm pathogen disease (新感溫病 *xīn gǎn wēn bìng*), which occurs upon the initial attack by a warm-heat pathogen, that is, the disease is characterized by the absence of an incubation period. The second is lurking warm pathogen disease (伏氣溫病 *fú qì wēn bìng*), which occurs following a period of incubation within the body.

Newly-contracted warm pathogen disease. A newly-contracted warm pathogen disease is characterized by the absence of an incubation period. Unlike a lurking warm pathogen disease, a newly-contracted warm pathogen disease initially affects the protective level, that is, the earliest manifestation is that of an exterior pattern. The signs and symptoms at the early stage of a newly-contracted warm pathogen disease include fever, aversion to cold, chills, little or no sweating, headache, cough, thin and white tongue coating, and a floating and rapid pulse. The disease progresses from the exterior to the interior, and from superficial levels of the body to deeper levels. In general, at the early stage it is mild and has a short course. The primary method for treating newly-contracted warm pathogen disease at the early stage is the elimination of exterior signs and symptoms by dispersing the warm-heat pathogen. The newly-contracted warm pathogen diseases include wind-warmth, autumn-dryness, summerheat-warmth, warm-toxin, and damp-warmth.

Lurking warm pathogen disease. Lurking warm pathogen disease refers to a warm pathogen disease that manifests following a period of incubation, that is, a significant time after the initial attack by either cold or summerheat.[23] This type of disease was first discussed in Chapter 3 of *Basic Questions:* "If the body is attacked by cold in winter, the person will suffer from a warm pathogen disease in spring."[24]

Several questions concerning lurking warm pathogen diseases have been raised and answered over the years:

- *Why does the pathogenic factor lurk, and why does it eventually emerge and transform into heat, whereupon it progresses from inside the body to the surface?*

  This is because the antipathogenic qi becomes so weak that it can no longer control the pathogen. According to Chapter 4 of *Basic Questions*, one's constitution must be considered when determining whether a person who has been attacked by cold in winter will suffer from a warm pathogen disease in spring: "If a person has sufficient essence, he will not suffer from a warm pathogen disease in spring, even though he has been attacked by cold in winter."[25] Kidney essence has always been regarded as one of the foundations of the body's ability to defend itself against pathogens. As previously noted, it was not until the late eighteenth century that Wu Tang suggested in *Systematic Differentiation of Warm Pathogen Diseases* that activities other than sex could lead to loss of essence. Using military metaphors, the mid-eighteenth century author Jiang Bao-Su (Jiang Wen-Zhai) in *Thirteen Chapter Precis of Medicine* (*Yī lüè shí sān piān*) elaborated upon the relationship between Kidney yang and external cold with respect to lurking cold:

  > When it encounters [a person with] exhaustion of Kidney qi such that the essence rattles around inside, and overwork of the bodily form such that sweat drains off on the outside, cold qi takes advantage [of the situation]. Similar types of qi search for each other [and so the cold] enters into the territory of the *shao yin* [Kidneys]. As the [Kidney] yang is again restrained, it is unable to attack [the cold] even if it advances, and the pores and interstices are conversely [overly] constricted [due to the cold]. When withdrawing, there is no way back, and so as [the cold] looks for something between advancing and withdrawing, it must follow the tactic of becoming forcibly entrenched in the aspect of the membrane source.[26]

- *In the case of spring-warmth, where does the cold lurk?* This has been the source of controversy for centuries. Among the most common answers are the muscles and skin,[27] muscles and bones,[28] *shao yang* level structures, including the membrane source,[29] and Kidney.[30] Ye Gui said that "Spring-warmth was caused by lurking cold in the Kidney due to Kidney yin deficiency. It manifests in the *shao yang* in spring because spring and the Gallbladder pertain to wood."[31] The late nineteenth-century author Lei Feng (Lei Shao-Yi) in *Discussion of Seasonal Diseases (Shí bìng lùn)* proposed a more flexible and useful approach. He stated that cold would lurk in different places in different people, depending on their constitutions. For example, the cold will lurk in the Kidney if the patient has Kidney deficiency, and in the muscles if the patient does physical work and has a strong physical constitution.[32] This has clinical significance.

• *Does the pathogenic factor emerge automatically?* No, it requires a secondary factor to induce its manifestation. Clinically, there are many factors that can induce a lurking warm pathogen disease to appear. Commonly, a secondary externally-contracted pathogenic factor (such as wind-heat during the spring, summer-heat during the summer, or dryness during the autumn or cold) attacks while the primary pathogen is lurking within the body. Alternatively, the consumption of improper foods, overstrain and stress, violent emotions, improper treatment, or excessive sexual activity can weaken the antipathogenic qi, which allows the lurking warm pathogen disease to emerge. This was stated clearly by the late nineteenth-century author Ye Lin (Ye Zi-Yu, active c. 1897): "Pathogens are congealed by cold weather in winter and lurk between the muscles and bones. They can be triggered by either wind-heat or emotional upset and manifest as a warm pathogen disease." [33]

• *How do we differentiate between newly-contracted warm pathogen disease and lurking warm pathogen disease?* While theoretically the two types of warm pathogen disease should be simple to distinguish, in practice it can be far from easy. Often it is difficult to determine if a warm-heat pathogen has lurked within the body, and whether that lurking pathogen is in fact the cause of the current warm pathogen disease. So is there anything peculiar about the presentation that may alert us to the fact that the patient has a warm pathogen disease due to a lurking warm-heat pathogen? Modern scholars have suggested that the practitioner carefully determine whether there are signs and symptoms of interior heat at the very onset of a warm pathogen disease. Their presence indicates a lurking warm pathogen disease.[34] This is a very practical method which, however, is somewhat limited in application. For example, both summerheat-warmth and damp-warmth may initially present with manifestations of interior heat, such as a strong thirst, sweating, fever, aversion to heat, scanty and dark urine, and a flooding and large pulse. Despite such limitations, this method is still quite useful.

Table 3.3	Newly-contracted and Lurking Warm Pathogen Diseases
Newly-contracted Warm Pathogen Diseases	**Lurking Warm Pathogen Diseases**
Wind-Warmth	Spring-Warmth
Autumn-Dryness	Lurking Summerheat
Damp-Warmth	
Summerheat-Warmth	
Warm-Toxin	

Theoretically, all kinds of warm-heat pathogens can lurk in the body if it is too weak to dispel them. However, it is the view of modern textbooks that only spring-warmth and lurking summerheat are regarded as lurking warm pathogen diseases (Table 3.3).[35]

The presentation of lurking warm pathogen disease has both negative and positive implications. On the one hand, it indicates that antipathogenic qi is not sufficiently strong to control the pathogen in the deeper levels of the body. On the other hand, once the lurking warm pathogen disease emerges, it draws attention to the presence of the illness. In addition, it makes it easier to discharge the disease from the body, since it will be closer to the surface. It is rather difficult to discharge when it is lurking in the deeper levels of the body. Moreover, according to Liu Bao-Yi (Liu Gu-Sen, c. 1900) in *Encountering the Sources of Warm-Heat Pathogen Diseases (Wēn rè féng yuán)*, "Pathologically speaking, it is a good sign when a lurking heat pathogen comes out from the interior to the exterior, and it is a bad sign when it remains in the interior and cannot reach the exterior."[36] This is because heat lurking in the interior of the body for a long time will exhaust the body's yin.

The onset of a lurking warm pathogen disease manifests as an interior heat pattern with such signs and symptoms as a hot sensation over the body, irritability, restlessness, thirst, dark yellow urine, maculas, hematemesis, epistaxis, and a red tongue with a yellow coating. If the lurking warm pathogen disease is induced to manifest by an externally-contracted pathogenic factor, exterior signs and symptoms, like aversion to cold, chills, and fever, will also be present. However, the major presentation will be the previously mentioned signs and symptoms associated with interior heat.

Wang Meng-Ying described the presentation of a lurking warm pathogen disease that is aroused from its latency stage by a non-externally-contracted pathogenic factor, for example, by the consumption of improper foods or violent emotions. Wang discussed the progression and treatment of lurking warm pathogen disease at some length in his book *Warp and Woof of Warm-Heat Pathogen Diseases (Wēn rè jīng wěi):*

Lurking warm pathogen disease progresses by moving from the interior to the exterior. It first progresses from the nutritive level to the qi level. Thus, at the first stage of the disease, the tongue is moist and has no coating. To identify the disease, the practitioner must feel for the soggy pulse, or a wiry or slightly rapid pulse, and look for irritability, restlessness, aversion to heat, and no increase in thirst. To treat this condition, one must use herbs to clear heat from the nutritive level. When the lurking warm-heat pathogen progresses from the nutritive level to the qi level, the tongue will begin to show a coating. One must then use herbs to clear heat from the qi level. If there is a severe lurking warm-heat pathogen, the patient will present with a deep-red tongue, dry throat, or a very submerged pulse and cold extremities. The strongest method for clearing a lurking warm-heat pathogen must be used immediately. After this treatment, a thick, sticky, turbid, and yellow tongue coating will gradually appear. These are the principal differences between lurking warm pathogen diseases and newly-contracted warm pathogen diseases in their onset and progression.[37]

There is another special case in lurking warm pathogen disease when a lurking warm-heat pathogen delves too deeply and cannot completely emerge. Even though the right treatment may be used, the tongue can become deep-red, with a dry and yellowish coating again, just a few days after the tongue has become slightly red and the yellowish tongue coating has gone. It is just like drawing a piece of silk from a silk cocoon. When pulling the thread, it almost seems as if there is no end in sight. This special progression is quite different from newly-contracted warm pathogen disease, where the warm-heat pathogen attacks from the outside and the pathogen progresses from the protective level to the qi level, and then from the qi level to the nutritive and blood levels.[38]

Generally speaking, in the early stage the symptoms of a lurking warm pathogen disease are relatively more severe than those of a newly-contracted warm pathogen disease. In addition, the course of the illness is usually longer for a lurking warm pathogen disease. This was succinctly stated by He Lian-Chen (He Bing-Yuan, 1860-1929) who summarized the difference between lurking warm pathogen disease and newly-contracted warm pathogen disease in terms of their progression and severity: "Compared with a newly-contracted warm pathogen disease, a lurking warm pathogen disease is more severe. It is much easier to treat the newly-contracted warm pathogen disease and harder to treat the lurking one."[39] In the early stage, the main method for treating a lurking warm pathogen disease is to clear the interior lurking heat; by contrast, the main method for treating the early stages of a newly-contract-ed warm pathogen disease is to disperse the externally-contracted warm-heat pathogen.[40] According to Wang Lü (Wang An-Dao, 1332-1391) in *Discourse on Tracing Back to the Medical Classics (Yī jīng sù huí jí)*, "The main treatment is to clear interior heat and to eliminate exterior signs and symptoms. Also, in some cases, exterior signs and symptoms will automatically disappear once the interior heat has been successfully cleared."[41] In the later stages, the treatment of lurking warm pathogen disease is similar to that of other warm pathogen diseases. Table 3.4 summarizes the differences between lurking warm pathogen disease and newly-contracted warm pathogen disease.

Table 3.4	Comparison Between Newly-Contracted and Lurking Warm Pathogen Diseases	
	Newly-Contracted Warm Pathogen Disease	**Lurking Warm Pathogen Disease**
ORIGINS	External warm-heat pathogens	Interior heat derived from lurking external pathogens
PRESENTATION IN THE EARLY STAGE	Exterior: aversion to cold, chills, body aches, nasal congestion, possible sweating	Interior: strong thirst, profuse sweating, high fever, aversion to warmth, scanty dark urine, flooding and large pulse
PROGRESSION	From exterior to interior, from protective to qi, nutritive, and blood levels	From interior to exterior, from nutritive to qi level, or to blood level
TREATMENT	Release the exterior and disperse warm-heat pathogen	Clear interior heat
SEVERITY OF DISEASE	Mild	Severe

Summary

This chapter has addressed the characteristics of five warm-heat pathogens in some detail. They are all hot in nature, give rise to heat signs and symptoms, readily injure the yin or fluids, and can attack the body through the skin as well as through the mouth and nose. To provide proper treatment, the practitioner should differentiate two subcategories: damp-heat diseases (summerheat-warmth, damp-warmth, and lurking summerheat) and warm-heat diseases (wind-warmth, spring-warmth, autumn-dryness, and warm-toxin).

In most cases, diseases caused by warm-heat pathogens manifest immediately after an attack. However, they can hide ('lurk') in the body for a period of time and emerge later as a full-blown disease. Thus, newly-contracted warm pathogen diseases and lurking warm pathogen diseases can be distinguished on the basis of their onset, that is, the length of time between the attack of the pathogen and the appearance of signs and symptoms. They can also be distinguished on the basis of their location, that is, the depth at which the pathogens are located in the body. Also look to differentiate them according to whether signs and symptoms of interior heat are present at the onset of the disease.

It is very difficult to predict how long a lurking warm-heat pathogen will remain in the interior before emerging. Nor is it clear why some warm-heat pathogens will lurk inside the body without ever inducing a disease. These issues have given rise to many arguments among scholars about the value of the theory of lurking warm pathogen diseases. Nevertheless, the theory is still useful because it can tell us the location of the disease and its severity. It can also be used to predict the progression of the disease, which is not only helpful for differentiation, but also for treatment. Western biomedicine has corroborated the existence of diseases that manifest after periods of incubation.

Since newly-contracted warm pathogen diseases and lurking warm pathogen diseases present and progress differently, the approach to treatment will also differ. Newly-contracted warm pathogen diseases are treated by releasing the exterior and dispersing the pathogen, while lurking warm pathogen diseases are treated by clearing the interior heat. If these differences are ignored, mistakes will be made. This is why lurking warm pathogen disease theory is still important today. However, no matter where the warm-heat pathogen resides, on the exterior or in the interior, the practitioner must bring it out, because it is a 'guest evil' or visitant pathogen (客邪 *kè xié*)[42] that does not belong in the body.

Endnotes

1. Anonymous, *Yellow Emperor's Inner Classic: Basic Questions (Huáng Dì nèi jīng sù wèn)*. Beijing: People's Health Publishing House, 1963: 256.

2. Lu Ting-Zhen, *Systematic Differentiation of the Six Etiologies (Liù yīn tiáo biàn)*, reproduced in *Collection of Rare Chinese Medical Books (Zhēn běn yī shū jí chéng)*. Beijing: Chinese Medicine and Pharmacology Publishing House, 1996: 722.

3. Anonymous, *Yellow Emperor's Inner Classic: Basic Questions*, 33.

4. Yang Shi-Yin, *Discussion of Formulas from Straight Directions from [Yang] Ren-Zhai (Rén-Zhāi zhí zhǐ)*. Shanghai: Shanghai Publishing House of Ancient Literature, 1991.

5. For further discussion of contained fever (身熱不揚 *shēn rè bù yáng)*, see Chapter 5 of the present volume.

6. Depression, known as *jīng shén yì yù* or *jīng shén yā yì*, refers to depression with an emotional component, as opposed to simple Liver qi constraint.

7. Song Zhao-Qi (Song You-Fu, c. 1878), *Distinguishing [Aspects] of Southern Diseases (Nán bìng bié jiàn)*. Shanghai: Shanghai Health Publishing House, 1958, Chapter 2: 10.

8. Anonymous, *Yellow Emperor's Inner Classic: Basic Questions*, 34.

9. Yu Chang, *Precepts for Physicians (Yī mén fǎ lǜ)*. Shanghai: Shanghai Science and Technology Publishing House, 1983: 157.

10. Chengdu College of Traditional Chinese Medicine, Warm Pathogen Diseases Teaching and Research Section, *Self-Study Textbook for Chinese Medicine: Warm Pathogen Diseases (Zhōng yī zì xué jiào cái: Wēn bìng xué)*. Chengdu: Chengdu College of Traditional Chinese Medicine, 1985: 109.

11. Meng Shu-Jiang et al., *Teaching Reference Books for Traditional Chinese Medical Colleges: Warm Pathogen Diseases (Gāo děng zhōng yī yuàn xiào jiào xué cān kǎo shū: wēn bìng xué)*. Beijing: People's Health Publishing House, 1989: 254.

12. Meng Shu-Jiang et al., *Warm Pathogen Diseases (Wēn bìng xué)*. Shanghai: Shanghai Science and Technology Publishing House, 1985: 95.

13. Anonymous, *Yellow Emperor's Inner Classic: Basic Questions*, 464.

14. Ibid., 581.

15. Zhao Xu-Chu et al., *Compendium of Modern Chinese Medicine Applications and Research: Warm Pathogen Diseases (Xiàn dài zhōng yī yào yìng yòng yǔ yán jiù dà xì: wēn bìng)*. Shanghai: Shanghai University of Chinese Medicine Publishing House, 1995: 54.

16. Wu Tang, *Systematic Differentiation of Warm Pathogen Diseases (Wēn bìng tiáo biàn)*. Beijing: People's Health Publishing House, 1963: 12.

17. He is currently teaching at the Chengdu University of Traditional Chinese Medicine.

18. Meng Shu-Jiang, *Warm Pathogen Diseases*, 706.

19. Wang Meng-Ying, *Warp and Woof of Warm-Heat Pathogen Diseases (Wēn rè jīng wěi)*. This title is contained in Lu Zhen, *Collected Rare Recent Books on Chinese Medicine: Warm Pathogen Disease Section (Jīn dài zhōng yī zhēn běn jí: wēn bìng fèn cè)*. Hangzhou: Zhejiang Science and Technology Publishing House, 1987: 136.

20. Zhang Jie-Bin [Zhang Jing-Yue], *Collected Treatises of [Zhang] Jing-Yue (Jǐng-Yuè quán shū)*, annotated by Zhao Li-Xun et al. Beijing: People's Health Publishing House, 1991: 281.

21. Chengdu College of Traditional Chinese Medicine, Warm Pathogen Diseases Teaching and Research Section, *Self-Study Textbook for Chinese Medicine: Warm Pathogen Diseases*, 128.

22. Xue Xue, *Systematic Differentiation of Damp-Heat (Shī rè tiáo biàn)*, found in Song Zhao-Qi (Song You-Fu), *Distinguishing [Aspects] of Southern Diseases (Nán bìng bié jiàn)*. Shanghai: Shanghai Health Publishing House, 1958, Chapter 2: 3.

23. The bulk of information in the classics that refers to lurking warm pathogen diseases addresses an initial attack by cold, which causes spring-warmth. Much less is said about lurking summerheat, at least prior to the publication of *Indispensable Tools for Pattern Treatment (Zhèng zhì zhǔn shéng)* by Wang Ken-Tang (Wang Yu-Tai, c. 1549-1619).

24. Anonymous, *Yellow Emperor's Inner Classic: Basic Questions*, 21.

25. Ibid., 24.

26. Jiang Bao-Su, *Thirteen Chapter Precis of Medicine (Yī lüè shí sān piān)*, reproduced in *Collection of Rare Chinese Medical Books (Zhēn běn yī shū jí chéng)*, Volume 2. Beijing: Chinese Medicine and Pharmacology Publishing House, 1996: 156.

27. Cold Damage Teaching and Research Section of the Nanjing College of Traditional Medicine, *Translation and Explanation of the Discussion of Cold Damage (Shāng hán lùn yì shì)*. Shanghai: Shanghai Science and Technology Publishing House, 1980: 268.

28. Chao Yuan-Fang, *Discussion of the Origins of Symptoms of Disease (Zhū bìng yuán hòu lùn)*. Beijing: People's Health Publishing House, 1992: 218.

29. Wu You-Xing, *Discussion of Warm Epidemics (Wēn yì lùn)*. Shenyang: Liaoning Science and Technology Publishing House, 1997: 4.

30. Yu Gen-Chu, *Revised Popular Guide to the Discussion of Cold Damage (Chóng ding tōng sú shāng hán lùn)*. Hangzhou: New Medicine Press, 1956: 242-243. Note that while Yu Gen-Chu wrote this book in 1776, the present edition was edited much later by He Lian-Chen and Xu Rong-Zhai. See also Meng Shu-Jiang et al., *Warm Pathogen Diseases*.

31. Meng Shu-Jiang, *Warm Pathogen Diseases*, 151.

32. Lei Feng, *Discussion of Seasonal Diseases (Shí bìng lùn)*. Beijing: People's Health Publishing House, 1956: 5.

33. Ye Lin, *Explanation of Lurking Pathogens (Fú qì jiě)*, reproduced in Cao Bing-Zhang (ed.), *Compendium of Medicine in China (Zhōng guó yī xué dà chéng)*. Shanghai: Shanghai Science and Technology Publishing House, 1990.

34. Meng Shu-Jiang, *Teaching Reference Books for Traditional Chinese Medical Colleges: Warm Pathogen Diseases*, 45.

35. Meng Shu-Jiang, *Warm Pathogen Diseases*, 52, 88.

36. Liu Bao-Yi, *Encountering the Sources of Warm-Heat Pathogen Diseases (Wēn rè féng yuán)*. Beijing: People's Health Publishing House, 1959: 75.

37. Wang Meng-Ying, *Warp and Woof of Warm-Heat Pathogen Diseases (Wēn rè jīng wěi)*, reproduced in Lu Zhen, *Collected Rare Recent Books on Chinese Medicine: Warm Pathogen Disease Section (Jīn dài zhōng yī zhēn běn jí: wēn bìng fēn cè)*. Hangzhou: Zhejiang Science and Technology Publishing House, 1987: 61.

38. Ibid.

39. He Lian-Chen, *Revised Expanded Discussion of Warm-Heat Pathogen Diseases (Chóng dìng guǎng wēn rè lùn)*. Beijing: People's Health Publishing House, 1960: 6.

40. Liu Bao-Yi, *Encountering the Sources of Warm-Heat Pathogen Diseases*, 60, 64.

41. Wang Lü, *Discourse on Tracing Back to the Medical Classics (Yī jīng sù huí jí)*. Nanjing: Jiangsu Science and Technology Publishing House, 1984: 5.

42. The term 'guest evil' means that it must be discharged as soon as possible because, like a guest in one's house, it should not stay forever. Clinically, we should try our best to quickly eliminate it from the body.

4 Differentiation of Patterns According to the Four Levels and Three Burners

T HE HUMAN BODY is a small ecosystem that is intimately connected to the external environment. Environmental fluctuations, such as dramatic changes in the weather, air pollution, and degradation of water quality, can give rise to warm-heat pathogens. Should the pathogen attack the body, it will disrupt or injure the qi, blood, yin and yang, channels and collaterals, and both the yin and yang organs. Clinical signs and symptoms associated with this dysfunction demarcate the progression of the disease.

According to traditional Chinese medicine, to effect a successful treatment the practitioner must perform an accurate and detailed differentiation of the illness, including its location, quality, and pathogenesis. Even after the distinction was made between diseases caused by cold pathogens and those caused by warm-heat pathogens, the question of how to differentiate diseases caused by warm-heat pathogens and measure their progress puzzled practitioners for some time. Ye Gui (Ye Tian-Shi, c. 1666–1745) and Wu Tang (Wu Ju-Tong, 1758–1836) unveiled two unique approaches to the differentiation and principles of transmission of warm pathogen diseases. These are based on grouping the signs and symptoms, and identifying, analyzing, and summarizing the relationships among warm pathogen disease patterns. This process, in turn, establishes a foundation for treatment. The first approach differentiates patterns according to the theory of the four levels, and the second approach according to the theory of the three burners.[1] While the two approaches are distinct, they also overlap and intertwine. A novice might be tempted to learn just one of these theories, but the lines between them are somewhat fuzzy, and both are useful in the clinic. It is much more helpful to study both carefully, and then to use them together.

73

Before elaborating upon each of the two theories, we will begin with a brief overview of the physical functions of the protective qi, qi, nutritive qi, and blood, and the Triple Burner. As you read this chapter, try to keep in mind the similarities and differences between the two approaches. A summary is presented at the end.

Differentiation of Patterns According to the Theory of Four Levels

In the late seventeenth and early eighteenth centuries, Ye Gui established the four-level differentiation (四分辨證 *sì fēn biàn zhèng)*, which is also called differentiation according to the protective, qi, nutritive, and blood levels (衛氣營血辨證 *wèi qì yíng xuè biàn zhèng)*. These terms are found throughout traditional Chinese medicine, not just in the four-level diagnostic scheme. But are they always used in an identical fashion? In most areas of Chinese medicine, 衛氣 *wèi qì* refers to protective qi, 營氣 *yíng qì* to nutritive qi, and 血 *xuè* to blood. Usually, these terms, as well as the word qi itself, refer to the activities and substance of the yin and yang organs. However, in the four-level diagnostic scheme, the words have specialized meanings which should not be confused with their more common usage.

PROTECTIVE QI, NUTRITIVE QI, AND BLOOD IN CHINESE MEDICINE

In traditional Chinese medicine, qi is the primordial material of the body. It maintains and supports the body's natural physiological functions. According to Chapter 30 of the *Divine Pivot (Líng shū)*, qi is what diffuses the flavors of food in the upper burner, warms the skin, fills out the body, and moistens the hair like a mist or dew.[2] Generally speaking, qi originates in the Kidney, receives support from the Spleen, and is distributed by the Lung, with the Liver controlling its movement. The condition of qi reflects the functions of the yin and yang organs. There are many types of qi, identified by their origin, location, and function.

Protective qi. The protective qi is the most yang aspect of qi. While other forms of qi circulate primarily inside the body, protective qi circulates between the blood vessels and the surface. It has a close relationship with the Lung. According to Chapter 43 of *Basic Questions (Sù wèn)*, the protective qi is formed from the transformation of food, and moves rapidly and smoothly. Because it cannot enter the vessels, it moves between the skin and subcutaneous tissues and the flesh, warms the membranes of the vital organs, and disperses throughout the chest and abdomen.[3] Chapter 47 of *Divine Pivot* says that the protective qi also warms and nourishes the skin, muscles, interstices, and pores, while controlling the opening and closing of the skin pores.[4] Thus, the protective qi guards the body against attack by externally-contracted pathogenic factors.

Nutritive qi. The nutritive qi is that which nourishes the body. Like protective qi, the nutritive qi is also derived from food. Yet, as a precursor to blood, it circulates in the vessels and nourishes the yin and yang organs. It is more yin in nature than is the protective qi, and has a close relationship to the Heart. Nutritive qi is used in the production of blood. As noted in chapter 43 of *Basic Questions*:

> The nutritive [qi] is the essential qi transformed from fluids and food. It regulates and harmonizes the five yin organs and disperses through the six yang organs, then enters into the vessels where it follows the course of the channels and vessels up and down. It has the function of permeating the five yin organs and connecting up the six yang organs.[5]

Chapter 71 of *Divine Pivot* observes: "The nutritive qi absorbs the fluids from food and allows it to seep it into the vessels. Both the fluids and the nutritive qi flow in the vessels and transform into blood."[6] Thus, nutritive qi not only nourishes the yin and yang organs, it is also used in the production of blood.

Blood. Blood is an important nutritive material for the organs of the body. It is formed from the nutritive qi and fluids and circulates in the vessels. According to Zhang Jie-Bin (Zhang Jing-Yue, c. 1636), the Spleen produces blood, the Heart moves it, the Liver regulates it, the Lung qi helps distribute it, and the Kidney essence supports it.[7]

In summary, the protective qi circulates between the vessels and the surface of the body. It protects the exterior and safeguards the body from attack by external pathogenic factors. The nutritive qi moves through the vessels; coupled with the fluids, it can be transformed into blood. Both nutritive qi and blood then circulate through the vessels.

With respect to location, the protective qi is found on the surface where it circulates outside of the vessels; it is the most superficial form of qi. Except for the protective qi, the qi travels within the yin and yang organs and channels, and is found inside the body. The other forms of qi are, therefore, located deeper in the body than is the protective qi. Both the nutritive qi and blood circulate in the vessels. Blood is located at a deeper level than nutritive qi because it is produced later than nutritive qi. Relatively speaking, in terms of depth, the order from the surface of the body to the organs and vessels is protective qi, qi, nutritive qi, and blood.

The protective and nutritive qi, and especially the relationship between them, plays an important role in the works of Zhang Ji. For example, Zhang noted in *Discussion of Cold Damage* that "When a *tai yang* disease [presents] with fever and sweating, it means that the nutritive is weak and the protective strong."[8] He also observed that "The problem with patients who frequently have spontaneous sweating is that the protective and nutritive qi do not work together in a congruent, harmonious manner."[9]

PROTECTIVE, QI, NUTRITIVE, AND BLOOD LEVELS IN FOUR-LEVEL DIFFERENTIATION

As previously noted, it was during the Qing dynasty that Ye Gui posited the theory of four-level differentiation of patterns for warm pathogen diseases. Based on references to warm pathogen diseases in the *Inner Classic (Nèi jīng)* and the clinical experiences of his predecessors, he realized that the function of the protective qi, qi, nutritive qi, and blood is impaired after an attack on the body by a warm-heat pathogen. In his theory, Ye assigned special meanings to the terms protective qi, qi, nutritive qi, and blood, which are different from those in earlier texts. In warm pathogen disease theory, these terms refer to the method of measuring and predicting the progress of a disease caused by warm-heat pathogens. This method is called the differentiation of patterns according to the theory of four levels. Again, the four levels are:

1. Protective level (衛分 *wèi fèn*)
2. Qi level (氣分 *qì fèn*)
3. Nutritive level (營分 *yíng fèn*)
4. Blood level (血分 *xuè fèn*)

With a few exceptions,[10] warm-heat pathogens initially attack the protective level, causing the qi to stagnate, and injuring the fluids. Following the initial attack, a disease may progress to the qi, nutritive, or blood level. From the perspective of eight-parameter differentiation, a disease in the protective level is regarded as an exterior disorder; once it progresses to the qi, nutritive, or blood level it becomes an interior disorder. As the severity of a disease increases, the strength of an individual's antipathogenic qi declines. Each level has its own characteristic manifestations. Understanding the manner in which warm-heat pathogens attack the body, and knowing how they manifest at each level, provides the skilled practitioner with strategies for preventing and treating these diseases.

Protective level patterns. The Lung governs the distribution of the protective qi, which is focused on the surface of the body, the nose, and the throat. When a warm-heat pathogen first attacks the body, it usually does so at the surface, nose, and throat, which are especially associated with the Lung. The function of the Lung in dispersing the protective qi is thereby impaired, which gives rise to a protective level pattern. The primary pathology of this pattern is stagnation of the protective qi due to the struggle between the protective qi and warm-heat pathogen, leading to failure of the Lung in dispersing the protective qi to the surface, nose, and throat. Clinical manifestations include:

- *Fever* as a result of the fierce struggle between the warm-heat pathogen and the protective qi.

- *Chills and slight aversion to cold* due to the failure of the protective qi to warm the surface. As previously mentioned, the function of the protective qi is to warm and nourish the skin, muscles, and interstices.

- *Slight or absent sweating*

- *Sneezing, nasal congestion, sinus drainage, sore throat, and cough,* which indicate that the Lung's functions of disseminating the qi and causing it to descend have been impaired.

- *Headache* may result from the warm-heat pathogen disrupting the movement of qi in the head.

- *Slightly increased thirst* shows that the warm-heat pathogen has just begun to injure the fluids. However, the patient does not drink much water because the fluids are only slightly affected.

- *A red-tipped tongue with a white and thin coating, and a floating and rapid pulse,* are part of the normal exterior presentation of a warm-heat pathogen.

Among these signs and symptoms, fever, slight aversion to cold, and slightly increased thirst are the cardinal symptoms that must be present to make a diagnosis of a protective level pattern. Some writers believe that fever, cough, and thirst are all necessary features of this presentation,[11] but my clinical experience suggests otherwise. Rather than a cough, patients with a protective level pattern will first present with such things as a swollen, red, and sore throat, red, itchy, and burning eyes, nasal discharge, sneezing, and a sensation of plugged ears. As the disease progresses deeper into the body, a cough will gradually develop. Also, while many textbooks state that an increase in the severity of thirst marks the entry of the pathogen into the interior, I have rarely found this to be the case.

It is important to note that while some of the signs and symptoms required to diagnose a protective, qi, nutritive, or blood level pattern differ somewhat depending on which of the specific warm-heat pathogens is involved, the general manifestations in each of the levels will be similar regardless of the resulting warm pathogen disease. Thus, the signs and symptoms listed above can theoretically occur in a protective level pattern associated with any warm pathogen disease.

Since a protective level pattern occurs in the most superficial level of the body, it is milder and has a shorter course than patterns in the other three levels. If the protective level pattern is treated in a timely fashion, the warm-heat pathogen can be eliminated from the body while it is still at the exterior. If it is not treated early, or if the warm-heat pathogen is very severe, the disease will progress to the qi level. However, the disease will progress directly from a protective level pattern to one affecting the Pericardium if any of the following occurs:

- The pathogen is extremely severe.
- There is constitutional yin deficiency.
- There is injury of the Heart yin or qi due to improper treatment.[12]

The disease would then be regarded as residing in the nutritive or blood level; this type of transmission is called abnormal or rebellious transmission. For further discussion of the abnormal or rebellious transmission of a warm pathogen disease to the Pericardium, see "Abnormal Progression" later in this chapter.

Qi level patterns. When a warm-heat pathogen penetrates from the outside to the inside of the body, it affects the physiological function and circulation of qi, causing it to stagnate, thereby producing heat. The result is a qi level pattern. Unlike the protective level, many internal organs, including the Lung and the Spleen, are involved in the qi level because qi circulates to so many of the internal organs. A qi level disease can therefore affect the Lung, Spleen, and all the yang organs.

Most qi level patterns evolve from protective level patterns that have deteriorated. However, some warm-heat pathogens, such as summerheat without dampness, can directly attack the Stomach in the qi level. Alternatively, a nutritive level pattern may regress to a qi level pattern, or a lurking warm pathogen disease may first manifest at the qi level as a result of a secondary pathogen.

The primary pathology of a qi level pattern—heat from excess and injury to the fluids—is a consequence of the severe struggle between antipathogenic qi and the warm-heat pathogen. Since qi level patterns can affect different yin and yang organs, the full range of clinical manifestations will vary. However, there are several common clinical features:

- *Vigorous fever*

- *Aversion to heat* (instead of aversion to cold). Since the warm-heat pathogen has progressed to the qi level, that is, it is now an interior condition, there is generally no chills or aversion to cold. However, there may be slight chills on the upper back due to injury of the Lung qi by heat from excess in the qi level. Since the qi of the Lung opens on BL-13 *(fèi shū)*, chills can occur in the area of BL-13 *(fèi shū)* when the Lung qi is weak or injured.

- *Profuse sweating* caused by extreme heat forcing fluids out of the body.

- *Thirst with a preference for cold beverages*

- *A yellow and dry tongue coating* is the primary manifestation of interior heat.

- *A flooding or slippery pulse* is caused by qi stagnation.

The key signs and symptoms of a qi level pattern are aversion to heat (instead of aversion to cold), thirst, and a yellow tongue coating.

In addition, there will be other signs and symptoms depending on which organs are involved. For example,

- *Accumulation of heat in the Lung,* which can lead to blockage of qi in the Lung, will result in a cough with thirst and a yellow tongue coating, coupled with wheezing.

- *Disturbance of the diaphragm by heat* can result in restlessness and insomnia.

- *Heat and dry stool in the Large Intestine* will manifest as tidal fever in the late afternoon, distention, hardness, and pain in the abdomen, dry hard stools or watery stools with a strong odor, and a dry and yellow tongue coating.

- *Heat from constraint in the Gallbladder* presents with a feverish body, bitter taste, thirst, nausea, restlessness, scant and yellow urine, red tongue with yellow coating, and a wiry, rapid pulse.

- *Accumulation of damp-heat in the Spleen* is marked by persistent fever even after sweating, dry mouth with a slight thirst, epigastric distention, nausea, vomiting, loose stools, yellow and greasy tongue coating, and a soggy, rapid pulse.

These patterns, along with many others, are discussed in Chapters 7 through 13.

The Lung is the only organ involved in both protective and qi level patterns. Which level a warm-heat pathogen attacks depends largely on the patient's underlying condition. When there is pre-existing phlegm-heat or Lung yin deficiency (common in smokers), warm-heat pathogens are more likely to progress quickly through the protective to the qi level, or even directly attack the Lung itself. If the Lung is functioning relatively well, the warm-heat pathogen will remain at the protective level and manifest primarily in terms of the superficial aspects of the Lung, that is, the skin, nose, and throat.[13] However, clinically, if the pathogen is not eliminated in a timely fashion, the disease can still progress and enter the Lung organ from the protective level. In the first and third examples, the pathology is said to be focused in the Lung. In the second example, however, only the external aspects of the Lung system are involved.

Qi level patterns occur deeper in the body than do protective level patterns; thus, the illnesses are more severe and last longer. In a qi level pattern, the antipathogenic qi is still strong enough to resist the warm-heat pathogen, so the illness can be cured if proper treatment is employed in a timely manner. However, without proper treatment, the disease will progress from the qi level to the nutritive or blood level.

Nutritive level patterns. When a warm-heat pathogen progresses from the protective or qi level to the nutritive level, it injures the yin and disturbs the spirit of the Heart. Nutritive level patterns are usually observed as a result of inward progression of protective or qi level patterns. However, if the warm-heat pathogen is severe or the antipathogenic qi weak, a warm-heat pathogen can directly attack the nutritive level.

In addition, a lurking warm pathogen disease can manifest first at the nutritive level.

According to the contemporary physician Hu Ding-Bang, blazing heat in the qi level requires that there be profuse sweating and damaged yin of the Heart as pre-conditions for a warm pathogen disease to progress from the qi level to the nutritive level.[14] This is because sweat is a Heart-related fluid,[15] and profuse sweating will injure both the qi and yin of the Heart, which renders it vulnerable to a warm-heat pathogen. Clinically, profuse sweating from any cause, including improper treatment, may induce a warm-heat pathogen to invade the nutritive level. The clinical features of a nutritive level pattern include:

- *Fever that worsens at night and a thin, rapid pulse* result from injury to the yin by the warm-heat pathogen in the nutritive level. The yin thereby cannot effectively balance the yang, especially at night when most of the yang qi moves deep within the body. Unlike the fever in the protective and qi level patterns, that seen in nutritive level patterns can either be objective, that is, measurable with a thermometer, or subjective, felt only by the patient. In addition, since the fever persists through the day but becomes progressively worse at night, it is different than the yin-deficient fever associated with an internal disorder, which occurs only in the late afternoon or during the night.

- *Insomnia, irritability, restlessness, occasional delirium or muddled consciousness, and a deep-red tongue* reflect the disturbance to the spirit of the Heart by the warm-heat pathogen. Since nutritive qi is part of the blood, the nutritive qi has a close relationship with the Heart, which opens on the tongue.

- *Thirst, but with little desire to drink,* results from the steaming up of yin by the warm-heat pathogen to the tongue. Here the patient may just have a dry mouth with no desire to drink, or feel only a bit thirsty. This type of thirst can be seen in nutritive level patterns with injury to the yin. When this occurs while the yin is injured enough to cause a dry mouth, the steaming effects of the heat at the nutritive level supply some moisture to the mouth, enough to reduce the patient's desire to drink. Of course, because the steaming is a by-product of a pathological process, it does not function in the same way as physiological yin.

- *Maculopapular rashes* result from the warm-heat pathogens invading the collaterals and forcing the blood out of the vessels.

The cardinal signs and symptoms of a nutritive level pattern are fever that worsens at night, irritability, restlessness, occasional delirium or muddled consciousness, and a deep-red tongue.

Clinically, the most commonly seen patterns are burning of the yin in the nutritive level by heat and veiling of the Pericardium by transmission of heat and phlegm. Burning of yin in the nutritive level by heat means a fever that worsens at night, restlessness, thirst with little desire to drink or no thirst at all, slight maculopapular rashes, and a deep-red tongue. Veiling of the Pericardium by transmission of heat and phlegm includes, in addition to the severe signs and symptoms of burning yin in the nutritive level, especially severe changes in consciousness such as muddled consciousness, delirium, or coma, along with stiffness of the tongue and cold extremities.

If the proper treatment is used in a timely fashion, the disease can be brought from the nutritive level back to the qi level, and will then improve. Otherwise, the disease will progress to the blood level and become critical.

Blood level patterns. A blood level pattern occurs when a warm-heat pathogen penetrates deeply and disturbs and exhausts the blood. Usually the disease progresses from the protective to the qi to the nutritive level, and then finally to the blood level. However, a warm-heat pathogen may occasionally attack the blood level directly. Blood level patterns are generally regarded as critical.

Extreme excess-type heat can force blood out of the vessels and cause it to congeal, producing blood stasis. This is the primary pathological feature of a blood level pattern. Other features include:

- *Fever*

- *Restlessness or delirium*

- *Muddled consciousness or coma*

- *Very deep-red tongue*

- *Loss of blood,* which includes vomiting blood, nosebleeds, bloody urine, and blood in the stools

- *Maculopapular rashes* over the entire body

The key signs and symptoms used to identify a blood level pattern are maculopapular rashes, bleeding, and a very deep-red tongue. The four most commonly seen blood level patterns are:

- *Extreme heat forcing blood out of the vessels:* restlessness, or coma and delirium, various forms of blood loss, maculopapular rashes, and a tongue which is very deep red, purple, or a combination of both

- *Burning of the qi and blood by heat:* vigorous fever, strong thirst, irritability, restlessness, deep-red tongue with yellow tongue coating, maculopapular rashes, and one of the various forms of bleeding

- *Stirring up of Liver wind by extreme heat:* feverish body, muddled consciousness, convulsion, stiffness of neck or even arched back rigidity (opisthotonos), upstaring eyes, closed eyes, very deep-red tongue, and a wiry, rapid pulse

- *Combination of blood stasis and heat:* constipation with dry, black stools, hardness, distention, and pain in the lower abdomen, dry mouth, normal urination, purple tongue or purple spots over the tongue, and a submerged and forceful or choppy pulse.

The blood level pattern is the most severe form of warm pathogen disease since it is located in the deepest level of the body. If the strength of the warm-heat pathogen is not reduced, and if the antipathogenic qi becomes exhausted, the condition will become critical. Only if the practitioner immediately follows the proper course of treatment can the patient be saved.

Progression of patterns in the four levels. Protective level patterns occur at an early stage of warm pathogen disease and constitute exterior heat patterns. Since they affect the protective qi and the Lung, protective level patterns are superficial and relatively mild in nature. Qi level patterns represent an intermediate stage and constitute interior heat patterns; they are mostly excessive in nature, with the exception of those in which the warm-heat pathogen injures the yin or qi. Qi level patterns can affect many different parts of the body including the chest, diaphragm, Lung, Stomach, Spleen and Large Intestine. They are deeper and more severe than protective level patterns. When a warm-heat pathogen invades the nutritive level, it injures the yin and disturbs the spirit of the Heart. A blood level pattern is the final stage of warm pathogen disease. Here the heat severely disturbs blood circulation and exhausts the blood. It is the most severe and critical stage of the illness.

Note that while nutritive level conditions are generally less severe than those in the blood level, this is not always the case. One example is the nutritive level pattern of veiling of the Pericardium, which can be very severe and even critical. This is because it can lead to collapse of the yang qi and even death. Some of the blood level patterns are not nearly as serious.

According to four-level differentiation, the typical progression of a warm pathogen disease is transverse, from the exterior to the interior, rather than vertical (see Table 4.1). Following is a description of the two mechanisms involved in the progression of warm pathogen diseases.

1. *Newly-contracted warm pathogen diseases* usually begin at the protective level, and, if left untreated or if treated improperly, progress to the qi level, then to the nutritive and finally to the blood level. This is only a general guideline as there are many variations seen in the clinic. Some warm pathogen diseases, including summerheatwarmth and damp-warmth, will typically invade the qi level directly. In addition, it is very common for patients to present with conditions that overlap more than one level. When this occurs it is important that we understand how they should be treated. Qin Bo-Wei (Qin Zhi-Ji, 1900–1970), a well-known traditional physician and teacher, pointed out that a critical stage is the transmission from the qi to the nutritive level. When this occurs, treatment should be urgently focused on bringing the disease back to the qi level, where it is much less dangerous. Qin noted that transmission to the nutritive level is her-

Table 4.1	Four-Level Differentiation	
Pathology	**Signs and Symptoms**	**Key Points for Identification**
▶ PROTECTIVE LEVEL		
Protective qi stagnation due to struggle with a warvm-heat pathogen, leading to the failure of the Lung to disperse the protective qi to the surface, nose, and throat	Fever, slight aversion to cold, chills, slight or absent sweating, sneezing, nasal congestion, sore throat, cough, headache, slight thirst, red- tipped tongue with a thin and white coating, floating and rapid pulse	Fever, slight aversion to cold, chills, cough, slight thirst, red-tipped tongue with a thin and white coating, floating and rapid pulse
▶ QI LEVEL		
Warm-heat pathogen penetrates to the interior affecting the circulation of qi, causing it to stagnate and produce heat	Vigorous fever, aversion to heat,* profuse sweating, thirst for cold beverages, yellow and dry tongue coating, flooding and slippery pulse	Vigorous fever, profuse sweating, thirst for cold beverages, yellow tongue coating, flooding and slippery pulse
(SAMPLE QI LEVEL PATHOLOGIES)		
Accumulation of heat in the Lung	Cough, wheezing, distending pain in the chest with thirst, restlessness, slippery, rapid pulse, yellow tongue coating	Vigorous fever, cough, wheezing, severe sweating, restlessness, thirst
Disturbance of the diaphragm by heat	Fever, thirst, restlessness, insomnia, slightly yellow tongue coating	Restlessness and insomnia with tossing and turning in bed, slightly yellow tongue coating
Heat from constraint in the Gallbladder	Feverish body, bitter taste, thirst, nausea, restlessness, scant, dark and yellow urine, red tongue with yellow coating, and wiry, rapid pulse	Fever, bitter taste, nausea, thirst, scanty and yellow urine

* There can also be a slight feeling of cold in the upper back.

83

Table 4.1, cont.		
▶ NUTRITIVE LEVEL		
Heat injures the yin and disturbs the spirit of the Heart	Fever that worsens at night, insomnia, restlessness, occasional delirium, thirst with little desire to drink, deep-red tongue, thin and rapid pulse. There may be maculopapular rashes.	Fever that worsens at night, restlessness, occasional delirium or muddled consciousness, deep-red tongue
▶ BLOOD LEVEL		
Warm-heat pathogen penetrates deeply and disturbs and exhausts the blood	Feverishness, restlessness or delirium, muddled con-sciousness or coma, very deep-red tongue, bleeding, maculopapular rashes over the entire body	Various kinds of bleeding, muddled consciousness or coma, feverishness, very deep-red tongue

alded by restlessness together with a deep-red tongue and dark-yellow coating that is becoming dry.[16] In a recent article, two physicians at Nanjing University of Traditional Chinese Medicine proposed that a sudden onset, severe presentation, and persistently high temperature are indications that a warm pathogen disease is likely to progress from the qi level to the nutritive level.[17]

2. *Lurking warm pathogen diseases,* where the warm-heat pathogen has been lurking for some time within the body—spring-warmth and lurking summerheat, for example—may occur initially at the nutritive level. If it later regresses to the qi level, this means that the disease is improving and will soon be cured. There is also a peculiar progression that can occur when certain warm-heat pathogens attack individuals with pre-existing constitutional disharmonies, such as qi or yin deficiency, or excess-type dampness. While a cursory look at the symptoms may suggest to the unwary practitioner that this is the result of an internal disorder, in fact the problem is due to an external warm-heat pathogen that has been lurking for some time within the body. Lurking heat can be a difficult concept to grasp. The following case study may help make it clearer.

Case study: lurking warm pathogen disease

Mr. Luo, 62 years old

First visit: The patient has a constitutional Spleen yang deficiency. He had been camping on the beach in late summer. During the early part of September he began to feel fatigued and lost a little weight. His pulse was slightly rapid and he had a low-grade fever. After taking antibiotics for a few days, his low-grade fever changed to a high fever of 40°C. He experienced nausea, vomiting, and distention in the chest and abdomen, along with six or seven attacks of diarrhea a day. The patient had cool extremities but a hot sensation in his abdomen and on the front of his head. He complained of slight sweating and frequent urination, with pain in his penis. His joints were sore. At the distal position, his pulse was slightly floating and rapid, and at the right middle position, deep and rapid. At the left middle position it was wiry and rapid, and at the proximal positions, submerged and soggy. His tongue was red with a thin, greasy coating.

He was diagnosed with lurking summerheat with dampness and heat in the Triple Burner. The treatment method was to clear summerheat and drain dampness with bitter, acrid, and bland herbs: Pogostemonis/Agastaches Herba *(huò xiāng)* (6g), Armeniacae Semen *(xìng rén)*(4.5g), Moslae Herba *(xiāng rú)* (3g), Poria *(fú líng)* (9g), Scutellariae Radix *(huáng qín)* (4.5g), Talcum *(huá shí)* (9g), Coicis Semen *(yì yǐ rén)* (15g), *fáng jǐ* (Stephaniae/Cocculi/etc. Radix) (4.5g), Polyporus *(zhū líng)* (4.5g), Lophatheri Herba *(dàn zhú yè)* (4.5g), Tetrapanacis Medulla *(tōng cǎo)* (4.5g), and Nelumbinis Folium *(hé yè)*(6g). The patient received two packets of the formula.

Second visit: His fever had come down and the vomiting and painful urination were resolved. The soreness in his joints had diminished. However, he was still having four or five bouts of diarrhea a day, and he continued to be fatigued, and to have a poor appetite. His pulse was deep and thin at the distal positions, deep and slippery at the middle positions, and deep and slow at the proximal positions. Although the strength of the disease had slackened, the damp-heat persisted and the Stomach qi had not yet fully recovered. The treatment method was modified to harmonize the Stomach qi, clear heat, and drain dampness. Moslae Herba *(xiāng rú)*, Armeniacae Semen *(xìng rén)*, Scutellariae Radix *(huáng qín)*, and *fáng jǐ* (Stephaniae/Cocculi/etc. Radix) were removed from the fomula, and Artemisiae scopariae Herba *(yīn chén)* (6g), Citri reticulatae Pericarpium *(chén pí)* (4.5g), Magnoliae officinalis Cortex *(hòu pò)* (3g), Sojae Semen germinatum *(dà dòu juǎn)* (9g), and Amomi Fructus rotundus *(bái dòu kòu)* (2.4g) were added. The patient received two packets of herbs. After they were finished, he experienced a slight sweat over his body and the fever was gone. His urination was normal, and he had two bowel movements a day. However, his appetite was still poor, and he felt slight abdominal bloating after eating. He experienced one episode of breaking into a cold sweat. His pulse was deep, thin, rapid, and faint. His tongue was red, but the greasy coating was gone. The damp-heat signs were resolved, but the Stomach qi remained weak. The treatment method was then to tonify the Stomach qi and enrich the Stomach yin until all signs and symptoms were resolved, then to discontinue treatment and follow dietary therapy for several months. Following this strategy, the patient recovered completely.[18]

Commentary: At first glance it might seem that this patient suffered from an internal disorder. However, from a yin and yang organ perspective, it is quite hard to explain why a patient with underlying Spleen yang deficiency would develop signs and symptoms of damp-heat such as high fever, nausea, vomiting, chest and abdominal distention, hot sensation in the abdomen and penis, diarrhea, and a red tongue with a white and greasy tongue coating. Could this damp-heat come from Spleen yang deficiency? While it was theoretically possible that some heat in the Stomach could be produced secondary to heat from constraint due to the weak flow of yang qi, that would not explain the intensity and widespread nature of the symptoms in this case.

The only way that this case can be understood is that the patient, who had Spleen yang deficiency, contracted summerheat, which had been lurking in the body due to weakness of antipathogenic qi. In the autumn, the lurking summerheat emerged due to the improper use of bitter, cold antibiotics which further damaged the Spleen yang and antipathogenic qi. This led to a full-blown case of lurking summerheat with dampness in the Triple Burner. While some sources suggest that only secondary pathogenic factors like wind-heat or wind-cold can induce a lurking pathogen to emerge, this case is a good example of another possibility.

Differentiation of Patterns According to Three-Burner Theory

Differentiation of patterns according to three-burner theory (三焦辨證 *sān jiāo biàn zhèng*) is also known as three-burner differentiation. As noted in Chapter 1, Zhang Ji was the first to use the three burners as a tool for differentiating disease. While many physicians subsequently worked to develop this type of differentiation, it did not become a mature system until the publication of *Systematic Differentiation of Warm Pathogen Diseases* by Wu Tang in 1798. Still, however, many modern practitioners have been puzzled about the relationship between three-burner differentiation and the yang organ Triple Burner, as well as how and why the three burners were chosen as the organizing principle for differentiation. It may therefore be helpful to introduce this section by reviewing the functions of the Triple Burner and its relationship to three-burner differentiation, before proceeding with our discussion of three-burner differentiation itself.

The Triple Burner (三焦 *sān jiāo*) was first described in the *Inner Classic*. Since then, scholars and physicians have developed the following ideas concerning its location and function.

Location of the Triple Burner. Classical Chinese medicine commonly refers to the body in symbolic terms, referring to natural phenomena as a basis for understanding. According to Chinese philosophy, the universe is divided into three parts. Heaven is in the upper reaches, the earth in its lower confines, and human beings are in between. The human body is likewise divided into three parts (burners). As noted in Chapter 18 of *Divine Pivot*:

> The upper burner emerges from the upper mouth of the Stomach and ascends with the esophagus, passing through the diaphragm and spreading through the chest. ... The middle burner also comes out of the Stomach and emerges behind the upper burner. ...The lower burner separates from the Large Intestine and pours [to cover] the Bladder and seeps into it.[19]

Obviously, according to the *Inner Classic,* the Triple Burner is a large organ that is comprised of the upper, middle, and lower parts of the trunk of the body. The upper burner refers to the part located above the diaphragm, containing the Heart and Lung. The middle burner refers to the part located below the diaphragm and above the umbilicus, containing the Spleen, Stomach, and part of the Large and Small Intestines. The lower burner refers to the part located below the umbilicus and above the external genital organs, and is thought to include the Kidney, Liver, Bladder, and part of the Large and Small Intestines.

Function of the Triple Burner. Functionally, the Triple Burner is regarded as one of the six yang organs. Chapter 31 of *Difficult Questions (Nán jīng)* observes that "The Triple Burner is the pathway for water circulation and food transportation and transformation. It is the beginning and end of the qi circulation."[20] Chapter 8 of *Basic Questions* says that "The Triple Burner promotes the transformation and transportation of water and fluids throughout the body."[21] From this description, physicians and scholars attributed certain functional qualities to the Triple Burner, regarding it as a pathway in the body for qi, blood, water, and fire. According to Chapter 18 of *Divine Pivot,* the function of the upper burner is to disperse qi and distribute blood that has been transformed from digested food in the form of vapor; the function of the middle burner is to grind, transform, and transport food in the form of foam (which arises from the fermentation or ripening process); and the function of the lower burner is to separate the clear from the turbid, and to discharge the turbid like a sluice.[22]

In summary, the Triple Burner is a pathway for the circulation of qi, blood, water, and fire. Its function is closely related to the transportation and transformation of food, distribution of qi and blood, and discharge of waste from the body. Its meaning also has some overlap with a vertical division of the body, which is divided up into upper, middle, and lower burners. It is this vertical division that allowed practitioners to use the three burners as a tool to locate and differentiate disease. This evolved into the differentiation of patterns according to the theory of three burners.

Zhang Ji expanded upon these concepts and described their relation to disease in Chapter 11 of *Essentials from the Golden Cabinet (Jīn guì yào luè)* where he noted:

> If heat is in the upper burner, it can lead to cough and then develop into Lung atrophy; if heat is in the middle burner, it can lead to dry and hard stools; if heat is in the lower burner, it can lead to bloody urine and disturbance and retention of urine.[23]

Later on, Liu Wan-Su (Liu Shou-Zhen, 1110–1200) in *Collection of Writings on the Mechanism of Disease, Suitability of Qi and Safeguarding of Life as Discussed in Basic Questions (Sù wèn bìng jī qì yí bǎo míng jí)* pointed out that "Maculopapular rashes cannot be purged when they appear at the onset of a disease that is located in the upper burner, nor at the end when it is located in the lower burner."[24] Thus, the location of the disease in a particular burner was seen to have clinical significance.

Yu Chang (Yu Jia-Yan, c. 1585–1664) made a cogent argument for using the three burners in the location and treatment of warm pathogen diseases.[25] He observed:

- Warm epidemics attack the body through the mouth and nose, then first invade the middle burner, and from there progress to the upper burner or lower burner.

- Lifting and dispersing are good methods for treating diseases located in the upper burner because the upper burner functions to create vapors.

- Promoting qi circulation is a good method for treating disease in the middle burner because the middle burner functions to ferment or ripen food to create foam.

- Purging stool and promoting urination are good methods for treating disease in the lower burner because the lower burner functions as a sluice.

Although Ye Gui is known for devising the four-level differentiation, he also commented extensively on the location of warm pathogen diseases in the individual burners in his books *Discussion of Warm-Heat Pathogen Disorders (Wēn rè lùn)*[26] and *Case Records as a Guide to Clinical Practice (Lín zhèng zhǐ nán yī àn)*.[27] However, as previously noted, the fully-developed theory of three-burner differentiation did not emerge until the publication of Wu Tang's *Systematic Differentiation of Warm Pathogen Diseases (Wēn bìng tiáo biàn)* in 1798. Wu based his theory on an understanding of the Triple Burner organ gleaned from the *Inner Classic*, a synthesis of ideas from previous scholars, and his own experience.

UPPER BURNER PATTERNS

Upper burner patterns occur early in a warm pathogen disease, and the symptoms are those of an attack on the Lung and/or Pericardium. Although upper burner patterns are in general considered to be mild disorders, those affecting the Pericardium are not. When a warm-heat pathogen progresses directly to the Pericardium, the disease is very serious and the patient is likely to die unless he receives immediate treatment.

Lung patterns. Lung patterns most often occur when an attack on the protective level progresses to the Lung. The period for this transmission can vary from hours to days. In children, patients with a weak physical constitution, or those with preexisting Lung problems, the transmission can occur in a few hours. Therefore, by the time you see them in the clinic, a patient may present with only a Lung pattern. However, when there is dampness associated with the pathogen, or if the patient has a strong constitution, it will take a few days or longer for the warm-heat pathogen to progress to the Lung. The Lung patterns are:

- *Failure of the Lung to disseminate the qi and cause it to descend as a result of an attack on the Lung and protective qi by a warm-heat pathogen.* Warm-heat pathogens first attack the skin, nose, and mouth. The Lung opens on the nose, distributes protective qi, and governs the skin. Therefore, when a warm-heat pathogen attacks the Lung, the protective qi will stagnate and the Lung will fail to properly disseminate the qi and cause it to descend. The signs and symptoms are fever, slight aversion to cold, chills, slight or absent sweating, headache, cough, thin and white tongue coating, red tip and edge of the tongue, and a floating and rapid pulse. Because of the Lung's modes of resistance, Lung patterns can be subdivided into two types, depending on whether the disease is situated more on the skin or in the Lung:

  1. Stagnation of protective qi on the skin, which manifests with a high fever, chills, aversion to cold, slight or absent sweating, and a headache.
  2. Failure of the Lung to disseminate the qi and cause it to descend, with slight stagnation of protective qi on the skin, which manifests with a mild fever, aversion to cold, and severe cough.

Nasal congestion, sneezing, and sore throat are commonly seen in both types. According to four-level differentiation theory, both types of Lung patterns are found at the protective level and will lead to one of three outcomes: it can be cured if it is properly treated; it can leave the protective level and become lodged entirely in the Lung; or it can progress from the protective level and the Lung to the Pericardium, which is a critical condition.

- *Blockage of qi in the Lung due to an accumulation of heat in the Lung.* If the warm-heat pathogen in the protective level and Lung is not eliminated by the body or through proper treatment, it will progress from the exterior (the protective level) to the interior (the qi level), leading to an accumulation of heat and blockage of qi in the Lung. This will present with fever, sweating, cough with yellow or greenish sputum, wheezing, chest pain or tightness, increased thirst, red tongue with a yellow coating, and a rapid pulse. If the heat injures the collaterals of the Lung causing the blood to leave the vessels, the sputum may be bloody. If phlegm-heat in the Lung is cleared and resolved, the disease will be cured. If not, the pattern can progress vertically from the Lung in the upper burner to the Stomach and Large Intestine in the middle burner,[28] leading to heat from excess in the Stomach, or constipation with dry stool and heat in the Large Intestine. Another possibility is that the disorder may progress transversely from the Lung to the Pericardium.

- *Stagnation of protective qi, failure of the Lung to disseminate the qi and cause it to descend, and stagnation of the Spleen qi by damp-heat.* The two previous patterns are caused by a warm-heat pathogen without dampness. When dampness is associated with the pathogen, the damp-heat will attack the body via the nose, mouth, skin, and muscles. At the beginning, heat signs and symptoms are not remarkable. In addition to stagnation of the protective qi and failure of the Lung to disseminate the qi and cause it to descend (see the first Lung pattern above), there will also be Spleen qi stagnation. The patient will present with aversion to cold, slight sweating, contained fever, a feeling like the head is wrapped in a bandage, heaviness and aching of the body, cough, difficult breathing, chest and epigastric distention, poor appetite, white and greasy tongue coating, and a soggy and moderate pulse. This disorder is actually a combination of protective and qi level patterns (four-level differentiation), or upper and middle burner patterns (three-burner differentiation). There will be one of two outcomes: if the dampness is resolved and the heat is cleared, the disorder will be cured; otherwise it may move on entirely to the Spleen and Stomach.

Pericardium patterns. Patterns involving the Pericardium are the result of either a direct attack on the Pericardium by summerheat, or the transmission of the disease from the protective level and Lung. If dampness is involved, these patterns can arise from an attack on the Pericardium by phlegm-heat in which phlegm, which is produced by the steaming-up of damp-heat in the qi level, predominates.

- *Blockage of the Pericardium by invasion of heat.* According to four-level differentiation theory, the organ most closely associated with the nutritive level is the Pericardium. Heat in the Pericardium can progress either from the Lung and protective level, from the sinking of the disorder from the qi level to the nutritive level, or from summerheat directly attacking the Pericardium. Clinical manifestations include:

— Muddled consciousness and delirium, or a lethargic state where the individual does not speak, results from the blockage of the spirit of the Heart. The Heart is the sovereign organ that pumps the blood and houses the spirit; the Pericardium is the organ that surrounds and protects the Heart and takes its place as controller of all the other organs. When a warm-heat pathogen attacks the Heart, it does so by attacking the Heart's protector, the Pericardium, leading to blockage of the spirit of the Heart.

— Retraction of the tongue with difficulty speaking is a result of the warm-heat pathogen congealing the fluids into phlegm. The phlegm-heat blocks the qi from reaching the tongue.

— Cold extremities result from the warm-heat pathogen blocking the qi from reaching the extremities.

— Fever, deep-red tongue, and a thin and rapid pulse result from the yin burning in the nutritive level.

These patterns can lead to one of three outcomes: The warm-heat pathogen can be resolved and the antipathogenic qi restored; blockage of the Pericardium can lead to collapse of yang qi; or the disease can progress to the lower burner.

• *Veiling of the Pericardium by phlegm and damp-heat.* This is actually a qi level pattern that is progressing slightly to the nutritive level. Steaming of damp-heat in the qi level, which produces phlegm, leads to veiling of the Pericardium. Clinical manifestations include:

— Constant fever that improves in the morning and worsens in the evening, yellow and greasy tongue coating, and a slippery and rapid pulse. All of these result from damp-heat in the qi level.

— Clear thinking alternating with confusion and delirium are caused by the 'veiling' of the Pericardium by damp-heat and phlegm.

These patterns can lead to one of two outcomes: they can be successfully treated if the heat is cleared, dampness and phlegm are resolved, and the orifice is opened, or they can progress to collapse of yang qi.

MIDDLE BURNER PATTERNS

Patterns of the middle burner include those in the *yang ming,* that is, the Stomach and Large Intestine, and in the Spleen. These patterns usually represent the progression of an illness that began in the Lung in the upper burner, or a direct attack of summer-heat with dampness on the Spleen and Stomach. In accordance with five-phase theory, dampness, as well as the Spleen (yin) and Stomach (yang), correspond to earth. Therefore, if there is more yang (heat), damp-heat will attack the Stomach, and may progress further to the Large Intestine. If there is more yin (dampness), damp-heat will attack the Spleen.

Yang ming patterns

- *Heat from excess in the Stomach.* This pattern is the same as the main pattern in the qi level. It usually progresses from the Lung in the upper burner as a result of the failure to clear the warm-heat pathogen from that organ. It can also be caused by a direct attack from summerheat. Signs and symptoms include vigorous fever, aversion to heat instead of cold, red face and eyes, thirst, rough breathing, yellow and dry tongue coating, and a flooding or slippery pulse. This pattern can have one of three outcomes: it can be successfully treated if the heat is cleared; it can progress to the Large Intestine; or it can progress to the lower burner, injuring the yin of the Liver and Kidney.

- *Obstruction of qi in the Large Intestine by dry stool and heat, with severe constipation.* This pattern is usually due to invasion of the Large Intestine by a warm-heat pathogen, leading to a mixture of heat and dry stool and injury to the fluids. It manifests with:

  — Fever that reaches its zenith between 3-7 P.M. According to traditional Chinese medicine, the qi in the *yang ming* is strongest at this time. When there is heat coupled with dry stool in the Large Intestine, the qi becomes more stagnant; consequently, the patient feels that the fever is worse at this time.

  — Constipation and concentrated urine are due to blockage of qi in the Large Intestine, coupled with injury to the fluids by heat.

  — A yellow, black, and dry tongue coating and a submerged and excessive pulse reflect interior dryness and heat from excess.

These patterns can have one of several outcomes. If the heat and dry stool are discharged by purging, the condition will be cured. The heat from excess can disturb the spirit in the Heart and/or stir up Liver wind. The heat can transform into toxin, injuring the collaterals and leading to bleeding or maculopapular rashes. Or the patterns will progress to the lower burner, injuring the Liver and Kidney yin.

Clinically, excessive *yang ming* heat can lead to mental changes such as muddled consciousness and delirium, which is similar to the blockage of the Pericardium by the invasion of heat. Mental changes related to *yang ming* heat are not as severe as those associated with the Pericardium. Differentiation is made easier by their presentations: vigorous fever, thirst, abdominal bloating, constipation, red tongue with *yang ming* heat; cold extremities, difficulty in speaking and a deep-red tongue with blockage of the Pericardium.

Spleen and Stomach patterns. These patterns result either from a transmission of damp-heat in the upper burner to the Spleen and Stomach, or a direct attack by summerheat with dampness on the Spleen and Stomach. They tend to be situated more in the Spleen than in the Stomach, unlike the *yang ming* patterns, which will be found in the Stomach and Large Intestine. Manifestations include:

- *Contained fever* that is reduced slightly, but does not completely disappear, even after sweating. This is usually accompanied by a sensation of heaviness in the body and lassitude. Heat is trapped by the dampness, and dampness is steamed by the heat, leading to qi stagnation that can produce further dampness and heat. If untreated, the struggle between the damp-heat and antipathogenic qi will continue. Therefore, contained fever that is not remarkably reduced even after sweating, coupled with obstruction of qi in the channels, gives rise to the sensation of a heavy body and lassitude.

- *Distention in the chest and epigastrium, and nausea,* are caused by stagnant qi in the middle burner. This in turn leads to rebellion of the Stomach qi.

- *Loose stools* are caused by the inability of the Spleen to properly do its job of transforming and transporting food. It is usually accompanied by abdominal bloating.

- *A greasy tongue coating and a soggy and moderate pulse* are typical of the tongue and pulse signs caused by dampness.

These patterns can be cured if the heat is cleared and dampness is resolved. Otherwise the dampness will transform into heat and progress to the lower burner. Because disorders of the middle burner are intermediate between those of the upper and lower burners, it is important that they be properly dealt with. If the heat or damp-heat can be expeditiously discharged from the body via the stool or urine, the progress of the disease can be stopped.

LOWER BURNER PATTERNS

The Kidney stores the essence and the Liver stores the blood. The two are mutually dependent, and together form the basis for all the yin of the body. When a warm-heat pathogen progresses to the lower burner, it can injure the yin and blood. Besides the obvious problems that yin and blood deficiency entail, this can lead to a stirring-up of Liver wind and to disharmony between the Heart and Kidney.

Kidney patterns. These are usually the result of severe injury to the fluids and yin in the upper and middle burners. Signs and symptoms include:

- *Listlessness, dry mouth and throat, diminished hearing, and a deficient pulse.* The Kidney stores yin and essence, and when the Kidney yin is exhausted, the body and organs will be deprived of nourishment. This is especially true of the throat, through which the Kidney channel travels, and the ears, through which the Kidney opens.
- *Fever, malar flushing, and relatively warm palms and soles.* The face is located in the upper part of the body and is associated with yang. When Kidney yin is exhausted, the yang will become excessive on the yin aspects of the body, such as the soles and palms, or it may even float on the surface and upper part of the body, leading to fever, malar flushing, and relatively hot soles and palms. These patterns can be cured if the Kidney yin is restored. Otherwise, they may progress to the Liver, leading to the stirring-up of Liver wind.

Liver patterns. These patterns usually appear as a result of the exhaustion of Kidney yin, as this will eventually lead to Liver yin deficiency and malnutrition of the sinews. The outcome is spasm of the sinews and the production of internal wind. Manifestations include trembling of the fingers, tonic-clonic convulsions, listlessness, violent palpitations with an empty sensation in the chest, dry, atrophied, and deep-red tongue, and a frail pulse.

The violent palpitations with empty sensation in the chest is the result of water (yin) in the Kidney becoming so weak that it cannot reach the Heart to nourish and balance the Heart fire, which thereupon becomes more aggressive. Wu Tang explained this pathology in *Systematic Differentiation of Warm Pathogen Diseases*:

> Convulsions and trembling come from failure of the Kidney to nourish the Liver due to deficiency of water in the Kidney. And convulsions and trembling show that water in the Kidney is so weak that it cannot be supplied quickly, depriving the spirit of the Heart of an anchor. This results in violent palpitations with an empty sensation in the chest.[29]

These patterns can be cured if the Kidney and Liver yin recover. But they may be terminal if the Kidney and Liver yin become exhausted.

PROGRESSION OF PATTERNS IN THE THREE BURNERS

Unlike four-level differentiation, three-burner differentiation focuses more on the injury to the yin of the organs, and mostly describes a vertical transmission through the body over the course of a disease, rather than a transverse one. Three-burner differentiation and treatment are more useful for those diseases involving yin deficiency and dampness.

Table 4.2	Three-Burner Differentiation		
Affected Organ	**Pathology**	**Signs and Symptoms**	**Key Points for Identification**
▶ UPPER BURNER			
Lung: warm-heat pathogen located in the protective and qi levels simulta-neously	Failure of the Lung to disseminate the qi and cause it to descend due to attack on the Lung and protective qi by warm-heat pathogen	Fever, slight aversion to cold, chills, headache, slight thirst, cough, thin and white tongue coating, floating and rapid pulse	Fever, slight aversion to cold, chills, slight thirst, cough, floating and rapid pulse
Lung: warm-heat pathogen found solely in the qi level	Blockage of qi in Lung due to accu-mulation of heat in Lung	Cough, labored breathing, fever, thirst, yellow tongue coating, rapid pulse	Cough, labored breathing, fever, thirst, yellow tongue coating
Pericardium	Confusion of the spirit of the Heart due to invasion of Pericardium by heat	Deep-red tongue, muddled consciousness, delirium, retraction of the tongue, coldness of the extremities, nonspeaking, lethargic state	Muddled consciousness, delirium, coldness of the extremities
▶ MIDDLE BURNER			
Stomach	Excess-type heat in the Stomach steaming upward	High fever, profuse sweating, aversion to heat, flushed face, red eyes, thirst with a need to drink a lot, coarse breathing, dry and yellow tongue coating, flooding pulse	High fever, profuse sweating, thirst with a need to drink a lot, dry and yellow tongue coating, flooding pulse
Large Intestine	Obstruction of qi in the Large Intestine by dry stools and heat	Fever that is worse between 3-7 P.M., constipation, concentrated urine, dry yellow, gray, or black tongue coating, and submerged and excessive pulse	Fever that is worse between 3-7 P.M., con-stipation, dry yellow, gray, or black tongue coating, submerged and excessive pulse

Table 4.2, cont.			
▶ MIDDLE BURNER, cont.			
Spleen	Disturbance of the Spleen and stagnation of qi due to attack by damp-heat	Contained fever even after sweating, chest and epigastric distention, nausea, heavy body, lassitude, greasy tongue coating, soggy pulse	Contained fever, chest and epigastric distention, greasy tongue coating
▶ LOWER BURNER			
Kidney	Exhaustion of Kidney yin due to prolonged exposure to warm-heat pathogen	Fever, malar flush, diminished hearing, sensation of greater warmth in the soles and palms than in the top of foot and back of hand, dry mouth and throat, listlessness, deficient pulse	A sensation of greater warmth in the soles and palms than in the top of the foot and back of the hand, dry mouth and throat, listlessness, deficient pulse
Liver	Stirring of Liver wind due to deficiency of Kidney yin, which thereby fails to nourish the Liver	Trembling of fingers, tonic-clonic convulsions, listlessness, violent palpitations with an empty sensation in the chest, dry, atrophied, deep-red tongue, frail pulse	Trembling of fingers, clonic convulsions, dry, atrophied, deep-red tongue, frail pulse

Upper burner patterns occur early in the development of a warm pathogen disease, and include symptoms which affect the Lung and Pericardium. Middle burner patterns are situated at a deeper or more critical level, and affect the Stomach, Large Intestine, and Spleen. The deepest or most critical level of a warm pathogen disease is the lower burner, with patterns affecting the Liver and Kidney. Related signs and symptoms are set forth in Table 4.2.

In *Systematic Differentiation of Warm Pathogen Diseases*, Wu Tang summarized the course of transmission of warm pathogen diseases. Warm-heat pathogens attack the body through the nose and mouth, which pertain to the Lung and the Stomach respectively. From here, if not properly treated, they will either progress transversely to the Pericardium, or vertically to the middle burner. If left untreated, or if treated improperly in the middle burner, the disease will progress to the lower burner.[30]

However, the progression of patterns in the three burners does not always proceed in this order. Sometimes a pattern will appear in the middle burner before it has fully disappeared from the upper burner. Examples include:

- Summerheat pathogen without dampness often attacks the Stomach in the middle burner in the early stage of summerheat-warmth.

- The early stages of damp-warmth affect the Spleen.

- Summerheat can directly attack the Pericardium or Liver.

- Lurking summerheat can progress from the lower burner to the middle burner.

In addition, a warm pathogen disease may appear in two or three burners simultaneously, as in the following examples:

- Because the Lung pairs with the Large Intestine, phlegm-heat in the Lung can lead to stagnation of qi in the Large Intestine, producing heat there and resulting in a combination of phlegm-heat in the Lung and heat in the Large Intestine.

- Because the Lung normally produces water for the Kidney, a warm-heat pathogen that impairs the water-producing capacity of the Lung will result in both Kidney and Lung yin deficiency.

- Because both the Large Intestine and Stomach pertain to the *yang ming*, and because the collaterals of the Stomach connect with the Heart, severe heat in the Large Intestine can invade the Pericardium through their interconnected channels. The result is a combination of invasion of the Pericardium by heat as well as heat in the Large Intestine.

- Because both the Large Intestine and Kidney are found in the lower burner, extreme heat in the Large Intestine can severely injure the Kidney yin, leading to heat from excess in the Large Intestine as well as Kidney yin deficiency.

Normal and Abnormal Transmission in Warm Pathogen Diseases

In the theory of warm pathogen diseases there are alternative explanations for the transmission or progression of disease: normal transmission (順傳 *shùn chúan*)—literally, 'smooth transmission'—and abnormal transmission (逆傳 *nì chuán*)—literally, 'rebellious/reverse transmission.' Because an understanding of the natural history of a disorder is an important part of knowing how to effectively treat it, these are significant clinical paradigms.

NORMAL TRANSMISSION

One type of normal transmission is the superficial to deep progression outlined in four-level differentiation: protective level to qi level to nutritive level and finally to blood level. This idea originated with Ye Gui.[31] Another meaning of normal transmission is defined by progression from one organ to another, specifically from the Lung to the Stomach and Large Intestine.[32] One relatively recent interpretation is that it refers to a warm-heat pathogen moving from the interior to the exterior of the body as the condition improves.[33] In all these cases the transmission is regarded as normal because this is what occurs when the patient has no particular weakness or vulnerability.

In the normal course of transmission a warm-heat pathogen progresses from the protective level to the qi level, mostly affecting the Lung, Stomach, and Large Intestine. It is easy to understand why the Lung is susceptible to warm-heat pathogens since it is the most superficial of all the yin organs; the classics often refer to the Lung as the 'delicate organ.' Yet why do warm-heat pathogens so readily attack the Stomach and Large Intestine? First, the muscles and flesh are associated with the Spleen and Stomach, while the skin pertains to the Lung and Large Intestine. When warm-heat pathogens progress from the skin to the muscles and flesh, they will directly affect the Stomach. Moreover, the Lung, Large Intestine, and Stomach channels are all closely related. Chapter 10 of *Divine Pivot* notes that the Lung channel originates in the middle burner, descends to connect with the Large Intestine, circles the opening of the Stomach, and then ascends to reach the Lung.[34] In addition, since the Lung is paired with the Large Intestine, an attack of a warm-heat pathogen on the skin or the Lung can readily progress to the Large Intestine. All of these factors facilitate the transmission of the warm-heat pathogen from the Lung to the Stomach and Large Intestine.

A full understanding of the transmission of a warm-heat pathogen requires familiarity with common qi level patterns caused by an attack of wind-heat. One of these patterns is heat from excess in the Stomach, with vigorous fever, profuse sweating, thirst with a preference for cold beverages, and a flooding and big pulse. Another pattern is the clumping of dry stool and heat in the Large Intestine, manifesting as tidal fever, delirium, severe constipation or dry and hard stool in the Large Intestine that leads to a discharge of foul water, a black-yellow tongue coating, and a submerged and forceful pulse. In addition, when wind-heat invades the interior, the wind automatically transforms into heat; this is because wind obstructs the circulation of qi, which causes qi stagnation and thereby heat. Therefore, when wind-heat invades the qi level, the heat may injure the yin of the Lung and Stomach, resulting in cough with little sputum, dry throat and mouth, thirst, and a red tongue with less than normal coating. If the heat is not quickly dispelled, it may invade the lower burner and exhaust the yin of the Liver and Kidney.

However, a patient with a qi level pattern will not necessarily manifest any of these signs and symptoms at the very onset of the illness. Thus, in the clinic it is extremely important to detect the initial signs and symptoms in order to identify transmission from the protective level to the qi level as early as possible. In general, if the patient is thirsty and prefers cold beverages, and has a yellow tongue coating, the illness is progressing from the protective level to the qi level. One should not wait for the full presentation of each pattern before initiating treatment. Otherwise the heat will have already injured the yin or fluids, and the treatment regimen will thus be more difficult and lengthy.

ABNORMAL TRANSMISSION

There are three types of abnormal transmission. In the first, heat progresses directly from the protective level to the nutritive or blood level. In the second, a warm-heat pathogen moves from the exterior to the interior of the body as the condition gets worse.[35] In the third, heat progresses from the Lung to the Pericardium or Heart. In *Discussion of Warm-Heat Pathogen Disorders,* Ye Gui first noted this kind of abnormal transmission when discussing the progression of the warm-heat pathogen from the Lung to the Pericardium.[36] Why did Ye think this was abnormal? In *A Stick to Awaken Physicians (Yī mén bàng hè),* Zhang Nan (Zhang Xu-Gu, c. 1825) explained it in terms of five-phase theory. Zhang noted that the Pericardium covers the Heart like a set of clothes and is therefore intimately related to that organ. The Heart pertains to fire and the Lung to metal, and this type of transmission is considered abnormal because, according to five-phase theory, a problem in the Heart should progress to the Lung, instead of the other way around.[37]

Often, in cases of transmission of a warm-heat pathogen from the Lung to the Pericardium, the transition time is very short. If this is an abnormal transmission, why does the warm-heat pathogen so readily invade the Pericardium? One reason, suggested by Ye Gui, is that "If a patient has a constitutional weakness of the Heart coupled with phlegm, once a warm-heat pathogen attacks the body, it will attack this weak place, leading to blockage of the Pericardium by transmission of heat."[38] In this case, weakness of the Heart refers to deficiency of Heart qi or yin. Yang Zhao-Li (Yang Su-Yuan, dates unknown) referred to the physical closeness of these organs as a reason when he observed that "The Lung is connected to the Heart, and heat in the Lung readily invades the Heart."[39] Another possibility is that when Lung heat becomes extreme, the Heart has no defense against it. One astute observation made by the contemporary scholar Hu Ding-Bang is that abnormal transmission occurs when the warm-heat pathogen is simply unable to progress normally. This occurs when there is no interior heat or retention of food in the Stomach or Large Intestine.[40] Among these explanations, Heart yin or qi deficiency plays the greatest role in abnormal transmission.

Another example of an abnormal transmission is the onset of rashes or coughing up blood as a result of heat invading the collaterals of the Lung; in this case, heat is forcing the blood out of the vessels. There are two different presentations of this disorder. In the first, there is no cough present, only bleeding in the form of papules or nosebleeds. In the second, there is cough coupled with bleeding and thirst. Generally, the presence of papules, which relate to the Lung, or maculas, which relate to the Stomach, reveals a qi level pattern. However, the presence of bleeding indicates that the pattern is at the blood level. This is regarded as an abnormal transmission because there is bleeding without any other Stomach signs or symptoms (except for maculas).

What significance does the identification of normal and abnormal transmissions have in the clinic? While it is never a good sign when a disease progresses from the outside of the body to the inside, there are differences in severity. Part of the difference with respect to warm pathogen diseases has to do with fundamental differences between the yin and yang organs. As noted in Chapter 11 of *Basic Questions,* the yin organs store qi, blood, and essence while the yang organs transport food and discharge waste.[41] Another characteristic of the yang organs is that their qi naturally moves downward and toward the outside. For this reason, they are often relied upon clinically to discharge pathogens via the stool or urine. From this perspective, it is clear that the body will sustain relatively less damage when a warm-heat pathogen affecting the protective level or the Lung progresses downward to a yang organ, such as the Stomach or Large Intestine, than when it progresses to a yin organ, such as the Pericardium, Liver, or Kidney. Because it is relatively easy to dispel warm-heat pathogens from the yang organs, when a warm pathogen disease progresses from the Lung (upper burner) to the Stomach and the Large Intestine (middle and lower burner, respectively), it is less serious than if it progresses instead to any of the yin organs, where the condition could easily become life-threatening. From this point of view, the prognosis is better with a normal transmission than with an abnormal transmission.

Relationship between Four-Level and Three-Burner Differentiation

Four-level and three-burner differentiation intersect in the following ways:

- *Four-level differentiation intersects three-burner differentiation.* The protective level pattern overlaps with the upper burner pattern of the failure of the Lung to disseminate the qi due to an attack on the Lung and protective qi. The qi level pattern overlaps with the upper burner pattern of the Lung, and the middle burner patterns of the Stomach, Large Intestine, and Spleen. The nutritive level pattern is similar to the Pericardium pattern of the upper burner.
- *Three-burner differentiation intersects four-level differentiation.* The upper burner patterns include the protective level and qi level patterns of the Lung, and the nutritive level patterns of the Pericardium and Heart. These include the

failure of the Lung to disseminate the qi and cause it to descend subsequent to an attack affecting the Lung and protective qi; accumulation of heat in the Lung; and blockage of the spirit of the Heart due to invasion of the Pericardium by heat. The middle burner patterns include those affecting the Large Intestine, Spleen, and Stomach, all of which pertain to the qi level. The lower burner pattern, however, is unique and is not equivalent to any pattern of the protective, qi, nutritive, or blood levels.

The two theories of differentiation have different foci. In contrast to three-burner differentiation, four-level differentiation attaches great importance to the *transverse* transmission in the development of a warm pathogen disease, that is, from the superficial level to the deep levels of the body. By contrast, three-burner differentiation pays more attention to the *vertical* transmission of a warm pathogen disease among the yin and yang organs, that is, from the upper burner to the middle burner, and finally to the lower burner.

In the clinic it is often not sufficient just to correctly identify a pattern's level and provide proper treatment according to four-level differentiation theory. Rather, the clinician must also identify and treat the affected organ(s). Actually, regardless of the treatment method, the clinician must work on regulating the function of the yin and yang organs. Without paying attention to the health of the organs, treatment will not be properly focused.

If a practitioner differentiates the patterns and provides treatment based solely upon four-level differentiation, the treatment method and herbs may not be entirely suitable. Moreover, even though three-burner differentiation pays more attention to the yin and yang organs involved in the development of a warm pathogen disease, it does not include all of the yin and yang organ patterns, especially those of the Gallbladder and Bladder. In addition, the transmission of patterns in the theory of three-burner differentiation is not as clear as in four-level differentiation. Thus, neither theory by itself can provide sufficient information to differentiate the patterns and guide the course of clinical treatment. They should therefore be combined. Contemporary writers and practitioners in China are moving toward the idea that three-burner differentiation is the more appropriate method for warm pathogen diseases related to damp-heat and/or injured yin.

Summary

Four-level and three-burner differentiation offer unique methods for differentiating warm pathogen diseases caused by warm-heat pathogens. They help the practitioner analyze the pathology, location, severity, and transmission of warm pathogen diseases, and provide detailed recommendations for treatment. Although each has its own special focus, they often complement one another and are commonly combined in the clinic to provide a thorough differentiation of patterns.

Endnotes

1. We use the term 'three burner' rather than Triple Burner in order to clearly show that what is being described here are areas of the body and not the functions of a particular yang organ.

2. Anonymous, *Yellow Emperor's Inner Classic: Divine Pivot (Huáng Dì nèi jīng líng shū)*. Beijing: People's Health Publishing House, 1963: 71.

3. Anonymous, *Yellow Emperor's Inner Classic: Basic Questions (Huáng Dì nèi jīng sù wèn)*. Beijing: People's Health Publishing House, 1963: 245.

4. Anonymous, *Yellow Emperor's Inner Classic: Divine Pivot*, 89.

5. Anonymous, *Yellow Emperor's Inner Classic: Basic Questions*, 244.

6. Anonymous, *Yellow Emperor's Inner Classic: Divine Pivot*, 126.

7. Zhang Jie-Bin (Zhang Jing-Yue), *Collected Treatises of [Zhang] Jing-Yue (Jǐng-Yuè quán shū)*. Beijing: People's Health Publishing House, 1991: 820.

8. Zhang Ji, *Discussion of Cold Damage (Shāng hán lùn)*. Shanghai: Shanghai Science and Technology Publishing House, 1983: 25..

9. Ibid., 16-17.

10. Summerheat-warmth without dampness can directly attack the *yang ming* (Stomach), damp-warmth can directly attack the Spleen and Stomach, and lurking summerheat can begin at either the qi or nutritive level. See Chapters 11, 12, and 13 for further details.

11. Meng Shu-Jiang et al., *Warm Pathogen Diseases (Wēn bìng xué)*. Shanghai: Shanghai Science and Technology Publishing House, 1985: 54.

12. Examples of improper treatment here include prescriptions that are too acrid and warm, which create excessive heat inside the body, or that are too bitter and cold, which traps heat inside the body.

13. Based on my understanding and experience, the nose and throat, like the skin, are parts of the exterior aspect of the Lung. Even though they can be thought of as being inside the body, they are open to the air and are included in the structures to which protective qi is distributed, along with the skin and subcutaneous tissues. For this reason, they have been called the 'clear pathways' (清道 qīng dào). This is why acute nose and throat symptoms from an attack of a warm-heat pathogen should be considered protective level disorders.

14. Hu Ding-Bang, "Initial discussion on the onset and progression principles of warm pathogen diseases (Shi lun wen re bing fa bing ji chuan bian gui lu)," in Beijing College of Traditional Chinese Medicine, *Selected Papers for the Thirty Year Anniversary of the Foundation of Beijing College of Traditional Chinese Medicine (Beijing zhong yi xue yuan san shi nian lun wen xuan)*. Beijing: Chinese Ancient Medical Literature Publishing House, 1986: 100.

15. Anonymous, *Yellow Emperor's Inner Classic: Basic Questions*, 152.

16. Qin Bo-Wei, *Medical Lecture Notes of [Qin] Qian Zhai (Qian zha yi xue jiang gao)*. Shanghai: Shanghai Science and Technology Publishing House, 1964: 65.

17. Guo Wei-Feng and Zhou Zhong-Ying, "Identification and significance of qi [level] heat being transmitted to the nutritive [level] in exogenous febrile diseases with severe symptoms *(Wai gan re bing zhong zheng qi re chuan ying de bian shi ji qi yi yi)."* *Journal of Traditional Chinese Medicine,* 1999;40(8):457-59.

18. Chinese Academy of Traditional Chinese Medicine, *Case Studies from Pu Fu-Zhou (Pú Fǔ-Zhōu yī liǎo jīng yàn jí).* Beijing: People's Health Publishing House, 1972: 63.

19. Anonymous, *Yellow Emperor's Inner Classic: Divine Pivot,* 52.

20. Anonymous, *Classic of Difficulties (Nan jing),* annotated by Nanjing College of Traditional Chinese Medicine. Beijing: People's Health Publishing House, 1979: 79.

21. Anonymous, *Yellow Emperor's Inner Classic: Basic Questions,* 58.

22. Ibid., 52.

23. Zhang Ji, *Explanation of the Essentials from the Golden Cabinet (Jīn guì yào luè shì yì),* annotated by the Hubei College of Traditional Chinese Medicine. Wuhan: Hunan People's Publishing House, 1963: 110.

24. Liu Wan-Su, *Collection of Writings on the Mechanism of Disease, Suitability of Qi, and the Safeguarding of Life as Discussed in Basic Questions (Sù wèn bìng jī qì yí bǎo míng jí).* Shanghai: Shanghai Ancient Literature Publishing House, 1991: 94.

25. Yu Chang, *Writing on the Esteemed Discussion (Shàng lùn piān),* reproduced in *Collection of Famous Books on Discussion of Cold Damage, Essentials from the Golden Cabinet and Warm Pathogen Disease,* 217.

26. Tang Da-Lie, *Collection of Papers of Physicians from Wu (Wú yī huì jiǎng).* Shanghai: Shanghai Science and Technology Publishing House, 1983: 5-6. This book was first published in 1792.

27. Ye Gui, *Case Records as a Guide to Clinical Practice (Lín zhèng zhǐ nán yī àn).* Shanghai: Shanghai Science and Technology Publishing House, 1959: 332-36, 343-44, 351.

28. In most modern TCM textbooks, the Large Intestine is considered to be located in the lower burner, primarily due to what they consider its physical location. However, from the perspective of warm-pathogen disease practitioners it belongs in the middle burner. This is because the obstruction of the Large Intestine presents with not only abdominal pain and/bloating, but even nausea and a poor appetite. These are all manifestations of disruption in the qi dynamic of the middle burner.

29. Wu Tang, *Systematic Differentiation of Warm Pathogen Diseases,* 125.

30. Ibid., 60.

31. Tang Da-Lie, *Collection of Papers of Physicians from Wu,* 5.

32. Wang Shi-Xiong, *Cases Studies from Wang Meng-Ying (Wang meng-ying yi an).* Beijing: Chinese Traditional Medicine and Pharmacology Publishing House, 1999: 27

33. Chen Guang-Song (active early twentieth century), *Annotation and Correction of the Discussion of Warm-Heat Disorders (Wēn rè lùn jiān zhèng),* reproduced in *Collection of Rare Medical Books (Zhēn běn yī shū jí chéng),* vol. 2. Beijing: Chinese Medicine and Pharmacology Publishing House, 1996: 617.

34. Anonymous, *Yellow Emperor's Inner Classic: Divine Pivot*, 30.

35. Chen Guang-Song, *Annotation and Correction of the Discussion of Warm-Heat Disorders*, 617.

36. Tang Da-Lie, *Collection of Papers of Physicians from Wu*, 3.

37. Meng Shu-Jiang, *Warm Pathogen Diseases*, 60.

38. Tang Da-Lie, *Collection of Papers of Physicians from Wu*, 7.

39. Meng Shu-Jiang, *Warm Pathogen Diseases*, 59.

40. Hu Ding-Bang, "Initial discussion on onset and progression principle of warm pathogen diseases," 100.

41. Anonymous, *Yellow Emperor's Inner Classic: Basic Questions*, 77.

5 Diagnosing Warm Pathogen Diseases

WE HAVE SEEN how the concepts of warm pathogen disease, while rooted in the fundamental theories of Chinese medicine, possess their own distinctive characteristics. Similarly, diagnosing and differentiating warm pathogen diseases are based on such commonly used methods as observing the patient's signs, examining the tongue body and coating, palpating the pulse, and asking questions. Yet many of these methods are used in ways that are distinctive to warm pathogen disease. In addition, there are unique methods of diagnosis that have been developed specifically for warm pathogen disease, including observing the condition of the teeth and gums, and identifying maculas, papules, and miliaria alba.

Examining the Tongue

Tongue diagnosis has a long history in Chinese medicine.[1] As early as the *Inner Classic* tongues were described as stiff, curled, or atrophied. A yellow tongue coating was first recorded in this book, and the condition of the tongue was used to predict the course of a disease.[2] In the work of Zhang Ji (early third century), descriptions of the tongue are mentioned ten times. By the time of Chao Yuan-Fang (c. 610), the cited tongue characteristics include swollen, distended, and ulcerated, as well as those that move erratically out of the mouth and around the lips or were bleeding.[3]

The first book to focus specifically on tongue diagnosis was not published until the fourteenth century. It was written by an otherwise unknown author with the surname Ao. His *Golden Mirror Collection (Jīn jìng lù)* was discovered by Du Ben (Du Bi-Qing) who edited the book, expanded the number of tongue illustrations from twelve to thirty-six, and published it around the year 1341 under the title *Ao's Golden Mirror Collection (Aó shì jīn jìng lù)*. The next major extant book on tongues was written around 1668 by Zhang Deng (Zhang Dan-Xian) and called *Tongue Diagnosis for Cold Damage (Shāng hán shé jiǎn)*. Zhang presented one-hundred twenty tongue illustrations and discussed the significance of a number of tongue colors, as well as the color and consistency of tongue coatings. Although the book focused on tongues relating to cold damage, it included information on the body and coating of tongues associated with internal disorders and warm pathogen diseases.

The first systematic discussion of tongue diagnosis in the context of warm pathogen diseases can be found in *Discussion of Warm-Heat Pathogen Disorders (Wēn rè lùn)* by Ye Gui (Ye Tian-Shi, c. 1666–1745) and his student Gu Jin-Wen. In this short book of only thirty-seven paragraphs, seventeen were devoted to tongue diagnosis, including discussion of the clinical significance and treatment of red, deep red, and purple tongues as well as white, yellow, gray, and black tongue coatings. Ye paid special attention to the tongue body color and coating in the differentiation of warm pathogen diseases. Unfortunately, the book was not illustrated, which made it difficult for a beginner to follow. This omission was remedied during the past century. In 1917, Cao Bing-Zhang (Cao Chi-Dian, 1877–1955) published *Guide to Distinguishing Tongues (Biàn shé zhǐ nán)*, which contained one-hundred twenty color illustrations of tongues, mostly related to warm pathogen diseases. In 1998 the first book specifically devoted to tongue diagnosis in warm pathogen diseases was published. This book contains over one-hundred fifty photographs of tongues grouped according to types of warm pathogen disease.[4]

In traditional Chinese medicine the tongue, which is closely associated with the internal organs, reflects the state of health or disease within the body. Channels of the Heart, Spleen, Kidney, and Liver reach to the root of the tongue, as do collaterals of the Bladder and Gallbladder channels. Among the organs, the Heart, Spleen, and Stomach are most closely associated with the tongue because the Heart opens onto the tongue, the Spleen affects the capacity for taste, and Stomach qi forms the tongue coating. By observing the condition of the tongue, the practitioner can:

- Determine the status of the antipathogenic qi (正氣 *zhèng qì*)
- Determine the location of the disease
- Assess the quality of a disease
- Determine the extent to which the fluids or yin have been damaged
- Help confirm the presence or absence of dampness
- Predict the progression and prognosis of the illness according to four-level or three-burner differentiation

Clinically, the main things to look for are the color and quality of the tongue coating and body, which must be combined and analyzed. In general, for hot disorders, the color of the tongue body is more reliable than the quality of the coating, and for damp disorders, just the opposite. Similarly, changes observed in the coating are particularly helpful for tracing the progress of warm-heat pathogens in the protective and qi levels, while changes in the body color are more helpful for tracking the progress of disease in the nutritive and blood levels.

TONGUE COATING

When observing the tongue coating, the primary characteristics are color, moisture, and thickness. Generally, a thin coating indicates that a disease is at an early stage or that it is in the exterior, while a thick coating indicates that the disease has entered the organs, and hence its location is deeper. As previously noted (Chapter 4), a disease in the protective level is superficial and is located on the surface, while a disease in the qi level shows organ involvement and is deeper. Changes in the tongue coating may therefore reflect a pathological progression in a warm pathogen disease. Specifically, a change from white to yellow shows progression from the protective level to the qi level, and a change from thin to thick reflects a progression from exterior to interior. In general, changes in the color of the tongue coating from white to yellow, yellow to gray, and gray to black indicate that the disease has moved deeper and has worsened. On the other hand, the moisture in the tongue coating reflects the condition of the fluids: a moist coating indicates that the fluids have not been injured by the warm-heat pathogen, while a dry coating or one that has horizontal cracks indicates that the fluids have been injured.

White tongue coating. A white coating is seen in protective level and some qi level patterns. There are two basic types of white tongue coating: thick and thin. A thin white coating suggests an exterior pattern at an early stage of a warm pathogen disease, that is, a mild and superficial illness that occurs mostly in the protective level. A thick white coating implies an interior pattern, which most often appears in the qi level and is mostly caused by dampness or phlegm. Based on its thickness, color, and degree of moisture, a white tongue coating can be subdivided into several types.

A thin white coating with normal saliva suggests that the fluids have not yet been injured. A thin white coating with a red tip and edge indicates that the warm-heat pathogen is attacking the protective level or the Lung, while a thin, white, and dry coating denotes injury to the fluids. In *Discussion of Warm-Heat Pathogen Disorders*, Ye Gui noted "If the tongue coating is white and thin, but looks dry, this indicates injury to the fluids in the Lung, and one should use light herbs like Ophiopogonis Radix *(mài mén dōng)*, Lonicerae Floris Distillatum *(jīn yín huā lù)*,[5] and Phragmitis Rhizomatis Succus *(lú gēn zhī)*;[6] that is, use light herbs to treat problems in the upper burner."[7] This is a warning against using herbs such as Rehmanniae Radix preparata *(shú dì huáng)* and Dendrobii Herba *(shí hú)* which are cloying and could trap the warm-heat pathogen and prolong the course of the disease.

A white and thin tongue coating that becomes so thick that the bottom of the tongue cannot be seen indicates that the warm pathogen disease has progressed from the exterior to the interior, especially to the qi level. Clinically, a white, thick, and dry tongue coating can reflect two pathologies:

1. One possibility is that, not only has the warm-heat pathogen reached the qi level, it has also injured the Stomach fluids and qi. According to Ye Gui, Glycyrrhizae Radix *(gān cǎo)*, which can slightly tonify the Stomach qi, should be added to those herbs that support the Stomach fluids.[8]

2. Another possibility is a pattern of damp-heat in the Spleen. In such cases the tongue coating is not only caused by injury to the Stomach fluids, but also by dampness blocking the Spleen and Stomach qi and preventing it from bringing fluids to the tongue. This often happens when dampness predominates; aromatic herbs such as Pogostemonis/Agastaches Herba *(huò xiāng)* and Eupatorii Herba *(pèi lán)* should be included in the treatment.

How does a practitioner distinguish between these two pathologies that have such similar presentations? Other signs and symptoms should be used to aid in the differentiation. For example, in the first case the patient will often be restless and/or have a thirst for cold beverages. And in the second case, the patient will often have a dry mouth with no desire to drink (or a desire for only a few sips), chest and epigastric distention, nausea, and/or vomiting.

A white, thick, and greasy coating indicates an accumulation of dampness in the qi level. If the damp-warmth has more dampness than heat, the patient will also experience contained fever *(shēn rè bù yáng)*,[9] heaviness and aches over the body and head, normal thirst, chest and epigastric distention, abdominal bloating, loose stools, and scanty urine. According to Ye Gui in *Discussion of Warm-Heat Pathogen Disorders*:

> A white, greasy coating is associated with thick saliva, and there is a sweet taste in the mouth. This is called Spleen singularity disease,[10] which is caused by an accumulation of damp-heat in the Spleen, leading to steaming-up of damp-heat and grain qi. One should use Eupatorii Herba *(pèi lán)*, which is aromatic, to transform dampness.[11]

Ye also noted that if a white, thick, and greasy coating is coupled with a deep-red tongue body, it indicates that heat is trapped by dampness.[12] Zhao Shao-Qin of the Beijing University of Traditional Chinese Medicine wrote in *Length and Breadth of Warm Pathogen Disease [Differentiation] (Wēn bìng zòng héng)* that this shows that there is heat in the nutritive level and dampness in the Spleen and Stomach. Treatment should first eliminate dampness from the Spleen and Stomach using acrid and bitter herbs. After the dampness is eliminated and the function of the Spleen and Stomach is restored, the heat in the nutritive level will be easily dispersed.[13]

A white, thick, greasy, and slippery tongue coating that looks like a white powder over the tongue is a special presentation of accumulation of dampness in the membrane source *(mò yuán)*.[14] If it is associated with a deep-red tongue body, it indicates heat in the nutritive level and dampness in the membrane source. The condition is severe and is apt to progress deeper because the heat in the nutritive level is being trapped by dampness in the membrane source, which is at the qi level. According to Wu Zhen in *Thorough Understanding of Cold Damage (Shāng hán zhǐ zhǎng)*, written in 1796, the formula Reach the Source Drink *(dá yuán yǐn)*[15] should be used together with guiding herbs for the *tai yang* (Notopterygii Rhizoma seu Radix *[qiāng huó]*), *yang ming* (Puerariae Radix *[gé gēn]*), and *shao yang* (Bupleuri Radix *[chái hú]*).[16]

Other relatively rare white tongue coatings include:

- A white tongue coating that looks like an 'alkali desert'[17] indicates, according to Ye Gui, that there is dampness associated with food retention in the Stomach.[18] Treatment should transform dampness, promote digestion, and eliminate food retention.

- A white tongue coating that looks dry and hard like sandpaper indicates that the warm-heat pathogen has progressed to the Stomach and quickly injured its fluids, that is, before it could make the tongue coating turn yellow. According to Wu You-Xing, this type of coating is also called a 'crystal coating' (水晶苔 *shuǐ jīng tāi)*. The purging method should be used as soon as possible.[19]

- A white and moldy layer over the tongue, which may sometimes spread through the mouth, indicates that the damp-heat is severe and that the yin in the Kidney and Stomach is damaged.[20]

In summary, a white tongue coating indicates that the warm pathogen disease is located in either the protective or qi level. This tongue coating is often seen in the early and middle stages of a warm pathogen disease, and shows that the pathogen is relatively superficial. Thus, the patient has a relatively good prognosis. (See Table 5.1.)

Yellow tongue coating. A yellow tongue coating indicates that the disease has progressed to the qi level, that is, to a middle stage. One must distinguish whether the yellow coating is thick or thin, moist or dry, or in combination with a white coating.

Usually, a yellow tongue coating indicates an interior pattern with heat from excess. A moist coating shows that there is no injury to the fluids. By contrast, a dry coating shows that the fluids have been impaired, and the dryer the yellow coating, the more severe the injury to the fluids. A thin coating implies that the disease is relatively superficial. By contrast, a thick coating suggests that the disease is situated at a deeper level; the thicker the yellow coating, the deeper the disease. A yellow, thick, and dry coating is seen in the pattern of heat from excess in the Stomach and Large Intestine with injury to the fluids, which implies the presence of severe constipation with dry stools and heat in the Large Intestine. A yellow, thick, and greasy coating reflects stagnation of damp-heat. Generally speaking, a yellow tongue coating represents a progression from a white coating and means that the warm-heat pathogen

Table 5.1	Classification and Clinical Significance of a White Tongue Coating		
Tongue Coating	**Concurrent Signs and Symptoms**	**Stage and Location**	**Comments**
Thin and white	Normal saliva; tongue body may have red tip and edges	Protective level or in the Lung	No injury to the fluids
Thin and white	Dry coating	Protective level or in the Lung	Injury to the fluids
Thick, white, and dry	Thirst for cold beverages, vigorous fever, restlessness	Qi level	Injury to the Stomach fluids
Thick, white, and dry	Dry mouth, but either no desire to drink or a desire to just sip, chest and epigastric distention, nausea, vomiting	Qi level	Dampness blocking qi in the Spleen and Stomach, the qi of which fails to bring fluids to the tongue
Thick, white, and greasy	Contained fever, heaviness and aches over the body and head, normal thirst, chest and epigastric distention, loose stool, scanty urine	Qi level	Accumulation of dampness predominates over heat
Thick, white, and greasy	Deep-red tongue body	Nutritive level	Heat in the nutritive level and dampness in the Spleen and Stomach
Thick, white, greasy, and slippery	Coating looks like white powder over the tongue	Qi level (membrane source)	Accumulation of dampness in the membrane source
Thick, white, greasy, and slippery	Deep-red tongue body	Nutritive and qi level (membrane source)	Heat in the nutritive level and dampness in the membrane source
White like an alkali desert		Qi level	Dampness associated with food retention in the Stomach

Table 5.1, cont.			
White like hard and dry sandpaper		Qi level	Heat in the Stomach has rapidly injured its fluids
White and moldy layer over the tongue		Qi level	Severe damp-heat has exhausted the Stomach and Kidney yin

has reached the qi level. When the coating is both yellow and white, it means that both the protective and qi levels are involved. According to Wu Zhen in *Thorough Understanding of Cold Damage*, if the coating has even a hint of whiteness, the pattern is still partially exterior. Only a purely yellow tongue coating indicates that the warm-heat pathogen has completely left the protective level and reached the qi level.[21]

Table 5.2	Classification and Clinical Significance of a Yellow Tongue Coating		
Tongue Coating	**Concurrent Signs and Symptoms**	**Stage and Location**	**Comments**
Thin, yellow, moist	No thirst for cold beverages	Early stage of qi level	No injury to fluids
Thin, yellow, dry	Thirst for cold beverages	Qi level	Injury to fluids by extreme heat from excess
Yellow and white	Aversion to cold, vigorous fever, thirst for cold beverages, slippery and rapid pulse	Warm-heat pathogen progressing to qi level, but still showing protective level symptoms	Combined exterior and interior pattern
Brownish-yellow	Dry with 'thorns' or cracks on tongue body, dry and hard stools, constipation	Qi level	Heat from excess with injury to fluids in the Large Intestine
Yellow and greasy	Abdominal distention and loose stools	Qi level	Stagnation of damp-heat

Gray tongue coating. A gray tongue coating commonly indicates that there is an interior heat pattern, which may be either excessive or deficient. However, it is usually seen when a yellow coating begins to progress to a black coating. It mainly appears in the qi level, although some nutritive and blood level patterns can present with a gray coating as well. It generally appears in the middle stage of a warm pathogen disease.

A gray tongue coating can also be seen in excessive or deficient, cold or hot, and phlegm-damp patterns. To differentiate the pattern in the clinic the practitioner should consider the level of dryness or moisture in the coating and the accompanying signs and symptoms elsewhere in the body.

Table 5.3	Classification and Clinical Significance of a Gray Tongue Coating		
Tongue Coating	**Concurrent Signs and Symptoms**	**Stage and Location**	**Comments**
Gray and dry	Constipation, hard and dry stools, tidal fevers, profuse sweating, distending pain in the abdomen	Qi level	Heat from excess in the Large Intestine with injury to the fluids
Gray and greasy	Chest and epigastric distention, thirst with a preference for warm beverages, or vomiting of clear fluids	Qi level	Stagnation of phlegm and dampness
Gray and slippery, watery, or very moist	Cold extremities, thin pulse, or vomiting and diarrhea	Qi level	Interior cold or interior cold and dampness due to yang deficiency

Black tongue coating. In general, a black tongue coating that was previously yellow or gray marks a critical change in the disease. It is often seen in the pattern of injury to yin due to heat from excess, and appears in the later stage of a warm pathogen disease. (See Table 5.4.)

TONGUE BODY

The tongue is the mirror of the Heart, and one of the Heart's functions is to govern the circulation of blood in the vessels. If the Heart can move enough blood through the body, including the tongue, the color of the tongue body will be slightly red and

Table 5.4	Classification and Clinical Significance of a Black Tongue Coating		
Tongue Coating	**Concurrent Signs and Symptoms**	**Stage and Location**	**Comments**
Black and dry	Shriveled tongue, constipation, dry and hard stools	Qi level	Exhaustion of yin and fluids due to extreme heat and toxin in the Large Intestine
Black, dry, scorched	Atrophied, dark, deep-red tongue, diminished hearing, hot sensation in the soles and palms	Lower burner	Warm-heat pathogen invading the lower burner and exhausting the Kidney yin
Black and moist	Fever, chest congestion, thirst with a preference for warm beverages	Qi level	Warm-heat pathogen associated with phlegm
Black and dry	Pale tongue and massive bleeding	Nutritive and blood levels	Exhaustion of both yin and yang

show good shape, luster, and movement. When a warm-heat pathogen invades the nutritive and blood levels, which are closely associated with the Heart, the tongue body will change accordingly. Therefore, observing the tongue body is crucial in identifying nutritive or blood level patterns and in determining the condition of the blood circulation.

Red tongue body. A red tongue body indicates either that a disease has gradually invaded the nutritive level or that there is heat from excess in the protective or qi levels. How do you differentiate between these different levels? First, during a pro-tective-level disease the redness only appears on the tip of the tongue, while in a qi-level disease the entire tongue body is red. Both types of red tongues are always associated with a coating. By contrast, the red tongue associated with a nutritive-level disease is deep red over the entire tongue, with little or no coating.

The color of the tongue when the heat is in the nutritive level may look similar to that seen in a patient with a constitutional deficiency of yin, that is, red, peeled, shiny, and geographic. However, the overall presentation in the two disorders is different. In a patient with a warm pathogen disease, the disease is acute. In a yin-deficient patient, the problem is of a more chronic nature, and there will be clear accompanying signs and symptoms of yin deficiency.

In traditional Chinese medicine, the tip of the tongue body is associated with the upper burner, which includes the Lung and Heart. A diagnosis of flare-up of Heart fire can be made when there is a red tongue with bright red dots on the tip, especially when the spirit of the Heart is disturbed, with symptoms such as irritability, restlessness, or insomnia.

To summarize, both excess and deficiency can produce a red tongue in diseases caused by a warm-heat pathogen. A bright red tongue body shows that the warm-heat pathogen is located in the Heart and/or nutritive level, and that it is a pattern of excess. A tongue body that is pinkish and lacks luster indicates a pattern of qi and blood deficiency in the Spleen and Heart.

Table 5.5	Classification and Clinical Significance of a Red Tongue Body		
Tongue Body	**Concurrent Signs and Symptoms**	**Stage and Location**	**Comments**
Red with cracks or bright red spots in middle	Fever that worsens at night	Nutritive level	Heat from excess heat and toxin in the nutritive level that has badly damaged the fluids
Red and tender without coating	Appearance of profuse saliva, but tongue feels dry to the touch	Nutritive level	Severity of warm-heat pathogen has been significantly reduced, but the fluids have not yet recovered
Pinkish and dry without luster	Palpitations, insomnia, fatigue, poor appetite	Upper and middle burners	Warm-heat pathogen is gone, but qi and yin have not recovered, and qi and blood deficiency in the Heart and Spleen

Deep-red tongue body. Deep-red tongues often follow red tongues, and the deep-red color indicates that the warm-heat pathogen has progressed to the nutritive level. The pathological significance of red and deep-red tongues is almost identical, however the deep-red tongue reflects a more severe disease. According to Ye Gui, "A deep-red tongue will be present when the warm-heat pathogen reaches the nutritive level."[22] In general, there is no coating or less coating on a deep-red tongue body. A coating that emerges or increases following treatment indicates that the warm-heat pathogen has left the nutritive level and has returned to the qi level.

Ye described the treatment for various kinds of deep-red tongues in *Discussion of Warm-Heat Pathogen Disorders:*

> A deep-red tongue with a greasy coating is caused by heat accompanied by dampness in the nutritive level; add aromatic herbs to transform dampness to a formula which treats heat in the nutritive level. If a deep-red tongue is so stiff that it cannot be extended from the mouth, it indicates obstruction of the tongue by phlegm-heat and stirring-up of Liver wind.[23] If a deep-red tongue shines like a mirror, the Stomach yin has been badly damaged; use sweet and cool herbs.[24] A deep-red tongue without saliva shows that heat from excess in the nutritive level has badly damaged the yin; use herbs that reduce fire and cool blood.[25] If there is a deep-red tongue with big red spots, it indicates that heat toxin is attacking the Heart; use Coptidis Rhizoma *(huáng lián)* and Succus Faecalis Aureus *(jīn zhī).*[26] A deep-red, atrophied, and dry tongue indicates that the Kidney yin is running out; one must give the patient Asini Corii Colla *(ē jiāo),* egg yolks *(jī zǐ huáng),* Rehmanniae Radix *(shēng dì huáng),*[27] and Asparagi Radix *(tiān mén dōng)* immediately.[28]

In summary, a deep-red tongue signifies that the warm-heat pathogen has progressed to the nutritive level. When observing a deep-red tongue, the practitioner should focus on whether there is a coating and whether the condition is one of excess or deficiency. Generally speaking, a deep-red tongue with luster indicates that the warm-heat pathogen has invaded the Pericardium. A dry and deep-red tongue shows extreme heat or fire from excess and injury to the yin. An atrophied and deep-red tongue without luster, or a deep-red tongue without any coating, suggests exhaustion of yin and fluids; the prognosis for the disease is poor. A deep-red tongue with a yellow and white coating indicates that part of the warm-heat pathogen is still in the qi level, that is, a pattern of excess. A deep-red tongue with a greasy coating indicates the presence of phlegm or dampness from excess.

Table 5.6	Classification and Clinical Significance of a Deep-Red Tongue Body		
Tongue Body	**Concurrent Signs and Symptoms**	**Stage and Location**	**Comments**
Deep red with luster	Coma, delirium, or muddled consciousness	Pericardium	Warm-heat pathogen invades the Pericardium
Deep red and dry	Insomnia	Nutritive level	Fire in nutritive level has injured the yin
Deep red with yellow and white coating	Fever that worsens at night, sweating, thirst for cold beverages	Qi and nutritive levels	Warm-heat pathogen has invaded nutritive level before leaving the qi level completely

Table 5.6, cont.			
Deep-red and mirror-like tongue	Thirst for cold beverages, nausea	Qi level (Stomach)	Stomach yin is exahused
Deep-red tongue with a greasy coating	Confusion of the mind, contained fever	Nutritive level	Dampness, heat, and phlegm in nutritive level, and veiling of the Pericardium by a combination of heat, phlegm, and dampness
Dry, atrophied, and dark deep-red tongue	Ringing in ears, diminished hearing	Lower burner (Kidney)	Kidney yin is significantly injured

Purple tongue body. Purple tongue bodies often arise from deep-red tongues, and the purple tongue often indicates that extreme heat and toxin are present in the nutritive and blood levels. The purple color signifies a disease that is more severe than that represented by a deep-red tongue.

When you see a purple tongue, attention should be focused on distinguishing whether it reflects a pattern of excess or deficiency, and cold or heat. A purple tongue with 'thorns' indicates the presence of extreme heat and toxin. A dry, atrophied purple tongue is a sign of yin exhaustion. A purple and dark tongue that looks normal but feels moist signifies blood stasis. According to Ye Gui, when there is blood stasis with a warm-heat pathogen, it is useful to add Succinum *(hǔ pò)*, Salviae miltiorrhizae Radix *(dān shēn)*, Persicae Semen *(táo rén)*, and Moutan Cortex *(mǔ dān pí)* to the formula to promote blood circulation.[29] Note that not all purplish tongues are due to heat. For example, a *slightly* purplish tongue with a slippery and moist coating is a sign of cold from deficiency, rather than heat from excess. (See Table 5.7.)

Shape and Movement of the Tongue

As mentioned above, through their channel connections the Heart, Liver, Kidney, and Spleen have a close relationship to the tongue. The flow of qi and blood in these channels, and the status of the qi, blood, yin, and yang in these organs, will directly affect not only the color of the tongue body and tongue coating, but also the movement and shape of the tongue body. Therefore, by observing the shape and movement of the tongue body, the practitioner can deduce the type of pathology affecting the organs and channels and the condition of the qi, blood, yin, and yang.

Table 5.7	Classification and Clinical Significance of a Purple Tongue Body		
Tongue Body	**Concurrent Signs and Symptoms**	**Stage and Location**	**Comments**
Dry, thorny, and purple	Dizziness, tinnitus, distending headache	Lower burner (Liver)	Extreme heat and toxin leads to bleeding or stirring of Liver wind
Dry, dark, and purple	Hot sensation in the palms and soles, dizziness, diminished hearing	Lower burner (Liver and Kidney)	Exhaustion of the Kidney and Liver yin
Dark, blue, and purple that looks normal but feels moist to the practitioner	Stabbing pain in the chest and abdomen	Upper or middle burner	Warm-heat pathogen with blood stasis

Table 5.8	Classification and Clinical Significance of the Shape and Movement of the Tongue Body		
Tongue Body	**Concurrent Signs and Symptoms**	**Stage and Location**	**Comments**
Rigid tongue	Pale tongue without coating, difficulty speaking	Lower burner (Liver)	Liver wind or deficiency of qi and fluids
Short tongue	Purple tongue with thick coating, difficulty speaking	Lower burner (Liver)	Interior obstruction of phlegm and stirring of Liver wind
Rolling tongue	Contraction of the scrotum	Lower burner (Liver)	Warm-heat pathogen invades Liver
Atrophied and flabby tongue	Hot sensation in soles and palms, dizziness	Lower burner (Liver and Kidney)	Kidney and Liver yin are becoming exhausted
Trembling tongue	Dizziness and convulsions	Lower burner (Liver)	Stirring of Liver wind
Swollen and big tongue	Yellow and greasy tongue coating	Qi level	Damp-heat transforms into toxin

CHANGES IN THE TONGUE AND THE PROGRESSION OF WARM PATHOGEN DISEASES

The tongue body and coating often change as warm pathogen diseases evolve. Paying close attention to these alterations in both the tongue body and coating will help you detect and understand the direction of the progression of a warm pathogen disease.

Changes in the tongue coating. In general, a change in the color of the tongue coating from white to yellow to gray to black indicates that a warm pathogen disease is progressing from the exterior to the interior, and is becoming more severe. For example, when a yellow and thin tongue coating (from a warm-heat pathogen invading the qi level) becomes dry, it indicates that heat in the qi level is becoming more intense. In addition, the dryness of the coating is an important sign of the severity of injury to the yin or fluids. During the early stage of a warm pathogen disease, when injury to the yin or fluids is not severe, the tongue coating will be just slightly less moist than normal. As the disease progresses, injury to the fluids or yin will become more marked, and the coating will become drier. It will also become thinner, cracked, and either partially or completely peeled. Once the Kidney yin is exhausted, the tongue body can atrophy. Clinically, a dry coating can also be seen in the accumulation of dampness in the Spleen. This is because dampness can block the qi mechanism, impairing the qi's function of distributing fluids to the tongue.

Changes in the thickness of the tongue coating and its color are important in gauging the severity of dampness and heat in damp-heat diseases. The thicker the coating, the more intense the dampness. For example, a white, thick, greasy tongue coating is commonly seen when damp-heat accumulates in the Spleen. If the heat becomes more intense, the coating will become yellow, thick, and greasy and may even become turbid. Also, it is very important to observe whether a thick tongue coating is rooted. A thick coating that is rooted on the tongue means that the dampness will be harder to eliminate, because it is retained at a relatively deep level of the body due to weakness of the antipathogenic qi, or it has become firmly mixed with other pathogenic factors. If a thick coating is loose or looks like it is floating on the body of the tongue, the dampness will be relatively easy to treat. Thus, a rooted and thick coating that becomes loose or superficial is an indication that the dampness is gradually diminishing. However, if a thick coating suddenly disappears completely and leaves a mirror tongue that feels dry, the fluids in the Stomach have been exhausted and the prognosis is poor.

The tongue coating can also indicate the transmission of disease. For example, a white, thick, greasy, and slippery tongue coating that looks as if white powder has been scattered over the tongue may gradually change into a yellow coating, starting from the root and progressing forward toward the center. This indicates that the damp-heat has progressed from the membrane source to the Stomach. According to Wu You-Xing, the color of the coating under these circumstances can change three times over the course of a single day (from white to yellow to black). He recommends adding Rhei Radix et Rhizoma *(dà huáng)* to Reach the Source Drink *(dá yuán yǐn)*[30] when the color of this type of coating changes from white to yellow, and using Major Order the Qi Decoction *(dà chéng qì tāng)*[31] when the color changes from yellow to black.[32]

Changes in the tongue body. Generally speaking, redness confined to the tip of the tongue reflects a protective level disorder; a red tongue body with little coating signifies that a warm pathogen disease has initially invaded the nutritive level; and a deep-red tongue means that a warm pathogen disease has progressed to the nutritive level. A very deep-red or purple tongue indicates a warm pathogen disease at the blood level. However, invasion of the Pericardium by heat can also present with a bright-red tongue. After heavy bleeding due to heat in the blood level, a very deep-red or purple tongue can change into a pale tongue without luster, because the qi is injured from blood loss. Likewise, a pale tongue without luster can present in the pattern of yang collapse following blockage of the Heart by heat. The luster of the tongue body is an important indicator of the severity of injury to the yin, especially the Kidney yin. When the tongue body loses its luster and becomes dull and shriveled, this indicates exhaustion of the Kidney yin.

Lurking warm pathogen diseases are a special case due to their progression from the interior to the exterior. According to Wang Shi-Xiong:

> [Lurking warm pathogen diseases] first progress from the nutritive level to the qi level. Thus, in the first stage of the disease the tongue is moist and has no coating. To identify the disease, the practitioner must feel for the soggy pulse or a wiry or slightly rapid pulse, and look for irritability, restlessness, aversion to heat, and no increase in thirst. To treat this condition, one must use herbs to clear heat from the nutritive level. When the lurking warm-heat pathogen progresses from the nutritive level to the qi level, the tongue will begin to show a coating. Then one must use herbs to clear heat from the qi level. If there is a severe lurking warm-heat pathogen, the patient will present with a deep-red tongue, a dry throat, or an extremely submerged pulse and cold extremities. The strongest method to clear a lurking warm-heat pathogen must be used immediately. After such treatment, a thick, greasy, turbid, and yellow tongue coating will gradually present itself. These are the principal differences between lurking warm pathogen disease and newly-contracted warm pathogen disease in their onset and progression.[33]

Dyed Tongues

It is not uncommon in the clinic to see patients whose tongues have been dyed by food or drink in such a way that they mimic diseased tongues. For example, drinking orange juice or coffee can turn the coating yellow; certain types of candy or chewing gum can turn the coating or body red, deep red, or purple; eating blueberries can make the coating or body blue; eating blackberries or smoking cigarettes can make the coating black, and so on. Likewise, a thick coating can become thin after eating or brushing the teeth. In addition, some patients scrape their tongues before seeing a practitioner. Therefore, before accepting a tongue at face value, it is important to ensure the absence of such confounding factors.

Examining the Teeth and Gums

In traditional Chinese medicine the teeth reflect the condition of the Kidney, while the gums receive nourishment from the channels of the Stomach. In *Discussion of Warm-Heat Pathogen Disorders*, Ye Gui noted that a warm-heat pathogen is apt to injure the fluids of the Stomach and the yin of the Kidney.[34] Therefore, examining the condition of the teeth and gums can help identify the severity of the heat and the health of the fluids and yin.

DRY TEETH

Dry teeth result from a lack of nourishment due to exhausted fluids. In the clinic, the incisors are the most important teeth to examine.

Table 5.9	Classification and Clinical Significance of Dry Teeth		
Teeth	**Concurrent Signs and Symptoms**	**Stage and Location**	**Comments**
Dry with luster (like pebbles)	Nausea, poor appetite, dry mouth	Middle burner (Stomach)	Injury to Stomach yin
Dry without luster (like withered bones)	Tinnitus, diminished hearing	Lower burner (Kidney)	Exhaustion of Kidney yin

In general, when examining for dry teeth the practitioner should focus on the degree of luster. According to Chapter 17 of *Basic Questions,* the quality of the essence and qi will affect the luster of the skin and teeth.[35] In a warm pathogen disease, the health of the Kidney yin determines the quality of luster seen on dry teeth. When the teeth have no luster or gloss, they are said to be dry. This means that the warm-heat pathogen has injured the Kidney yin, which is then unable to properly nourish the teeth.

Bleeding Gums

The practitioner should pay attention to whether swelling and pain accompany the bleeding gums. The presence of swelling, pain, and bright-red blood is an indication of injury to the Stomach channel by blazing Stomach fire. The absence of swelling and pain suggests a flare-up of fire from deficiency as a result of the Kidney yin deficiency.

Table 5.10	Classification and Clinical Significance of Bleeding Gums		
Gums	**Concurrent Signs and Symptoms**	**Stage and Location**	**Comments**
Bleeding with swelling and pain	Bleeding is significant and red, with intense thirst for cold beverages	Middle burner (Stomach)	Injury to the Stomach channel by blazing Stomach fire
Bleeding without swelling or pain	Lower back weakness and soreness, night sweats	Lower burner (Kidney)	Flare-up of fire from Kidney yin deficiency

Identifying Maculas, Papules, and Miliaria Alba

Identifying the color, shape, and distribution of maculas, papules, and miliaria alba can help the practitioner determine the severity, depth, and prognosis of a warm pathogen disease.

Maculas and Papules

Identifying maculas and papules. In Chinese, maculas are called 斑 *bān* while papules are called 疹 *zhěn*. Both are skin eruptions that occur during the progression of a warm pathogen disease, and both are important signs for differentiating patterns. Although they are terms for different types of eruptions, since they may emerge concurrently they were always referred to collectively as 斑疹 *bān zhěn*, or maculopapular rashes, in the classical literature. They are first mentioned in Zhang Ji's *Essentials from the Golden Cabinet (Jīn guì yào luè)* around the third century, where they are described as a manifestation of yang toxin.[36] Chao Yuan-Fang (c. 610) in *Discussion of the Origins of Symptoms of Disease (Zhū bìng yuán hòu lùn)* pointed out that lurking cold and toxin or epidemic qi can produce maculas owing to the failure of the toxin to be dispersed.[37] In 1642, Wu You-Xing in *Discussion of Warm Epidemics (Wēn yì lùn)* pointed out that maculas are caused by epidemic qi in the blood level, and signify that qi is leaving the body.[38] Ye Gui also systematically discussed how to observe maculo-papular rashes and explained their clinical significance.[39]

The appearance of maculas and papules is both a positive and negative sign. On the one hand, their occurrence indicates that the warm-heat pathogen has progressed to either the nutritive or blood level, and that the disease has therefore penetrated deeper. On the other hand, their expression on the skin indicates that there is still a chance for the warm-heat pathogen to exit the body via this route.

Differences in shape between maculas and papules. Although maculas and papules manifest as red spots on the skin, they are clinically quite different from each other in shape and pathological mechanism. Maculas manifest as many red spots that connect to each other, the color of which does not change when pressure is applied. The entire area surrounding the spots may become red, and although the color can be clearly *seen*, there is no difference in the texture of the skin to the touch. The affected area looks like embroidery, in the sense that, while different pictures can be seen on silk clothing, there is no difference in the texture when you touch the material. Thus, although several separate patches can be seen on the skin, it nevertheless feels whole to the touch. In addition, the skin does not flake when the maculas resolve.

Papules also manifest as red spots, but are smaller than maculas, about the size of a grain of millet. However, unlike maculas, papules protrude from the skin surface. Thus, they can be felt, and the skin flakes after the rash has disappeared.

Pathological mechanism of maculas and papules. Generally speaking, maculas result from an invasion by a warm-heat pathogen reaching the nutritive and blood levels. Papules result from an invasion of the nutritive level by a warm-heat pathogen. However, maculas and papules have distinct pathologies: They are associated with different yin and yang organs, and with diseases that are located at different levels of the body.

Maculas result from blood leaving the vessels following an attack on the nutritive and blood levels by heat from excess in the Stomach. Because the tissue associated with the Stomach is muscle tissue, maculas originate in the muscles, that is, deeper than the skin.[40] Clinically, a thirst for cold beverages, and the presence of dry and hard stools, are often associated with maculas. From the perspective of four-level differentiation, in addition to the nutritive and blood levels, there is also some involvement of the qi level. This is because some of the accompanying signs and symptoms mentioned above pertain to the qi level. The presence of blood outside of the vessels shows that the blood level is involved.

On the other hand, papules result when blood leaves the vessels following an attack on the nutritive level by constrained wind-heat in the Lung.[41] Clinically, it is very common to see papules in conjunction with chills, aversion to cold, sore throat, and cough.[42]

The appearance of maculas or papules indicates that the warm-heat pathogen is moving outward. When this occurs, one should observe their color, shape, and distribution, and the accompanying signs and symptoms, to determine the mildness or severity of the disease, and to select the correct treatment principle.

Table 5.11	Differences between Maculas and Papules in Shape and Pathological Mechanism	
Shape	**Pathological Mechanism**	
MACULAS		
Red spots connected with each other, forming a red area that can be seen but not felt; color is not diminished with pressure	Results from blood leaving the vessels following an attack on the nutritive and blood levels by heat from excess in Stomach	
PAPULES		
Small millet-sized red spots that protrude from the skin and can be seen and felt; color is diminished with pressure	Results from blood leaving the vessels following an attack on the nutritive level by stagnant wind-heat in Lung	

Prodromal symptoms signaling the onset of maculas and papules. In general, before maculas and papules emerge on the skin, one will feel feverish, restless, and thirsty, and there will be a deep-red tongue with a yellow coating and a rapid pulse. If these signs and symptoms are accompanied by distention in the head, diminished acuity of hearing, and a feverish body, it indicates that maculas will soon appear. On the other hand, if these signs and symptoms are accompanied by chest distention and cough, it suggests that papules will soon appear.

Observing the colors of the maculas and papules. Red maculas or papules with luster are signs of the smooth circulation of blood and the outward movement of a warm-heat pathogen. Bright-red maculas or papules show that there is an excess of heat and toxin in the blood. Deep-red maculas or papules indicate that there is intense heat and toxin in both the nutritive and blood levels, and that the disease is deep and severe. Black maculas or papules show that excessive amounts of heat and toxin are present and that the disease is critical. Maculas or papules that are black yet have luster suggest that the qi and blood are still strong, and that the disease can be cured if proper treatment is administered. Maculas or papules that are black and are encircled with a *red* corona indicate that fire is stagnant in the body, but that the qi and blood are still strong; in fact, the black color may turn red following the use of herbs of a cool and light nature. Maculas or papules that are black and dull, without luster, suggest that the heat and toxin are adhering to the inside of the body due to exhaustion of source qi.

To summarize, an increase in the darkness of maculas or papules implies that the condition is worsening: red signifies mild, deep red more severe, and black the most severe.

Observing the shape of the maculas and papules. Maculas or papules that look superficial, with only tiny bumps protruding above the skin, indicate that the heat and toxin are superficial, and that the warm-heat pathogen is moving outward and dispersing. In this case, the prognosis is good. On the other hand, if they appear to be rooted in the skin (like an arrow that has penetrated its target), this suggests that the heat and toxin are trapped inside the body and are reluctant to leave. In that case, the prognosis is poor.

Observing the density of maculas and papules. The distribution of maculas and papules reflects the severity of a disease. If they are few in number and scattered about, the heat and toxin are located at a superficial level, and the prognosis is good. Should they be numerous and dense, however, this suggests that the heat and toxin are located at a deep level, the illness is severe, and the prognosis is poor. As Ye Gui observed in *Discussion of Warm-Heat Pathogen Disorders*, "It is a favorable sign for maculas or papules to occur, but not in great number."[43] If maculas or papules are too prolific, the underlying heat and toxin will cause excessive damage to the blood and qi.

Observing concurrent signs and symptoms. If the maculas or papules appear concurrently with a reduction in fever and increased clarity of thought, this is a sign that the warm-heat pathogen has resolved, the heat is clearing, and the function of the yin and yang organs is returning to normal. If the maculas or papules appear concurrently with a vigorous fever, muddled consciousness, or coldness of the extremities, or if they become dull in color soon after their expression, this suggests that the toxin and fire are trapped inside the body as a result of the inability of the weak antipathogenic qi to resist the warm-heat pathogen.

Treatment principles for maculas and papules. Maculas pertain to the Stomach channel and organ and are due to an attack on the nutritive and blood levels by heat in the Stomach. Papules pertain to the Lung and result from an attack on the nutritive level by constrained wind-heat in the Lung. Because of this basic difference in etiology, treatment of the two is quite different (see Table 5.12).

If maculas are associated with papules, the main treatment principle should be transforming maculas, combined with venting papules. Should maculas or papules be accompanied by severe constipation with dry stools and heat in the Large Intestine, one should use the purging method. This was explained by Wu You-Xing:

> When the pathogen resides in the blood level, the interior qi becomes clogged
> and obstructed such that the lurking pathogen cannot be vented to the outside
> and [thereupon] forms maculas. If the patient is purged, the clogged qi and the
> protective qi will then flow smoothly … and the pathogen can [by this means]
> be released externally.[44]

Table 5.12	Differences in Organ of Origin, Pathology, and Treatment of Maculas and Papules	
Organ of Origin	**Pathology**	**Treatment**
MACULAS		
Stomach	Attack on the nutritive and blood levels by heat in the Stomach	Clear heat from the Stomach, cool the blood, and transform maculas
PAPULES		
Lung	Attack on the nutritive level by stagnant wind-heat in the Lung	Disperse the Lung, dispel wind-heat, clear heat in the nutritive level, and vent papules

If papules appear on the skin and are caused by an attack on the nutritive level by
constrained wind-heat in the Lung, and it is more superficial than maculas, then acrid, cool, and light herbs should be used to clear and vent heat from the nutritive level
and the Lung. To transform maculas at the muscular level, which are deeper than
papules, one should clear heat, cool blood, and clean toxin with acrid, bitter, and cold
herbs, or purge heat and toxin with bitter, salty, and cold herbs.

Contraindications in treating maculas and papules. Three contraindications in the
treatment of maculas or papules should be remembered:

1. *In the early stages of macule or papule formation, do not rely solely on bitter and
   cold herbs, as they can congeal the warm-heat pathogen within the body.* Instead,
   use herbs that clear and disperse heat. Constipation due to accumulation of heat
   in the Large Intestine may impair the flow of qi on the surface, retarding the expression of maculas or papules. In this case, the practitioner should purge gently and only for a brief time. According Wu Tang in *Systematic Differentiation of
   Warm Pathogen Diseases*:

If maculas or papules appear in association with a *yang ming* pattern, leading to stagnation of heat and dryness in the Large Intestine and slow eruption, use Regulate the Stomach and Order the Qi Decoction *(tiáo wèi chéng qì tāng)* [45] to slightly purge heat and direct the Large Intestine qi downward. Once the stool moves smoothly, such treatment should be stopped or severe purging will injure the qi, resulting in failure of the heat to exit, and the maculas or papules will move deeper.[46]

2. *Do not use ascending and warm herbs.* Again, according to Wu Tang:

If only warm and ascending herbs are used, the heat will increase, and maculas and papules will worsen. This can even lead to nosebleeds, cough due to heat attacking the Lung, and muddled consciousness or coma due to sinking of heat into the Pericardium.[47]

3. *Do not use tonifying and warm herbs if there is only heat from excess without qi deficiency* because this could exacerbate the warm-heat pathogen by producing qi constraint and stagnation, or even lead to a stirring of Liver wind if the heat is extreme.

Miliaria Alba

Identifying miliaria alba. Miliaria alba (白㾦 *bái péi*) manifest as small vesicles that look like crystals. In general, they are round in shape and range in size from 0.1–1.5mm. The smallest are no larger than the tip of a needle, and the biggest are the size of a grain of millet. They can be palpated. They are soft to the touch and cause no pain. They are most commonly found on the neck, chest, and abdomen. Thin flakes are left on the skin after they disappear.

Pathological mechanism of miliaria alba. Miliaria alba result from damp-heat adhering to and steaming out of the qi level to the skin. Correctly identifying them can help a practitioner to make a judgement about the quality of the underlying disease and the condition of the patient's fluids and qi. In general, miliaria alba are most commonly seen in damp-related diseases, such as damp-warmth, summer-heat-warmth with dampness, and lurking summerheat, especially if the practitioner either:

- Fails to transform and leach out dampness and disperse heat
- Uses cloying herbs to enrich the yin, leading to the steaming of dampness by heat.

Generally speaking, the appearance of miliaria alba indicates that the warm pathogen disease has a strong damp-heat component, is located at the qi level, and reflects a tendency for the damp-heat to exit the body through the skin.

Prodromal symptoms signaling the onset of miliaria alba. Before the appearance of miliaria alba, a patient may develop a fever and feel a sense of distention in the chest. Once they appear, the chest distention will go away because the interior dampness has moved to the exterior, and the qi can circulate smoothly in the chest again. Clinically, miliaria alba may appear several times following sweating and a fever because damp-heat is characterized by stickiness and stagnation and cannot emerge to the surface all at once.

Classification of miliaria alba and their clinical significance. There are two categories of miliaria alba, differentiated on the basis of the presence of fluid in the vesicle and the luster of the vesicle itself. As previously noted, examining the miliaria alba will help the practitioner assess the quality of a pathogen and the condition of the qi and fluids. If the miliaria alba are sparkling and full of clear water, referred to as shining miliaria (晶痦 *jīng péi*), and if the fever is diminishing and the clarity of thought is returning, this indicates that the damp-heat is moving out of the body. This is occurring because the fluids and qi are apparently strong enough to dispel the damp-heat. Miliaria alba that are shrinking or contain no fluid, and are not sparkling, are called withered miliaria (枯痦 *kū péi*). If this is coupled with persistent fever and mental confusion, it indicates that damp-heat is sinking further into the body. This means that the fluids and qi are so weak that they are unable to eliminate the damp-heat.

Table 5.13	Classification and Clinical Significance of Vesicles
Manifestations	**Pathology**
Vesicles are full of clear fluid and sparkling, fever is declining, and the mind is clear	Damp-heat is being expelled from the body
Vesicles are not filled with fluid and lack luster, the fever persists, and there may be muddled consciousness	Damp-heat is progressing deeper into the body

Treatment principle for miliaria alba. The treatment principle for miliaria alba is to disperse heat, resolve dampness, and promote qi circulation.

- *For shining miliaria,* treatment should focus on the warm-heat pathogen, that is, it should disperse heat, leach out dampness, and promote qi circulation. According to Wu Tang, "The isolated use of acrid and cool herbs to disperse dampness on the surface, or bitter and cold herbs to clear interior heat, should be avoided; acrid, cool, and bland herbs are the right choice."[48] This is because the use of acrid and cool herbs alone will work to disperse the heat, but will not help much with the turbid dampness. Bitter and cold herbs can actually trap the dampness. The best treatment is to vent heat and promote qi circulation through the skin with acrid and cool herbs, and to allow dampness to exit through the urine by using bland herbs to promote urination.

- *For withering miliaria that result from both qi and fluid exhaustion,* consider enriching the yin and tonifying the qi. Since miliaria alba are caused by damp-heat, and are located in the qi level rather than the protective level, it is forbidden to use herbs with an acrid and warm nature in isolation.

Differentiation of Common Signs and Symptoms

Fever

Fever, which is a cardinal sign of a warm pathogen disease, shows that the entire body is reacting to a warm-heat pathogen. Fever results from the struggle between antipathogenic qi and the warm-heat pathogen. Fever can be either good or bad for the body. It is good if there is sufficient antipathogenic qi to fend off the warm-heat pathogen, but bad if the struggle between the warm-heat pathogen and the antipathogenic qi injures the qi as well as the fluids. Clinically, if antipathogenic qi overcomes the warm-heat pathogen, the fever will disappear; otherwise, the prolonged fever will injure the qi as well as the fluids, or even lead to death from the exhaustion of yin and collapse of yang.

Fever in warm pathogen diseases can be divided into two types, excessive and deficient. If it occurs in the early stage of a warm pathogen disease, it is a sign of excess that indicates strong protective qi and a superficial and mild pattern. In the middle stage of a warm pathogen disease, fever is also a sign of excess and signifies that there is a severe struggle between the antipathogenic qi and the warm-heat pathogen. The intensity of the struggle is a result of the strength of both the antipathogenic qi and the warm-heat pathogen. In later stages of a warm pathogen disease, a prolonged fever is always associated with injury to the yin and fluids, and is a sign of deficiency.

Differences between the fever of warm pathogen disease and the fever of internal disharmonies. Fever is a common sign in warm pathogen diseases, but it is also associated with internal disharmonies. The practitioner must identify the differences between these two types of fever. Generally speaking, a fever due to an internal disharmony has a slow onset and a prolonged course, while a fever due to a warm-heat pathogen has a rapid onset and results from an acute attack. The signs and symptoms associated with the two types of fever also vary. Fevers due to internal disharmonies are persistent and low-grade and are associated with a hot sensation in the soles and palms, night sweats, spontaneous sweats, dizziness, and chronic fatigue. By contrast, fevers associated with chills and aversion to cold that are due to a warm-heat pathogen show signs and symptoms pertaining to the protective level. If the pathogen is in the qi level, the fever will be accompanied by thirst with a preference for cold beverages, a yellow tongue coating, and a slippery pulse. If the pathogen is in the nutritive level, the fever will be accompanied by insomnia, irritability, restlessness, and a deep-red tongue. If the pathogen is found in the blood level, the fever will be accompanied by bleeding symptoms.

Types of fever in warm pathogen diseases and their clinical significance. There are eight common types of fever associated with a warm-heat pathogen that are seen in the clinic. They can be divided into two categories, excess and deficiency.

Excess category. Within this group are five types of fever:

1. *Concurrent fever and chills* (發熱惡寒 *fā rè wū hán*). In the early stages of a warm pathogen disease, fever accompanied by chills indicates that the warm-heat pathogen is attacking the protective level. This is caused by stagnation of the protective qi due to the struggle between the warm-heat pathogen and the protective qi. This has two effects. First, the protective qi stagnates, which produces fever. Second, because the protective qi is so busy fending off the pathogen, and has become stagnant, it is unable to warm the exterior. This leads to chills and aversion to cold. Usually, the fever is accompanied by sore throat, runny nose, sneezing, headache, slight thirst, red tongue tip and edge, and a floating and rapid pulse. However, when summerheat attacks the Stomach, it steams the fluids out of the body and injures both the qi and fluids, impairing the ability of the protective qi to warm the surface. In this case, the patient may also have fever with chills. When that happens, the patient will first experience a vigorous fever and profuse sweating, then feel chills (usually mild) on the back accompanied by irritability, thirst for cold beverages, a dry and yellow tongue coating, and a big pulse at the superficial level, but weak at the deep level.

2. *Alternating fever and chills* (寒熱往來 *hán rè wǎng lái*). Fever that alternates with chills indicates heat from constraint in the Gallbladder and/or Triple Burner. A bitter taste in the mouth, dry throat, dizziness, plugged-up ears, distention in the hypochondriac region, nausea, and a thin and yellow tongue coating often accompany this type of fever. If just the Gallbladder is involved, there will only be heat. If the Triple Burner is involved, there will not only be heat, but also dampness, because, according to classical teachings, the Triple Burner is a pathway for the circulation of water, fire, qi, and blood. When the warm-heat pathogen invades the Triple Burner, water circulation will be affected and dampness will be produced. Also, when damp-heat in which dampness

is predominant attacks the membrane source, the patient will experience alternating fever and chills. Other signs and symptoms include distention in the epigastrium and abdomen, and a white, thick, greasy, and slippery tongue coating that looks like white powder. These are the distinguishing signs and symptoms of damp-heat in the membrane source.

3. *Vigorous fever* (壯熱 *zhuàng rè*). A vigorous fever is a high fever in which there is not only no aversion to cold, but possibly an aversion to heat. This indicates an invasion of the qi level, especially the Stomach, by the warm-heat pathogen. It is caused by a severe struggle between the warm-heat pathogen and antipathogenic qi, indicating that the disease is in the Large Intestine and Stomach. This type of fever is accompanied by profuse sweating, a strong thirst for cold beverages, yellow tongue coating, and a slippery and rapid or big and rapid pulse.

According to Dong Jian-Hua of the Beijing University of Traditional Chinese Medicine, there is another type of excessive fever called one kick fever *(yī jiǎo rè)* that is similar to vigorous fever. It manifests with high fever (more than 39°C) that rises very quickly (like a kick) at the onset, usually accompanied by an aversion to heat, profuse sweating, strong thirst, red face, yellow tongue coating, and a superficial and flooding pulse. It persists for a long time, and the fluctuation in the fever is less than one degree per day. The etiology of this type of fever is heat in the Lung at the qi level. Dong suggests using modified White Tiger Decoction *(bái hǔ tāng)*[49] to treat this type of fever.[50]

4. *Afternoon fever* (日晡潮熱 *rì bū cháo rè*). This type of fever is worse in the afternoon, generally between 3–7 P.M., but is also present at other times. Typically, the fever is accompanied by severe constipation with dry stools and heat in the Large Intestine, which pertains to the qi level. It is theorized that the fever peaks at this time because the qi in the *yang ming* reaches its zenith between 3–7 P.M., and is accompanied by a severe struggle between the antipathogenic qi in the *yang ming* and the warm-heat pathogen. Since the presentation of this fever is like a wave in the sea, it is also called tidal fever (潮熱 *cháo rè*), as it returns at a predictable time, just like the tide. Clinically, this type of fever is accompanied by a hard and painful abdomen, constipation with hard and dry stools, or yellow diarrhea with a strong, foul odor, a dry, thorny, and brownish-yellow tongue coating, and a deep and forceful pulse.

5. *Contained fever* (身熱不揚 *shēn rè bù yáng*). This type of fever may persist for a long time. The patient feels hot, and the skin may feel warm to the touch, but the temperature may not be elevated as measured by a thermometer. This term also refers to a fever that is relieved (or reduced) for a while and then returns, indicating a damp-heat disease in the qi level. The contained fever is caused by the steaming of damp-heat, in which heat is trapped by dampness. Clinically,

distention in the epigastrium and abdomen, heavy sensation throughout the body, lassitude, dry mouth but an aversion to drink, greasy tongue coating, and a soggy and moderate pulse often accompany this type of fever.

Deficiency category. Within this group are three types of fever:

1. *Low-grade fever* (低熱 *dī rè*). A low-grade fever, especially when the palmar surfaces of the feet and hands feel warmer than the dorsal aspects, is a sign of Kidney and Liver yin deficiency. It occurs in a late stage of a warm pathogen disease and is caused by yin deficiency of the Liver and Kidney, giving rise to heat from deficiency. Clinically, this type of fever is often accompanied by malar flush, dry mouth and throat, fatigue, diminished hearing, slight trembling of the hands and feet, a dark, deep-red tongue with subnormal coating, or dry and atrophied tongue, and a weak pulse. According to Professor Dong, this type of fever can be caused by injury to the Lung and Stomach fluids in the later stages of a warm pathogen disease (accompanied by thirst and cough), or by an attack on the protective level and Lung by wind-heat (accompanied by slight aversion to cold, chills, and cough).[51]

2. *Elevated fever at night* (身熱夜甚 *shēn rè yè shèn*). A fever that progressively worsens at night is a sign of injury to the yin in the nutritive level. It results from an invasion of the nutritive level by a warm-heat pathogen. During the night the yin of the body is supported by the yin that is present in nature, both of which increase in strength during this time. Together, they struggle with the warm-heat pathogen; hence, an elevated fever at night. Clinically, this type of fever is accompanied by irritability, restlessness, insomnia, dry mouth but an aversion to drink, faint skin maculas and papules, deep-red tongue, and a rapid and thin pulse. According to Wu You-Xing, the invasion of the blood level by heat can also present with this type of fever.[52]

3. *Nighttime fever followed by morning coolness* (夜熱早涼 *yè rè zǎo liáng*). A fever that manifests with night sweats and a cessation of sweating the next morning is due to heat that remains in the Kidney and injures the Kidney yin during the later stages of a warm pathogen disease. As previously mentioned, at night the yin of the body is reinforced by the yin in nature, and the combination of the two struggles with the warm-heat pathogen, leading to fever. But in the morning, the yin of the body is again weak due to the waning support from the yin in nature, leading to a disappearance of the fever. Also, because the warm-heat pathogen is located in the Kidney, the protective qi on the surface is not affected, leaving it to do its job of controlling the opening and closing of the pores on the skin. Thus, there is an absence of sweating which accompanies the disappearance of the fever. Clinically, we often see this type of fever in thin people with a red tongue that has little coating, and a rapid and thin pulse. According to Wu Tang, the combination of heat and blood stasis in the lower burner may also present with this type of fever.[53]

Professor Dong Jian-Hua has written that there is another type of fever associated with warm pathogen diseases called fluctuating fever, which rises and falls but never drops to normal. It is usually caused by damp-heat or lurking summerheat.[54]

Abnormal Sweating

According to Chapter 7 of *Basic Questions*, sweating occurs when the yang qi steams the yin,[55] which exits the body through the pores on the surface of the skin. The normal secretion of sweat depends upon an adequate supply of yin and yang and the smooth circulation of qi. Therefore, according to the early nineteenth-century author Zhang Nan (Zhang Xu-Gu) in *A Stick to Awaken Physicians (Yī mén bàng hè)*, the practitioner can gather information about the condition of the fluids and the circulation of qi by inquiring about and observing the patient's sweating.[56] Four types of abnormal sweating are commonly seen in diseases caused by warm-heat pathogens:

1. *Absence of sweating*. Absence of sweating will occur when the disease is either in the protective or nutritive levels. However, the pathology and accompanying signs and symptoms will be quite different at each level. If the disease is in the protective level, the absence of sweating is due to a damp-related warm-heat pathogen in which dampness predominates, attacking the exterior and blocking qi circulation between the muscles and skin. Lurking heat inside the body, associated with an attack on the protective level by exogenous cold, is also marked by the absence of sweating. A lack of sweating due to damp-heat in the protective level always presents with chills, fever, headache, feeling of heaviness, stiffness, and generalized body aches. A lack of sweating due to lurking heat, associated with cold attacking the protective level, will present with fever, slight aversion to cold, thirst, cough, sore throat, a mixed yellow and white tongue coating, and a rapid pulse. If the disease is in the nutritive level, the pathology is due to injury to the yin from heat. Since the source of fluids has been damaged, sweat will not be produced. In this case, the absence of sweating is accompanied by a fever that worsens at night and a deep-red tongue.

2. *Sweating at irregular intervals*. Sweating from time to time is symptomatic of a damp-heat disease in the qi level. Usually, the sweating will diminish for a while due to heat leaving the body with the sweat, but it soon returns owing to the dampness, which has not been fully eliminated by the sweating. Instead, the dampness blocks the qi and produces heat. Thus, the sweating will return in force. A fluctuating fever, chest and epigastric distention, nausea, and a yellow and greasy tongue coating often coexist with this type of sweating.

3. *Profuse sweating*. Profuse sweating is usually seen when the disease is in the qi

level, especially when extreme heat forces the fluids to effuse. Such cases are always accompanied by vigorous fever, irritability, restlessness, and a strong thirst for cold beverages. However, there are two types of profuse sweating due to deficiency that are often seen in the clinic. One is due to yin collapse and manifests as dry lips and teeth, red tongue without saliva, loss of consciousness, and a big pulse without any force. The second is caused by yang collapse and presents with cold extremities, pale face, low and weak voice, pale tongue without luster, and a feeble pulse.

4. *Sweating after shivering.* Sweating which follows shivering is symptomatic of the presence of a warm-heat pathogen in the qi level, and a vigorous struggle between the antipathogenic qi and the warm pathogen, during which the antipathogenic qi tries to expel the warm-heat pathogen from the body. Generally speaking, cold extremities, purple nails, and a very deep pulse are the accompanying signs and symptoms. In such cases, the primary focus should be on palpating the patient, particularly the pulse. If the body feels warm and calm, the fever is receding, and the pulse is not fast, this indicates that the antipathogenic qi has overcome the warm-heat pathogen, and that the deficiency of antipathogenic qi will soon return to normal; the prognosis is good. If the patient feels feverish and is restless, has a cold body with sweating, and a very fast pulse, this indicates that the antipathogenic qi has been overcome by the warm-heat-pathogen, and a collapse of yang is imminent.

According to Professor Dong, there are three other types of abnormal sweating in warm pathogen diseases. The first is called slight sweating and is marked by generalized but slight sweating accompanied by fever, either slight or no aversion to cold, cough, thirst, headache, a white, thin, and dry or slightly yellow tongue coating, red tongue tip, and a rapid pulse. It is caused by an attack on the protective level and the Lung by wind-heat in the early stage of a warm pathogen disease. The second type is called stinky sweating in which the sweat smells sour. It is usually seen in cases of damp-warmth accompanied by fluctuating fever, chest distention, nausea, or loose stools, miliaria alba on the neck, chest, and abdomen, a yellow, white, and greasy tongue coating, and a soggy and hesitant pulse. In this case the sweat is persistent, but does not emerge uniformly over the entire body at the same time. Damp-heat steaming in the Liver and Gallbladder can lead to a sour-smelling sweat that is accompanied by thirst with no desire to drink, edema of the extremities, a yellow and greasy tongue coating, and a deep and slippery pulse. The third type is called sticky sweating in which the sweating is oily and profuse. It is a sign that the illness has reached a critical stage due to the failure of the yin to attract yang and the imminent separation of yin and yang. It is usually accompanied by cold extremities, weakness and shortness of breath, extreme fatigue, a curling tongue with subnormal saliva, and a feeble or big but weak pulse.[57]

THIRST

Thirst, which results from an injury to the fluids by heat or impaired distribution of the fluids, is a common symptom of a warm pathogen disease. Differentiating the two types of thirst will help the practitioner assess the distribution of the fluids, the quality of the heat, and the extent of injury to the fluids.

1. *Thirst with a desire to drink.* This is a manifestation of injury to the fluids by heat from excess. If the warm-heat pathogen attacks the protective level, there will be mild thirst with a slight desire to drink because the injury is not too severe. If the warm-heat pathogen invades the qi level and the fluids in the Stomach are badly injured due to heat from excess in the Stomach, there will be marked thirst with a preference for cold beverages, coupled with a vigorous fever and profuse sweating.
2. *Thirst without a desire to drink.* This type of thirst can be caused by stagnation of dampness in the Spleen, which obstructs the qi mechanism and impairs the Spleen's ability to raise the qi and distribute the fluids. In such cases, associated signs and symptoms include contained fever, chest and epigastric distention, and a white and greasy tongue coating. Alternatively, this type of thirst can be seen in cases of injury to the yin due to invasion of the nutritive level by a warm-heat pathogen. Here the patient may just feel a dry mouth with no desire to drink, or feel thirst with a desire to drink only a little. The latter results from the nutritive yin, which is steamed upward to the tongue by the warm-heat pathogen. Additionally, if the thirst is accompanied by a bitter taste, this indicates that there is a flare-up of fire in the Gallbladder as well as injury to the fluids.

IMPAIRED CONSCIOUSNESS

In five-phase theory, fire is associated with the Heart. Normally, the fire found in nature promotes human growth. Fire in the human body aids in the digestion of food; this is called 'fire producing earth.' When fire is at a normal level, it will not be harmful to the Heart. However, should the fire be extreme, it will give rise to pathological heat or fire that becomes a warm-heat pathogen capable of injuring the body and affecting Heart function.

According to traditional Chinese medical theory, the main function of the Heart is to house the spirit. Thus, once a warm-heat pathogen caused by abnormal fire invades the Heart, the function of the Heart in housing the spirit will be impaired, and there will be signs and symptoms of impaired consciousness. Clinically, disturbance or blockage of the Heart spirit by a warm-heat pathogen manifests as irritability, restlessness, muddled consciousness, coma, and delirium. In warm pathogen diseases, there are eight types of impaired consciousness that can be found in the clinic (see Table 5.14).

Table 5.14	Impaired Consciousness and its Clinical Significance in Warm Pathogen Disease	
Type	**Concurrent Signs and Symptoms**	**Clinical Significance**
Occasional delirium	Restlessness and a deep-red tongue without coating	Disturbance of the Heart spirit by heat in the nutritive level
Coma and delirium manifesting as mania	Blood symptoms, such as maculas and papules, and hematemesis	Blockage of the Heart spirit by heat in the blood level
Coma	Feverish trunk, cold extremities, inability to talk, and deep-red tongue	Blockage of the Heart spirit and veiling of the Pericardium by invasion of heat
Coma and delirium	Tidal fever, constipation (dry stool or diarrhea with yellow stool and foul odor), pain, distention, and hardness of the abdomen, dry and yellow tongue coating	Severe dry stools and heat in the Large Intestine, and blockage of the Heart spirit by heat in the Stomach via its channel
Uncontrollable drowsiness	Sometimes waking up and sometimes losing conscious- ness with delirium, a yellow and greasy tongue coating, and a soggy and slippery pulse	Disturbance of the Heart spirit and veiling of the Pericardium by heat and phlegm, which comes from damp-heat in the qi level
Sudden loss of consciousness	Prolonged overexposure to sun or working in front of a furnace in a factory, sudden loss of consciousness, delirium, and a stiff tongue with difficulty speaking or sudden coma with cold extremities, fever, restlessness, labored breathing, yellow urine, and rapid pulse	Direct invasion of the Pericardium by summerheat, leading to veiling of the Pericardium
Lethargic stupor	Inability to speak	Heat veiling the Pericardium; extremely serious
Coma, or muddled consciousness, mania, and delirium	Hardness, distention, and pain in the lower abdomen, black stools, and dark and purple tongue color	Blockage of the Heart spirit by a mixture of heat and blood stasis due to retention of blood in the lower burner

SPASMS, TREMORS, AND CONVULSIONS

Like coma, spasms, tremors, and convulsions are critical signs in any warm pathogen disease; they reflect the stirring of Liver wind. The Liver stores the blood and governs the sinews. If the blood in the Liver is sufficient, the sinews will be nourished and the movement of the muscles will be normal. A warm-heat pathogen can injure the yin of the Liver or Kidney, leading to Liver yin deficiency, and eventually to the stirring of Liver wind. As a result, the sinews will be malnourished and spasms, tremors, or convulsions of the muscles will occur. In general, there are two types of Liver wind caused by warm-heat pathogens:

1. *Liver wind due to heat from excess.* Since both the Liver and Pericardium pertain to *jue yin*, a warm-heat pathogen can easily stir up the Liver wind when it invades the Pericardium, leading to convulsions. Thus, it is common in warm pathogen diseases for a coma to appear first, followed by convulsions. Generally speaking, the onset of convulsions is quick, and the patient will present with frequent convulsions of the arms and legs, stiffness of the neck, clenching of the jaws, arched back rigidity (opisthotonus), staring upward, cold extremities, coma, deep-red tongue, and a rapid and wiry pulse. If the heat from excess in the Stomach and Large Intestine stirs up Liver wind, there will also be a vigorous fever or tidal fever, strong thirst for cold beverages, profuse sweating, dry and hard stools, and a yellow tongue coating.
2. *Liver wind due to deficiency of the Liver and Kidney yin.* This type of Liver wind appears in the late stage of a warm pathogen disease. In such cases, the Kidney yin has been injured by a warm-heat pathogen, leading to yin deficiency of the Liver and Kidney, malnutrition of the sinews, and a stirring of Liver wind. Clinically, this type of Liver wind is quite different from that due to heat from excess. It manifests as small movements of the hands and feet with malar flush, low-grade fever, dry throat and mouth, listlessness, diminished hearing, palpitations or panic attack, a dry, atrophied, deep-red tongue, and a thin and rapid pulse.

Summary

Among the diagnostic methods used for analyzing warm pathogen diseases, examination of the tongue body and coating, teeth, maculas and papules, and miliaria alba is very important. Not only does this provide objective information for pattern differentiation based on the theories of the four levels and three burners, it also provides guidance in the prognosis of warm pathogen disease. Fever and its associated symptoms, such as chills, are also important for identifying the location of the disease in the body. Thirst and sweating provide useful information about the condition of the antipathogenic qi and of the yin and fluids, both of which are prone to injury from heat. Impaired consciousness indicates the condition of the spirit of the Heart, and spasms, tremors, and convulsions reflect involvement of the Liver. Clinically, without knowing the location of the disease and the condition of the antipathogenic qi, it is very difficult to correctly diagnose, and consequently, to determine the proper treatment. Therefore, in order to effectively treat warm pathogen diseases, one must master these diagnostic methods.

Endnotes

1. Chen Ze-Lin, Chen Mei-Fang, *Research on Tongue Diagnosis (Shé zhěn yán jiù)*. Shanghai: Shanghai Science and Technology Publishing House, 1982: 1-3.

2. Anonymous, *Yellow Emperor's Inner Classic: Basic Questions (Huáng Dì nèi jīng sù wèn)*. Beijing: People's Health Publishing House, 1963: 184, 188; Anonymous, *Yellow Emperor's Inner Classic: Divine Pivot (Huáng Dì nèi jīng líng shū)*. Beijing: People's Health Publishing House, 1963: 36.

3. Research and Study Section on Basic Theory of Beijing College of Traditional Chinese Medicine, *Tongue Diagnosis in Traditional Chinese Medicine (Zhōng yī shé zhěn)*. Beijing: People's Health Publishing House, 1980: 2.

4. Zhang Zhi-Wen, Liu Bi-Qing, ed., *Atlas of Tongue Diagnosis in Warm Pathogen Diseases (Wēn bìng shé zhěn tú pǔ)*. Beijing: People's Health Publishing House, 1998.

5. This is sweet and cold and enters the Lung, Stomach, Heart and Spleen channels. This is the fluid distilled from Lonicerae Flos *(jīn yín huā)*. Its actions are similar to the flower itself, but it has the added ability to cool summerheat while remaining quite gentle to the Stomach. It is excellent for treating children's heat rash as well as toxic sores.

6. This is the juice of Phragmitis Rhizoma *(lú gēn)*. It has a stronger action in clearing heat and producing fluids than does the root. It is therefore used for such problems as severe damage to the fluids by heat, leading to cough with sticky sputum and a dry mouth.

7. Tang Da-Lie, *Collection of Papers of Physicians from Wu (Wú yī huì jiǎng)*. Shanghai: Shanghai Science and Technology Publishing House, 1983: 6.

8. Ibid.

9. Contained fever is discussed at some length under "Differentiating Common Signs and Symptoms" below.

10. The word that we translate as 'singularity' (瘅 *dàn*) is found in the *Inner Classic* with a variety of meanings. Often it means 'singularly hot,' as in Chapter 35 of *Basic Questions* where a singular malarial disorder (瘅瘧 *dàn nuè*) is said to exhibit fever but no chills. However, Ye is referring to an entry in Chapter 47 of *Basic Questions* that describes Spleen singularity (脾瘅病 *pí dàn bìng*) as a problem that results from the overeating of sweet foods that leads to obesity and then to a form of wasting and thirsting disorder.

11. Tang Da-Lie, *Collection of Papers of Physicians from Wu*, 6.

12. Ibid.

13. Zhao Shao-Qin, Hu Ding-Bang, Liu Jing-Yuan, *Length and Breadth of Warm Pathogen Disease [Differentiation] (Wēn bìng zòng héng)*. Beijing: Beijing College of Traditional Chinese Medicine, 1979: 251

14. For more information on this structure, see Chapter 6, n. 26.

15. This formula was first recorded in *Discussion of Warm Epidemics (Wēn yì lùn)*. It contains Arecae Semen *(bīng láng)* (6g), Magnoliae officinalis Cortex *(hòu pò)* (3g), Magnoliae officinalis Cortex *(hòu pò)* (1.5g), Anemarrhenae Rhizoma *(zhī mǔ)* (3g), Paeoniae Radix alba *(bái sháo)* (3g), Scutellariae Radix *(huáng qín)* (3g), and Glycyrrhizae Radix *(gān cǎo)* (1.5g). See Chapter 12 for further information.

16. Wu Zhen, *Thorough Understanding of Cold Damage (Shāng hán zhǐ zhǎng)*. Shanghai: Shanghai Science and Technology Publishing House, 1959: 31.

17. In Ye Gui's book, *Discussion of Warm-Heat Disorders,* the original sentence was "If the tongue coating looks like alkali [鹸 *jiǎn*]." According to my understanding, alkali here means that the tongue coating looks white, dry, thick, and rough in consistency.

18. Tang Da-Lie, *Collection of Papers of Physicians from Wu*, 6.

19. Wu You-Xing, *Discussion of Warm Epidemics (Wēn yì lùn)*. Shenyang: Liaoning Science and Technology Publishing House, 1997: 21. This text was originally published in 1642.

20. Shi Shou-Tang, *Bases of Medicine (Yī yuán)*. Nanjing: Jiangsu Science and Technology Publishing House, 1983: 49.

21. Wu Zhen, *Thorough Understanding of Cold Damage*, 8.

22. Tang Da-Lie, *Collection of Papers of Physicians from Wu*, 7.

23. Ye Gui did not mention any herbs in the case of phlegm-heat stirring up Liver wind. See Tang Da-Lie, *Collection of Papers of Physicians from Wu*, 8. According to Zhao Shao-Qin, the following herbs will be helpful in this situation: Saigae tataricae Cornu *(líng yáng jiǎo)*, Fritillariae cirrhosae Bulbus *(chuān bèi mǔ)*, Uncariae Ramulus cum Uncis *(gōu téng)*, and Bambusae Succus *(zhú lì)*. See Zhao Shao-Qin et al., *Length and Breadth of Warm Pathogen Disease [Differentiation]*, 248.

24. According to Zhao Shao-Qin, Ophiopogonis Radix *(mài mén dōng)*, Polygonati odorati Rhizoma *(yù zhú)*, and Trichosanthis Radix *(tiān huā fěn)* can be used in treating this condition. See Zhao Shao-Qin et al., *Length and Breadth of Warm Pathogen Disease [Differentiation]*, 248.

25. In my experience, Rehmanniae Radix *(shēng dì huáng)*, Rhinocerotis Cornu *(xī jiǎo)*, Forsythiae Fructus *(lián qiào)*, and Moutan Cortex *(mǔ dān pí)* can be used in treating this condition.

26. This is made by putting human stool (loose stool) in a clay pot and sealing it. Bury the clay pot underground for three years and take it out. The clear water in the clay pot is called 'golden liquid' (金汁 *jīn zhī*). It strongly clears heat and resolves toxicity. While not used at present, I have seen my father prescribe this substance in his practice more than thirty years ago. Coptidis Rhizoma *(huáng lián)* or Isatidis Folium *(dà qīng yè)* can be substituted in this formula.

27. The source text does not specify the preferred form of the herb. Clinically, either Rehmanniae Radix *(shēng dì huáng)* or Rehmanniae Radix preparata *(shú dì huáng)*, or both, could be used. However, in this situation, Rehmanniae Radix preparata *(shú dì huáng)* would be preferable due to its stronger action in enriching Kidney yin.

28. Tang Da-Lie, *Collection of Papers of Physicians from Wu*, 8.

29. Ibid.

30. Wu You-Xing, *Discussion of Warm Epidemics*, 2. See Chapter 12 for further details.

31. This formula was first recorded in *Discussion of Cold Damage (Shāng hán lùn)* and consists of Rhei Radix et Rhizoma *(dà huáng)* (12g), Natrii Sulfas *(máng xiāo)* (9-12g), Aurantii Fructus immaturus *(zhǐ shí)* (12-15g), and Magnoliae officinalis Cortex *(hòu pò)* (24g).

32. Wu You-Xing, *Discussion of Warm Epidemics*, 5.

33. Wang Shi-Xiong, *Warp and Woof of Warm-Heat Pathogen Diseases (Wēn rè jīng wěi)*. This title is contained in Lu Zhen, *Collected Rare Recent Books on Chinese Medicine: Warm Pathogen Disease Section (Jīn dài zhōng yī zhēn běn jí: wēn bìng fèn cè)*. Hangzhou: Zhejiang Science and Technology Publishing House, 1987: 61

34. Tang Da-Lie, *Collection of Papers of Physicians from Wu*, 9-10.

35. Anonymous, *Yellow Emperor's Inner Classic: Basic Questions*, 99.

36. Zhang Ji, *Essentials from the Golden Cabinet (Jīn guì yào luè fāng lùn)*, ed. Hubei College of Traditional Chinese Medicine. Beijing: People's Health Publishing House, 1963: 39.

37. Chao Yuan-Fang, *Discussion of the Origins of Symptoms of Disease*. Beijing: People's Health Publishing House, 1992: 326.

38. Wu You-Xing, *Discussion of Warm Epidemics*, 6-7.

39. Tang Da-Lie, *Collection of Papers of Physicians from Wu*, 9.

40. According to Lu Ting-Zhen, "Maculas are caused by heat and toxin in the Stomach." See Lu Ting-Zhen, *Systematic Differentiation of the Six Etiologies (Liù yīn tiáo biàn)*, in *Collection of Rare Chinese Medical Books (Zhēn běn yī shū jí chéng)*. Beijing: Chinese Medicine and Pharmacology Publishing House, 1996: 724.

41. "Papules are caused by wind-heat in the Lung." Ibid.

42. Compared to maculas, papules are actually involved in both the protective and nutritive levels, and are more superficial than maculas, because some of the accompanying signs and symptoms mentioned above belong to the protective level.

43. Tang Da-Lie, *Collection of Papers of Physicians from Wu*, 9.

44. Wu You-Xing, *Discussion of Warm Epidemics*, 7.

45. This formula was first recorded in *Discussion of Cold Damage (Shāng hán lùn)*. It contains Rhei Radix et Rhizoma *(dà huáng)* (12g), Natrii Sulfas *(máng xiāo)* (9-12g), and honey-toasted Glycyrrhizae Radix preparata *(zhì gān cǎo)* (6g). See Chapter 7 for further details.

46. Wu Tang, *Systematic Differentiation of Warm Pathogen Diseases (Wēn bìng tiáo biàn)*. Beijing: People's Health Publishing House, 1963: 72.

47. Ibid.

48. Ibid., 98.

49. White Tiger Decoction *(bái hǔ tāng)* was first recorded in *Discussion of Cold Damage.* It contains Gypsum fibrosum *(shí gāo)* (30g), Anemarrhenae Rhizoma *(zhī mǔ)* (9g), Nonglutinous rice *(gěng mǐ)* (9-15g), and honey-toasted Glycyrrhizae Radix preparata *(zhì gān cǎo)* (3g). See Chapter 7 for further details.

50. Dong Jian-Hua, "Features, range, and clinical differentiation of warm pathogen diseases *(Wen bing te dian, fan wei ji qi lin chuang jian bie)*" in Fang Yao-Zhong, Xu Jia-Song (eds.), *Collection of Lectures on Warm Pathogen Diseases (Wēn bìng huì jiǎng)*. Beijing: People's Health Publishing House, 1986: 56.

51. Ibid.

52. Wu You-Xing, *Discussion of Warm Epidemics,* 8.

53. Wu Tang, *Systematic Differentiation of Warm Pathogen Diseases,* 128.

54. Dong Jian-Hua, "Features, range, and clinical differentiation of warm pathogen diseases," 56-57.

55. Anonymous, *Yellow Emperor's Inner Classic: Basic Questions,* 56.

56. Meng Shu-Jiang et al., *Warm Pathogen Diseases (Wēn bìng xué)*. Shanghai: Shanghai Science and Technology Publishing House, 1985: 26.

57. Dong Jian-Hua, "Features, range, and clinical differentiation of warm pathogen diseases," 57-58.

6 Treatment Methods for Warm Pathogen Diseases

B Y THE EARLY eighteenth century, Ye Gui's *Discussion of Warm-Heat Disorders* had established the four basic principles for treating illness based on the four-level differentiation of disease.[1] These principles have since been widely used in the treatment of warm pathogen diseases.

1. *Treat warm pathogen disease patterns in the protective level by inducing sweating.* Here, Ye was not referring to the use of acrid and warm herbs, as this would merely serve to add more heat to the body, like throwing gasoline on a fire. Rather, for warm pathogen disease patterns in the protective level, the practitioner must release the exterior condition by inducing sweating with acrid and cool herbs such as Arctii Fructus *(niú bàng zǐ)* and Menthae haplocalycis Herba *(bò hé)*. The purpose of inducing sweating is to provide the warm-heat pathogen with a 'substrate' to which it can adhere, and by which it can exit the body.

   Some modern writers believe that the emphasis on inducing sweating is misleading, if not actually incorrect. According to Zhao Shao-Qin, a professor at the Beijing University of Traditional Chinese Medicine, Ye Gui did not mean to say that the goal of treatment here is to induce sweating. What he actually meant was that acrid, cool, and light herbs that clear and release heat and vent pathogens should be used. Since the problem here is that a warm-heat pathogen is constrained in the protective level and Lung, these types of herbs can eliminate the warm-heat pathogen, harmonize the nutritive and protective qi, and distribute the fluids, resulting in slight sweating and thus a cure of the disease. The sweating itself is merely a by-product of the process, and not the reason

141

for treatment.[2] While this idea helps us remember that the sweating Ye Gui was referring to is different from that induced by such acrid and warm herbs as Ephedrae Herba *(má huáng)* and Cinnamomi Ramulus *(guì zhī)* which can injure the yin and fluids, it ignores the important role that sweat plays in providing a vehicle to which the warm-heat pathogens can adhere and exit the body. Dai Tian-Zhang (Dai Lin-Jiao, 1644–1722) in *Discussion of Widespread Warm Epidemics (Guǎng wēn yì lùn)* noted that "Without sweating, there is no way for the warm-heat pathogen to exit. Therefore, inducing sweating is one of the important treatment methods for warm pathogen disease."[3]

The question arises: Should we always induce sweating in the treatment of a warm pathogen disease in the protective level, or for an exterior pattern in a warm pathogen disease?[4] According to Meng Shu-Jiang, the key point is whether the patient is already sweating. Generally speaking, if a patient with a protective level disorder is not sweating, the interstices and pores are more or less closed, and sweating should be induced. However, if a patient is already sweating, even slightly, one should not induce further sweating.[5]

2. *Treat warm pathogen disease patterns in the qi level by clearing heat with acrid and cold, acrid and cool, or bitter and cold herbs.* According to Ye Gui, "Clearing heat is suitable for patterns that have reached the qi level."[6] There are three sets of herbs for this purpose:

- acrid and cool herbs
- acrid and cold herbs
- bitter and cold herbs

The first two sets of herbs focus on dispersing heat transversely from the body through the Lung or skin. By contrast, the third set, which includes herbs such as Coptidis Rhizoma *(huáng lián)*, Scutellariae Radix *(huáng qín)*, Phellodendri Cortex *(huáng bǎi)*, and Gardeniae Fructus *(zhī zǐ)*, draws heat downward to exit the body via the stool or urine. According to Zhao Shao-Qin, purging herbs with bitter and cold properties like Rhei Radix et Rhizoma *(dà huáng)*, Sennae Folium *(fān xiè yè)*, and Aloe *(lú huì)*, and those with sweet and cold properties like Glehniae/Adenophorae Radix *(shā shēn)*, Ophiopogonis Radix *(mài mén dōng)*, Dendrobii Herba *(shí hú)*, and Trichosanthis Radix *(tiān huā fěn)*, produce fluids and clear heat; they can also be used to clear heat from qi level patterns of warm pathogen diseases.[7]

3. *Treat warm pathogen disease patterns in the nutritive level by cooling the nutritive level and clearing heat.* This is accomplished with bitter and cold herbs, which clear heat by drawing it downward. At the same time, the practitioner should

seek to expel heat from the nutritive level via the qi level with acrid, light, and cold herbs. Because nutritive qi is still a form of qi, it is thought to be closer to the qi level than it is to the blood level. This is an example of a common method of treatment in Chinese medicine: Whenever possible, provide more than one route for pathogens to exit the body. Acrid, light, and cold herbs are used to transversely disperse heat from the nutritive level to the qi level. Ye Gui noted that when heat reaches the nutritive level, "there is still a chance of bringing the warm-heat pathogen back to the qi level."[8] Herbs like Rhinocerotis Cornu *(xī jiǎo)*, Saigae tataricae Cornu *(líng yáng jiǎo)*, and Scrophulariae Radix *(xuán shēn)*, which are bitter, salty, and cold, would seem to be inappropriate since they only serve to move the heat downward instead of outward. Contemporary practitioners agree that the appropriate formula here would combine those herbs with Lophatheri Herba *(dàn zhú yè)*, Forsythiae Fructus *(lián qiào)*, and Lonicerae Flos *(jīn yín huā)*. Monitoring changes in the tongue is essential for determining whether or not the warm-heat pathogen has returned to the qi level. If the tongue has changed from a deep-red color with less than normal coating (or no coating) to just red with a yellow coating, the warm-heat pathogen has reverted to the qi level.

4. *Treat warm pathogen disease patterns in the blood level by cooling the blood and dispersing blood stasis.* Ye Gui said that "When a warm-heat pathogen invades the blood level, it can injure the blood and force it out of the vessels [leading to blood stasis]."[9] Herbs like Rehmanniae Radix *(shēng dì huáng)*, Paeoniae Radix rubra *(chì sháo)*, Moutan Cortex *(mǔ dān pí)*, and Asini Corii Colla *(ē jiāo)* should be used to cool and disperse blood. Cooling the blood when a warm-heat pathogen invades the blood level would seem to be the obvious course of treatment for the blood level, but it is not so obvious in the context of blood stasis:

- Herbs that cool blood are cold or cool in nature and can readily congeal the blood and produce blood stasis.

- Heat generated by a warm-heat pathogen can congeal the blood and produce blood stasis.

- Existing blood stasis can block the movement of qi in the blood and give rise to heat, leading to further bleeding.

Therefore, in order to treat the warm-heat pathogen and prevent formation of further blood stasis and bleeding, the practitioner must simultaneously use herbs that can cool blood and disperse stasis. While Ye Gui did mention tonification methods, such as the use of Asini Corii Colla *(ē jiāo)* and Rehmanniae Radix *(shēng dì huáng)* for blood level disorders in *Discussion of Warm-Heat Disorders*, most practitioners tend to focus exclusively on the excessive aspects of heat and blood stasis in the blood level and ignore the deficient aspect, that is, injury to the yin and fluids. According to a contemporary warm pathogen disease specialist, Meng Shu-Jiang, blood level patterns may involve injury to the yin and fluids.[10] To avoid this, Rehmanniae Radix preparata *(shú dì huáng)*, Paeoniae Radix alba *(bái sháo)*, and Salviae miltiorrhizae Radix *(dān shēn)* can be added to the herbs listed above.

About fifty years after the publication of Ye Gui's book, Wu Tang wrote *Systematic Differentiation of Warm Pathogen Diseases (Wēn bìng tiáo biàn)*, which established three basic methods for treating diseases based on three-burner differentiation. Like the four methods described above, these methods are also effective in treating warm pathogen disease:

1. *Treat patterns in the upper burner by dispersing the warm-heat pathogen via the skin, nose, and mouth.* Patterns occurring in the upper burner are considered superficial and represent the first stage of a warm pathogen disease. In order to treat patterns in the upper burner, use light herbs to disperse and release the warm-heat pathogens. Wu Tang described this method as using herbs that are as light as the feathers of a bird.[11]

2. *Treat patterns in the middle burner by supporting the Spleen's lifting and the Stomach's descending actions.* The middle burner is a bridge that connects the upper and lower burners, bringing qi in the lower burner upward and causing qi in the upper burner to descend. The Spleen's function of lifting, and the Stomach's function of causing qi to descend, are crucial to this task. Injury to the Stomach yin by heat, and the presence of dampness in the Spleen, commonly hamper these functions. Therefore, eliminating dampness through transformation, drying, and draining will support and restore the Spleen's lifting function. Likewise, enriching the Stomach yin and clearing heat from the Stomach will support and restore its descending function. Wu Tang likened these methods to calibrating a scale that must always be kept in balance. This can be done with herbs that are neither too light nor too heavy, and cause neither too much descending nor too much ascending.[12]

3. *Treat patterns in the lower burner by enriching the Kidney and Liver yin.* When a warm pathogen disease reaches the lower burner, both Kidney and Liver yin will become badly injured; the practitioner must use heavy and cloying herbs like Rehmanniae Radix preparata *(shú dì huáng)*, Trionycis Carapax *(biē jiǎ)*, and Asini Corii Colla *(ē jiāo)* because only they can reach the lower burner and are strong enough to enrich the Kidney and Liver yin. Wu Tang described this method as adding a heavy weight to a scale to tip the balance.[13]

Clinically, it is common to find the disease in two levels (or burners) at the same time. When this occurs, it is important to assess the relative degree of disease in each level or burner and treat accordingly.

Since the time that Ye Gui and Wu Tang first set down the principles for treating patterns of warm pathogen disease in the four levels and three burners, practitioners have made additional refinements. For example, the contemporary physician Zhang Zhi-Wen has expressed his version of these principles as follows:[14]

1. In the early stage of a warm pathogen disease, release the exterior condition with acrid and cool herbs such as Menthae haplocalycis Herba *(bò hé)*, Arctii Fructus *(niú bàng zǐ)*, Sojae Semen preparatum *(dàn dòu chǐ)*, Lonicerae Flos *(jīn yín huā)*, Mori Folium *(sāng yè)*, and Forsythiae Fructus *(lián qiào)*.

2. In the middle stage of a warm pathogen disease, either (a) clear the heat and vent it, with acrid and cold herbs such as Trichosanthis Pericarpium *(guā lóu pí)*, Phragmitis Rhizoma *(lú gēn)*, Pyri Exocarpium *(lí pí)*,[15] Lophatheri Herba *(dàn zhú yè)*, and Forsythiae Fructus *(lián qiào)*, or (b) drain the interior heat with bitter and cold herbs such as Coptidis Rhizoma *(huáng lián)*, Scutellariae Radix *(huáng qín)*, Phellodendri Cortex *(huáng bǎi)*, and Gardeniae Fructus *(zhī zǐ)*. When Forsythiae Fructus *(lián qiào)* is used to clear and vent the heat, consider not only its acrid flavor and cold nature, but also its light property.

3. In the later stage of a warm pathogen disease, generate fluids and enrich the yin with cold substances that are either sweet or salty such as Rehmanniae Radix *(shēng dì huáng)*, Asini Corii Colla *(ē jiāo)*, Trionycis Carapax *(biē jiǎ)*, Scrophulariae Radix *(xuán shēn)*, Ophiopogonis Radix *(mài mén dōng)*, Polygonati odorati Rhizoma *(yù zhú)*, and Glehniae/Adenophorae Radix *(shā shēn)*.

Regardless of the stage, for all warm pathogen diseases the main thrust of treatment should be to eliminate the warm-heat pathogens, rather than to support the antipathogenic qi. It is the pathogen that causes the disease and injures the yin or fluids, or causes other problems such as phlegm and blood stasis; yet these consequences are of secondary concern, even if important. The details of treatment will of course vary from one type of warm pathogen disease to another, as will be discussed in the following chapters.

At present, the consensus is that there are eleven methods of treatment for warm pathogen diseases:

1. Release exterior conditions
2. Clear and dispel heat from the qi level
3. Harmonize
4. Dispel dampness
5. Purge
6. Clear heat from the nutritive level
7. Cool the blood
8. Open the orifices

9. Extinguish wind
10. Enrich the yin
11. Secure abandoned disorders

Only clearing heat from the nutritive level and cooling the blood are treatment methods which are peculiar to warm pathogen diseases. The other strategies are used in the treatment of a variety of diseases. In this chapter we will consider each of these methods, basically in the order of the severity of the disease, from mild to severe.

Release Exterior Conditions

The first method of treatment is to release the exterior (解表 *jiě biǎo*), which eliminates pathogenic factors through the exterior, that is, through openings in the pores on the surface of the body and the muscular layer. Since this method disseminates the Lung qi, promotes the circulation of protective qi, and opens up the pores, it often induces sweating. Some practitioners refer to this method as 'diaphoresis.' However, it must be emphasized that the purpose of this form of treatment is not to induce sweating. As discussed above, in some ways, sweating may be thought of as merely a side effect. In the early stage of a warm pathogen disease, sweating shows that the protective qi is strong and is capable of pushing the warm-heat pathogen out of the body. In reality, not every patient will sweat during treatment. However, it should always induce the protective qi to open up the pores and interstices, thereby dissipating and releasing the pathogen. What the patient actually feels is a diminishment in body aches, fever, and aversion to cold. The patient may or may not sweat.

In the clinic, the release of an exterior condition is accomplished with formulas that contain acrid, cool, and dispersing herbs. These are suitable for exterior patterns located in the protective level and Lung in the upper burner at an early stage of a newly-contracted warm pathogen disease. This method can also be used in treating a lurking warm pathogen disease that is activated by an attack from a secondary external pathogenic factor.

Dispelling exterior wind and dispersing exterior heat is an important method of treatment for the early stage of a warm pathogen disease. One example of this method is releasing the exterior with acrid and cool herbs. This method is used in treating an attack on the protective level and the Lung by wind-heat at an early stage of wind-warmth. The main indications are fever, mild chills and aversion to cold, slight or no sweating, slight thirst, cough, red tip and edges of the tongue with a thin and white tongue coating, and a floating and rapid pulse. Formulas commonly used to facilitate this method are Mulberry Leaf and Chrysanthemum Drink (*sāng jú yǐn*) and Honeysuckle and Forsythia Powder (*yín qiào sǎn*).[16] Theoretically, only acrid and cool herbs meet these criteria, but clinically, one should add one or two acrid and warm herbs to prevent the possible side effects that are often experienced from using too many cool herbs, such as congealing of the protective qi and closing of the pores. Obviously, if the protective qi is stagnant and the pores are closed, there is no way for a warm-heat pathogen to exit the body. The warm-heat pathogen may then progress to the qi or even the nutritive or blood levels, and the disease will accordingly deteriorate. It is important to note that there are several different warm-heat pathogens, each with its own indications, methods of treatment, and appropriate formulas.

Table 6.1	Release the Exterior	
Treatment Methods	**Indications**	**Formulas**
Disperse wind and drain heat (*shū fēng xiè rè*), also known as releasing the exterior, with acrid and cool herbs (*xīn liáng jiě biǎo*)	Attack on the protective level and Lung by wind-heat at an early stage of warm pathogen disease: fever, slight aversion to cold, chills, slight or absent sweating, slight thirst, cough, red tip and edges of the tongue with thin, white coating, floating and rapid pulse	Mulberry Leaf and Chrysanthemum Drink (*sāng jú yǐn*), Honeysuckle and Forsythia Powder (*yín qiào sǎn*)
Vent the exterior and resolve summer-heat (*tòu biǎo jiě shǔ*) with acrid, cool, warm, aromatic, and bitter herbs	Accumulation of summer-heat with an attack of cold in the muscles and exterior: headache, uncomfortable body that is stiff or slightly sore, fever, absence of sweating, thirst, restlessness	Newly Augmented Mosla Drink (*xīn jiā xiāng rú yǐn*)
Dissipate the exterior and transform damp[-heat] (*xuān biǎo huà shī*) with aromatic, warm, and cold herbs	Attack on the protective level by damp-heat at an early stage of damp-warmth: aversion to cold, generalized heaviness, slight fever, chest and epigastric distention, white tongue coating, soggy and moderate pulse	Patchouli/Agastache, Magnolia Bark, Pinellia, and Poria Decoction (*huò pò xià líng tāng*)
Disperse the exterior and moisten dryness (*shū biǎo rùn zào*) with acrid, cool, and moist herbs	Attack on the protective level and the Lung by dry-heat: headache, fever, slight aversion to cold, cough with little sputum, sore and dry throat, dry nose and lips, thin and white tongue coating with scanty saliva, red tip and edges of tongue	Mulberry Leaf and Apricot Kernel Decoction (*sāng xìng tāng*)

CONSIDERATIONS WHEN RELEASING EXTERIOR CONDITIONS

Underlying or constitutional issues. For optimal results the practitioner should bear in mind the following considerations:

- *Patients whose fluids are injured by a warm-heat pathogen.* Many practitioners mistakenly use cloying herbs such as Asini Corii Colla *(ē jiāo)*, Rehmanniae Radix preparata *(shú dì huáng)*, and Dendrobii Herba *(shí hú)* in treating patients whose fluids are injured by a warm-heat pathogen, especially by dry-heat during the fall, or those with underlying yin deficiency with a dry mouth, throat, and nose. This, however, is a mistake as these herbs will trap the pathogen inside the body. Instead, one should use herbs like Rehmanniae Radix *(shēng dì huáng)* and Ophiopogonis Radix *(mài mén dōng)*. It is also recommended that the patient eat pears or water chestnuts during the course of treatment to enrich the yin. When rechecking the patient, pay close attention to both the degree of dryness and the strength of the pathogen, and adjust the herbs accordingly.

- *Patients with deficiency of both the qi and yin or fluids.* Avoid using herbs such as Ginseng Radix *(rén shēn)* and Rehmanniae Radix preparata *(shú dì huáng)* in patients who have both qi and yin or fluid deficiency. Not only do these herbs tonify qi, generate fluids, or enrich the yin, they can also exacerbate the heat or trap warm-heat pathogens within the body. Instead, one should use Pseudostellariae Radix *(tài zǐ shēn)* because it slightly enriches the yin and tonifies the qi without trapping the warm-heat pathogen and exacerbating the heat. After eliminating the warm-heat pathogen, the practitioner can wait and judge the severity of the qi and yin deficiency, and then use stronger herbs as indicated.

- *Women who have recently given birth.* Avoid using strong dispersing herbs such as Menthae haplocalycis Herba *(bò hé)* and Artemisiae annuae Herba *(qīng hāo)*, which induce strong sweating, in women who have recently given birth. This is because both the qi and blood are deficient in these women, and such herbs can injure the qi and blood. This precaution also applies to women immediately following menstruation, especially after heavy bleeding. According to Ye Gui,[17] the warm-heat pathogen can readily attack the blood chamber (血室 *xuè shì*)[18] during or after menstruation, leading to a complex of warm-heat pathogen and blood stasis. This may disturb or even block the spirit of the Heart. Should the spirit of the Heart be disturbed, the resulting pattern is mild and the patient will present with irritability, insomnia, lack of concentration, and fuzzy thinking. But if it blocks the spirit of the Heart, the pattern is severe with poor memory and delirium, or even coma.[19]

  According to Wang Shi-Xiong (Wang Meng-Ying, 1806-1866), a warm-heat pathogen can invade the blood chamber in three ways:[20]

1. At the onset of menstruation, which leads to blood stasis. The treatment is to invigorate the blood.[21]

2. Immediately following the conclusion of menstruation, because of the resulting emptiness of the blood chamber. The treatment is to nourish the blood and enrich the yin, clear heat, and cool the blood.

3. By attacking the blood chamber and inducing early menstruation, with heavy bleeding. The treatment is to clear heat to normalize the movement of blood.

Based on his own experience and that of his colleagues, the contemporary physician Zhao Shao-Qin in *Length and Breadth of Warm Pathogen Disease [Differentiation]* described the herbs that should be used in each of the three types of invasion of the blood chamber by a warm-heat pathogen. For the first type, use a modified Minor Bupleurum Decoction *(xiǎo chái hú tāng)*, that is, one that omits Ginseng Radix *(rén shēn)* and Jujubae Fructus *(dà zǎo)*, but contains Rehmanniae Radix *(shēng dì huáng)*, Persicae Semen *(táo rén)*, Crataegi Fructus *(shān zhā)*, and Moutan Cortex *(mǔ dān pí)* or Rhinocerotis Cornu *(xī jiǎo)*. For the second type, use Rehmanniae Radix *(shēng dì huáng)*, Scrophulariae Radix *(xuán shēn)*, Salviae miltiorrhizae Radix *(dān shēn)*, Paeoniae Radix rubra *(chì sháo)*, and Paeoniae Radix alba *(bái sháo)*. And for the third type, use Rehmanniae Radix *(shēng dì huáng)*, Sanguisorbae Radix *(dì yú)*, Paeoniae Radix rubra *(chì sháo)*, Bubali Cornu *(shuǐ niú jiǎo)*, and Moutan Cortex *(mǔ dān pí)*.[22]

- *Children.* The practitioner must consider two pathological aspects when treating children who have been attacked by a warm-heat pathogen:

  1. A warm-heat pathogen will progress faster in children than in adults because children, by their very nature, are more yang than adults. It is common for children who contract a warm-heat pathogen to experience abnormal progression (逆傳 *nì chuán)*. For example, pneumonia or acute bronchitis can easily progress to delirium or even coma in one or two days. It is accordingly very important that you treat the child's illness as soon as possible with a method that is strong enough to halt the progression. This does not mean using a large dosage or a large number of herbs. Rather, you should increase the frequency of treatment. For example, a patient normally takes three doses of a decoction each day. However, children with high fever, severe sore throat, and a cough with yellow sputum should take a dose every two hours, or even hourly.

  2. Children will almost always present with food retention in connection with an attack of a warm-heat pathogen. Food retention may exist either before the child contracts the pathogen due to intake of improper foods, or it may de-

149

velop after the child contracts the pathogen. In either case, it can slow down the digestive process. Whenever the tongue coating is thick or greasy, the practitioner should add herbs to the decoction that promote digestion, such as Massa medicata fermentata *(shén qū)*, dry-fried Hordei Fructus germinatus *(chǎo mài yá)* or dry-fried Setariae (Oryzae) Fructus germinatus *(chǎo gǔ yá)*.

Herbal issues. Consider the following points when using herbal formulas to release exterior conditions:

- *Inappropriate use of only acrid and warm herbs to induce sweating.* The use of only acrid and warm herbs to induce sweating to release a warm pathogen disease from the exterior is contraindicated, as this will give rise to the production of fire. However, it is a good idea to include one or two acrid and warm herbs, such as Schizonepetae Herba *(jīng jiè)* or Sojae Semen preparatum *(dàn dòu chǐ)*, prepared with Ephedrae Herba *(má huáng)*. Including such herbs in the context of a formula made up primarily of acrid and cool herbs will enhance its dispersing function. It will also prevent the pores and interstices from closing, which would slow the process of eliminating the warm-heat pathogen.

- *Producing too vigorous a diaphoretic response.* To prevent injury to the fluids by inducing too vigorous of a diaphoretic response, it is best to induce only slight sweating, that is, just like the drizzle of a summer shower, rather than the torrent of a heavy downpour. In addition, this method should be terminated as soon as the exterior condition nears resolution. The degree of resolution depends upon the patient's constitution, for example, seventy to eighty percent resolved in a healthy individual, or ninety percent resolved in an elderly patient. The remainder should be left to the antipathogenic qi's natural ability to fight illness.

- *Combining with other types of herbs.* It is common for patients with underlying yin deficiency to present with a protective level warm pathogen disease. In these cases, some yin-enriching herbs must be included in the prescription, as there will otherwise not be enough fluids to permit sweating. Under these circumstances, acrid and cool herbs should be combined with others such as Rehmanniae Radix *(shēng dì huáng)*, Ophiopogonis Radix *(mài mén dōng)*, and Polygonati odorati Rhizoma *(yù zhú)*. If there is both qi and yin deficiency, add Panacis quinquefolii Radix *(xī yáng shēn)*. While in theory one should avoid the use of bitter and cold herbs to disperse a warm-heat pathogen, this is only a relative contraindication. Wu Tang himself added one or two such herbs to his formula Mulberry Leaf and Chrysanthemum Drink *(sāng jú yǐn)*. In addition, it is not uncommon for wind-heat in the protective level to be accompanied by toxin, or to quickly transform into toxin, with such symptoms as high fever and a red, swollen, painful throat. For this reason, bitter, cold herbs that resolve toxicity, such as Isatidis Folium *(dà qīng yè)*, Isatidis/Baphicacanthis Radix *(bǎn lán gēn)*, or Taraxaci Herba *(pú gōng yīng)*, are frequently added to prescriptions for treating protective level conditions.

• *Preserving the nature of the herbs.* Most herbs used in this treatment method are acrid and light. It is therefore suitable to cook them for only a short time (approximately seven minutes) in order to maintain their light and acrid qualities for dispersing warm-heat pathogens.

Clear and Dispel Heat from the Qi Level

The second treatment method is to clear heat (清热 *qīng rè*). In warm pathogen disease theory, this method is used to clear and dispel heat located in the qi level. As previously noted, in qi level patterns there is a fierce struggle between antipathogenic qi and the warm-heat pathogen. If not properly treated in a timely manner, a warm-heat pathogen without form may combine with the formed fecal material and take up residence in the Large Intestine. Alternatively, it may invade the nutritive or blood levels, or injure and exhaust the yin of the Kidney and Liver, leading to the stirring of internal wind. Thus, the qi level is a key stage in warm pathogen diseases, and since the inception of warm pathogen disease theory, practitioners have attached great importance to treating diseases at this level.

This method serves to clear interior heat directly, while easing irritability, generating fluids, and relieving thirst indirectly. It is especially suitable when heat progresses from the protective level to the Lung and Stomach. As with protective level patterns, there are many different qi level patterns. There are also many indications, methods of treatment, and formulas used for clearing and dispelling heat from the qi level which should be taken under consideration. To clear and dispel heat from the qi level, acrid and cold herbs, or bitter and cold herbs, are utilized. Various treatment methods should be utilized in accordance with the depth and quality of the disease. (See Table 6.2.)

In order to properly use these methods, one should carefully consider the following slight differences among them:

• *Lightly clearing heat and disseminating the Lung qi with light and cold herbs* is directed at a warm-heat pathogen located in the qi level of the upper burner, especially in the chest and diaphragm. Light herbs such as Lonicerae Flos *(jīn yín huā)*, Forsythiae Fructus *(lián qiào)*, Lophatheri Herba *(dàn zhú yè)*, Gardeniae Fructus *(zhī zǐ)*, Trichosanthis Pericarpium *(guā lóu pí)*, and Phragmitis

Table 6.2	Clear and Dispel Heat from the Qi Level	
Treatment Methods	**Indications**	**Formulas**
Lightly clear [heat] and disseminate the [Lung] qi (*qīng qīng xuān qì*) with light and cold herbs	Qi stagnation in chest and diaphragm due to heat from constraint: fever, slight thirst, insomnia, thin and yellow tongue coating	Gardenia and Prepared Soybean Decoction (*zhì zǐ chǐ tāng*)
Clear [heat in the] qi [level] with acrid and cold herbs (*xīn hán qīng qì*)	Heat from excess in Stomach: vigorous fever, restlessness, thirst, dry and yellow tongue coating, flooding and rapid pulse	White Tiger Decoction (*bái hǔ tāng*)
	Stagnation of heat in the Lung: cough labored breathing, fever, restlessness, thirst, rapid pulse	Ephedra, Apricot Kernel, Gypsum, and Licorice Decoction (*má xìng shí gān tāng*)
Clear heat and drain fire (*qīng rè xiè huǒ*) with bitter and cold herbs	Fire or heat from constraint in the qi level: fever, bitter taste, thirst, dark and yellow urine, restlessness, red tongue with yellow coating	Scutellaria Decoction (*huáng qín tāng*)

Rhizoma *(lú gēn)* should be chosen to disperse the warm-heat pathogen from the qi level to the protective level, and then to vent it through the surface of the body.

- *Clearing heat from the qi level with acrid and cold herbs* will slowly disperse heat from the exterior as well as clear heat from the Lung and Stomach. This method also serves to slightly induce sweating with acrid herbs, such as Gypsum fibrosum *(shí gāo)*, that reach the Lung and disseminate the qi. Therefore, the patient may experience slight sweating that carries heat out of the body. This method is different from the one below in that the herbs are not as light as those used to reach the Lung in the upper burner.

- *Clearing heat and draining fire with bitter and cold herbs* draws heat and fire down from organs like the Heart, Lung, Liver, Stomach, Large Intestine, Gallbladder, and Triple Burner, and passes it out of the body via urination. Theoretically, when bitter and cold herbs like Coptidis Rhizoma *(huáng lián)*, Scutellariae Radix *(huáng qín)*, and Gardeniae Fructus *(zhī zǐ)* are used to treat qi level heat in the chest, diaphragm, Lung, and Stomach, they will congeal and trap the warm-heat pathogen within the body. However, *if* it is severe, the use of bitter and cold herbs is not absolutely contraindicated when treating heat in these locations. In such cases, include a small dose of a bitter and cold herb in an otherwise acrid, light, and cold herbal formula. Zhang Zhi-Wen, who currently teaches at Chengdu University of Traditional Chinese Medicine, prefers using Platycodi Radix *(jié gěng)*, Glycyrrhizae Radix *(gān cǎo)*, Menthae haplocalycis Herba *(bò hé)*, Scutellariae Radix *(huáng qín)*, Gardeniae Fructus *(zhī zǐ)*, Forsythiae Fructus *(lián qiào)*, and Lophatheri Herba *(dàn zhú yè)* for treating heat from constraint in the diaphragm with irritability, insomnia, and a red tongue with a yellow coating.[23] He also likes to add Artemisiae annuae Herba *(qīng hāo)*, Citrulli Exocarpium *(xī guā pí)* and Nelumbinis Folium *(hé yè)* for patterns that are summerheat-related. For phlegm-heat in the chest leading to cough, irritability, and insomnia, he suggests the addition of Talcum *(huá shí)*, Tetrapanacis Medulla *(tōng cǎo)*, Armeniacae Semen *(xìng rén)*, Poriae Cutis *(fú líng pí)*, and Eriobotryae Folium *(pí pá yè)* to provide two avenues by which heat can exit the body, that is, via the Lung and the Bladder.

The treatment methods described above are intended to serve only as a broad outline of this method. In the clinic, one must apply the methods in accordance with the vagaries of the different patterns. Several examples follow.

- If a warm-heat pathogen attacks the qi level, but remnants remain in the protective level, consider simultaneously

  — Adding herbs like Menthae haplocalycis Herba *(bò hé)* and Lonicerae Flos *(jīn yín huā)* to expel the warm-heat pathogen from the exterior. For example, the eighteenth-century physician Yu Gen-Chu recommended the addition of Lophatheri Herba *(dàn zhú yè)*, Nelumbinis Folium *(hé yè)*, and Menthae haplocalycis Herba *(bò hé)* to White Tiger Decoction *(bái hǔ tāng)*[24] for treating warm-heat in the qi level before the condition in the protective level has fully resolved. It is said that this formula has the advantage of clearing heat from constraint without congealing the heat.[25]

  — Expelling interior heat and promoting the circulation of qi in the chest and diaphragm with herbs like Aurantii Fructus *(zhǐ ké)* and Trichosanthis Pericarpium *(guā lóu pí)*.

- If the heat in the qi level is so severe that it has injured the yin and fluids, clearing heat from the qi level should be combined with enriching yin and generating fluids. Herbs for this purpose include Glehniae/Adenophorae Radix *(shā shēn)*, Ophiopogonis Radix *(mài mén dōng)*, Trichosanthis Radix *(tiān huā fěn)*, and Dendrobii Herba *(shí hú)*. These herbs are sweet, but cold. They serve to generate fluids, enrich yin, and clear heat.

- If both the qi and yin are injured by heat, a combination of sweet, cold, astringent, and slightly warm herbs like Ginseng Radix *(rén shēn)*, Ophiopogonis Radix *(mài mén dōng)*, and Schisandrae Fructus *(wǔ wèi zǐ)* are indicated. If both the qi and the fluids are injured by summerheat, Panacis quinquefolii Radix *(xī yáng shēn)*, Dendrobii Herba *(shí hú)*, Ophiopogonis Radix *(mài mén dōng)*, and nonglutinous rice *(gěng mǐ)* should be selected. In Chinese herbal theory, it is routine to use a combination of sweet and cold herbs for treating the yin or fluids in the Lung and Stomach as well as for clearing heat from the qi level. However, this combination cannot be used for severe heat from constraint, where it may lead to fire if neither the yin nor the fluids has been injured. Instead, bitter and cold herbs like Scutellariae Radix *(huáng qín)*, Coptidis Rhizoma *(huáng lián)*, Phellodendri Cortex *(huáng bǎi)*, and Gentianae Radix *(lóng dǎn cǎo)* should be used. He Lian-Chen (He Bing-Yuan, 1860-1929) observed that in these circumstances, if only herbs like Rehmanniae Radix *(shēng dì huáng)*, Scrophulariae Radix *(xuán shēn)*, and Ophiopogonis Radix *(mài mén dōng)* are used for severe heat from constraint and fire, the fire will become stronger. In addition, this will aggravate the adverse changes in consciousness, as the fluids generated from the sweet and cold herbs will congeal into cloying phlegm from the intense fire. In severe cases the resulting phlegm can lead to blockage of the Heart spirit with cold extremities, muddled consciousness, or even interior blockage and exterior collapse.[26] However, when used judiciously, bitter and sweet herbs can be used together, as Wu Tang recommended in combining Scutellariae Radix *(huáng qín)*, Coptidis Rhizoma *(huáng lián)*, Phellodendri Cortex *(huáng bǎi)*, Ophiopogonis Radix *(mài mén dōng)*, Rehmanniae Radix *(shēng dì huáng)*, and Scrophulariae Radix *(xuán shēn)* for treating scanty urine due to heat from excess and injury to the flu-ids.[27] It is the cloying herbs that must be avoided.

- If there is blockage of qi in the Lung due to heat from constraint, besides herbs that clear heat in the qi level, add others like Platycodi Radix *(jié gěng)*, Trichosanthis Pericarpium *(guā lóu pí)*, and Armeniacae Semen *(xìng rén)* to disseminate and direct the Lung qi downward.

- If heat and toxins accumulate in a certain area on the skin, there will be inflammation, swelling, and pain in that area in addition to fever and thirst. Thus, herbs to clear heat and drain fire must be combined with others to resolve toxicity and subdue swelling such as Lonicerae Flos *(jīn yín huā)*, Forsythiae Fructus *(lián qiào)*, Isatidis/Baphicacanthis Radix *(bǎn lán gēn)*, and Isatidis Folium *(dà qīng yè)*.

- If there is severe constipation with dry stools and heat in the Large Intestine, use the purging method with bitter and cold herbs like Rhei Radix et Rhizoma *(dà huáng)*, Natrii Sulfas *(máng xiāo)*, Aloe *(lú huì)*, and Sennae Folium *(fān xiè yè)* to provide an avenue for the warm-heat pathogen to exit the body via the stool.

Considerations when Clearing and Dispelling Heat from the Qi Level

Contraindications. This method is contraindicated under the following conditions:

- *When the warm-heat pathogen has not yet attacked the qi level.* This method should not be used when the pathogen has yet to reach the qi level. Otherwise, it will drive the exterior symptoms deeper into the body.
- *Clearing heat and draining fire when the heat has not yet transformed into fire.* At the point when the patient experiences burning chest, irritability, restlessness, and insomnia, the heat is on the verge of transforming into fire. You should then disperse interior heat and promote the circulation of qi in the chest and diaphragm. Appropriate acrid and cool herbs for this purpose include Gardeniae Fructus *(zhī zǐ)*, Sojae Semen preparatum *(dàn dòu chǐ)*, Lophatheri Herba *(dàn zhú yè)*, and Trichosanthis Pericarpium *(guā lóu pí)*. At this point it is too early to clear heat and drain fire with bitter and cold herbs; to do so would actually accelerate the intensity of the interior heat. This is because they may constrain the qi and thus generate heat. Signs and symptoms associated with transformation into fire include headache, red eyes, tinnitus, a burning tongue, canker sores, and nosebleeds.

Other factors. Keep the following things in mind when using this method:

- *Damp-heat patterns in the qi level.* For these patterns, combine the method above with the transformation of dampness by using herbs like Atractylodis Rhizoma *(cāng zhú)*, Pogostemonis/Agastaches Herba *(huò xiāng)*, and Eupatorii Herba *(pèi lán)*.
- *Patients with underlying yang deficiency.* Do not use large doses of bitter and cold herbs like Scutellariae Radix *(huáng qín)*, Coptidis Rhizoma *(huáng lián)*, Phellodendri Cortex *(huáng bǎi)*, and Gentianae Radix *(lóng dǎn cǎo)* in patients with yang deficiency, even if there is heat in the qi level. This may aggravate the injury to the yang. In addition, as the heat diminishes, the use of bitter, cold herbs should be reduced, and as soon as the heat is eliminated, discontinued entirely.
- *Using too many herbs to promote urination, or those which strongly promote urination.* When the warm-heat pathogen enters the qi level the urine will become dark and scanty. This indicates that the heat has injured the fluids and also that the heat is leaving the body through the urine. While it is appropriate

to support this process with a few herbs that both conduct heat downward and out of the body through the urine while also clearing heat and generating fluids, one must do so with caution. If urination is promoted too forcefully, or for too long, it will further exhaust the fluids. The appropriate herbs in this situation are Phragmitis Rhizoma *(lú gēn)* and Lophatheri Herba *(dàn zhú yè)*.

Harmonize

The third method of treatment is to harmonize (和解 *hé jiě*), which can be used in both a broad and narrow sense. In the broad sense, harmonizing means a variety of treatment methods that work simultaneously on two different but interrelated parts of the body. Examples include the simultaneous treatment of the exterior and interior, tonifying deficiency while draining excess, or combining cold and warm herbs.

In its narrow sense, harmonizing in terms of warm pathogen disease refers to the treatment of a warm-heat pathogen that is neither in the exterior nor in the interior, for example, the Stomach or Large Intestine. In this context, we harmonize the half-exterior and half-interior aspect of the body, resolving dampness and phlegm, promoting qi circulation in the Triple Burner and Gallbladder, venting heat, and clearing heat from the Triple Burner, Gallbladder, and membrane source.[28] This method is used if the pathogen has invaded and accumulated in the Gallbladder, Triple Burner, or membrane source. It serves to disperse heat to the outside and to improve the circulation of qi so that the warm-heat pathogen can be expelled from the exterior and the circulation of qi in the yang organs can be normalized.

Note, however, that since patterns involving the Gallbladder, Triple Burner, and membrane source are different, the indications, methods of treatment, and formulas used to treat each of them will also differ. (See Table 6.3.)

It is very important to distinguish between the method of harmonizing the *shao yang* and the method of harmonizing in the context of a warm pathogen disease, even though both are types of half-exterior and half-interior patterns. One harmonizes the *shao yang* when a *shao yang* pattern, as described in *Discussion of Cold Damage (Shāng hán lùn)*, is observed. A *shao yang* pattern is caused by wind-cold transforming into heat without form, which is regarded as a transitional stage between the *tai yang* and *yang ming* stages. In the *shao yang* stage the qi, especially of the Stomach and Spleen, is no longer strong. This calls for the use of herbs that clear and disperse heat from constraint in the Gallbladder, such as Bupleuri Radix *(chái hú)* and Scutellariae Radix *(huáng qín)*, as well as qi tonics such as Ginseng Radix *(rén shēn)*, Jujubae Fructus *(dà zǎo)*, and honey-toasted Glycyrrhizae Radix preparata *(zhì gān cǎo)*. By contrast, all three of the warm pathogen disease harmonizing methods described here are used for treating pathogens *with* form, for example, dampness and/or phlegm. Herbs like

Table 6.3	Harmonize	
Treatment Methods	**Indications**	**Formulas**
Clear and drain the *shao yang* [Gallbladder] (*qīng xiè shào yáng*) with acrid, bitter, and cold herbs	Heat from constraint in the Gallbladder with phlegm and dampness: alternating fever and chills, bitter taste, hypochondriac and costal pain, restlessness, thirst, yellow urine, epigastric distention, nausea, red tongue with yellow and greasy coating, wiry and rapid pulse	Sweet Wormwood and Scutellaria Decoction to Clear the Gallbladder (*hāo qín qīng dǎn tāng*)
Divide and reduce while moving and draining [dampness, phlegm, and heat in the Triple Burner] (*fēn xiāo zǒu xiè*) with acrid, bitter, bland, cold, and warm herbs	Accumulation of phlegm-heat in the Triple Burner: fever and chills that wax and wane, distention in chest and abdomen, scanty urine, greasy tongue coating	Warm the Gallbladder Decoction (*wēn dǎn tāng*)
Open and bring damp-heat out from the membrane source (*kāi dá mó yuán*) with aromatic and slightly warm herbs	Damp-heat stagnating in the membrane source and blocking the qi: intense chills and slight fever, distention in chest and abdomen, white and greasy tongue coating that looks like white powder over tongue, bright- or deep-red tongue	Lei's Formula to Disseminate and Vent [Dampness and Heat] from the Membrane Source (*Léi shì xuān tòu mó yuán fāng*), Reach the Source Drink (*dá yuán yǐn*)

Citri reticulatae Pericarpium *(chén pí)*, Bambusae Caulis in taeniam *(zhú rú)*, Tsaoko Fructus *(cǎo guǒ)*, Magnoliae officinalis Cortex *(hòu pò)*, Poria rubra *(chì fú líng)*, and Talcum *(huá shí)* are used to eliminate dampness or resolve phlegm. Also, because of the presence of dampness or phlegm, which are yin pathogens with form that readily cause qi to stagnate, herbs such as Arecae Semen *(bīng láng)*, Magnoliae officinalis Cortex *(hòu pò)*, Aurantii Fructus *(zhǐ ké)*, Platycodi Radix *(jié gěng)*, and Citri reticulatae Pericarpium *(chén pí)* are added to move the qi.

It should be noted that there are slight differences among the three warm pathogen disease harmonizing methods:

- *Clearing and draining the shao yang* focuses on the Gallbladder and Stomach: clearing heat from constraint in the Gallbladder, resolving phlegm and dampness, and causing the Stomach qi to descend with herbs such as Artemisiae annuae Herba *(qīng hāo)*, Scutellariae Radix *(huáng qín)*, Pinelliae Rhizoma preparatum *(zhì bàn xià)*, Bambusae Caulis in taeniam *(zhú rú)*, and Talcum *(huá shí)*. This is because, when there is heat from constraint in the Gallbladder, the heat is likely to block qi circulation, leading to stagnation of fluids and attack on the Stomach by the Gallbladder (wood attacking earth). This results in the production of dampness and phlegm, as well as rebellious Stomach qi.

• *Dividing and reducing while moving and draining dampness, phlegm, and heat in the Triple Burner* focuses on the Triple Burner. It involves the use of herbs like Platycodi Radix *(jié gěng)* and Armeniacae Semen *(xìng rén)* to disseminate the Lung qi in the upper burner and cause it to descend; Magnoliae officinalis Cortex *(hòu pò)* and Amomi Fructus rotundus *(bái dòu kòu)* to transform dampness and promote Spleen qi circulation; and Poria *(fú líng)* and Talcum *(huá shí)* to leach out dampness from the Bladder in the lower burner. The circulation of water and qi is the primary physical function of the Triple Burner; the production of dampness and stagnation of qi will be the chief pathology when a warm-heat pathogen, especially one related to dampness, attacks the Triple Burner. Attention should therefore be paid to promoting the movement of qi. If the qi moves well, the dampness will be drained and transformed, and no new dampness will be generated.

• *Opening and bringing damp-heat out from the membrane source* focuses on the membrane source with herbs such as Magnoliae officinalis Cortex *(hòu pò)*, Arecae Semen *(bīng láng)*, Tsaoko Fructus *(cǎo guǒ)*, Pogostemonis/Agastaches Herba *(huò xiāng)*, and Pinelliae Rhizoma preparatum *(zhì bàn xià)*. In this pattern, dampness and heat are tightly bound together, although dampness predominates. This is a relatively rare condition, and little is written about it in the Ming and Qing era books on warm pathogen disease.

CONSIDERATIONS WHEN HARMONIZING

• The herbs used to clear heat from constraint from the Gallbladder are not as strong as those used to clear interior heat from excess in the Stomach at the qi level. It is therefore suitable to apply the harmonizing method in treating heat from constraint in the Gallbladder and Triple Burner, but not when there is heat from excess in the Stomach.

• The method of opening and bringing damp-heat out from the membrane source focuses more on resolving phlegm and dampness than on clearing heat. If there is heat from excess and the patient is thirsty and drinks a lot, other treatment methods, such as clearing heat, should be substituted.

• Most of the herbs used in opening and bringing damp-heat out from the membrane source are dry and warm in nature. The practitioner should be careful when prescribing them, particularly in a high dosage, for a patient with underlying yin deficiency.

• When most of the dampness has been eliminated and heat predominates, do not use either of the two harmonizing methods of opening and bringing damp-heat out from the membrane source, or dividing and reducing dampness, phlegm, and heat in the Triple Burner. Otherwise, the herbs that are dry and warm in nature will increase the internal heat, injure the yin, or even stir up internal wind.

Dispel Dampness

The fourth method for treating a warm pathogen disease is to dispel dampness (驅 濕 *qū shī*). This method seeks to dry up, transform, and leach out dampness with bitter, aromatic, and bland herbs, respectively. It is used to improve qi circulation, activate the Spleen and harmonize the Stomach, and promote urination (the method by which dampness is eliminated from the body).

Dispelling dampness can be subdivided into four distinct methods based on the condition and location of the dampness. For best results, it is crucial to iden- tify whether dampness or heat predominates, and to select the method for dispelling dampness accordingly. You must also focus not only on drying, transforming, and draining dampness, but on promoting qi circulation. This is because interior damp- ness is primarily caused by stagnation of qi in the organs. Dampness blocks qi circu- lation and produces further dampness or even Liver qi stagnation and blood stasis. Based on my own understanding and experience, qi not only commands the move- ment of blood, it also commands the movement of fluids. Once qi circulation nor- malizes in the organs, especially in the Spleen, dampness will no longer be produced. Therefore, no matter where the dampness is located, promoting qi circulation is an indispensable method for treating dampness.

The four methods for dispelling dampness (Table 6.4) are:

1. *Disseminating qi and transforming dampness* focuses on promoting qi circu- lation in the upper burner with herbs like Amomi Fructus rotundus (*bái dòu kòu*), Pogostemonis/Agastaches Herba (*huò xiāng*), and Armeniacae Semen (*xìng rén*), which are light and work together to disseminate and cause the Lung qi to descend. According to Wu Tang in *Systematic Differentiation of Warm Pathogen Diseases*, normal qi circulation in the Lung is crucial:

   All formulas that treat dampness in the Triple Burner should focus on the up- per burner.[29] … Only Three-Nut Decoction (*sān rén tāng*)[30] with its light herbs can cause the Lung qi to disseminate and descend. This is important because the Lung governs qi circulation over the body, and dampness will be transformed when qi circulation in the Lung is normal.[31]

Table 6.4	Dispel Dampness	
Treatment Methods	**Indications**	**Formulas**
Disseminate qi and transform dampness (*xuān qì huà shī*) with aromatic, bland, cold, and warm herbs	Stagnation of qi mechanism due to heat from accumulation of dampness at early stage of damp-warmth: fever that worsens in the afternoon and remains after sweating, slight aversion to cold, chest and epigastric distention, scanty urine, white and greasy tongue coating, soggy and moderate pulse	Three-Nut Decoction (*sān rén tāng*)
Dry up dampness and drain heat (*zào shī xiè rè*) with acrid, bitter, cold, and warm herbs	Dampness gradually transforming into heat and accumulating in the middle burner: fever, thirst but only able to drink a little, epigastric and abdominal distention, nausea with urge to vomit, bitter taste, yellow and greasy tongue coating	Coptis and Magnolia Bark Drink (*lián pò yǐn*)
Transform dampness (*fāng xiāng huà shī*) with aromatic and warm herbs	Damp-heat (dampness predominant) in middle burner affecting the upper and lower burners: fever that remains after sweating, distention in the chest and abdomen, dry mouth with no desire to drink, nausea or vomiting, loose stools with sensation of incomplete evacuation, turbid urine, gray, white, thick, and greasy tongue coating	Lei's Fragrant and Aromatic Formula to Transform Turbidity (*Léi shì fāng xiāng huàa zhuó fāng*), Third Modification of Rectify the Qi Powder (*sān jiā jiǎn zhèng qì sǎn*)
Separate and drain out damp-heat (*fēn lì shī rè*) with bland and cold herbs	Accumulation of dampness in lower burner: scanty or absent urine, distention in head, thirst, white tongue coating	Poria Peel Decoction (*fú líng pí tāng*)

2. *Drying up dampness and draining heat* focuses on eliminating damp-heat from the middle burner by promoting qi circulation in the Spleen and Stomach. Acrid herbs like Acori tatarinowii Rhizoma *(shí chāng pǔ)* and Sojae Semen preparatum *(dàn dòu chǐ)* support the lifting function of qi in the Spleen, while bitter herbs like Coptidis Rhizoma *(huáng lián)* and Magnoliae officinalis Cortex *(hòu pò)* help the descending function of qi in the Stomach. The formula should also include herbs that are cold in nature, such as Coptidis Rhizoma *(huáng lián)* and Scutellariae Radix *(huáng qín)*, that act to clear heat and dry dampness.

3. *Transforming dampness with aromatic herbs* can arouse the Spleen and promote qi circulation when the Spleen's function is suppressed by the accumulation of dampness. Also, according to the modern master Qin Bo-Wei, they can transversely disperse damp-heat in the qi level from the body.[32]

4. *Separating and draining out damp-heat* focuses on dampness in the lower burner and facilitates its departure from the body via the urine. According to the thirteenth-century writer Li Gao, in his *Discussion of the Spleen and Stomach (Pí wèi lùn)*: "When treating dampness, one cannot but promote uri-nation."[33] From this point of view, draining dampness via urination is used for dampness anywhere in the body.

Considerations when Dispelling Dampness

• Do not dispel dampness after it has transformed into dry-heat.

• Be careful when dispelling dampness in a patient with underlying yin deficiency. It is common to see patients who have both damp-heat and yin deficiency concurrently. For example, the patient with ulcerative colitis who is receiving the pharmaceutical prednisone will show both damp-heat and yin deficiency. In this situation, it is very hard for a practitioner to choose a treatment method. Drying, transforming, and draining dampness will exacerbate the yin deficiency; while enriching the yin with cloying herbs will increase the dampness. It is recommended that one follow three steps in selecting herbs to deal with dampness in such cases:

  1. Identify the proportion of dampness, heat, and yin deficiency and choose the proper ratio of herbs for each condition.

  2. Choose mild herbs, such as Poria *(fú líng)* and Pogostemonis/Agastaches Herba *(huò xiāng)*, if the dampness itself is mild.

  3. When the patient returns for a follow-up visit, check to see if the yin deficiency has been exacerbated and adjust the herbs and dosage accordingly.

Purge

The fifth method for treating a warm pathogen disease is to purge it from the body (下 *xià* or 通下 *tōng xià*), literally, to move or unblock downward. The function of this method in the context of warm pathogen diseases is to discharge the heat or damp-heat, retention of food, and blood stasis by means of catharsis. It is appropriate for patterns such as severe constipation with dry stools and heat in the Large Intestine, accumulation of damp-heat, retention of food, and accumulation of blood stasis in the lower burner. Herbs with a bitter and salty flavor and cold nature are used because the bitter and salty flavors cause the qi to descend, which is the normal direction of qi movement in the Stomach and Large Intestine. There are four distinct treatment methods for purging (see Table 6.5):

1. *Unblocking the yang organs (Intestines) and draining the heat* is the most commonly used approach in the clinic. It is also called using bitter and cold herbs to purge downward. In traditional Chinese medicine the Stomach is viewed as a container that receives food while the Large Intestine is a vehicle for transporting waste. According to Liu Bao-Yi in *Encountering the Sources of Warm-Heat Pathogen Diseases (Wēn rè féng yuán)*, "When a warm-heat pathogen invades the Stomach [and Large Intestine], it will not [readily] be further transmitted. When the heat of a warm pathogen disease clumps in the Stomach and yang organs [Large Intestine], in six or seven out of ten cases, it will be resolved if purged."[34] Thus, purging heat and dry stool with bitter, salty, and cold herbs plays a very important role in the treatment of warm pathogen diseases. Actually, the purpose of purging heat and dry stool with bitter, salty, and cold herbs is not just to eliminate the warm-heat pathogen, but also to prevent injury to the yin and fluids, since the warm-heat pathogen readily injures them as it progresses. Therefore, according to warm pathogen disease theory, once a warm-heat pathogen reaches the Large Intestine, purging should be used.

Some practitioners argue that one can use the purging method even though there are still exterior signs and symptoms. According to Dai Tian-Zhang in *Discussion of Widespread Warm Epidemics (Guǎng wēn yì lùn)*, "Whether or not there are exterior signs and symptoms, the purging method should be used when there are signs and symptoms of interior heat."[35] Zeng Gui-Fang, recently retired from Chengdu University of Traditional Chinese Medicine, strongly suggested that Rhei Radix et Rhizoma *(dà huáng)* be used in treating high fever due to wind-heat in children, even when they exhibit exterior signs.[36] In my own clinical experience, I have also noticed that in some cases, adding Rhei Radix et Rhizoma *(dà huáng)* to a formula reduces a high fever more quickly than by simply using acrid and cool herbs.

Table 6.5	Purge	
Treatment Methods	**Indications**	**Formulas**
Unblock the yang organs [Intestines] and drain heat (*tōng fǔ xiè rè*) with bitter, salty, and cold herbs	Severe constipation with dry stools and heat in Large Intestine: tidal fever, delirium, hard abdomen, distending pain in abdomen that worsens with pressure, constipation, dark-yellow or dry, dark, and thorny tongue coating, submerged and excessive pulse	Major Order the Qi Decoction (*dà chéng qì tāng*), Regulate the Stomach and Order the Qi Decoction (*tiáo wèi chéng qì tāng*)
Conduct out stagnation and unblock the stool (*dǎo zhì tōng biàn*) with bitter, cold, and slightly warm herbs	Damp-heat combined with retained food in Stomach and Large Intestine: epigastric and abdominal distention, nausea, vomiting, loose stools accompanied by discomfort and a sense of incomplete evacuation, yellow and sour-smelling stools, and a thick, yellow, and turbid tongue coating	Unripe Bitter Orange Pill to Guide out Stagnation (*zhǐ shí dǎo zhì wán*)
Enrich fluids while unblocking and purging (*zēng yè tōng xià*) with sweet, bitter, salty, and cold herbs	Severe injury of fluids from accumulation of heat in Large Intestine: prolonged fever, dry mouth, cracked lips, constipation, and dry tongue coating	Increase the Fluids and Order the Qi Decoction (*zēng yè chéng qì tāng*)
Unblock stagnation and break up clumps (*tōng yú pò jié*) with bitter, salty, cold, and slightly warm herbs	Heat combined with blood stasis in lower burner: fever, hard and painful distention in lower abdomen, constipation or mania, purple and deep-red tongue, submerged and excessive pulse	Peach Kernel Decoction to Order the Qi (*táo rén chéng qì tāng*)

2. *Conducting out stagnation and unblocking the stool* focuses on damp-heat combined with food retention in the Stomach and Large Intestine. Actually, this is a very complex treatment method. It entails the use of bitter, cold, and slightly warm substances to purge heat and dry stool while also transforming dampness, strengthening the Spleen, and promoting digestion. This is necessary since the condition here is a combination of damp-heat plus retention of food in

the Stomach and Large Intestine. The key point is that heat is associated with dampness and food retention. To treat this condition, purging must be done slowly because dampness is characterized by turbidity and takes time to discharge. Thus, unlike purging heat and dry stool with bitter, salty and cold herbs, in which purging for a day or two will be enough to discharge the heat, purging damp-heat with food retention requires more time. Both the patient and the practitioner must not be in a hurry. If the practitioner uses a harsh treatment like that used for purging heat and dry stool, it may quickly discharge the heat. However, the dampness will not be discharged completely, and more dampness will be produced due to the injury suffered by the Spleen qi as a result of the harsh purgative. Also, the diarrhea will worsen due to the harm caused to the transformative and transportive functions of the Spleen. Moreover, the dampness will block the circulation of qi and end up generating heat. So, at what point can one stop the type of purging that is appropriate for damp-heat and food stagnation, and what yardstick can be used to determine when to stop treatment? According to Ye Gui in *Discussion of Warm-Heat Disorders*, "Once the stools become firm, one should be careful and not purge anymore."[37] This is because well-formed stools indicate that there is no longer any dampness.

3. *Generate the fluids while unblocking and purging* focuses on the deficiency of yin and fluids, as well as the accumulation of heat in the Large Intestine. This method combines the use of sweet and cold herbs to increase the fluids, and bitter, salty, and cold herbs to purge heat. The logic of this treatment method can be understood by thinking of the stool in the Large Intestine as a boat on a river. Without enough water to surround it, the boat cannot travel smoothly. Wu Tang, in *Systematic Differentiation of Warm Pathogen Diseases*, calls this method "adding water to help float the boat."[38]

4. *Unblock stagnation and break up clumps* focuses on a mixture of heat and blood stasis in the lower burner. Some purging herbs are used in this method, but their purpose is not only to discharge heat, but also to provide a way to eliminate blood stasis.

There are two other common systems for describing purging methods. The first is to delineate the purging according to the organ involved, as was done by Wu Tang in *Systematic Differentiation of Warm Pathogen Diseases.* [39]

- If there is concurrent phlegm-heat in the Lung and accumulation of heat in the Large Intestine, treatment involves disseminating the Lung qi and causing it to descend, transforming phlegm, and purging heat from the Large Intestine. Herbs like Armeniacae Semen *(xìng rén)*, Gypsum fibrosum *(shí gāo)*, Trichosanthis Pericarpium *(guā lóu pí)*, and Rhei Radix et Rhizoma *(dà huáng)* can be used.

- If there is phlegm-heat in the chest associated with accumulation of heat in the Large Intestine, the appropriate treatment method is to unbind the chest (開 胸 *kāi xiōng*) and unblock the Intestines to drain the heat. Herbs like Coptidis Rhizoma *(huáng lián)*, Aurantii Fructus immaturus *(zhǐ shí)*, Trichosanthis Semen *(guā lóu rén)*, Pinelliae Rhizoma preparatum *(zhì bàn xià)*, Rhei Radix et Rhizoma *(dà huáng)*, and Natrii Sulfas *(máng xiāo)* can be used.[40]

- If the heat is located only in the Large Intestine, treatment involves unblocking the bowels and draining heat and dry stool by purging the Large Intestine. Herbs like Rhei Radix et Rhizoma *(dà huáng)*, Natrii Sulfas *(máng xiāo)*, and honey-toasted Glycyrrhizae Radix preparata *(zhì gān cǎo)* would be appropriate.

- If there is blockage of the Pericardium by phlegm-heat associated with accumulation of heat in the Large Intestine, the appropriate treatment calls for opening the orifices and purging heat from the Large Intestine. Usually, the formula Calm the Palace Pill with Cattle Gallstone *(ān gōng niú huáng wán)*[41] with the addition of Rhei Radix et Rhizoma *(dà huáng)* can be used for this purpose.

- If heat has accumulated in both the Large Intestine and Small Intestine, the appropriate treatment calls for draining heat through the Small Intestine and purging heat from the Large Intestine. This can be done with Paeoniae Radix rubra *(chì sháo)*, Rehmanniae Radix *(shēng dì huáng)*, Coptidis Rhizoma *(huáng lián)*, Phellodendri Cortex *(huáng bǎi)*, Rhei Radix et Rhizoma *(dà huáng)*, and Natrii Sulfas *(máng xiāo)*.

The second system involves combining the method of purging with other treatment methods:

- Combine purging with clearing and dispelling heat from the qi level for the combination of severe constipation with dry stools and heat in the Large Intestine with heat in the upper burner. According to Yu Gen-Chu, the appropriate formula is Augmented Cool the Diaphragm Powder *(jiā wèi liáng gé sǎn)*.[42]

- Combine purging with clearing and dispelling heat from the qi level for severe constipation with dry stools and heat in the Large Intestine and heat in the Stomach. According to Yu Gen-Chu, the appropriate formula is White Tiger to Order the Qi Decoction *(bái hǔ chéng qì tāng)*.[43]

- Combine purging with clearing and dispelling heat from the qi level for severe constipation with dry stools and heat in the Large Intestine with heat and toxin. According to Yu Gen-Chu, the best formula for these cases is Resolve Toxicity and Order the Qi Decoction *(jié dú chéng qì tāng)*, which includes a combination of herbs to clear heat, drain fire, and resolve toxicity.[44]

- Combine purging with cooling blood for accumulation of heat in the Large Intestine that has progressed to the blood level. According to He Lian-Chen in his 1907 book *Revised and Expanded Discussion of Warm-Heat Pathogen Diseases*, the formula of choice for this situation is Best Rhinoceros Horn and Rehmannia Decoction *(bá cuì xī jiǎo dì huáng tāng)*, which combines purging herbs with others that cool blood.[45]

- Combine purging with tonifying the qi and enriching the yin for accumulation of heat in the Large Intestine with deficiency of qi and yin. According to Wu Tang in *Systematic Differentiation of Warm Pathogen Diseases*, the formula recommended for this situation is Newly Augmented Yellow Dragon Decoction *(xīn jiā huáng lóng tāng)*, which combines herbs for tonifying qi, enriching yin, and purging heat.[46]

CONSIDERATIONS WHEN PURGING

Contraindications. Purging is contraindicated for the following conditions:

- Do not use the purging method when there are no factors of excess in the Large Intestine or in the lower burner, that is, severe constipation with dry stools and heat, damp-heat, retention of food, or blood stasis.
- At a later stage of a warm pathogen disease, constipation is mostly caused by exhaustion of fluids in the Large Intestine. Purging with bitter and cold herbs is contraindicated at that time.

Other factors. When using the purging method, keep the following in mind:

- Theoretically, the purging method is contraindicated when there is an exterior condition. Clinically, however, the purging method can be used in treating exterior conditions as long as the signs and symptoms of heat or damp-heat in the Large Intestine are more emergent and severe. However, herbs to relieve exterior conditions should be used concurrently.
- If the excess pathogenic factors return following purging, one should repeat this method, but the practitioner must be careful not to injure the qi and yin.
- If there is underlying yin deficiency or severe injury to the fluids or yin, combine the purging method with the enriching yin method in order to generate fluids and enrich the yin.

Clear Heat from the Nutritive Level

The sixth treatment method is to clear heat from the nutritive level (清營 *qīng yíng*). This is a unique method for treating warm pathogen diseases. Its function is to clear heat from the nutritive level and to vent heat to the qi level. Its indication is therefore heat in the nutritive level. (See Table 6.6.)

Table 6.6	Clear Heat from the Nutritive Level	
Treatment Methods	**Indications**	**Formulas**
Clear heat from the nutritive level and drain heat (*qīng yíng xiè rè*) with bitter, sweet, salty, and cold herbs	Invasion of the nutritive level: fever that worsens at night, restlessness, occasional delirium, faint eruptions and rashes, deep-red tongue	Clear the Nutritive Level Decoction (*qīng yíng tāng*)
Clear heat from both the qi and nutritive levels (*qì yíng liáng qīng*) with acrid, bitter, sweet, and cold herbs	Intense heat in both the qi and nutritive levels: vigorous fever, thirst, restlessness (or skin eruptions), deep-red tongue with yellow coating, excessive pulse	Modified Jade Woma Decoction (*jiā jiǎn yù nǔ jiān*), Transform Maculas Decoction (*huà bān tāng*)

When a warm-heat pathogen invades the nutritive level, two kinds of pathologies will occur. On the one hand, there is heat from excess in the nutritive level. On the other hand, the heat will injure the yin. Formulas for clearing heat from the nutritive level address these two problems:

1. The formulas for clearing heat from the nutritive level contain more or less the same herbs that are used to clear and dispel heat from the qi level. This is not coincidental.

2. Herbs that clear heat from the nutritive level can also enrich the yin directly.

But why must we clear and dispel heat from the qi level after a warm-heat pathogen invades the nutritive level? And should the warm-heat pathogen be dispelled through sweating or discharged through the stool or urine? According to the principles set forth by Ye Gui in *Discussion of Warm-Heat Disorders*, one must vent heat to transmit it to the qi level (透熱轉氣 *tòu rè zhuǎn qì*)[47] where it can be discharged through the urine or stool. The only way to do this is to combine herbs that clear and dispel heat from the qi level with others that clear heat and enrich the yin in the nutritive level.[48]

As previously noted, there are several ways to clear and dispel heat from the qi level. Which one is appropriate in this instance? Of the three methods for clearing heat from the qi level, two of them—lightly clearing heat and disseminating the Lung qi, and clearing heat from the qi level with acrid and cold herbs—can be properly used here. The first method is used for invasion of the nutritive level by heat, and relies on herbs like Lonicerae Flos (*jīn yín huā*), Forsythiae Fructus (*lián qiào*), Lophatheri Herba (*dàn zhú yè*), and Sojae Semen preparatum (*dàn dòu chǐ*). The second method is used for intense heat in both the qi and nutritive levels, using herbs like Gypsum fibrosum *(shí gāo)* and Anemarrhenae Rhizoma *(zhī mǔ)*. Because both methods rely on acrid or light herbs, which have a dispersing action, they can vent heat from the nutritive level out to the qi level. However, the first method is stronger than the second due to its reliance on both light and acrid herbs. The third method for clearing and dispelling heat from the qi level—clearing heat and draining fire—uses bitter and cold herbs such as Coptidis Rhizoma *(huáng lián)* and Scutellariae Radix *(huáng qín)*, and has no dispersing action to vent heat from the nutritive level to the qi level. This method, in fact, may congeal the heat in the nutritive level.

Zhao Shao-Qin is of a similar opinion, and treats warm-heat pathogens in the nutritive level by cooling and clearing heat while venting heat to the qi level. Zhao has a slightly different view about the pathology, however. In these cases the qi has become stagnant, leaving the heat with no avenue to exit from the body. This sets up a vicious circle: heat in the nutritive level causes the qi to become stagnant, and the stagnant qi in turn keeps the heat at this level. Thus, any formula that helps provide an exit for the heat in the nutritive level can be referred to as 'venting' heat to the qi level, even if none of the ingredients has the function of venting.[49] Zhao describes four approaches for accomplishing this purpose:[50]

1. For pure heat from constraint, the appropriate treatment method is to disperse and expel heat from the nutritive level to the qi level with acrid and cool herbs like Mori Folium *(sāng yè)*, Chrysanthemi Flos *(jú huā)*, Lonicerae Flos *(jīn yín huā)*, Forsythiae Fructus *(lián qiào)*, and Lophatheri Herba *(dàn zhú yè)*. For severe heat from constraint, add Bombyx batryticatus *(bái jiāng cán)*, Cicadae Periostracum *(chán tuì)*, and Saposhnikoviae Radix *(fáng fēng)*.

2. For stagnant damp-heat located in the upper burner, the appropriate method is to disperse dampness, separately resolve dampness and heat, and free the heat from the clinging dampness. The overall goal is to expel the heat to the qi level with aromatic herbs such as Pogostemonis/Agastaches Herba *(huò xiāng)*, Eupatorii Herba *(pèi lán)*, Sojae Semen preparatum *(dàn dòu chǐ)*, Armeniacae Semen *(xìng rén)*, and Amomi Fructus rotundus *(bái dòu kòu)*.

3. For stagnant damp-heat in the middle burner, the appropriate method is to promote qi circulation and transform dampness, which will free heat from the clinging dampness. The overall goal is to expel the heat to the qi level with a combination of bitter, acrid, and aromatic herbs such as Perillae Caulis *(zǐ sū gěng)*, Pinelliae massa fermentata *(bàn xià qū)*,[51] Magnoliae officinalis Cortex *(hòu pò)*, Citri reticulatae Pericarpium *(chén pí)*, and Amomi Fructus rotundus *(bái dòu kòu)*.

4. For the patient who has been improperly treated with too many cloying herbs, or with cloying herbs too soon in the course of treatment, thereby trapping the warm-heat pathogen in the nutritive level, the appropriate method is to

promote digestion, disseminate the Lung qi, and resolve phlegm-heat in the Lung. Suggested herbs include Hordei Fructus germinatus *(mài yá)*, Setariae (Oryzae) Fructus germinatus *(gǔ yá)*, Gigeriae galli Endothelium corneum *(jī nèi jīn)*, Curcumae Radix *(yù jīn)*, Trichosanthis Pericarpium *(guā lóu pí)*, and Armeniacae Semen *(xìng rén)*, and the formula Preserve Harmony Pill *(bǎo hé wán)*.[52] These can repair the injury caused by improper treatment and help re-solve the heat from food retention and/or phlegm and bring it back to the qi level.

Based on his fifty years of clinical experience, Zhao believes that improvement in the patient's consciousness is a good marker for indicating that the heat has been vent-ed to the qi level. This would include improvement in such symptoms as irritability, restlessness, muddled consciousness, and delirium. Another important marker is the tongue body, which will change from deep red to red as the heat in the nutritive level is vented to the qi level.[53]

CONSIDERATIONS WHEN CLEARING HEAT FROM THE NUTRITIVE LEVEL

- Do not use this method if the warm-heat pathogen is still in the qi level and has not yet reached the nutritive level, regardless of the severity of the heat. Otherwise, application of this method will serve to guide the warm-heat pathogen into the nutritive level.

- The focus of treatment should be on venting heat to the qi level as well as clearing heat from the nutritive level. Thus, not only should the treatment rely on cold or cool and bitter herbs, such as Rehmanniae Radix *(shēng dì huáng)* and Scrophulariae Radix *(xuán shēn)*, to clear heat from the nutritive level, but also cool and cold herbs, such as Lophatheri Herba *(dàn zhú yè)* and Lonicerae Flos *(jīn yín huā)*, which have a light quality and can disperse heat and vent it to the qi level. If you only use cold and bitter herbs, especially those with cloying qualities such as Rehmanniae Radix *(shēng dì huáng)* and Scrophulariae Radix *(xuán shēn)*, this will trap the warm-heat pathogen and allow it to penetrate deeper and deeper into the body.

Cool the Blood

The seventh method for treating warm pathogen disease, cooling the blood (凉血 *liáng xuè)*, is actually a subcategory of the clearing-heat method described above.

This method is appropriate for treating heat from excess in the blood level as a result of invasion of heat and toxins. Its function is to cool blood, resolve toxicity, break up blood stasis, and invigorate the blood. It is therefore suitable for dealing with heat, toxins, and blood stasis in the blood level. However, since the nutritive level is more superficial than the blood level, the methods used for treating the two levels are different. Unlike the treatment for the nutritive level, herbs such as Rehmanniae Radix (*shēng dì huáng*), Scrophulariae Radix (*xuán shēn*), and Paeoniae Radix rubra (*chì sháo*) must be used. These herbs resolve toxicity, break up blood stasis, and invigorate the blood in order to restore tranquility to the spirit and arrest the bleeding.

Table 6.7	Cool the Blood	
Treatment Methods	**Indications**	**Formulas**
Cool blood and disperse blood stasis (*liáng xuè sàn xuè*) with sweet, salty, and cold herbs	Reckless movement of blood due to invasion of blood level by heat and toxin: high fever, restlessness (or even delirium and mania), many maculas and papules, blood in stool, vomiting blood, purple or very deep-red tongue	Rhinoceros Horn and Rehmannia Decoction (*xī jiǎo dì huáng tāng*)
Strongly clear heat and toxin from the qi and blood levels (*dà qīng qì xuè*) with sweet, bitter, salty, and cold herbs	Heat and toxin from excess in qi and blood levels: vigorous fever, restlessness, thirst, foul-smelling breath, coma, delirium, severe headache and body pain, dark-purple spots on skin (or vomiting blood), hematuria, very deep-red and purple tongue with dry yellow or dry black coating	Clear Epidemics and Overcome Toxin Drink (*qīng wēn bài dú yǐn*)

Invigorating the blood is an important method for treating warm pathogen diseases in the blood level. At first glance, it may seem that by focusing on the heat in the blood (and the use of herbs to cool blood) would be sufficient to prevent heat from forcing the blood out of the vessels. However, this viewpoint is too narrow and could lead to disastrous results. One must look at a secondary pathogenic factor that emerges after bleeding: blood stasis. Blood stasis emerges right after bleeding since blood outside the vessels can neither nourish nor flow. Instead, the blood has become static, and if it is not treated with herbs that invigorate the blood *and* remove blood stasis, the stasis will block qi circulation and produce more heat, which in turn will lead to further bleeding. Thus, the effort that was taken to clear heat will be for naught. Furthermore, it is possible that blood stasis already exists prior to the bleeding, as a result of congealing of the blood by heat in the vessels. Invigorating the blood and removing blood stasis not only addresses the existing blood stasis, but also prevents further bleeding and the production of more heat. In addition, herbs that cool the blood are cold and can readily cause the blood to congeal if they are not accompanied by herbs that invigorate the blood. For these reasons, herbs that invigorate the blood and remove stasis are included to counteract the cold nature of the blood-cooling herbs; the combination prevents the development of new blood stasis.

In addition to the above, strongly clearing heat from the qi and blood levels is regarded as one type of cooling the blood method.[54] The indications are heat from excess and toxin in the qi, nutritive, and blood levels. Thus, the method of strongly clearing heat and toxin from the qi and blood levels is made up of several therapeutic methods grouped together:

- Clearing heat from the qi level with acrid and cold herbs

- Clearing heat, draining fire, and resolving toxicity with bitter and cold herbs

- Cooling blood with bitter and cold herbs

- Dispersing blood stasis with acrid, bitter, and cold herbs

The treatment is multifaceted because the condition itself is not only hot, but also toxic, and is not only in the blood level, but also in the qi and nutritive levels. The practitioner must therefore use a combination of methods and a complex formula. Clinically, cooling the blood is often combined with two other methods discussed below: opening the orifices and extinguishing internal wind.

Considerations when Cooling the Blood

- Do not use this method if the warm-heat pathogen has not yet invaded the blood level.

- Use this method with caution when heat is accompanied by dampness. Dampness is a turbid, yin pathogenic factor. Using only cold or cool herbs to cool the blood will trap dampness within the body. It is therefore important to assess the extent of the dampness, especially the proportion of dampness to heat in any case of damp-heat, and use some slightly warm herbs that dry dampness, such as Atractylodis Rhizoma (*cāng zhú*) and Pinelliae Rhizoma preparatum (*zhì bàn xià*), along with the cool or cold herbs.

Open the Orifices

The eighth treatment method, opening the orifices (開竅 *kāi qiào),* when used in the context of a warm pathogen disease, is usually combined with other treatment methods. This method is indicated for veiling of the Pericardium or blockage of the Heart spirit by heat or phlegm-heat, leading to loss of consciousness, and serves to restore consciousness by clearing heat from the Heart and Pericardium, resolving phlegm, removing the blockage from the Heart, and removing blood stasis from the Heart and Pericardium.[55] To open the orifices in the clinic, herbs with an aromatic flavor which act to restore consciousness are used. Examples include Bovis Calculus *(niú huáng),* Moschus *(shè xiāng),* Borneolum *(bīng piàn),* Curcumae Radix *(yù jīn),* and Acori tatarinowii Rhizoma *(shí chāng pǔ).*

Table 6.8	Open the Orfices	
Treatment Methods	**Indications**	**Formulas**
Clear the Heart [Pericardium] and open the orifices *(qīng xīn kāi qiào)* with acrid, aromatic, bitter, and cold herbs	Invasion of Pericardium by warm-heat pathogen leading to blockage of Heart: delirium and coma, fever, coldness of extremities, stiff tongue with speech difficulty or lethargic state with inability to speak, bright- or deep-red tongue with luster, thin and rapid pulse	Calm the Palace Pill with Cattle Gallstone *(ān gōng niú huáng wán),* Greatest Treasure Special Pill *(zhì bǎo dān),* Purple Snow Special Pill *(zǐ xuě dān)*
Transform blood stasis to open the orifices *(huà yú kāi qiào)* with acrid, aromatic, salty, cold, and warm herbs	Blockage of Heart by blood stasis: coma or muddled consciousness coupled with lethargy and speech difficulty, purple and deep-red tongue, purple nails and face, very dark spots on the skin	Rhinoceros Horn and Succinum Greatest Treasure Special Pill *(xī pò zhì bǎo dān)*
Transform phlegm to open the orifices *(huō tán kāi qiào)* with aromatic, bitter, acrid, and warm herbs	Veiling of Pericardium by damp-heat and phlegm: muddled consciousness or lethargy without speaking, occasional delirium, red tongue with yellow or white greasy coating, soggy, slippery, and rapid pulse	Acorus and Curcuma Decoction *(chāng pǔ yù jīn tāng)*

Varying levels of phlegm exist in all three of the conditions listed in Table 6.8. This is because:

- Heat can congeal the fluids in the Pericardium into phlegm.
- When blood stasis is present, there is stagnation of fluids that can, over time, produce phlegm.
- Damp-heat can produce phlegm.

However, the three methods used for treating the phlegm are quite different from each other. The first condition is marked by more severe pathological heat, and as a result, cold herbs should be used. The latter two conditions are relatively colder in nature because not just phlegm, but also dampness or blood stasis, both of which are yin pathogenic factors, are involved. They accordingly require warm herbs to deal with the dampness or blood stasis. Thus, if the treatment method of resolving phlegm to open the orifices (which requires warm herbs) is used for the pattern of invasion of the Pericardium by heat and blockage of the Heart (which requires cold herbs), more heat will be added to the Pericardium. If the treatment method of clearing and dispersing heat from the Pericardium and opening the orifices is used for the pattern of veiling of the Pericardium due to the steaming of damp-heat and the production of phlegm, the cold herbs will exacerbate the phlegm.

CONSIDERATIONS WHEN OPENING THE ORIFICES

Contraindications. This method would be inadvisable under the following conditions:

- If there is no alteration in consciousness, even if the warm-heat pathogen has invaded the nutritive level
- If the alteration in consciousness has not resulted from blockage of the Heart by heat from excess or veiling of the Pericardium by phlegm-heat
- If the alteration in consciousness is caused by the collapse of yang and scattering of the spirit.

Other factors. Keep the following considerations in mind:

- Each of these three treatment methods has its own indications, and they should not be used as the primary treatment when the reason for the blockage of the Heart is clear. For example, if there is a coma due to excess heat in the Large Intestine that steams upward and blocks the Heart, the heat from excess in the Large Intestine must be purged with bitter and cold herbs rather than just acrid and aromatic herbs, which would raise the heat up and could aggravate the coma.

- Opening the orifices is intended only for treating emergency conditions of impaired consciousness. It is appropriate that it be used in conjunction with other methods such as clearing heat from the nutritive level, cooling blood, and extinguishing internal wind.
- Veiling of the Pericardium by phlegm-heat is not the only process in warm pathogen diseases that impairs consciousness. Two other common causes are disturbance of the Heart spirit due to heat steaming from the Stomach, and a combination of heat and blood stasis in the lower burner. As always, treatment should be directed at the root of the problem. To treat the former, clear and purge heat, and for the latter, clear heat and also dispel blood stasis.

Extinguish Wind

The ninth method for treating warm pathogen diseases is to extinguish wind (熄風 *xī fēng*) to arrest convulsions. This method acts to subdue endogenous wind by cooling the Liver, enriching the yin of the Liver and Kidney, and calming hyperactive Liver yang. It is therefore used for treating the internal stirring of Liver wind due to heat from excess, or the perturbation of internal wind from deficiency due to exhaustion of yin in the Liver and Kidney.

Table 6.9	Extinguish Wind	
Treatment Methods	**Indications**	**Formulas**
Cool the Liver and extinguish wind (*liáng gān xī fēng*) with bitter, salty, and cold herbs	Stirring of Liver wind due to excess interior heat: fever, cold extremities, convulsions (or even trismus, opisthotonos, or coma), clenched teeth, red tongue with yellow coating, wiry and rapid pulse	Antelope Horn and Uncaria Decoction (*líng jiǎo gōu téng yǐn*)
Enrich the yin and extinguish wind (*zī yīn xī fēng*) with sweet, cloying, and cold herbs	Stirring of Liver wind secondary to Kidney and Liver yin deficiency at a late stage of warm pathogen disease: tremors or even convulsions, listlessness, dry and atrophied deep-red tongue, rapid and weak pulse	Major Arrest Wind Pearls (*dà dìng fēng zhū*)

It is very important to distinguish between internal wind that results from excess and that which results from deficiency. For excess, much more attention should be placed on cooling the Liver, and for deficiency, on enriching the Liver and Kidney yin. It is strongly recommended that one combine methods of clearing heat in the qi level, cooling blood, opening the orifices, and purging in order to extinguish internal wind, since the internal wind can be caused by problems of both heat from excess in the qi and blood levels, as well as veiling of the Pericardium or blockage of the Heart.

Clinically, the stirring of Liver wind can be caused by many kinds of excess-type interior heat patterns, and since there are different causes for the stirring of Liver wind, the treatment methods must be selected accordingly. Examples of excess-type heat patterns that lead to Liver wind include:

- *Stirring of Liver wind from blazing heat in the Stomach.* Manifestations include vigorous fever, strong thirst, profuse sweating, cold extremities, and convulsions. The treatment for this condition is a combination of clearing and dispelling heat from the qi level, with extinguishing internal wind and relieving convulsions by clearing heat and cooling the Liver. According to the late-Qing author He Lian-Chen, the best formula for treating this condition is White Tiger Decoction with Rhinoceros Horn and Antelope Horn *(xī líng bái hǔ tāng).*[56]

- *Stirring of Liver wind due to heat from excess in the Large Intestine.* Manifestations include cold extremities, convulsions, tidal fever, delirium, constipation or watery stools with a strong, foul odor, a dry and yellow tongue coating, and a slippery and forceful pulse. The recommended formula is Regulate the Stomach and Order the Qi Decoction *(tiáo wèi chéng qì tāng)*[57] with the addition of Uncariae Ramulus cum Uncis *(gōu téng)*, Chrysanthemi Flos *(jú huā)* and Saigae tataricae Cornu *(líng yáng jiǎo).*

- *Stirring of Liver wind due to heat from excess in the nutritive level and the Pericardium.* Manifestations include cold extremities, convulsions, irritability, restlessness, intermittent delirium, faint skin eruptions, deep-red tongue, and a thin and rapid pulse. According to Wu Tang in *Systematic Differentiation of Warm Pathogen Diseases*, the ideal formula for this pattern is Clear the Nutritive Level Decoction *(qīng yíng tāng)*[58] with the addition of Moutan Cortex *(mǔ dān pí)*, Saigae tataricae Cornu *(líng yáng jiǎo)*, and Uncariae Ramulus cum Uncis *(gōu téng).*

Clinically, blood stasis and phlegm often accompany the stirring of Liver wind. When this occurs, the practitioner should use herbs that remove blood stasis and resolve phlegm such as Bovis Calculus *(niú huáng)*, Pinelliae Rhizoma preparatum *(zhì bàn xià)*, and Salviae miltiorrhizae Radix *(dān shēn)*. After the stirring of Liver wind has subsided, the convulsions will disappear. But this does not mean that the heat that gave rise to the Liver wind is completely cleared. Residual heat may remain and mix with the blood stasis, leading to obstruction of the channels and to low-grade fever and paralysis. For this situation, Wu You-Xing recommended Three-Shell Powder *(sān jiǎ sǎn).*[59]

CONSIDERATIONS WHEN EXTINGUISHING WIND

- Avoid injuring the fluids and yin when using herbs that are acrid and warm to extinguish internal wind and relieve convulsions, particularly animal products like Scolopendra *(wú gōng)* and Scorpio *(quán xiē).*
- Avoid using herbs that enrich the yin of the Liver and Kidney when the Liver wind is caused by heat from excess. Otherwise, the effect will be to retain the warm-heat pathogen.
- Children may experience convulsions when the disease is located in the protective and qi levels due to extreme heat stirring up internal wind. Under these circumstances, much more attention should be placed on venting and clearing the heat, and only a few herbs should be added to extinguish internal wind. This is because once the heat is gone, the wind will subside and the convulsions will be relieved. It is therefore inappropriate to rely primarily on herbs that extinguish internal wind under these conditions.

Enrich the Yin

The tenth method for treating warm pathogen diseases is to enrich the yin (滋陰 *zī yīn)*, a form of tonification (補 *bǔ).* Here the yin is supplemented to generate fluids in order to maintain a healthy balance between yin and yang. This method enriches the yin, supplies the fluids, directly moistens dryness, and indirectly reduces fire. It is therefore suitable for a pattern of injury or exhaustion of fluids or of yin by a warm-heat pathogen, especially in the lower burner. According to the early twenti-eth-century physician Liu Bao-Yi, in a lurking warm pathogen disease, the pathogen lurks in the *shao yin* (Kidney). As such, the more severe the Kidney yin deficiency, the more severe the disease. Thus, by enriching the Kidney yin, one can, under certain circum-stances, help dispel the warm-heat pathogen.[60]

Clinically, severe yin deficiency most often occurs when a warm-heat pathogen invades the lower burner. However, as previously noted (Chapter 2), it may also oc-cur in the early stage of a warm pathogen disease. The underlying condition of the yin and fluids can determine the prognosis for a warm pathogen disease. According to the early twen-tieth-century physician Wu Xi-Huang, "If the yin or fluids are not badly injured, the opportunity to treat a disease still exists and the prognosis is good."[61] Otherwise, the prognosis will be poor. Therefore, once they have been injured, it is very important to enrich the yin and supply the fluids as soon as possible. (See Table 6.10.)

Table 6.10	Enrich the Yin	
Treatment Methods	**Indications**	**Formulas**
Enrich and nourish the Lung and Stomach (*zí yǎng fèi wèi*) with sweet, cool, and moist herbs	Deficiency of Lung yin or Lung and Stomach yin and fluids resulting from failure to recover from a warm pathogen disease: dry throat, nose, and mouth, dry cough with little sputum, poor appetite, dry tongue coating or red tongue with little coating	Glehnia/Adenophora and Ophiopogonis Decoction (*shā shēn mài mén dōng tāng*), Benefit the Stomach Decoction (*yì wèi tāng*)
Enrich the fluids and moisten the Intestines (*zēng yè rùn cháng*) with sweet, cold, and salty herbs	Dryness in Large Intestine due to exhaustion of fluids after a warm pathogen disease: dry throat and mouth, constipation, dry and hard stools, red and dry tongue	Increase the Fluids Decoction (*zēng yè tāng*)
Replenish the Kidney yin (*tián bǔ shèn yīn*) with salty, cloying, heavy, and cold herbs	Prolonged heat in lower burner leading to exhaustion of Kidney yin: low grade fever, flushed face, hot soles and palms, dry throat and mouth, listlessness, constantly tired, violent palpitations, deep-red tongue with little coating, thin and weak or irregular pulse	Modified Restore the Pulse Decoction (*jiā jiǎn fù mài tāng*)

CONSIDERATIONS WHEN ENRICHING THE YIN

- When there is injury to the yin and fluids coupled with interior heat from excess, the treatment protocol is a combination of enriching the yin and clearing heat, using sweet and cold herbs with bitter and cold or acrid and cool herbs.

- For Lung and Stomach yin deficiency, one should also pay attention to promoting qi circulation. When they are yin-deficient, these organs often fail to properly direct their qi downward, which can lead to qi stagnation.

- When in the course of a warm pathogen disease the Intestines become dry, they should be moistened. However, if there is an accumulation of dry-heat in the Large Intestine, the yin-enriching herbs should be combined with purgatives.

- Exercise care when using this method in patients who have both yin deficiency and dampnetss. For this condition, one should enrich the yin in a way that will not cause retention of dampness, and eliminate the dampness in a way that will not injure the yin. In order to do this, avoid the use of bitter and warm herbs, such as Tsaoko Fructus (*cǎo guǒ*), Atractylodis Rhizoma (*cāng zhú*), and Magnoliae officinalis Cortex (*hòu pò*), and herbs that may be too cloying, such as Testudinis Plastrum (*guī bǎn*), Trionycis Carapax (*biē jiǎ*), Asini Corii Colla (*ē jiāo*), and Rehmanniae Radix preparata (*shú dì huáng*).

Secure Abandoned Disorders

The eleventh treatment method for warm pathogen diseases is to secure abandoned disorders (固脱 *gù tuō*). This is used in emergencies for dealing with patterns of collapse. It is mostly used to treat collapse of qi and yin, and collapse of yang. Generally speaking, a warm-heat pathogen readily injures the yin and fluids. The pathogen may induce excessive sweating, which can badly injure the yin and lead to the depletion of the base to which the yang can attach. The result is not only yin collapse, but qi and yang collapse as well. (See Table 6.11.)

CONSIDERATIONS WHEN SECURING ABANDONED DISORDERS

- When this is the appropriate treatment method, it must be used as quickly as possible. At the present time, due to legal and ethical issues, patients with abandoned disorders should be sent directly to the emergency room. However, it is still helpful to be prepared to treat these patients if necessary.
- The proper decoction, dosage, and modification of the herbs used in this method are crucial. Generally speaking, one should cook the formula for 30 minutes, decoct it with a small amount of water, and include herbs that can arrest collapse quickly. Administer small but frequent portions of the decoction to the patient (every hour or half hour).
- Once the yang qi is restored, look for signs of fire and exhaustion of the yin, and treat accordingly.

Considerations when Treating
Warm Pathogen Diseases

Warm pathogen diseases can be divided into two principal groups: those caused by warm-heat without dampness and those caused by warm-heat with dampness. Not only are the treatments different, but also the cautions and contraindications.

Table 6.11	Secure Abandoned Disorders	
Treatment Methods	**Indications**	**Typical Formulas**
Secure abandoned disorders by augmenting the qi (*yì qì gù tuō*) with sweet, sour, warm, and cold herbs	Injury of qi and yin with collapse of antipathogenic qi: sudden decrease in fever, profuse sweating, shortness of breath, listlessness and general lassitude, weak and scattered pulse, 'mirror' tongue without coating	Generate the Pulse Powder (*shēng mài sǎn*)
Revive the yang and rescue from rebellion (*huí yáng jiù nì*) with sweet, acrid, astringent, and hot herbs	Sudden collapse of yang qi: cold extremities after profuse sweating, listlessness, lassitude, pale face, pale and very moist tongue, indistinct and weak pulse	Ginseng, Aconite Accessory Root, Dragon Bone and Oyster Shell Decoction (*shēn fù lóng mǔ tāng*)

TREATING A WARM-HEAT PATHOGEN WITHOUT DAMPNESS

Contraindications. The following are contraindications that the practitioner must keep in mind when treating illnesses caused by a warm-heat pathogen without dampness:

- *Do not use formulas consisting primarily of acrid and warm herbs.* Because a warm-heat pathogen without dampness is a yang pathogenic factor that readily injures the yin and fluids, it is absolutely contraindicated to use a formula consisting primarily of acrid and warm herbs, such as Ephedrae Herba (*má huáng*) and Cinnamomi Ramulus (*guì zhī*), to induce sweating. If this is done, it will aggravate the heat, badly injure the yin or fluids, and cause the disease to penetrate more deeply into the body.

- *Herbs that promote urination should be used with extreme caution.* Clinically, the practitioner will see patients who have scanty urine or who are not urinating at all because of injury to the yin or fluids from the heat. In this situation, clearing heat and enriching yin or fluids are the methods of choice. Do not use herbs that strongly promote urination, such as Polyporus (*zhū líng*) and Alismatis Rhizoma (*zé xiè*). However, to successfully eliminate the heat, the practitioner must occasionally use mild diuretics that are light and gentle, such as Lophatheri Herba (*dàn zhú yè*), to disperse and drain heat via the urine.

- *Be cautious in using cloying herbs to enrich the yin.* As previously noted, patterns of yin or fluid deficiency can be seen in the early stage of a warm pathogen disease because a warm-heat pathogen, especially one without dampness, readily injures the yin or fluids. For treatment, much more attention should be placed on clearing the heat, which is the root of yin and fluid deficiency, than on enriching the yin. This can be done by using slightly sweet and cold herbs to enrich the yin and fluids, such as Polygonati odorati Rhizoma *(yù zhú)*, Ophiopogonis Radix *(mài mén dōng)*, and Phragmitis Rhizoma *(lú gēn)*. If cloying herbs to enrich the yin or fluids are used, such as Rehmanniae Radix preparata *(shú dì huáng)*, Trionycis Carapax *(biē jiǎ)*, and Testudinis Plastri Colla *(guī bǎn jiāo)*, they will trap the warm-heat pathogen inside the body.

- *Be careful with bitter and cold herbs.* To treat extreme heat, bitter and cold herbs are sometimes needed. In most cases, however, acrid and cool herbs are the first choice, not only because they clear heat, but also because they disperse heat and qi without also causing the qi to stagnate. If treatment with bitter and cold herbs leads to qi stagnation, dryness will be generated even if the warm-heat pathogen has been treated effectively. Because the acrid quality disperses, and the cool quality clears heat, they can do this without trapping the warm-heat pathogen inside the body. In some cases, even when bitter and cold herbs are necessary, they should be combined with acrid herbs to prevent the side effects of the bitter and cold herbs.

Treating a Warm-Heat Pathogen with Dampness

Contraindications. The following are contraindications to remember when treating illnesses caused by a warm-heat pathogen with dampness:

- *Do not induce profuse sweating.* The sweating method is used to clear exogenous pathogenic factors, including damp-related factors such as damp-heat and summerheat, from the exterior. However, the ideal method is to slowly induce slight sweating, with acrid and aromatic herbs, because dampness is turbid and difficult to eliminate. Using an herb that induces strong sweating, such as Cinnamomi Ramulus *(guì zhī)* and Ephedrae Herba *(má huáng)*, will not only dispel dampness inefficiently, it will also injure both the qi and yin after the profuse sweating has ended, or even steam dampness to veil the Pericardium, leading to muddled consciousness.

- *Do not purge strongly when there is more dampness than heat.* Since dampness is turbid and cannot be easily eliminated, the use of strong purgatives, such as Rhei Radix et Rhizoma *(dà huáng)* and Natrii Sulfas *(máng xiāo)*, will not only fail to eliminate dampness, but will also injure the yang of the Spleen and Stomach. When these organs function poorly, they will produce even more dampness, as they will be unable to cause the qi to descend and to transform and transport food. The food will ferment into dampness.

- *Be cautious when enriching the yin.* Herbs used to enrich the yin are mostly cloying and readily promote dampness. Clinically, a patient with dampness may present with thirst and fever in the afternoon. This is similar to the presentation seen in individuals with yin deficiency. However, with damp-heat, the excess internal dampness, which is a yin pathogenic factor, will suppress the desire to drink more water. At the same time, the excess internal dampness can block the qi and affect distribution of fluids to the tongue. Thus, these patients will feel thirsty but drink very little water, or none at all. They will also feel feverish in the afternoon but present with a thick or greasy tongue coating, instead of a less than normal coating or none at all, as would be the case with a pattern of yin deficiency.

- *Be cautious when warming and tonifying the qi.* Clinically, the patient with dampness, especially when dampness is predominant, will present with cold extremities, pale face, and fatigue because the qi or yang is obstructed by the dampness and thus cannot properly function to warm the body. As a result, the qi and yang do not reach the face and extremities. However, the use of warm or hot herbs such as Ginseng Radix *(rén shēn)*, Astragali Radix *(huáng qí)*, Epimedii Herba *(yín yáng huò)*, and Morindae officinalis Radix *(bā jǐ tiān)* in such cases should be avoided. Otherwise, more heat will be produced, due to the warm and tonifying nature of the herbs.

OTHER FACTORS

The information above describes the general treatment methods for diseases caused by warm-heat pathogens. However, the practitioner should focus not only on the warm-heat pathogen, which is the initial pathogenic factor, but also on secondary pathogenic factors such as phlegm, food retention, qi stagnation, and blood stasis, which may arise from dysfunction of the yin and yang organs due to an attack by the warm-heat pathogens. How does a warm-heat pathogen cause such secondary factors to arise? The warm-heat pathogen is heat-related. Besides injuring the yin, imagine what else happens after it attacks the body. If it were only a heat-related pathogen, it may affect the circulation of qi in an organ, interfering, for example, with the disseminating and descending functions of the Lung, or the ascending and descending functions of the Spleen and Stomach. The upshot in these cases would be the production of phlegm in the Lung or food retention in the Stomach, respectively. Heat itself can also congeal the fluids in the Lung into phlegm, and cause blood stasis in the vessels. In addition, according to Chapter 5 of *Basic Questions*, extreme fire (heat) will exhaust the qi.[62] For this reason, qi deficiency can arise following an attack by a warm-heat pathogen.

When damp-heat attacks the body, it will likely obstruct the circulation of qi in the Spleen and Liver. This leads to the production of phlegm and Liver qi stagnation.

In those cases where heat predominates, the effects are similar, but milder, to those of a purely warm-heat pathogen. If there is more dampness than heat, the pathogen will more likely injure the qi of the Spleen.

It may be difficult to understand why dampness can give rise to Liver qi stagnation. According to five-phase theory, the relationship between the Liver and Spleen reflects the relationship between wood and earth. They are mutually supportive. That is, decaying wood enriches the earth, and the earth generates healthy wood. If too much dampness resides in the earth, wood cannot flourish. Clinically, patients with dampness are likely to have Liver qi stagnation. Even in the normal and healthy person, humid weather may lead to Liver qi stagnation and feelings of depression or constraint.

These pathogenic factors are not only induced by a warm-heat pathogen. In some cases, they may be present before the attack of the warm-heat pathogen. For example, children who suffer from cough, sore throat, and high fever may have preexisting food retention or phlegm, which can occur if they have a history of consuming too much candy and chocolate, making the digestive system sluggish, and resulting in conditions such as food retention. If the practitioner only pays attention to the warm-heat pathogen without fully considering these other pathogenic factors, especially those with form like phlegm, blood stasis, and food retention, these ignored factors may then act as a 'substrate' to which a warm-heat pathogen can adhere. It may then be very difficult to achieve satisfactory treatment results. Therefore, the following methods are used to treat these four associated pathogenic factors:

1. *Treatment for phlegm.* If an attack of wind-heat or dry-heat congeals the fluids in the Lung, causing phlegm-heat in the Lung with cough, a thick, yellow sputum, and a yellow, greasy tongue coating, add Citri reticulatae Exocarpium rubrum (*jú hóng*), Trichosanthis Pericarpium (*guā lóu pí*), Fritillariae thunbergii Bulbus (*zhè bèi mǔ*), Bambusae Caulis in taeniam (*zhú rú*), and Meretricis/Cyclinae Concha (*gé qiào*) into a formula like Mulberry Leaf and Chrysanthemum Drink (*sāng jú yǐn*)[63] or Mulberry Leaf and Apricot Kernal Decoction (*sāng xìng tāng*),[64] for wind-heat and dry-heat, respectively. For invasion of the Pericardium by extreme heat, leading to stirring of Liver wind and blockage of the spirit of the Heart, as well as congealing of fluids into phlegm with convulsions, coma, a rigid tongue with difficulty speaking, drooling or a rattling sound in the throat, and a deep-red tongue with a yellow and greasy coating, add *Bambusae Concretio silicea* (*tiān zhú huáng*), Bambusae Succus (*zhú lì*), Acori tatarinowii Rhizoma (*shí chāng pǔ*), and Curcumae Radix (*yù jīn*) to a formula to clear heat, extinguish wind, and open the orifices.

2. *Treatment for food retention.* Food retention can occur in two ways:

- It may exist prior to an attack of a warm-heat pathogen. This usually occurs in children or adults who often eat large meals late in the evening.
- It can occur when a patient eats his customary amount of food even after contracting a warm-heat pathogen. Because most of the body's qi is fighting the warm-heat pathogen and the patient stays in bed and is inactive, any food that is eaten will not be fully digested.

The practitioner must determine where the food is retained and choose the appropriate treatment method. If the food is retained in the Stomach and the patient shows distention in the chest and epigastric region, nausea, belching with a foul smell or vomiting of sour, undigested food, epigastric pain, a thick tongue coating, and a slippery pulse, add Crataegi Fructus *(shān zhā)*, Massa medicata fermentata *(shén qū)*, dry-fried Setariae (Oryzae) Fructus germinatus *(chǎo gǔ yá)*, dry-fried Hordei Fructus germinatus *(chǎo mài yá)*, Raphani Semen *(lái fú zǐ)*, Citri reticulatae Pericarpium *(chén pí)*, and Aurantii Fructus *(zhǐ ké)* to a formula that treats the warm-heat pathogen. If the food is retained in the Large Intestine and the patient has distending pain in the abdomen, abdominal bloating, borborygmus, gas, constipation or loose stools with a sour smell, add Arecae Semen *(bīng láng)*, Raphani Semen *(lái fú zǐ)*, Aurantii Fructus *(zhǐ ké)*, Magnoliae officinalis Cortex *(hòu pò)*, and Rhei Radix et Rhizoma *(dà huáng)* to a formula that treats the warm-heat pathogen.

3. *Treatment for Liver qi stagnation.* The signs and symptoms of Liver qi stagnation are sighing, depression, anxiety, and distention in the chest or hypochondriac region. Add *Citri reticulatae viride Pericarpium (qīng pí)*, Aurantii Fructus *(zhǐ ké)*, Bupleuri Radix *(chái hú)*, Cyperi Rhizoma *(xiāng fù)*, Curcumae Radix *(yù jīn)*, and Hordei Fructus germinatus *(mài yá)* to a formula that treats the warm-heat pathogen.

4. *Treatment for blood stasis.* Blood that congeals is a common cause of blood stasis. It may exist prior to an attack by a warm-heat pathogen, or it may be caused, for example, by heat invading the blood chamber during menstruation, or by heat invading the blood vessels. The signs and symptoms of blood stasis are stabbing pain in the chest, hardness and distending pain in the lower abdomen, or purple spots on the skin. If it is located in the chest or hypochondriac region, add *Carthami Flos (hóng huā)*, Salviae miltiorrhizae Radix *(dān shēn)*, Paeoniae Radix rubra *(chì sháo)*, and Moutan Cortex *(mǔ dān pí)* to a formula that treats the warm-heat pathogen. If it is located in the lower burner and the patient experiences a hard and distending pain in the lower abdomen, confusion, and a purple tongue, add Rhei Radix et Rhizoma *(dà huáng)*, Persicae Semen *(táo rén)*, and Moutan Cortex *(mǔ dān pí)* to purge blood stasis and invigorate the blood.

Early in the twentieth century, He Lian-Chen listed several treatments for Spleen qi deficiency in his book *Revised and Expanded Discussion of Warm-Heat Pathogen Diseases.* He said that warm pathogen diseases are most difficult to treat in those with Spleen deficiency:

> Warm-heat [pathogens] are resolved after sweating, clearing, or purging. In those with Spleen deficiency, the exterior cannot make sweat while the interior cannot withstand purging. Or, if they do manage to sweat, the qi will follow the sweat out and be lost; and if they do withstand purging, the qi will go out below and be lost. So if you only use clearing and draining [methods], the middle qi cannot bear it. Frequently the colder the herbs, the more likely it is that the pathogen will remain.[65]

According to He, it is necessary to induce sweating, but it is not necessary to induce much sweating. The practitioner should combine the methods of releasing the exterior with tonifying the Spleen qi, using such herbs as Ginseng Radix *(rén shēn)* and Atractylodis macrocephalae Rhizoma *(bái zhú)*. Also, the use of purging in a patient with Spleen qi deficiency should be done with care. If it is necessary to purge in this situation, this method should be combined with herbs that tonify the Spleen qi, such as Ginseng Radix *(rén shēn)* and Atractylodis macrocephalae Rhizoma *(bái zhú)*. Clearing heat should be combined with herbs like Panacis quinquefolii Radix *(xī yáng shēn)*, Ophiopogonis Radix *(mài mén dōng)*, and honey-toasted Glycyrrhizae Radix preparata *(zhì gān cǎo)* to tonify the qi and enrich the yin.

Also, for best results, consider the patient's diet. Make clear to the patient that foods that add heat to the body, such as deep-fried, spicy, and hot foods, as well as alcohol, must be avoided. Foods that add dampness to the body, such as dairy and raw vegetables, should also be avoided. Cooling foods that support the fluids, such as pears, water chestnuts, and sugar cane juice, are highly recommended. Also, the patient should avoid big meals soon after recovering from a warm pathogen disease because Spleen and Stomach function may not yet be fully back to normal. Eating too much food will cause food retention, creating a substrate to which any residual warm-heat pathogen can attach.

Summary

In this chapter, eleven methods were described for treating warm pathogen diseases. The practitioner should pay particular attention to differentiating and diagnosing the illness before choosing a method of treatment. Accompanying tables set forth the indications and related formulas for each method. Information to assist in using these methods and avoiding side effects was also provided. Finally, general considerations and contraindications that the practitioner should keep in mind when treating warm pathogen diseases (with or without dampness) were noted. These are crucial to clinical success.

Endnotes

1. Tang Da-Lie, *Collection of Papers of Physicians from Wu (Wú yī huì jiǎng)*. Shanghai: Shanghai Science and Technology Publishing House, 1983: 5.

2. Zhao Shao-Qin, "'Sweating for the protective level' is not a method to induce sweating *(Zài wèi hàn zhī kě yě bìng fēi yíng yòng hàn fǎ)*," in Fang Yao-Zhong and Xu Jia-Song (eds.), *Collection of Lectures on Warm Pathogen Diseases (Wēn bìng huì jiǎng)*. Beijing: People's Health Publishing House, 1986: 65. See also Zhao Shao-Qin, Hu Ding-Bang, Liu Jing-Yuan, *Length and Breadth of Warm Pathogen Disease [Differentiation] (Wēn bìng zòng héng)*. Beijing: Beijing College of Traditional Chinese Medicine, 1979: 235.

3. Dai Tian-Zhang, *Discussion of Widespread Warm Epidemics (Guǎng wēn yì lùn)*, in Cao Bing-Zhang (ed.), *Compendium of Medicine in China (Zhōng guó yī xué dà chéng)*. Shanghai: Shanghai Science and Technology Publishing House, 1990, Chapter 4: 1.

4. Inducing sweating here is a treatment approach and is not a result of the treatment.

5. Meng Shu-Jiang et al., *Teaching Reference Books for Traditional Chinese Medical Colleges: Warm Pathogen Diseases (Gāo děng zhōng yī yuàn xiào jiào xué cān kǎo shū: wēn bìng xué)*. Beijing: People's Health Publishing House, 1989: 101.

6. Tang Da-Lie, *Collection of Papers of Physicians from Wu*, 5.

7. Zhao Shao-Qin et al., *Length and Breadth of Warm Pathogen Disease [Differentiation]*, 235.

8. Tang Da-Lie, *Collection of Papers of Physicians from Wu*, 5.

9. Ibid.

10. Meng Shu-Jiang, "Discussion of several issues on warm pathogen disease *(Dui wen bing xue zhong you guan wen it de tao lun)*," in Fang Yao-Zhong and Xu Jia-Song (eds.), *Collection of Lectures on Warm Pathogen Diseases*, 145.

11. Wu Tang, *Systematic Differentiation of Warm Pathogen Diseases (Wēn bìng tiáo biàn)*. Beijing: People's Health Publishing House, 1963: 176.

12. Ibid.

13. Ibid.

14. Zhang Zhi- Wen, personal communication, 1980.

15. The Asian pear peel is sweet, astringent, and cool and enters the Lung and Heart channels. It clears heat from the Heart and moistens the Lungs while also generating fluids. It is used for thirst and restlessness due to attacks of summerheat along with cough, vomiting of blood, carbuncles, and boils. The dosage of the dried product is 9-15g; for the fresh product it is 30-60g.

16. Both of these formulas are discussed in Chapter 7.

17. Tang Da-Lie, *Collection of Papers of Physicians from Wu*, 11.

18. The term 'blood chamber' first appeared in paragraph 148 of *Discussion of Cold Damage*. The real meaning of blood chamber as used in this classic is uncertain, and is controversial to this day. It is clear that it is located in the lower burner and is somehow related to

menstruation. Three interpretations are most commonly accepted. The first is by the Ming dynasty writer Zhang Jie-Bin (Zhang Jing-Yue, 1563-1640), who wrote in *Appendices to the Classified Classic (Lèi jīng fù yì)* that the blood chamber referred to the Womb. The second interpretation is by Ke Qin (Ke Yun-Bo), who wrote in his late seventeenth-century book *Collected Writings on Renewal of the Discussion of Cold Damage (Shāng hán lái sū jí)* that the term referred to the Liver. The third interpretation is by Xiao Gen-Liu (Xiao Shen-Zhai), who wrote in his 1684 book *Records of Experiences with Women's Diseases (Nǔ kē jīng lùn)* that the term was synonymous with the Penetrating vessel, because the Penetrating vessel is also called the 'sea of blood.'

19. This complex can also result in a sudden cessation of menstruation, if it occurs during menstruation, or delirium or muddled consciousness with distending pain in the lower abdomen and a purple and deep-red tongue. In such cases, the practitioner can use a modification of Minor Bupleurum Decoction *(xiǎo chái hú tāng)* which clears heat, cools blood, and promotes blood circulation. This was formulated by Tao Hua, author of *Six Texts on Cold Damage (Shāng hán liù shū)*, and contains Bupleuri Radix *(chái hú)*, Pinelliae Rhizoma preparatum *(zhì bàn xià)*, Scutellariae Radix *(huáng qín)*, Zingiberis Rhizoma recens *(shēng jiāng)*, honey-toasted Glycyrrhizae Radix preparata *(zhì gān cǎo)*, Rehmanniae Radix *(shēng dì huáng)*, Persicae Semen *(táo rén)*, Crataegi Fructus *(shān zhā)*, and Moutan Cortex *(mǔ dān pí)* or Rhinocerotis Cornu *(xī jiǎo)*.

20. Wang Shi-Xiong, *Warp and Woof of Warm-Heat Pathogen Diseases (Wēn rè jīng wěi)*, reproduced in Lu Zhen, *Collected Rare Recent Books on Chinese Medicine: Warm Pathogen Disease Section (Jīn dài zhōng yī zhēn běn jí: wēn bìng fēn cè)*. Hangzhou: Zhejiang Science and Technology Publishing House, 1987: 80.

21. I would have to disagree with this, as in these situations the first thing to be done is to clear the heat.

22. Zhao Shao-Qin et al., *Length and Breadth of Warm Pathogen Disease [Differentiation]*, 271.

23. Class notes from Chengdu College of Traditional Chinese Medicine, 1980.

24. Yu Gen-Chu, *Revised Popular Guide to the Discussion of Cold Damage (Chóng ding tōng sú shāng hán lùn)*. Hangzhou: New Medicine Press, 1956: 94. See Chapter 7 for further discussion of White Tiger Decoction *(bái hǔ tāng)*.

25. Ibid., 95.

26. He Lian-Chen, *Revised and Expanded Discussion of Warm-Heat Pathogen Diseases (Chóng dìng guǎng wēn rè lùn)*. Beijing: People's Health Publishing House, 1960: 161.

27. Wu Tang, *Systematic Differentiation of Warm Pathogen Diseases*, 74.

28. The term membrane source (膜原 *mó yuán*) has two meanings. The first refers to the place between the pleura and diaphragm, as recorded in Chapter 39 of *Basic Questions (Sù wèn)*. The second is a special term that refers to a half-exterior and half-interior condition in a warm pathogen disease. This second meaning emerged in *Discussion of Warm Epidemics (Wēn yì lùn)*, written by Wu You-Xing. However, it was still used ambiguously until Xue Xue explained it further in his book *Systematic Differentiation of Damp-Heat (Shī rè tiáo biàn)*: "The membrane source is located between the Stomach and the muscle layer. It reaches the muscles externally and the Stomach internally, and is the gate of the Triple Burner...It is in the half-exterior and half-interior part of the body." This passage can

be found in Song Zhao-Qi, *Distinguishing [Aspects] of Southern Diseases (Nán bìng bié jiàn)*. Shanghai: Shanghai Health Publishing House, 1958: 3. Interestingly enough, while all of these texts provide a name and location for the membrane source and discuss its pathology, they are silent as to its physiologic functions.

29. Wu Tang, *Systematic Differentiation of Warm Pathogen Diseases*, 102.

30. Ibid., 40. See Chapter 12 for further details.

31. Ibid.

32. Qin Bo-Wei, *Medical Lecture Notes of [Qin] Qian-Zhai (Qiān-Zhāi yī xué jiǎng gǎo)*. Shanghai: Shanghai Science and Technology Publishing House, 1964: 68.

33. Ye Chuan et al., *Collection of the Famous Works by Four Outstanding Physicians of the Jin and Yuan Dynasties (Jīn Yuán sì dà yī xué jiā míng zhù jí chéng)*. Beijing: China Publishing House of Traditional Chinese Medicine, 1995: 444.

34. Liu Bao-Yi, *Encountering the Sources of Warm-Heat Pathogen Diseases (Wēn rè féng yuán)*. Beijing: People's Health Publishing House, 1959: 66.

35. Dai Tian-Zhang, *Discussion of Widespread Warm Epidemics (Guǎng wēn yì lùn)*, reproduced in Cao Bing-Zhang (ed.), *Compendium of Medicine in China (Zhōng guó yī xué dà chéng)*. Shanghai: Shanghai Science and Technology Publishing House, 1990: 3-4.

36. Class notes, Chengdu College of Traditional Chinese Medicine, 1980.

37. Tang Da-Lie, *Collection of Papers of Physicians from Wu*, 6.

38. Wu Tang, *Systematic Differentiation of Warm Pathogen Diseases*, 65.

39. Ibid., 64, 70.

40. The first two methods treat a similar problem, which is simultaneous phlegm-heat in the upper burner and accumulation of heat in the Large Intestine. However, there is a slight difference. In the first method the phlegm-heat is located in the Lung, and in the second method in the chest.

41. See Chapter 7 for further details.

42. Yu Gen-Chu, *Revised Popular Guide to the Discussion of Cold Damage*, 68. This formula consists of Natrii Sulfas *(máng xiāo)* (3g), Kansui Radix *(gān suì)* (2.4g), Lepidii/ Descurainiae Semen *(tíng lì zǐ)* (4.5g), Menthae haplocalycis Herba *(bò hé)* (4.5g), Rhei Radix et Rhizoma *(dà huáng)* (3g), Sinapis Semen *(bái jiè zǐ)* (2.4g), Gardeniae Fructus *(zhī zǐ)* (9g), Forsythiae Fructus *(lián qiào)* (4.5g), Aurantii Fructus immaturus *(zhǐ shí)* (4.5g), Bambusae Succus *(zhú lì)* (two spoonfuls), Zingiberis Rhizomatis Succus *(jiāng zhī)* (two drops). For more information about Cool the Diaphragm Powder *(liáng gé sǎn)* on which this is based, see Chapter 7.

43. Ibid., 64. This formula consists of Gypsum fibrosum *(shí gāo)* (24g), Rhei Radix et Rhizoma *(dà huáng)* (9g), Glycyrrhizae Radix *(gān cǎo)* (2.4g), Anemarrhenae Rhizoma *(zhī mǔ)* (12g), Natrii Sulfas *(máng xiāo)* (6g), and nonglutinous rice *(gěng mǐ)* (9g).

44. Ibid., 65. This formula consists of Lonicerae Flos *(jīn yín huā)* (9g), Gardeniae Fructus *(zhī zǐ)* (9g), Coptidis Rhizoma *(huáng lián)* (3g), Phellodendri Cortex *(huáng bǎi)* (3g), Forsythiae Fructus *(lián qiào)* (9g), Scutellariae Radix *(huáng qín)* (6g), Aurantii Fructus immaturus *(zhǐ shí)* (6g), Rhei Radix et Rhizoma *(dà huáng)* (9g), Natrii Sulfas *(máng xiāo)* (1.5g), Succus Faecalis Aureus *(jīn zhī)* (30g), and Pheretima *(dì lóng)* (two pieces).

45. He Lian-Chen, *Revised and Expanded Discussion of Warm-Heat Pathogen Diseases*, 88. This formula consists of Rhinocerotis Cornu *(xī jiǎo)* (3g), Rehmanniae Radix *(shēng dì huáng)* (45g), Rhei Radix et Rhizoma *(dà huáng)* (9g), Coptidis Rhizoma *(huáng lián)* (3g), and Scutellariae Radix *(huáng qín)* (6g). At present, Bubali Cornu *(shuǐ niú jiǎo)* (18g) should be substituted for Rhinocerotis Cornu *(xī jiǎo)*.

46. Wu Tang, *Systematic Differentiation of Warm Pathogen Diseases*, 68. See Chapter 8 for further details.

47. Tang Da-Lie, *Collection of Papers of Physicians from Wu*, 5.

48. Warm Pathogen Disease Teaching and Research Section of Chengdu College of Traditional Chinese Medicine, *Self-Study Textbook for Chinese Medicine: Warm Pathogen Diseases (Zhōng yī zì xué jiào cái: Wēn bìng xué)*. Chengdu: Chengdu College of Traditional Chinese Medicine, 1985: 38.

49. Zhao Shao-Qin, "On the treatment for venting heat from the nutritive level to the qi level *(Lùn rù yíng yǒu kě tòu rè zhuǎn qì)*," in Fang Yao-Zhong and Xu Jia-Song (eds.), *Collection of Lectures on Warm Pathogen Diseases (Wēn bìng huì jiǎng)*. Beijing: People's Health Publishing House, 1986: 72.

50. Zhao Shao-Qin et al., *Length and Breadth of Warm Pathogen Disease [Differentiation]*, 236.

51. This is made by fermenting a combination of Pinelliae Rhizoma preparatum *(zhì bàn xià)*, wheat flour, and fresh ginger juice, Zingiberis Rhizomatis Succus *(jiāng zhī)*. It is bitter, acrid and neutral. It resolves phlegm, stops vomiting, and promotes digestion for food retention.

52. Zhu Zhen-Heng, *Teachings of [Zhu] Dan-Xi (Dān-Xī xīn fǎ)*, reproduced in *Collection of Works from [Zhu] Dan-Xi (Dān-Xī yī jí)*. Beijing: People's Health Publishing House, 1993: 349. This formula consists of Crataegi Fructus *(shān zhā)* (18g), Massa medicata fermentata *(shén qū)* (6g), Pinelliae Rhizoma preparatum *(zhì bàn xià)* (9g), Poria *(fú líng)* (9g), Citri reticulatae Pericarpium *(chén pí)* (3g), Forsythiae Fructus *(lián qiào)* (3g), and Raphani Semen *(lái fú zǐ)* (3g).

53. Zhao Shao-Qin, "On the treatment for venting heat from the nutritive level to the qi level," 75.

54. Warm Pathogen Disease Teaching and Research Section of Chengdu College of Traditional Chinese Medicine, *Self-Study Textbook for Chinese Medicine: Warm Pathogen Diseases*, 39.

55. Currently, this method is also being widely applied in China to treat dementia caused by blood stasis and phlegm, wind-stroke due to stirring of Liver wind with phlegm and blood stasis, and severe epileptic attack.

56. He Lian-Chen, *Revised and Expanded Discussion of Warm-Heat Pathogen Diseases*, 125. It contains Gypsum fibrosum *(shí gāo)* (18g), Anemarrhenae Rhizoma *(zhī mǔ)* (12g), Chrysanthemi Flos *(jú huā)* (9g), Uncariae Ramulus cum Uncis *(gōu téng)* (4.5g), Glycyrrhizae Radix *(gān cǎo)* (1.8g), nonglutinous rice *(gěng mǐ)* (9g), Rhinocerotis Cornu *(xī jiǎo)* (3g), and Saigae tataricae Cornu *(líng yáng jiǎo)* (4.5g).

57. Zhang Ji, *Discussion of Cold Damage (Shāng hán lùn)*. Beijing: People's Health Publishing House, 1983: 10. This formula consists of Rhei Radix et Rhizoma *(dà huáng)* (12g),

Glycyrrhizae Radix *(gān cǎo)* (6g), and Natrii Sulfas *(máng xiāo)* (9-12g). See Chapter 7 for further details.

58. Wu Tang, *Systematic Differentiation of Warm Pathogen Diseases*, 22. This formula consists of Rhinocerotis Cornu *(xī jiǎo)* (9g), Rehmanniae Radix *(shēng dì huáng)* (9g), Scrophulariae Radix *(xuán shēn)* (9g), Lophatheri Herba *(dàn zhú yè)* (3g), Ophiopogonis Radix *(mài mén dōng)* (9g), Salviae miltiorrhizae Radix *(dān shēn)* (6g), Coptidis Rhizoma *(huáng lián)* (4.5g), Lonicerae Flos *(jīn yín huā)* (9g), and Forsythiae Fructus *(lián qiào)* (6g). See Chapter 7 for further details.

59. According to Zhang Zhi-Wen, a professor at Chengdu University of Traditional Chinese Medicine, this formula is also useful for treating the sequelae of encephalitis B. (Class notes, 1980). Three-Shell Powder *(sān jiǎ sǎn)* was first recorded in Wu You-Xing, *Discussion of Warm Epidemics (Wēn yì lùn)*. Liaoning: Liaoning Science and Technology Publishing House, 1997: 23. See Chapter 11 for further details.

60. Liu Bao-Yi, *Encountering the Sources of Warm-Heat Pathogen Diseases*, 64, 65.

61. Meng Shu-Jiang et al., *Warm Pathogen Diseases (Wēn bìng xué)*. Shanghai: Shanghai Science and Technology Publishing House, 1985: 35.

62. Anonymous, *Yellow Emperor's Inner Classic: Basic Questions (Huáng Dì nèi jīng sù wèn)*. Beijing: People's Health Publishing House, 1963: 33.

63. Wu Tang, *Systematic Differentiation of Warm Pathogen Diseases*, 18. This formula consists of Armeniacae Semen *(xìng rén)* (6g), Forsythiae Fructus *(lián qiào)* (4.5g), Menthae haplocalycis Herba *(bò hé)* (2.4g), Mori Folium *(sāng yè)* (7.5g), Chrysanthemi Flos *(jú huā)* (3g), Platycodi Radix *(jié gěng)* (6g), Glycyrrhizae Radix *(gān cǎo)* (2.4g), and Phragmitis Rhizoma *(lú gēn)* (6g). See Chapter 7 for further details.

64. Wu Tang, *Systematic Differentiation of Warm Pathogen Diseases*, 45. This formula consists of Mori Folium *(sāng yè)* (3g), Armeniacae Semen *(xìng rén)* (4.5g), Glehniae/Adenophorae Radix *(shā shēn)* (6g), Fritillariae thunbergii Bulbus *(zhè bèi mǔ)* (6g), Sojae Semen preparatum *(dàn dòu chǐ)* (3g), Gardeniae Epicarpium *(shān zhī pí)* (3g), and Pyri Exocarpium *(lí pí)* (3g). See Chapter 9 for further details.

65. He Lian-Chen, *Revised and Expanded Discussion of Warm-Heat Pathogen Diseases*, 45.

Differentiation and Treatment of Warm Pathogen Diseases

Section A – Warm-Heat Pathogen Diseases

A S NOTED IN Chapter 2 of Part One, warm pathogen diseases can be divided into two categories:

1. Warm-heat pathogen diseases caused by a warm-heat pathogen without dampness
2. Damp-heat diseases caused by a warm-heat pathogen with dampness.

Generally speaking, warm-heat pathogen diseases tend to injure the yin or fluids and readily invade the nutritive and blood levels. By contrast, damp-heat diseases tend to present with qi stagnation, water retention, and accumulation of dampness in one or more of the burners. Clinically, it is uncommon for a patient with a damp-heat disease to present with a purely protective level condition in its early stage. Similarly, nutritive and blood level patterns will usually not occur unless the damp-heat transforms into dry-heat. Therefore, while it is wise to use the different diagnostic schemes flexibly and in concert, it is quite common for practitioners to rely primarily on four-level differentiation for warm-heat pathogen diseases, and three-burner differentiation for damp-heat diseases.

Warm-heat pathogen diseases include wind-warmth, spring-warmth, autumn-dryness, and warm-toxin. In general, we can use cool or cold herbs to treat these disorders. It is important, however, that you choose a treatment method based on four-level differentiation. Overall, for protective level patterns, use acrid and cool herbs to disperse warm-heat pathogens. For qi level patterns, use sweet and cold or bitter and cold herbs to clear the interior heat. For nutritive level patterns, clear the heat, cool the blood, and enrich the yin with herbs that vent heat from the nutritive level. And for blood level patterns, cool the blood, promote the circulation of blood, and enrich the yin. For additional information on the selection of treatment methods, see Chapter 6.

7 Wind-Warmth

W IND-WARMTH (風溫 *fēng wēn*) is caused by an attack of the wind-heat pathogen (風熱 *fēng rè*) during the spring or winter.[1] Initially, it is characterized by signs and symptoms related to the protective level and the Lung including fever, slight chills, aversion to cold, cough, and slight thirst. If it occurs in winter, usually due to unseasonably warm weather, it is referred to as winter-warmth (冬溫 *dōng wēn*). Biomedical diseases such as influenza, lobar pneumonia, and acute bronchitis overlap somewhat with the Chinese medical diagnosis of wind-warmth, and can be treated with the same methods.

Etiology and Pathology

The etiology of wind-warmth is an attack on the body by an exogenous wind-heat pathogen. Both wind and heat are yang pathogens characterized by upward and outward dispersion. The nose and mouth are situated in the upper or yang aspect of the body, and are thus prone to attack by wind-heat. The Lung opens through the nose and is therefore the first yin organ that is subject to attack. Because the Lung governs the protective qi and the skin and hair, an invasion of the Lung by wind-heat will necessarily involve the surface of the body, resulting in stagnation of the protective qi as well as the Lung qi.

Practically speaking, there are actually two pathologies and two distinct clini-

193

cal manifestations in early-stage disease: sometimes the wind-heat mainly attacks the protective level and sometimes it mainly attacks the Lung. In the first case, wind-heat attacks the protective layer, leading to stagnation of the protective qi. This, in turn, leads to a struggle between antipathogenic qi and wind-heat resulting in fever, slight chills, aversion to cold, headache, absent or slight sweating, and a floating, rapid pulse. In the second case, the disease is located in both the exterior and the Lung, but is focused in the Lung. The pathology is failure of the Lung qi to disseminate and descend as a result of an attack by wind-heat. Cough is the main symptom, coupled with slight fever and chills.

Factors for Identifying Wind-Warmth

There are three important factors to consider in identifying wind-warmth:

1. *Time of year.* If a warm pathogen disease appears in the spring or winter, the practitioner should consider the presence of wind-warmth.

2. *Signs and symptoms.* The main signs and symptoms relate to the Lung and protective level. In the early stage these include fever, aversion to cold, chills, cough, thirst, and a floating and rapid pulse. These may be followed by the appearance of a qi level pattern, such as accumulation of heat in the Lung, and at an even later stage by injury to the Lung and Stomach yin.

3. *Correct diagnosis of the illness.* Carefully differentiate between wind-warmth and spring-warmth since they share certain traits. (See Chapter 8 for further discussion of spring-warmth.)

Since so many organs can be involved in wind-warmth, once a diagnosis is made, it is very important to pinpoint its location. Otherwise there will be no clear target, and treatment will be ineffective.

As noted, in the early stage of wind-warmth only the protective qi and Lung are involved, leading to chills, aversion to cold, fever, sneezing, nasal congestion, headache, and cough. The practitioner must determine the predominant site of the attack. If it is the protective qi, exterior signs and symptoms (chills, aversion to cold, fever) will be paramount. Conversely, if the main focus of attack is the Lung, cough will be paramount. In some cases the Triple Burner or Gallbladder channels may be involved, leading to ear problems such as itching, pain, a plugged sensation, or diminished hearing.

If the pathogen has reached the qi level, one must identify whether the Lung, Stomach, or Large Intestine is involved. If it is the Lung, the main manifestations will be cough and wheezing or dyspnea. If it is the Stomach, the main manifestations will be irritability, profuse sweating, and thirst because heat opens the pores and forces fluids out through the skin. If it is the Large Intestine, the main manifestations will be tidal fever and either constipation with hard and dry stools or a discharge of intensely foul-smelling liquid.

Should heat progress directly to the Pericardium, one must determine if it is causing an interior blockage of the Heart or an exterior collapse of yang qi. Interior blockage of the Heart will present with muddled consciousness, stiffness of the tongue with difficulty speaking, and a feverish chest and abdomen. Exterior collapse of yang qi may present with muddled consciousness (or, if severe, coma), cold extremities, profuse cold sweat, weak voice, and a very submerged and faint pulse.

Progression of Wind-Warmth

Once correctly diagnosed, the next important step is to determine the progression. Two distinct pathogenic factors cause wind-warmth: wind and heat. Since they are both yang pathogenic factors, wind-warmth progresses rather quickly. It is important to understand how the disease is progressing so that treatment can be provided in a timely manner, thereby preventing further progression. There are two modes of progression for wind-warmth: normal and abnormal (see also Chapter 4).

NORMAL PROGRESSION

In the normal progression, the wind-heat pathogen progresses from the protective to the qi level, primarily affecting the Lung, Stomach, and Large Intestine. It is easy to understand why the Lung is susceptible to wind-heat since it is the most superficial of the yin organs, and is regarded as the 'delicate' organ in Chinese medicine. But why does wind-heat so easily attack the Stomach and Large Intestine? In traditional Chinese medical theory the tissue corresponding to the Stomach is muscle. When wind-heat progresses from the skin to the muscles and flesh, it will directly affect the Stomach, which is the organ associated with muscle tissue. Finally, since the Lung is paired with the Large Intestine, an attack by wind-heat on the skin or the Lung can readily progress to the Large Intestine.

To fully understand the progression of wind-warmth one must be familiar with common qi-level patterns caused by an attack of wind-heat. One pattern is heat from excess in the Stomach characterized by vigorous fever, profuse sweating, and thirst with a preference for cold beverages, and a flooding and big pulse. Another pattern is clumping of dry stool and heat in the Large Intestine, which manifests as tidal fever, delirium, dry and hard stool in the Large Intestine that leads to a discharge of foul water, a dark-yellow tongue coating, and a submerged and forceful pulse. In addition, when wind-heat reaches the interior of the body, wind transforms into heat.

This is because wind blocks qi circulation, and the resulting constraint leads to heat. Therefore, when wind-heat invades the qi level, the heat may injure the yin of the Lung and Stomach, resulting in cough with little sputum, dry throat and mouth, thirst, and a red tongue with less than normal coating. If the heat is not quickly dispelled, it may invade the lower burner and exhaust the Liver and Kidney yin.

But a note of caution: A patient with a qi-level pattern may not necessarily manifest any of these typical signs and symptoms at the very onset of the illness. It is therefore extremely important to detect the initial signs and symptoms in order to identify the progression from the protective to the qi level as early as possible. If this is done, the patient can be treated in such a way that the disease does not progress but resolves relatively quickly. In general, if the patient is thirsty and prefers cold beverages, and has a yellow tongue coating, the illness is progressing from the protective to the qi level. One should not wait for the full presentation of each pattern before initiating treatment. This will lead to poor results because heat will have already damaged the yin or fluids, and the treatment regimen will be more difficult and prolonged.

ABNORMAL PROGRESSION

In the abnormal progression, heat progresses directly from the protective to the nutritive or blood level, or from the Lung to the Pericardium or Heart, without first progressing to the qi level (here the qi level refers to organs other than the Lung). The signs and symptoms reflecting involvement of the Pericardium or Heart include muddled consciousness or coma, delirium, cold extremities, and stiffness of the tongue with difficulty speaking. In such cases the wind-heat pathogen stays in the Lung for only a very short time, and manifestations of the Lung qi's inability to descend and disseminate are present for only a day or two, especially in children. Why then does the wind-heat pathogen invade the Pericardium or the Heart so easily? According to Ye Gui in *Discussion of Warm-Heat Disorders,* "If a patient has constitutional weakness of the Heart coupled with phlegm, when a warm-heat pathogen attacks the body it will attack this weak place, leading to blockage of the Pericardium by transmission of heat."[2] In this case, weakness of the Heart refers to Heart qi or yin deficiency.

Another example of abnormal progression is the onset of rashes as a result of heat invading the collaterals of the Lung, forcing blood from the vessels. There are two different manifestations of this disorder. In the first there is no cough, just bleeding from rashes or the nose. In the second there is cough coupled with bleeding and thirst. Generally, the presence of papules, which relate to the Lung, or maculas, which relate to the Stomach, are indicative of a qi level pattern. However, the presence of bleeding indicates that the pattern is at the blood level (see Table 7.1).

Table 7.1	Progression and Clinical Manifestations of Wind-Warmth	
Transmission Type	**Sample Patterns**	**Clinical Manifestations**
NORMAL PROGRESSION		
Progression to the qi level	Heat from excess in the Stomach	Vigorous fever, profuse sweating, severe thirst, flooding pulse
	Clumping of dry stool, heat in the Large Intestine	Tidal fever, delirium, constipation or discharge of foul-smelling liquid per rectum, dark-yellow tongue coating, submerged, forceful pulse
ABNORMAL PROGRESSION		
Progression directly to the Pericardium	Veiling of the Pericardium by heat and phlegm	Muddled consciousness or coma, delirium, cold extremities, stiff, dark-red tongue with difficulty speaking

Treatment Principles

There are four treatment principles, each of which is based on a different stage in the progression of wind-warmth:

1. In the early stage the focus should be on dispersing wind-heat with acrid and cool herbs. Use the method of eliminating the exterior condition by dispelling exterior wind and dispersing exterior heat with such herbs as Lophatheri Herba *(dàn zhú yè)*, Arctii Fructus *(niú bàng zǐ)*, and Lonicerae Flos *(jīn yín huā)*. To prevent these cold herbs from causing the pores to congeal, add one or two mildly acrid and warm herbs, such as Schizonepetae Herba *(jīng jiè)* or Sojae Semen preparatum *(dàn dòu chǐ)*, when it is prepared with Ephedrae Herba *(má huáng)*.

2. In the middle stage it is desirable to combine three methods. The first is to clear heat from the qi level with acrid and cold herbs such as Gypsum fibrosum *(shí gāo)* and Phragmitis Rhizoma *(lú gēn)*. The second is to clear and drain fire with bitter and cold herbs such as Scutellariae Radix *(huáng qín)* and Coptidis Rhizoma *(huáng lián)*. The third is to drain the heat out through the bowels by purging with bitter and salty cold herbs such as Rhei Radix et Rhizoma *(dà huáng)* and Natrii Sulfas *(máng xiāo)*.

3. At a later stage, or when the patient is experiencing the "remnants of heat" (*yú rè*),[3] the practitioner should clear heat, enrich yin, and generate fluids with sweet and cold herbs[4] such as Glehniae/Adenophorae Radix *(shā shēn)*, Ophiopogonis Radix *(mài mén dōng)*, Rehmanniae Radix *(shēng dì huáng)*, and Scrophulariae Radix *(xuán shēn)*.

4. If the wind-heat has progressed directly to the Pericardium, the heat should be cleared and the orifices opened as quickly as possible with aromatic, bitter, and cold herbs such as Bovis Calculus *(niú huáng)*, Borneolum *(bīng piàn)*, Rhinocerotis Cornu *(xī jiǎo)*, Lophatheri Herba *(dàn zhú yè)*, Salviae miltiorrhizae Radix *(dān shēn)*, Coptidis Rhizoma *(huáng lián)*, and Forsythiae Fructus *(lián qiào)*.

Differentiation and Treatment of Wind-Warmth in the Protective Level

ATTACK ON THE PROTECTIVE LEVEL BY WIND-HEAT THAT SLIGHTLY AFFECTS THE LUNG

Manifestations. There are two concurrent aspects to this pattern:[5]

1. *Attack on the protective level and exterior by wind-heat* with fever, slight chills and aversion to cold, absent or slight sweating, slight thirst, headache, red tip and edge of the tongue with a thin, white coating, and a floating, rapid pulse.

2. *Failure of the Lung qi to disseminate and descend due to an attack of wind-heat* with cough.

NOTE: Among these signs and symptoms the fever, slight chills and aversion to cold, cough, red tip and edge of the tongue and white coating, and the floating, rapid pulse are the key points of identification for the pattern of attack on the protective level by wind-heat that slightly affects the Lung. Since this pattern is in certain respects similar to wind-cold attacking the *tai yang,* as described in *Discussion of Cold Damage (Shāng hán lùn)*, differentiating between the two is important (see Table 7.2).

Pathology. Wind-heat attacking the protective level leads to stagnation of the protective qi. In addition, the attack affects the Lungs slightly, leading to failure of the Lung qi to disseminate and descend. In this pattern, exterior signs and symptoms in the protective level predominate.

Table 7.2	Comparison of Wind-Heat Attacking Protective Level vs. Wind-Cold Attacking *Tai Yang*		
Pathology	**Common Signs & Symptoms**	**Differences**	**Treatment**
Stagnation of protective qi and failure of Lung qi to disseminate and descend due to attack of wind-heat	Fever, aversion to cold, absent or slight sweating, headache, floating pulse	Attack on protective level by wind-heat that slightly affects the Lung: fever predominates with mild chills, slight thirst, cough, red tongue tip, rapid pulse	Release the exterior with acrid and cool herbs, and disseminate Lung qi
Disharmony between protective and nutritive qi, obstruction of *tai yang* Bladder channel		Wind-cold attacking *tai yang*: chills predominate with no thirst, floating and moderate or tight pulse	Release the exterior with acrid and warm herbs, harmonize nutritive and protective qi, and promote sweating

Treatment principles. Release the exterior with acrid and cool herbs, and disseminate the Lung qi with herbs that are light in weight. Although there may be a cough, this pattern constitutes only a mild attack on the Lung. Therefore, treatment need only disseminate the Lung qi in order to distribute the protective qi to the exterior and alleviate the cough.

Formula:

HONEYSUCKLE AND FORSYTHIA POWDER *(yín qiào sǎn)*

SOURCE: *Systematic Differentiation of Warm Pathogen Diseases*

Lonicerae Flos *(jīn yín huā)* 30g
Forsythiae Fructus *(lián qiào)* 30g
Platycodi Radix *(jié gěng)* 18g
Menthae haplocalycis Herba *(bò hé)* 18g
Lophatheri Herba *(dàn zhú yè)* 12g
Glycyrrhizae Radix *(gān cǎo)* 15g
Schizonepetae Herba *(jīng jiè)* 12g
Sojae Semen preparatum *(dàn dòu chǐ)* 15g
Arctii Fructus *(niú bàng zǐ)* 18g
Phragmitis Rhizoma *(lú gēn)* 15–30g

ANALYSIS OF FORMULA: This important and popular formula treats attack on the exterior by wind-heat. Schizonepetae Herba *(jīng jiè)*, Sojae Semen preparatum *(dàn dòu chǐ)*, and Menthae haplocalycis Herba *(bò hé)* release the exterior through *slight* sweating. Lonicerae Flos *(jīn yín huā)*, Forsythiae Fructus *(lián qiào)*, and Lophatheri Herba *(dàn zhú yè)* clear heat and let it exit from the exterior following diaphoresis. Arctii Fructus *(niú bàng zǐ)*, Glycyrrhizae Radix *(gān cǎo)*, and Platycodi Radix *(jié gěng)* together disseminate the Lung qi. Phragmitis Rhizoma *(lú gēn)* is commonly used to generate fluids and alleviate thirst.

MODIFICATIONS: This is a very common disorder that presents with a multitude of permutations. The basic formula can be modified as follows:

- For exterior cold and interior heat (fever, chills, aversion to cold, severe headache, general body aches, lack of sweating, thirst, yellow urine, red tongue tip), add Ephedrae Herba *(má huáng)* if there is no sweating and Saposhnikoviae Radix *(fáng fēng)* for the general body aches. Together these herbs dispel exterior cold by opening the skin pores and thereby allowing it to exit the body. No more than 6g of either Ephedrae Herba *(má huáng)* and Saposhnikoviae Radix *(fáng fēng)* should be added. If too large a dosage is used, the sweating may be excessive, which can severely damage the fluids.

- For wind-heat attacking the Lung, Liver, and Gallbladder channels (runny nose, sneezing, nasal congestion, plugged sensation in the ears, itchy eyes), add Chrysanthemi Flos *(jú huā)*, Scutellariae Radix *(huáng qín)*, Magnoliae Flos *(xīn yí)*, and Bupleuri Radix *(chái hú)*.

- For wind-heat and dampness attacking the exterior (pain and a heavy sensation throughout the body), add Gentianae macrophyllae Radix *(qín jiāo)*, Mori Ramulus *(sāng zhī)*, and Atractylodis Rhizoma *(cāng zhú)* to eliminate exogenous dampness.

- For an attack of wind-heat on both the Lung and protective qi associated with stagnation of endogenous dampness in the middle burner (nausea or vomiting, chest distention, thick and greasy tongue coating), add Pogostemonis/Agastaches Herba *(huò xiāng)* and Curcumae Radix *(yù jīn)* to resolve the interior dampness.

- For combined exogenous and endogenous dampness (contained fever, chest and epigastric distention, yellow urine, greasy tongue coating), add Artemisiae annuae Herba *(qīng hāo)*, Pogostemonis/Agastaches Herba *(huò xiāng)*, Artemisiae scopariae Herba *(yīn chén)*, and Talcum *(huá shí)*.

- For an attack on the throat by heat and toxin that has transformed from wind-heat in the Lung and protective level (swelling and pain in the throat), add herbs to clear heat, resolve toxicity, and relieve the swollen throat, such as Lasiosphaera/Calvatia *(mǎ bó)* and Scrophulariae Radix *(xuán shēn)*. This method was formulated by Wu Tang in *Systematic Differentiation of Warm Pathogen Diseases (Wēn bìng tiáo biàn).*[6] Isatidis Folium *(dà qīng yè)* and Isatidis/ Baphicacanthis Radix *(bǎn lán gēn)* are also effective for treating sore throat due to heat and toxin. If the patient feels severe pain locally and the tonsils look red and swollen, add warm herbs with an acrid flavor to promote blood circulation. According to the early twentieth-century physician He Lian-Chen (He Bing-Yuan) in *Revised and Expanded Discussion of Warm-Heat Pathogen Diseases (Chóng dìng guǎng wēn rè lùn),* these types of herbs will prevent the stagnation of blood circulation that would otherwise be caused by acrid and cool or cold herbs.[7] In my experience, herbs that are useful for this purpose are Persicae Semen *(táo rén)* and *Carthami Flos (hóng huā).*

- For invasion of the blood by heat (out-of-control bleeding including epistaxis), avoid herbs that are either warm or ascending, such as Schizonepetae Herba *(jīng jiè),* Sojae Semen preparatum *(dàn dòu chǐ),* and Platycodi Radix *(jié gěng),* which may induce or exacerbate the epistaxis by increasing heat or pushing it toward the nose. Instead, add charred Gardeniae Fructus *(zhī zǐ),* Scutellariae Radix *(huáng qín),* or Imperatae Rhizoma *(bái máo gēn)* to clear heat, cool blood, and stop bleeding.

- For injury to the fluids by heat with significant thirst, add Trichosanthis Radix *(tiān huā fěn)* and increase the dosage of Phragmitis Rhizoma *(lú gēn)* to clear heat and generate fluids.

- For heat invading the collaterals of the Lung (papules), remove Sojae Semen preparatum *(dàn dòu chǐ),* which is warm when it is prepared with Ephedrae Herba *(má huáng),* and substitute charred Schizonepetae Herba *(jīng jiè)* for Schizonepetae Herba *(jīng jiè),* the function of which is to stop bleeding. In addition, add Rehmanniae Radix *(shēng dì huáng),* Moutan Cortex *(mǔ dān pí),* Scrophulariae Radix *(xuán shēn),* and Lophatheri Herba *(dàn zhú yè)* to cool blood, express eruptions and rashes, and facilitate the exit of heat from the body.

- For the initial stages of an abnormal progression of heat to the nutritive level from the protective level (restlessness, insomnia, red tongue), add herbs to cool the blood and enrich the yin, such as Rehmanniae Radix *(shēng dì huáng)* and Scrophulariae Radix *(xuán shēn).*

- For injury to the fluids by heat (reduced urination), add Anemarrhenae Rhizoma *(zhī mǔ),* Gardeniae Fructus *(zhī zǐ),* and Scutellariae Radix *(huáng qín)* to clear the heat, and Ophiopogonis Radix *(mài mén dōng)* and Glehniae/Adenophorae Radix *(shā shēn)* to enrich the yin. This treatment strategy, developed by Wu

Tang in *Systematic Differentiation of Warm Pathogen Diseases*, was based on his understanding of a statement in the *Inner Classic* that heat should be treated by combining bitterness and sweetness.[8]

• For carbuncles that manifest as red, swollen, and painful lumps, remove the warm herbs Schizonepetae Herba *(jīng jiè)* and Sojae Semen preparatum *(dàn dòu chǐ)*, but add Taraxaci Herba *(pú gōng yīng)*, Violae Herba *(zǐ huā dì dīng)*, Chrysanthemi indici Flos *(yě jú huā)*, Fritillariae thunbergii Bulbus *(zhè bèi mǔ)*, Angelicae dahuricae Radix *(bái zhǐ)*, Paeoniae Radix rubra *(chì sháo)*, and Trichosanthis Radix *(tiān huā fěn)* to clear heat, resolve toxicity, cool blood, and drain pus.

DECOCTION AND ADMINISTRATION: To facilitate the exit of wind-heat from the body, not only must one select light herbs, they must also be properly decocted and administered. Otherwise, the results will be less than optimal. Therefore, after differentiating the illness, and choosing an appropriate method of treatment and formula, one must select the proper method of decoction and administration.

Decocting. According to Wu Tang in *Systematic Differentiation of Warm Pathogen Diseases*, all the ingredients in the formula should be ground into powder, with the exception of Phragmitis Rhizoma *(lú gēn)*, which should be fresh. Soak the herbs in cold water in an earthen pot for 30 minutes, then bring the pot to a boil under a high flame for about eight minutes. Once the strong fragrance of herbs permeates the air, stop cooking the decoction.

Why should the herbs be decocted in this manner? Their function here is to disseminate the Lung qi and facilitate the exit of wind-heat from the body. For this purpose, it is the light nature and acrid flavor of the herbs, rather than their bitter flavor, that is needed. If the herbs are cooked for a longer period of time, their light nature and acrid flavor will be leached out with the steam, and only the bitter flavor will remain. Should this occur, their effect will be felt in the middle burner, rather than the upper burner, where they can disseminate the Lung qi and facilitate the exit of wind-heat.[9]

Dosage. As a general rule, the following method can be followed for determining the proper dosage of a Chinese herbal decoction:[10]

• Adults, over 14 years for females and 16 years for males,[11] should take one-half cup of the decoction two to three times daily.

• Children, ranging from one to 14 years for females and one to 16 years for males, should take two to three spoonfuls of the decoction three times daily.

- Infants less than a year old should take one to two spoonfuls of the decoction three times daily.

However, because here the formula Honeysuckle and Forsythia Powder (*yín qiào sǎn*) is being used to treat an acute attack, and the wind-heat must be dispersed as quickly as possible, I believe that the conventional dosage is inadequate. I therefore recommend that the dosage and frequency of this formula be increased as follows:

- Adults should take one-half cup of the decoction six times daily.

- Children can safely take three to five spoonfuls of the decoction six times daily.

- Infants can safely take two to three spoonfuls of the decoction six times daily.

Case study: Honeysuckle and Forsythia Powder (*yín qiào sǎn*)[12]

Four days previously, the patient, a 16-year-old male, overate during a meal and then hurried back home. That night he suffered from aversion to cold, chills, fever, headache, epigastric distention, and vomiting. The fever remained even after a period of sweating. Later still, the patient began to cough and developed chest pain. Following the appearance of these symptoms, he was hospitalized.

First visit. The patient presented with a fever, aversion to cold, chills, slight sweating, distended pain in the head, pain in the left side of the chest, cough followed by the expectoration of sticky, slightly yellow or brownish sputum, epigastric distention, and constipation, thirst for cold beverages, red tongue tip, white and slightly yellow tongue coating, and a floating, slippery, rapid pulse. He had a temperature of 41°C, pulse rate of 115 beats per minute, white blood cell count of 18,300/μl, and a sputum culture that was positive for *Streptococcus pneumoniae*. A chest x-ray revealed a focal area of consolidation in the left lower lobe. From a biomedical perspective, he was diagnosed with lobar pneumonia. A traditional Chinese doctor diagnosed it as wind-warmth affecting the Lung, coupled with retention of food in the Stomach. The patient was treated by relieving this exterior pattern with acrid and cool herbs, and others that promote digestion and eliminate food retention. The formula chosen was a modification of Honeysuckle and Forsythia Powder (*yín qiào sǎn*):

Sojae Semen preparatum (*dàn dòu chǐ*)	12g
Lonicerae Flos (*jīn yín huā*)	9g
Forsythiae Fructus (*lián qiào*)	9g
Mori Folium (*sāng yè*)	9g
Schizonepetae Herba (*jīng jiè*)	4.5g
Menthae haplocalycis Herba (*bò hé*)	3g (add at end)
Armeniacae Semen (*xìng rén*)	9g

Arctii Fructus *(niú bàng zǐ)* 9g

Platycodi Radix *(jié gěng)* 4.5g

Aurantii Fructus *(zhǐ ké)* 4.5g

Trichosanthis Pericarpium *(guā lóu pí)* 12g

Trichosanthis Semen *(guā lóu rén)* 12g

Eriobotryae Folium *(pí pá yè)* 9g

Second visit. After two days treatment with the decoction the patient's fever, chills, and aversion to cold abated, his epigastric distention decreased, and he had a bowel movement. He still had slight distending pain in the chest and a cough with sticky and yellow sputum. The doctor further modified the formula by removing Schizonepetae Herba *(jīng jiè)*, Sojae Semen preparatum *(dàn dòu chǐ)*, Trichosanthis Pericarpium *(guā lóu pí)*, Trichosanthis Semen *(guā lóu rén)*, and Eriobotryae Folium *(pí pá yè)*, and adding Peucedani Radix *(qián hú)* (6g), Gardeniae Fructus *(zhī zǐ)* (9g), and Scutellariae Radix *(huáng qín)* (4.5g) for another two days. Two days later all the signs and symptoms were gone, the chest x-ray was negative, and the white blood cell count was within normal limits at 7,200/μl.[13]

WIND-HEAT ATTACKING THE LUNG

Manifestations. There are two concurrent aspects to this pattern:

1. *Failure of the Lung qi to disseminate and descend due to an attack on the Lung by wind-heat* with severe cough.

2. *Attack on the protective level and exterior by wind-heat* with slight fever, slight increase in thirst, slight aversion to cold, a thin and white tongue coating, and a floating, rapid pulse.

NOTE: Unlike the previous pattern, this one stresses the attack on the Lung by wind-heat. There are milder exterior signs and symptoms. The key identifiers for this pattern are severe cough, fever, and slightly above-average thirst. (See Table 7.3 for a summary of the differences between wind-heat attacking the protective level and slightly affecting the Lung, and wind-heat attacking the Lung.)

Pathology. Failure of the Lung qi to disseminate and descend due to an attack on the Lung by wind-heat.

Treatment principles. Disperse and disseminate the Lung qi with acrid, cool, and light herbs, which are associated with eliminating exterior signs and symptoms, and direct the Lung qi downward with bitter herbs.

Table 7.3	Pathology and Clinical Manifestations of Early Stage Wind-Warmth
Pathology	**Signs and Symptoms**
WIND-HEAT ATTACKING THE PROTECTIVE LEVEL AND SLIGHTLY AFFECTING THE LUNG	
Stagnation of protective qi and exterior by attack of wind-heat, leading to struggle between antipathogenic qi and wind-heat	Fever, slight chills and aversion to cold, headache, absent or slight sweating, floating, rapid pulse
WIND-HEAT ATTACKING THE LUNG	
Stagnation of Lung qi by attack of wind-heat giving rise to failure of Lung qi to disseminate and descend	Cough (principal sign) with slight fever and aversion to cold

Formula:

MULBERRY LEAF AND CHRYSANTHEMUM DRINK *(sāng jú yǐn)*

SOURCE: *Systematic Differentiation of Warm Pathogen Diseases*

Mori Folium *(sāng yè)* 7.5g

Chrysanthemi Flos *(jú huā)* 3g

Menthae haplocalycis Herba *(bò hé)* 2.4g

Platycodi Radix *(jié gěng)* 6g

Forsythiae Fructus *(lián qiào)* 4.5g

Armeniacae Semen *(xìng rén)* 6g

Phragmitis Rhizoma *(lú gēn)* 6g

Glycyrrhizae Radix *(gān cǎo)* 2.4g

ANALYSIS OF FORMULA: This is a very important formula for treating cough due to wind-heat attacking the Lung. It is so easy to modify that it is often the first formula selected to treat cough due to wind-heat, even when accompanied by epistaxis, rhinitis, or sinusitis. In this formula, Mori Folium *(sāng yè)*, Chrysanthemi Flos *(jú huā)*, Menthae haplocalycis Herba *(bò hé)*, and Forsythiae Fructus *(lián qiào)* vent heat from the Lung. Platycodi Radix *(jié gěng)*, Glycyrrhizae Radix *(gān cǎo)*, and Armeniacae Semen *(xìng rén)* disseminate the Lung qi to direct it downward to relieve cough. Phragmitis Rhizoma *(lú gēn)* clears heat and generates fluids.

MODIFICATIONS: The basic formula can be modified as follows:

- For attack on the head by wind-heat (headache and dizziness), add Viticis Fructus *(màn jīng zǐ)*, Tribuli Fructus *(cì jí lí)*, and Bombyx batryticatus *(bái jiāng cán)* to disperse exterior wind and dispel exterior heat.
- For cough with sneezing, runny nose, nasal congestion, itchy eyes, and plugged ears, add Magnoliae Flos *(xīn yí)*, Scutellariae Radix *(huáng qín)*, and Bupleuri Radix *(chái hú)*, and increase the dosage of Chrysanthemi Flos *(jú huā)*.
- For red, itchy, and tearing eyes coupled with photophobia, add Cassiae Semen *(jué míng zǐ)* and Celosiae Semen *(qīng xiāng zǐ)*, and increase the dosage of Chrysanthemi Flos *(jú huā)* to dispel wind and brighten the eyes.
- For an invasion of the qi level by heat (cough coupled with some difficulty in breathing, profuse sweating, strong thirst, and a yellow tongue coating), add Gypsum fibrosum *(shí gāo)* and Anemarrhenae Rhizoma *(zhī mǔ)* to clear the heat from the qi level and to relieve the breathing difficulty.
- For blockage of the chest by phlegm-heat and wind-heat (cough with a large amount of yellow sputum and chest congestion), add Trichosanthis Pericarpium *(guā lóu pí)*, Houttuyniae Herba *(yú xīng cǎo)*, and Pinelliae Rhizoma preparatum *(zhì bàn xià)* to clear heat, resolve phlegm, and promote qi circulation in the chest.
- For cough with little sputum, add Glehniae/Adenophorae Radix *(shā shēn)* and Trichosanthis Pericarpium *(guā lóu pí)* to moisten the Lung and stop the cough.
- For constipation due to the Lung's failure to send qi down to the Large Intestine, increase the dosage of Armeniacae Semen *(xìng rén)* and add Trichosanthis Semen *(guā lóu rén)*.
- For severe nasal congestion with yellow and thick discharge, increase the dosage of Menthae haplocalycis Herba *(bò hé)* and Mori Folium *(sāng yè)*. In addition, add a relatively small amount (6–9g) of the warm herbs Angelicae dahuricae Radix *(bái zhǐ)* and Magnoliae Flos *(xīn yí)*.
- For failure of the Lung qi to disseminate (sore throat and hoarse voice), add Sterculiae lychnophorae Semen *(pàng dà hǎi)* and Oroxyli Semen *(mù hú dié)*. A throat that is swollen and filled with pustules indicates toxin. Otherwise, the sore throat is the result of qi stagnation; in that case, help the throat by simply disseminating the Lung qi and clearing heat.
- For cough with blood-tinged sputum or epistaxis, add Scutellariae Radix *(huáng qín)*, Agrimoniae Herba *(xiān hè cǎo)*, and Imperatae Rhizoma *(bái máo gēn)* to clear heat and stop bleeding.

DECOCTION AND ADMINISTRATION: Follow the instructions for Honeysuckle and Forsythia Powder *(yín qiào sǎn)* and do not cook for more than 12 minutes. For adults, take one-half cup of the decoction six times daily. For children, take three to five spoonfuls of the decoction six times daily, and for infants, one to two spoonfuls six times daily.

Case study: Mulberry Leaf and Chrysanthemum Drink *(sāng jú yǐn)*

The patient, a two-year-old boy, had been hospitalized due to high fever for three days. Physical examination and laboratory tests showed a white blood cell count of 27,400/μl and a temperature of 39.9°C. A Western medical physician determined that the fever was due to *Adenovirus pneumoniae.*[14] The patient received penicillin, streptomycin, and sintomycin, with no effect. A traditional Chinese doctor was then invited to treat the patient.

First visit. The patient still had a high fever but was not sweating. He was sleepy and thirsty, and had a cough coupled with slight wheezing. His tongue was red with a slightly yellow coating, and he had a floating, rapid pulse. The doctor diagnosed the condition as wind-heat attacking the Lung leading to obstruction of qi in the Lung, and the treatment method was to disperse wind-heat and disseminate the Lung qi with acrid and cool herbs. Mulberry Leaf and Chrysanthemum Drink *(sāng jú yǐn)* was selected for this purpose: Mori Folium *(sāng yè)* (3g), Chrysanthemi Flos *(jú huā)* (6g), Forsythiae Fructus *(lián qiào)* (4.5g), Armeniacae Semen *(xìng rén)*(4.5g), Platycodi Radix *(jié gěng)* (1.5g), Glycyrrhizae Radix *(gān cǎo)* (1.5g), Arctii Fructus *(niú bàng zǐ)* (4.5g), Menthae haplocalycis Herba *(bò hé)* (2.4g), Phragmitis Rhizoma *(lú gēn)* (15g), Lophatheri Herba *(dàn zhú yè)* (6g), and Allii fistulosi Bulbus *(cōng bái)* (7.5cm). The patient was given two packets to take over a period of two days.

Second visit. After taking the formula, the patient sweated slightly, and his temperature was somewhat reduced. He still had a productive cough with sputum, a red tongue with a yellow, thin coating, and a slippery, rapid pulse. His pores were opened, providing an opportunity for wind-heat to exit the body. However, remnants of wind-heat remained in the Lung, so it was then appropriate to disperse and clear heat, and resolve phlegm in the Lung. The formula was modified as follows: Perillae Folium *(zǐ sū yè)* (3g), Peucedani Radix *(qián hú)* (3g), Platycodi Radix *(jié gěng)* (2.4g), Mori Cortex *(sāng bái pí)* (3g), Scutellariae Radix *(huáng qín)* (2.4g), Trichosanthis Radix *(tiān huā fěn)* (6g), Lophatheri Herba *(dàn zhú yè)* (4.5g), Citri reticulatae Exocarpium rubrum *(jú hóng)* (3g), and Eriobotryae Folium *(pí pá yè)* (6g). The patient was given one packet for one day.

Third visit. The patient continued to sweat slightly, but the fever was gone. He had more energy and appeared more alert, although he still had a very slight cough. He had not had a bowel movement for two days. His tongue was slightly red with a slightly yellow and greasy coating, and he had a submerged, rapid pulse. These signs and symptoms indicated that the wind-heat was gone, but there was persistent dysfunction in the Lung and Large Intestine. The doctor removed Perillae Folium *(zǐ sū yè)* from the formula and added Aurantii Fructus immaturus *(zhǐ shí)* (3g), Raphani Semen *(lái fú zǐ)* (3g), and Hordei Fructus germinatus *(mài yá)* (3g).

Fourth visit. The patient's cough was now gone, but he still had not had a bowel movement. There was a greasy coating in the center of the tongue, and he had a slippery, rapid pulse. These indicated a disharmony of the Lung and Stomach, with slight dampness and food retention. The doctor altered the treatment method to adjust and harmonize the Lung and Stomach, leach out dampness, and promote digestion. He used the following herbs: Benincasae Semen *(dōng guā zǐ)* (12g), Armeniacae Semen *(xìng rén)*(6g), Coicis Semen *(yì yǐ rén)* (12g), Phragmitis Rhizoma *(lú gēn)* (15g), Aurantii Fructus immaturus *(zhǐ shí)* (4.5g), Raphani Semen *(lái fú zǐ)* (4.5g), Hordei Fructus germinatus *(mài yá)* (6g), fried Crataegi Fructus *(shān zhā)* (6g), and Massa medicata fermentata *(shén qū)* (6g). After taking two packets of this modified formula over two days, the patient's appetite, stool, and sleep returned to normal and he was discharged from the hospital.[15]

Comparison. Since Mulberry Leaf and Chrysanthemum Drink *(sāng jú yǐn)* and Honeysuckle and Forsythia Powder *(yín qiào sǎn)* share herbs like Menthae haplocalycis Herba *(bò hé)*, Forsythiae Fructus *(lián qiào)*, Glycyrrhizae Radix *(gān cǎo)*, Phragmitis Rhizoma *(lú gēn)*, and Platycodi Radix *(jié gěng)*, which disseminate the Lung qi and eliminate wind-heat, both are effective for treating wind-heat attacking the Lung and the protective level. However, in order to thoroughly understand these formulas so as to apply them precisely, the practitioner must understand the important differences between them. Mulberry Leaf and Chrysanthemum Drink *(sāng jú yǐn)* does not release the exterior as strongly as Honeysuckle and Forsythia Powder *(yín qiào sǎn)*, but focuses instead on the cough. It is suitable for treating an attack on the Lung by wind-heat, in which cough is the main manifestation. On the other hand, Honeysuckle and Forsythia Powder *(yín qiào sǎn)* is more effective for releasing the exterior and is therefore appropriate for treating an attack on the protective level by wind-heat that slightly affects the Lung (see Table 7.4).

NOTE: Both of these formulas are used for treating upper burner patterns. By understanding their use, the practitioner will see that it is very important when treating upper burner patterns to separate heat from wind and to vent the wind-heat upward and out of the body. Thus, both formulas include herbs that are light in nature to disperse both the wind and heat from the protective level and the Lung. To modify these formulas for specific presentations, it is helpful to discern the relative importance of wind and heat in the particular case.

Table 7.4	Comparison of Honeysuckle and Forsythia Powder vs. Mulberry Leaf and Chrysanthemum Drink		
Pathology	**Indications**	**Treatment Principles**	**Functions of Formula**
HONEYSUCKLE AND FORSYTHIA POWDER (*yín qiào sǎn*)			
Stagnation of protective qi	Fever and exterior signs and symptoms predominate	Dispel exogenous wind, separate heat from wind, and open the pores on the skin with acrid, cool, and acrid, slightly warm herbs	Focus is on separating heat from wind and dissipating both
Failure of Lung qi to disseminate and descend		Disseminate the Lung qi	Enhances the release of the exterior
MULBERRY LEAF AND CHRYSANTHEMUM DRINK (*sāng jú yǐn*)			
Failure of Lung qi to disseminate and descend	Cough predominates	Dispels exogenous wind-heat with acrid, cool, and light herbs. Disseminates the Lung qi and directs it downward	Focus is on disseminating Lung qi and directing it downward, thereby relieving cough

Differentiation and Treatment of Wind-Warmth in the Qi Level

ACCUMULATION OF HEAT IN THE LUNG AND STOMACH

Manifestations. There are two concurrent aspects to this pattern:

1. *Accumulation of heat in the Lung leads to the Lung's failure to disseminate its qi and direct it downward,* with cough and labored breathing or wheezing, and distending pain in the chest.
2. *Heat from excess in the Stomach* with vigorous fever, severe sweating, thirst, irritability, restlessness, a red tongue with yellow coating, and a full, rapid, or slippery, rapid pulse.

NOTE: The key distinguishing symptoms are vigorous fever, cough, wheezing, severe sweating, irritability, restlessness, and thirst. The others are common signs and symptoms that indicate that heat has progressed from the protective to the qi level. In severe cases, shortness of breath and flaring of the nostrils are seen.

Pathology. Lung qi blocked due to accumulation of heat in the Lung, associated with heat from excess in the Stomach.

Treatment principles. Clear heat from the Lung and Stomach, disseminate the Lung qi and direct it downward, and calm the wheezing.

Formula:

EPHEDRA, APRICOT KERNEL, GYPSUM, AND LICORICE DECOCTION
(má xìng shí gān tāng) [16]

SOURCE: *Systematic Differentiation of Warm Pathogen Diseases*

Ephedrae Herba *(má huáng)*..............................9g
Gypsum fibrosum *(shí gāo)*..............................9g
Armeniacae Semen *(xìng rén)*...........................9g
Honey-toasted Glycyrrhizae Radix preparata *(zhì gān cǎo)*.......6g

ANALYSIS OF FORMULA: Because of its acrid flavor and warm nature, Ephedrae Herba *(má huáng)* eliminates exterior conditions by opening the pores. With its acrid flavor and cold nature, Gypsum fibrosum *(shí gāo)* is good for clearing heat from the Lung and Stomach in the qi level. However, when the two herbs are combined, Ephedrae Herba *(má huáng)* promotes the Lung's function of disseminating by opening the pores on the skin, thereby providing an avenue for heat to exit the body.[17] Thus, Ephedrae Herba *(má huáng)* combined with Gypsum fibrosum *(shí gāo)* does not induce diaphoresis for eliminating exterior conditions, but rather opens the pores on the skin. In addition, this pair of herbs lacks the side effect of inducing too much diaphoresis.

Armeniacae Semen *(xìng rén)* is combined with Ephedrae Herba *(má huáng)* to relieve wheezing. Because of its descending function, Armeniacae Semen *(xìng rén)* enhances the function of Ephedrae Herba *(má huáng)* in disseminating the Lung qi. Honey-toasted Glycyrrhizae Radix preparata *(zhì gān cǎo)* harmonizes the functions of the other herbs.

MODIFICATIONS: The basic formula can be modified as follows:

- For heat combined with phlegm in the Lung that leads to obstruction of qi in the chest manifesting in severe cough with profuse, yellow sputum coupled with a stifling sensation in the chest, add Houttuyniae Herba *(yú xīng cǎo)*, Scutellariae Radix *(huáng qín)*, Fritillariae thunbergii Bulbus *(zhè bèi mǔ)*, and Trichosanthis Pericarpium *(guā lóu pí)* to resolve phlegm and promote circulation of qi in the chest.
- For heat-induced injury to the collaterals of the Lung with blood in the sputum, add herbs to cool blood and stop bleeding, including Gardeniae Fructus *(zhī zǐ)*, Imperatae Rhizoma *(bái máo gēn)*, and Platycladi Cacumen *(cè bǎi yè)*.

- For an acute attack of severe blockage of qi of the Lung with such intense difficulty in breathing that the patient cannot lie down, combine Perillae Fructus *(zǐ sū zǐ)* with Lepidii/ Descurainiae Semen *(tíng lì zǐ)* to direct the Lung qi downward and calm wheezing.

- For cough with nausea, add Bambusae Caulis in taeniam *(zhú rú)* and Pinelliae Rhizoma preparatum *(zhì bàn xià)* to direct the Stomach qi downward.

- For constipation, add Trichosanthis Semen *(guā lóu rén)*, which, together with Armeniacae Semen *(xìng rén)*, directs the Lung qi downward and promotes bowel movements.

- For heat and toxin that have damaged both the blood and the Lung with a cough that produces a large amount of foul-smelling, bloody pus and sputum, add Lonicerae Flos *(jīn yín huā)*, Forsythiae Fructus *(lián qiào)*, Taraxaci Herba *(pú gōng yīng)*, Houttuyniae Herba *(yú xīng cǎo)*, and Scutellariae Radix *(huáng qín)* to clear heat, resolve toxicity, and drain off the pus.

DECOCTION AND ADMINISTRATION: In this formula it is desirable to use the slightly acrid flavor of Ephedrae Herba *(má huáng)* to open the pores on the skin and disseminate the Lung qi. To achieve this result, Ephedrae Herba *(má huáng)* should be cooked alone for about 15 minutes. After removing the foam that accumulates on top of the decoction,[18] add the other herbs and continue cooking. Although Gypsum fibrosum *(shí gāo)* is often cooked for at least 30 minutes prior to adding the remainder of the decoction, in this formula Gypsum fibrosum *(shí gāo)* should be cooked for a shorter time than Ephedrae Herba *(má huáng)* to preserve its acrid flavor.

Case study: Ephedra, Apricot Kernel, Gypsum, and Licorice Decoction *(má xìng shí gān tāng)*

This one-year-old male patient was hospitalized a week after he began suffering from a cough with copious sputum and fever.

First visit. The patient's temperature was 39°C and his respiration rate was 60 breaths per minute. He breathed with great difficulty and looked tired, but was not sweating. He had a thin and white tongue coating. Chest x-ray revealed a consolidation in the lower lobe of the lung. The biomedical diagnosis was pneumonia. A traditional Chinese doctor diagnosed the patient with wind-heat attacking the Lung. He applied the treatment principles of dispersing and clearing heat from the Lung with acrid and cool herbs, and prescribed a modified version of Ephedra, Apricot Kernel, Gypsum, and Licorice Decoction *(má xìng shí gān tāng)*: Ephedrae Herba *(má huáng)* (3g), Armeniacae Semen *(xìng rén)*(9g), Glycyrrhizae Radix *(gān cǎo)* (6g), Gypsum fibrosum *(shí gāo)* (12g), Lonicerae Flos *(jīn yín huā)* (6g), Forsythiae Fructus *(lián qiào)* (9g), Platycodi Radix *(jié gěng)* (6g), Schizonepetae Herba *(jīng jiè)* (12g), and fresh Phragmitis Rhizoma *(lú gēn)* (30g).

Second visit. After taking one packet of the formula, the patient's fever was gone and his temperature returned to normal (36.7°C). His energy, cough, and breathing improved, and the sputum was reduced. He still had a poor appetite and his tongue coating was white, yellow, and greasy. The exterior pattern was resolved, but there were still remnants of heat. The doctor further modified the formula, removing Schizonepetae Herba *(jīng jiè)* and adding Aurantii Fructus *(zhǐ ké)*.

Third visit. The patient's cough and labored breathing continued to improve and his appetite gradually returned to normal. He had a thin, white tongue coating and a moderate pulse. The doctor prescribed Mulberry Leaf and Chrysanthemum Drink *(sāng jú yǐn)* to disseminate the Lung qi and disperse heat. The patient totally recovered and was discharged from the hospital after six days.[19]

Comparison. Both Ephedra, Apricot Kernel, Gypsum, and Licorice Decoction *(má xìng shí gān tāng)* and Mulberry Leaf and Chrysanthemum Drink *(sāng jú yǐn)* are designed for treating patterns of heat in the Lung. However, the major pathologies treated by the two formulas are quite different. Mulberry Leaf and Chrysanthemum Decoction *(sāng jú yǐn)* is designed for a more superficial condition that involves the protective level with such signs and symptoms as aversion to cold, chills, a thin, white tongue coating, and a floating, rapid pulse. The treatment approach is to disseminate the Lung qi and disperse wind-heat from the exterior with acrid, cool, and light herbs. By contrast, the pathology treated by Ephedra, Apricot Kernel, Gypsum, and Licorice Decoction *(má xìng shí gān tāng)* is accumulation of heat in the Lung leading to blockage of its qi along with heat in the Stomach. This is a qi level pattern, and the primary manifestations are accordingly severe cough with labored breathing or wheezing, thirst, profuse sweating, red tongue with a yellow coating, and a full or slippery, rapid pulse. Since the disorder is situated in the Lung and Stomach, the acrid, cool, and light herbs used to disperse wind-heat and disseminate the Lung qi are not sufficient. Instead, heavy, cool, and acrid herbs, such as Gypsum fibrosum *(shí gāo)*, are combined with light herbs, such as Ephedrae Herba *(má huáng)*, which can reach the Lung as well as the Stomach, and also bitter herbs, such as Armeniacae Semen *(xìng rén)*, which can disseminate the Lung qi and direct it downward (see Table 7.5).

HEAT FROM CONSTRAINT IN THE CHEST AND DIAPHRAGM

Manifestations. There are two concurrent aspects to this pattern:

Table 7.5	Comparison of Mulberry and Chrysanthemum Decoction vs. Ephedra, Apricot Kernal, Gypsum, and Licorice Decoction		
Pathology	**Common Signs and Symptoms**	**Differences**	**Treatment**
MULBERRY AND CHRYSANTHEMUM DECOCTION (*sāng jú yǐn*)			
Wind-heat attacks Lung, impairing dissemination of Lung qi; slight involvement of the protective level	Cough and signs of heat in the Lung and Stomach	Aversion to cold, thin and white tongue coating, floating, rapid pulse	Disseminate the Lung qi with light, acrid, and cool herbs, and dispel the mild exterior signs and symptoms
EPHEDRA, APRICOT KERNEL, GYPSUM, AND LICORICE DECOCTION (*má xìng shí gān tāng*)			
Obstruction of Lung qi due to accumulation of heat in the Lung and Stomach; only qi level involvement	Cough and signs of heat in the Lung	Severe cough with labored breathing or wheezing, or even flaring of nostrils, restlessness, thirst, profuse sweating, excessive or slippery, rapid pulse	Clear heat from the Lung and Stomach, disseminate the Lung qi and direct it downward, thereby calming the wheezing

1. *An initial invasion of the qi level with disappearance of exterior signs and symptoms* with fever, no aversion to cold, thirst, and a slightly yellow tongue coating.
2. *Disturbance of the spirit due to heat from constraint in the chest and diaphragm* with irritability and insomnia with tossing and turning in bed.

NOTE: The key identifiers for this pattern are irritability, restlessness, and insomnia with tossing and turning in bed, and a slightly yellow tongue coating. The irritability is due to heat in the qi level and is quite different from the restlessness seen when heat progresses to the nutritive level. In a qi-level pattern, the heat only slightly disturbs the spirit such that the person feels irritable and hot, while in nutritive-level disorders the problem is more severe, causing the body to move, as in restlessness, tossing and turning. In addition, a nutritive-level pattern is accompanied by a fever that worsens at night, and a deep-red tongue.

Pathology. Heat from constraint in the chest and diaphragm secondary to an invasion of the qi level by heat.

Treatment principles. Clear and disperse heat from the chest and diaphragm with light herbs.

213

Formula:

GARDENIA AND PREPARED SOYBEAN DECOCTION *(zhī zǐ chǐ tāng)*

SOURCE: *Discussion of Cold Damage*

Gardeniae Fructus *(zhī zǐ)* 12g
Sojae Semen preparatum *(dàn dòu chǐ)*. 9g

ANALYSIS OF FORMULA: According to Chapter 71 of *Basic Questions*, the best way to deal with fire (heat) from constraint is to disperse it.[20] Since this pattern involves interior heat from constraint located in the upper burner, treatment should disperse the heat and vent it from the upper burner. Sojae Semen preparatum *(dàn dòu chǐ)*, with its acrid flavor, disperses heat from constraint in the chest and diaphragm, while Gardeniae Fructus *(zhī zǐ)*, with its bitter flavor, clears interior heat directly.

MODIFICATIONS: The basic formula can be modified as follows:

- Where some exterior symptoms remain (chills, runny nose, sore throat), add Menthae haplocalycis Herba *(bò hé)* and Arctii Fructus *(niú bàng zǐ)*.

- For injury to the fluids by heat (thirst and a yellow, dry tongue coating), add Phragmitis Rhizoma *(lú gēn)*, Trichosanthis Radix *(tiān huā fěn)*, and Lophatheri Herba *(dàn zhú yè)*.

- For cough due to failure of the Lung qi to disseminate and descend, add Mori Folium *(sāng yè)*, Armeniacae Semen *(xìng rén)*, and Trichosanthis Pericarpium *(guā lóu pí)*.

- For phlegm-heat (chest distention, cough with thick sputum, and a yellow, greasy tongue coating), add Armeniacae Semen *(xìng rén)*, Coicis Semen *(yì yǐ rén)*, Talcum *(huá shí)*, Tetrapanacis Medulla *(tōng cǎo)*, Eriobotryae Folium *(pí pá yè)*, and Trichosanthis Pericarpium *(guā lóu pí)*.

- For stagnant qi in the Lung (chest distention), add Armeniacae Semen *(xìng rén)*, Trichosanthis Pericarpium *(guā lóu pí)*, and Curcumae Radix *(yù jīn)*.

- For damage to the qi by heat (shortness of breath), add Glycyrrhizae Radix *(gān cǎo)* (source text).

- For rebellion of Stomach qi due to heat from constraint (vomiting), add Zingiberis Rhizoma recens *(shēng jiāng)* (source text).

DECOCTION AND ADMINISTRATION: In order to disperse heat from constraint in the chest and diaphragm, choose herbs such as Sojae Semen preparatum *(dàn dòu chǐ)*, but also pay attention to the method of cooking. Here one must first cook Sojae Semen preparatum *(dàn dòu chǐ)* for about eight minutes, then add Gardeniae Fructus *(zhī *zǐ);* both are cooked together for an additional five minutes. This is because Gardeniae Fructus *(zhī zǐ)* has a bitter flavor that is apt to reach the middle and lower burners (as it can drain heat from all three burners). In addition, it is quite cold, which may be inappropriate for treating heat from constraint in the chest and diaphragm. By cooking for only five minutes, the effects of its bitter and cold nature are ameliorated, and its actions are then focused on the upper burner. The acrid flavor of Sojae Semen preparatum *(dàn dòu chǐ),* necessary for dispersing heat in the chest and diaphragm, will not be affected by cooking it for thirteen minutes or so. These two herbs, decocted specifically in this manner, are especially useful for treating heat from constraint in the upper burner.

Case study: Gardenia and Prepared Soybean Decoction *(zhī zǐ chǐ tāng)*

First visit (11/05/1983). The patient, a 13-year-old male, had been suffering from irritability, insomnia, and palpitations for five days. He had caught a cold and developed a fever a week earlier. His parents had given him medicine for a common cold and his condition improved. But five days ago the fever returned, and this time it would not go down after taking the same medicine. Instead, he developed irritability, restlessness, insomnia, and palpitations. He was diagnosed at a hospital with AV block due to viral myocarditis. Because he did not want to be hospitalized, he was treated at the out-patient department with antibiotics and vitamin C. But because there was no improvement after three days, he went to a traditional Chinese doctor for treatment.

The patient presented with fever, irritability, chest distention, insomnia, and palpitations. He also had poor appetite, nausea, and vomiting. His bowel movements and urination were normal. He had a thin, yellow tongue coating and a rapid pulse. The diagnosis was disturbance of the Heart by accumulation of interior heat. The treatment principles were to clear and disperse heat, calm the Heart, and relieve irritability. A modified form of Gardenia and Prepared Soybean Decoction *(zhī zǐ chǐ tāng)* was prescribed: Gardeniae Fructus *(zhī zǐ)* (10g), Sojae Semen preparatum *(dàn dòu chǐ)* (15g), Zingiberis Rhizoma recens *(shēng jiāng)* (3 slices), and Bambusae Caulis in taeniam *(zhú rú)* (6g). Three packets of the herbs were given to the patient.

Second visit (11/08/1983). The irritability, palpitations, nausea, and vomiting had improved. His sleep was normal. But he still had a poor appetite, a yellow, thin tongue coating, and slightly rapid pulse. The herbs Gigeriae galli Endothelium corneum *(jī nèi jīn)* (6g) and Dioscoreae Rhizoma *(shān yào)* (15g) were added to the formula. He was given two packets of the herbs.

Third visit (11/10/1983). The irritability, palpitations, nausea, and vomiting were gone. His appetite had gradually improved. He had a normal sinus rhythm on ECG and was given Dioscoreae Rhizoma *(shān yào)* to improve his appetite.[21]

STAGNATION OF PHLEGM AND HEAT IN THE CHEST AND EPIGASTRIUM

Manifestations. There are two concurrent aspects to this pattern:

1. *Heat from excess in the chest and epigastrium* with a flushed face, fever, thirst with a preference for cold beverages, and vomiting after drinking.

2. *Stagnation of phlegm and heat in the chest and epigastrium leading to a failure of Lung qi to descend into the Large Intestine* with chest and epigastric distention, pain on pressure in the chest and epigastrium, constipation, and a yellow, slippery tongue coating.

NOTE: Among the signs and symptoms, fever, thirst with a preference for cold beverages, and distention and pain on pressure in the chest and epigastrium are the key identifiers for this pattern. The Stomach is also involved, as is evident from the distending pain in the epigastrium and vomiting after drinking. In fact, this is a combination of upper and middle burner patterns.

Fever and thirst with a preference for cold beverages are also present in a pattern of heat from excess in the Stomach. However, vomiting after drinking water, and distention and pain in the chest and epigastrium, along with the yellow, slippery tongue coating indicate the presence of phlegm-heat in the chest and epigastrium. Constipation and fever may at first appear to be caused by the clumping of dry stool and heat in the Large Intestine, but if that were the case the patient would also have abdominal distention, abdominal pain aggravated by pressure, and a dry, yellow tongue coating.

Pathology. Stagnation of phlegm and heat in the chest and epigastrium.

Treatment principles. Resolve phlegm, and relieve stagnation of heat and phlegm, with bitter and acrid herbs.

Formula:

> **MINOR SINKING INTO THE CHEST DECOCTION PLUS UNRIPE BITTER ORANGE** *(xiǎo xiàn xiōng jiā zhǐ shí tāng)*
>
> SOURCE: *Systematic Differentiation of Warm Pathogen Diseases*[22]
>
> Coptidis Rhizoma *(huáng lián)* 6g
> Trichosanthis Fructus *(guā lóu)* 9g
> Pinelliae Rhizoma preparatum *(zhì bàn xià)* 15g
> Aurantii Fructus immaturus *(zhǐ shí)* 6g

ANALYSIS OF FORMULA: Bitter in flavor and cold in nature, Coptidis Rhizoma *(huáng lián)* clears heat and directs the Stomach qi downward. Pinelliae Rhizoma preparatum *(zhì bàn xià)* is a key herb for resolving phlegm and harmonizing the function of the Stomach. These functions work in concert to stop vomiting. Aurantii Fructus immaturus *(zhǐ shí)* directs the qi downward and disperses stagnation of heat in the chest. In this formula, both Trichosanthis Pericarpium *(guā lóu pí)* and Trichosanthis Semen *(guā lóu rén)* can be used concurrently, because the patient is suffering from distending pain in the chest and the epigastrium, coupled with constipation. Trichosanthis Pericarpium *(guā lóu pí)*, an acrid and cold herb, treats the distending pain in the chest and epigastrium by promoting qi circulation in the chest, while the moistening action of Trichosanthis Semen *(guā lóu rén)* treats constipation.

MODIFICATIONS: The basic formula can be modified as follows:

- For severe vomiting, increase the dosage of Pinelliae Rhizoma preparatum *(zhì bàn xià)* and add Bambusae Caulis in taeniam *(zhú rú)* and Zingiberis Rhizomatis Succus *(jiāng zhī)* - ginger juice.
- For dryness and heat in the Large Intestine (dry and hard stool and a dry, yellow tongue coating), add Rhei Radix et Rhizoma *(dà huáng)* and Magnoliae officinalis Cortex *(hòu pò)*.

DECOCTION AND ADMINISTRATION: In order to make use of the bitter taste of Aurantii Fructus immaturus *(zhǐ shí)* to direct the qi downward, cook it for at least 20 minutes before adding the other herbs.

BLOCKAGE OF THE LUNG BY PHLEGM AND HEAT COUPLED WITH CLUMPING OF STOOL AND HEAT IN THE LARGE INTESTINE

Manifestations. There are two concurrent aspects to this pattern:

1. *Blockage of the Lung by phlegm and heat leading to the failure of the Lung qi to disseminate and descend* with persistent cough, labored breathing, and profuse sputum.
2. *Clumping of stool and heat in the Large Intestine* with tidal fever, constipation, and a yellow, greasy tongue coating.

NOTE: Clinically, one must distinguish this pattern from stagnation of phlegm and heat in the chest and epigastrium. Here, cough and labored breathing are present because the Lung's functions of disseminating and descending have been impaired. However, in the case of stagnation of phlegm and heat in the chest and epigastrium, when pressure is applied there, distending pain will be felt because phlegm and heat are located in the chest and epigastrium instead of in the Lung.

The pattern discussed here is situated in both yin and yang organs in both the upper and lower burners, that is, heat in the Large Intestine as well as phlegm and heat in the Lung. However, the pathological root is in the Lung, and heat in the Large Intestine is transmitted from the Lung. Therefore, to correctly identify the pattern, much more attention should be paid to the Lung signs and symptoms. Only constipation and a yellow tongue coating is needed to diagnose heat in the Large Intestine. Constipation may present as either sluggishness of bowel movement with reduced frequency *or* dry and hard stool. It is not necessary to wait for dry and hard stool to manifest in order to diagnose the Large Intestine problem.

Pathology. Blockage of the Lung by phlegm and heat, leading to the failure of the Lung qi to disseminate and descend, and the transmission of heat to the Large Intestine. The latter leads to clumping of stool and heat in the Large Intestine.

Treatment principles. Disseminate the Lung qi and direct it downward, resolve phlegm, and clear heat by purging.

Formula:

DISSEMINATE THE WHITE AND ORDER THE QI DECOCTION
(xuān bái chéng qì tāng)

SOURCE: *Systematic Differentiation of Warm Pathogen Diseases*

Gypsum fibrosum *(shí gāo)* 15g
Rhei Radix et Rhizoma *(dà huáng)* 9g
Armeniacae Semen *(xìng rén)* 6g
Trichosanthis Pericarpium *(guā lóu pí)* 4.5g

ANALYSIS OF FORMULA: In five-phase theory the Lung corresponds to metal and the color white. 'Disseminate the white' *(xuán bái)* is another way of saying disseminate the Lung qi. Actually, this formula is based on a combination of White Tiger Decoction *(bái hǔ tāng)* and Order the Qi Decoction *(chéng qì tāng)*. Gypsum fibrosum *(shí gāo)* is a key herb in White Tiger Decoction *(bái hǔ tāng)*, and Rhei Radix et Rhizoma *(dà huáng)* is a key herb in Order the Qi Decoction *(chéng qì tāng)*.

Once heat has invaded the lower burner, as in the present pattern, Ephedrae Herba *(má huáng)*, which promotes the disseminating function of the Lung, should no longer be used. Instead, use Trichosanthis Pericarpium *(guā lóu pí)* and Armeniacae Semen *(xìng rén)* to resolve phlegm and unbind the chest, since the direction of the disease is downward and there is Large Intestine involvement. Also, Rhei Radix et Rhizoma *(dà huáng)* is substituted for Ephedrae Herba *(má huáng)* to purge heat through the discharge of stool from the Large Intestine. This provides an avenue for heat to exit via the interior instead of the exterior. Once the clumping of stool and heat in the Large Intestine is removed, the heat in the Lung is easily dissipated. Conversely, once the heat in the Lung has been eliminated, the Lung's function of disseminating and descending will be restored, and the qi will readily descend to the Large Intestine. Thus, three of the four herbs in this formula focus on the Lung because it is the root of the pathology.

Currently, the method of purging yang organs to treat yin organs is widely used in the clinic. For example, Wang En-Bao of the Beijing Friendship Hospital conducted a double-blind study on the treatment of pneumonia. The results show that the group treated with the herbs Rhei Radix et Rhizoma *(dà huáng)*, Natrii Sulfas *(máng xiāo)*, Glycyrrhizae Radix *(gān cǎo)*, Scrophulariae Radix *(xuán shēn)*, Taraxaci Herba *(pú gōng yīng)*, Patriniae Herba *(bài jiàng cǎo)*, Scutellariae barbatae Herba *(bàn zhī lián)*, and Polygoni cuspidati Rhizoma *(hǔ zhàng)* experienced a shorter duration of illness compared with the group treated with antibiotics.[23] The herbs Rhei Radix et Rhizoma *(dà huáng)* and Natrii Sulfas *(máng xiāo)* were used to expel heat and toxin from the body and the Lung.

MODIFICATIONS: The basic formula can be modified as follows:

- For heat, phlegm, and weak bowel movements, it is strongly recommended to combine Trichosanthis Pericarpium *(guā lóu pí)* and Trichosanthis Semen *(guā lóu rén)*.

- For severe phlegm and heat in the Lung with wheezing, add Houttuyniae Herba *(yú xīng cǎo)*.

- For heat and toxin with severe chest pain and high fever, add Taraxaci Herba *(pú gōng yīng)*, Sargentodoxae Caulis *(hóng téng)*, and Houttuyniae Herba *(yú xīng cǎo)*.

DECOCTION AND ADMINISTRATION: In this pattern there is heat in the Lung and impacted heat and stool in the Large Intestine. Here the heat in the Large Intestine is less intense than in the pattern for which Major Order the Qi Decoction *(dà chéng qì tāng)*[24] is indicated. For this reason, Rhei Radix et Rhizoma *(dà huáng)* can be cooked along with the other herbs, instead of added at or near the end; the purgative effect is correspondingly milder.

Comparison. To help the practitioner select an appropriate formula for wind-warmth, Table 7.6 compares Disseminate the White and Order the Qi Decoction *(xuān bái chéng qì tāng)* with Ephedra, Apricot Kernel, Gypsum, and Licorice Decoction *(má xìng shí gān tāng)*.

Table 7.6	Comparison of Disseminate the White and Order the Qi Decoction vs. Ephedra, Apricot Kernel, Gypsum, and Licorice Decoction		
Pathology	**Common Points**	**Signs and Symptoms**	**Treatment**
DISSEMINATE THE WHITE AND ORDER THE QI DECOCTION (*xuān baí chéng qì tāng*)			
Blockage of the Lung by phlegm and heat, leading to failure of Lung qi to disseminate and descend, coupled with clumping of stool and heat in Large Intestine	Qi level problems with wheezing	Tidal fever, persistent and labored breathing, constipation, yellow and greasy tongue coating	Disseminate the Lung qi and direct it downward, resolve phlegm, clear heat by purging
EPHEDRA, APRICOT KERNEL, GYPSUM, AND LICORICE DECOCTION (*má xìng shí gān tāng*)			
Blockage of Lung qi due to accumulation of heat in Lung and Stomach	Qi level problems with wheezing	Restlessness, profuse sweating, thirst, red tongue with yellow coating	Clear heat from Lung and Stomach, disseminate Lung qi and direct it downward, thereby calming the wheezing

REMNANTS OF HEAT AND INJURY TO THE LUNG AND STOMACH YIN

Manifestations. There are three concurrent aspects to this pattern:

1. *Remnants of heat* with fever.
2. *Injury to the Lung yin* with a dry cough and scanty, sticky sputum.
3. *Injury to the Stomach yin* with a dry mouth, thirst, red tongue with little coating, and thin pulse.

Pathology. Injury to Lung and Stomach yin coupled with the remnants of heat.

Treatment principles. Enrich the Lung and the Stomach yin with sweet and cold herbs.

Formula:

GLEHNIA/ADENOPHORA AND OPHIOPOGONIS DECOCTION
(*shā shēn mài mén dōng tāng*)

SOURCE: *Systematic Differentiation of Warm Pathogen Diseases*

Glehniae/Adenophorae Radix (*shā shēn*) 9g
Ophiopogonis Radix (*mài mén dōng*) 9g

Polygonati odorati Rhizoma *(yù zhú)* 6g
Mori Folium *(sāng yè)* 4.5g
Trichosanthis Radix *(tiān huā fěn)* 4.5g
Lablab Semen album *(bái biǎn dòu)* 4.5g
Glycyrrhizae Radix *(gān cǎo)* 3g

ANALYSIS OF FORMULA: This is a well-known formula used to enrich the yin of the Lung and Stomach. It can be used for Lung and Stomach yin deficiency regardless of the disease. In this formula, Glehniae/Adenophorae Radix *(shā shēn)*, Ophiopogonis Radix *(mài mén dōng)*, Polygonati odorati Rhizoma *(yù zhú)*, and Trichosanthis Radix *(tiān huā fěn)*, all of which have a sweet flavor and cold nature, enrich the yin of the Lung and the Stomach. Mori Folium *(sāng yè)* clears remnant heat from the Lung in order to stop the cough. Lablab Semen album *(bái biǎn dòu)* and Glycyrrhizae Radix *(gān cǎo)* harmonize and strengthen the qi of the Stomach.

MODIFICATIONS: The basic formula can be modified as follows:

- For injury to the qi by heat (shortness of breath and spontaneous sweating), add Panacis quinquefolii Radix *(xī yáng shēn)* and Schisandrae Fructus *(wǔ wèi zǐ)*.
- For yin deficiency with heat from deficiency in the Lung (prolonged dry cough and low-grade fever), add Lycii Cortex *(dì gǔ pí)* (source text).

TRANSMISSION OF HEAT TO THE LARGE INTESTINE FROM THE LUNG

Manifestations. There are two concurrent aspects to this pattern:

1. *Heat in the Lung* with fever, labored breathing, tight chest, and cough.
2. *Transmission of heat to the Large Intestine* with diarrhea (yellow, hot, and foul-smelling stool), burning sensation around the anus, yellow tongue coating, and rapid pulse.

NOTE: Among these signs and symptoms, the yellow, hot, and foul-smelling stool, burning sensation around the anus, yellow tongue coating, and rapid pulse are the key identifiers for this pattern.

Transmission of heat from the Lung to the Large Intestine does not indicate that the disease is getting worse. Rather, it shows that the function of the Lung in causing its qi to descend is normal, and that it is capable of bringing heat downward to its paired organ to be discharged from the body. Obviously, this is a good sign, for the disease will soon be cured. According to Wang Shi-Xiong (Wang Meng-Ying, 1806–1866) in *Case Studies From Wang Meng-Ying (Wáng Mèng-Yīng yī àn)*, "[The disease] progressing from the Lung to the Large Intestine shows that the body wants to find a way for pathogenic factors to exit. It is therefore a good sign of normal progression."[25]

This pattern is similar to that of clumping of dry stool and heat in the Large Intestine, coupled with watery discharge. However, because there is no dry stool accompanying the heat in the present pattern, there is no pressure-induced abdominal pain or discharge of foul-smelling liquid. So why is there no clumping of dry stool and heat in the Large Intestine in this pattern? This depends on whether there is dry stool or retention of food prior to the transmission of heat to the Large Intestine. If there is, heat is apt to combine with the stool. If not, there is nothing with which heat can combine, and there will be no clumping of stool and heat in the Large Intestine. Still, why would the heat in the Large Intestine give rise to diarrhea, instead of injuring the fluids and causing constipation? Since there is neither dry stool nor retention of food in the Large Intestine, heat, characterized by quick movement, forces the discharge of stool before it is well formed.

In addition, the present pattern and that of clumping of dry stool and heat in the Large Intestine may share the symptoms of burning sensation around the anus and foul-smelling stools. However, because the present pattern is caused by transmission of heat from the Lung to the Large Intestine, there must also be Lung signs and symptoms, such as cough or a tight chest. This is not the case with clumping of dry stool and heat in the Large Intestine.

The present pattern is also similar to the pattern of blockage of the Lung by phlegm and heat coupled with clumping of stool and heat in the Large Intestine. However, unlike that pattern, the pathological focus of this pattern is no longer in the Lung. Instead, it is centered in the Large Intestine. Therefore, except for cough, a little sputum, and slightly labored breathing—all evidence of some Lung involvement—the other signs and symptoms point to involvement of the Large Intestine. Nevertheless, both patterns are marked by problems with bowel movements.

Pathology. Heat transmitted from the Lung to the Large Intestine.

Treatment principles. Clear heat and stop the diarrhea with bitter and cold herbs.

Formula:

KUDZU, SCUTELLARIA, AND COPTIS DECOCTION
(gé gēn huáng qín huáng lián tāng)

SOURCE: *Discussion of Cold Damage*

Puerariae Radix *(gé gēn)* 15–24g
Scutellariae Radix *(huáng qín)* 9g
Coptidis Rhizoma *(huáng lián)* 9g
Honey-toasted Glycyrrhizae Radix preparata *(zhì gān cǎo)* 6g

ANALYSIS OF FORMULA: When Zhang Ji first introduced this formula it was recommended for treating heat that had sunk into the Large Intestine after the improper purging of an exterior pattern. Practitioners who specialize in treating warm pathogen diseases have found that the formula is also effective in treating the present pattern, transmission of heat to the Large Intestine from the Lung.[26]

Puerariae Radix *(gé gēn)*, which is acrid and cool, clears heat and lifts the qi in the middle burner to stop diarrhea. Scutellariae Radix *(huáng qín)* clears heat from the Lung and Large Intestine. Coptidis Rhizoma *(huáng lián)* also clears heat from the Large Intestine. Honey-toasted Glycyrrhizae Radix preparata *(zhì gān cǎo)* harmonizes the function of the Stomach and the Spleen.

MODIFICATIONS: The basic formula can be modified as follows:

- For heat from excess in the Lung (severe cough), add Chrysanthemi Flos *(jú huā)*, Mori Folium *(sāng yè)*, and Platycodi Radix *(jié gěng)* to clear heat and to promote the Lung's disseminating function.

- For an attack on the Stomach by heat (nausea or vomiting), add Pogostemonis/Agastaches Herba *(huò xiāng)* and Bambusae Caulis in taeniam *(zhú rú)* to harmonize the Stomach in order to quell the nausea and vomiting.

- For abdominal cramps, add Paeoniae Radix alba *(bái sháo)*.

- *Discussion of Cold Damage* advises cooking the Puerariae Radix *(gé gēn)* first. However, this practice is not commonly followed today, and I believe that it is unnecessary.

HEAT FROM EXCESS IN THE STOMACH

Manifestations. There are three concurrent aspects to this pattern:

1. *Injury to the Stomach fluids due to heat from excess in the Stomach* with vigorous fever, profuse sweating, thirst with a preference for cold beverages, and a full pulse.
2. *Disturbance of the Heart spirit* with irritability.
3. *Stomach heat attacking the Lung* with labored breathing.

NOTE: This pattern is similar to that of the *yang ming* channel pattern described in six-stage theory in the *Discussion of Cold Damage*. Among these signs and symptoms, vigorous fever, profuse sweating, thirst with a preference for cold beverages, and a full pulse are the key identifiers for this pattern.

Pathology. Heat from excess in the Stomach injuring the fluids.

Treatment principles. Clear heat with acrid and cold herbs, and generate fluids with sweet and cold herbs. The focus is on clearing heat, since once the heat is gone the fluids will readily recover.

Formula:

WHITE TIGER DECOCTION *(bái hǔ tāng)*

SOURCE: *Discussion of Cold Damage*

Gypsum fibrosum *(shí gāo)* 30g
Anemarrhenae Rhizoma *(zhī mǔ)* 9g
Nonglutinous rice *(gěng mǐ)* 9–15g
Honey-toasted Glycyrrhizae Radix preparata *(zhì gān cǎo)* 3g

---

ANALYSIS OF FORMULA: White Tiger Decoction *(bái hǔ tāng)* is commonly used to clear heat and generate fluids, and contains herbs with acrid, bitter, and sweet flavors and a moist nature. Gypsum fibrosum *(shí gāo)* and Anemarrhenae Rhizoma *(zhī mǔ)* clear and disperse heat from the Stomach. Honey-toasted Glycyrrhizae Radix preparata *(zhì gān cǎo)* and nonglutinous rice *(gěng mǐ)* tonify the qi of the Stomach and generate fluids. They can also prevent possible injury to the qi of the Stomach from the bitter and cold properties of Anemarrhenae Rhizoma *(zhī mǔ)*.

MODIFICATIONS: The basic formula can be modified as follows:

- For any residual signs and symptoms of an exterior pattern affecting the protective level, add Mori Folium *(sāng yè)* and Menthae haplocalycis Herba *(bò hé)*.

- For exterior cold such as body aches, absence of sweating, chills, and aversion to cold, add Allii fistulosi Bulbus *(cōng bái)* and Sojae Semen preparatum *(dàn dòu chǐ)*.

- For exterior dampness such as a heavy sensation in the body and the absence of sweating, add Atractylodis Rhizoma *(cāng zhú)*.

- To enhance the formula's action in clearing heat and generating fluids, add Lonicerae Flos *(jīn yín huā)*, Phragmitis Rhizoma *(lú gēn)*, and Dendrobii Herba *(shí hú)*.

- For badly injured Stomach yin with severe thirst and a mirror-like tongue, the patient should drink pear juice or Five Juice Drink *(wǔ zhī yǐn)*.[27] Five Juice Drink consists of the juice from pears, lotus node,[28] Phragmitis Rhizoma *(lú gēn)*, Ophiopogonis Radix *(mài mén dōng)*, and Eleocharitis Rhizoma *(bí qì)*.[29]

- For qi that has been damaged by extreme heat (chills in the upper back and a full but hollow pulse), immediately add Ginseng Radix *(rén shēn)* to tonify the qi and generate fluids. Normally, Ginseng Radix *(rén shēn)* should be separated from the other herbs, cooked, and then added to the strained decoction, or ground into powder and swallowed with the decoction. Clinically, damage of the qi can manifest with shortness of breath, fatigue, and a pulse that is either hollow or (more common) big at the superficial level, but weak at the deep level.

- For accompanying disharmony at the *shao yang* stage (alternating chills and fever), add Bupleuri Radix *(chái hú)* and Scutellariae Radix *(huáng qín)*.
- For extreme heat in the Stomach that stirs up Liver wind (convulsions), add Saigae tataricae Cornu *(líng yáng jiǎo)*, Uncariae Ramulus cum Uncis *(gōu téng)*, and Chrysanthemi Flos *(jú huā)*.

Contraindications. In *Systematic Differentiation of Warm Pathogen Diseases*, Wu Tang cited the following four contraindications to the use of White Tiger Decoction *(bái hǔ tāng):*

1. Do not use this formula by itself when there are still exterior signs and symptoms because the bitter flavor and cold nature of the formula will trap pathogens (e.g., wind-heat or wind-cold) in the exterior.
2. Do not use it when there is only slight interior heat. It is indicated only for severe heat.
3. Do not use it in the absence of thirst since a lack of thirst suggests that there is no heat from excess in the Stomach, and that the fluids are not damaged.
4. Do not use it when the pulse is submerged, which would indicate that there is either no avenue for the interior heat to exit, or that there is a deficiency of yang qi.

DECOCTION AND ADMINISTRATION: Cook until the rice is well done, then strain and ingest the liquid. Generally, Gypsum fibrosum *(shí gāo)* should be cooked for 30 minutes before adding the other herbs. However, in this particular formula, nonglutinous rice *(gěng mǐ)* takes 30–45 minutes to cook, so there is no need to extend the cooking time of Gypsum fibrosum *(shí gāo).*

CLUMPING OF DRY STOOL AND HEAT IN THE LARGE INTESTINE

Manifestations. There are two concurrent aspects to this pattern:

1. *Clumping of dry stool and heat in the Large Intestine* with tidal fever, constipation with hard and dry stool or diarrhea with a discharge of foul-smelling liquid, hard and distending pain in the abdomen, and a submerged and forceful pulse.
2. *Injury to the fluids* with a dry, yellow tongue coating that may be cracked.

Pathology. Clumping of dry stool and heat in the Large Intestine coupled with slight injury to the fluids.

Treatment principles. Soften hard stool and eliminate heat by purging with bitter, salty, and cold herbs in order to protect the yin and fluids. The same method is used even if there is diarrhea with discharge of foul-smelling liquid.

NOTE: Once there is clumping of dry stool and heat in the Large Intestine, the heat should be immediately eliminated by purging if the antipathogenic qi is strong enough. Otherwise, the heat will deplete the yin and fluids, resulting in a pattern of heat from excess and deficiency of antipathogenic qi.

Formula:

> REGULATE THE STOMACH AND ORDER THE QI DECOCTION
> *(tiáo wèi chéng qì tāng)*
>
> SOURCE: *Discussion of Cold Damage*
>
> Honey-toasted Glycyrrhizae Radix preparata *(zhì gān cǎo)*........6g
>
> Rhei Radix et Rhizoma *(dà huáng)*.........................12g
>
> Natrii Sulfas *(máng xiāo)* 9–12g

ANALYSIS OF FORMULA: In this formula, Natrii Sulfas *(máng xiāo)*, which is salty and cold, softens hard stool. Rhei Radix et Rhizoma *(dà huáng)*, with its bitter flavor and cold nature, clears heat by purging. Honey-toasted Glycyrrhizae Radix preparata *(zhì gān cǎo)* harmonizes the other herbs and ameliorates the strong purgative effects of Rhei Radix et Rhizoma *(dà huáng)* and Natrii Sulfas *(máng xiāo)*. Clinically, however, when a patient has a dry and yellow tongue coating, a strong purgative should be given as soon as possible to drain the heat from the body. In such cases, reduce the dosage of honey-toasted Glycyrrhizae Radix preparata *(zhì gān cǎo)* and increase the dosage of Natrii Sulfas *(máng xiāo)* to enhance the purging effect.

MODIFICATIONS: The basic formula can be modified as follows:

• Major Order the Qi Decoction *(dà chéng qì tāng)* and Minor Order the Qi Decoction *(xiǎo chéng qì tāng)*[30] are rarely used to deal with clumping of dry stool and heat in the Large Intestines in warm pathogen diseases, especially those caused just by heat. This is because these formulas contain a warm herb, Magnoliae officinalis Cortex *(hòu pò)*, and a drying herb, Aurantii Fructus immaturus *(zhǐ shí)*, which can aggravate the injury to the yin and fluids. However, if there is distending pain in the abdomen, a small dose of these two herbs may be used to promote the movement of qi in the Large Intestine and to relieve distending pain.

- For severe injury to the fluids, add Rehmanniae Radix *(shēng dì huáng)*, Scrophulariae Radix *(xuán shēn)*, and Ophiopogonis Radix *(mài mén dōng)* to generate fluids. These three herbs comprise the formula Increase the Fluids Decoction *(zēng yè tāng)*, first recorded in *Systematic Differentiation of Warm Pathogen Diseases*. Wu Tang referred to this as "adding water to help float the boat."[31] Just as a boat can sail smoothly on a river that has sufficient water, so too can stool move smoothly through the Large Intestine if there are enough fluids to nourish the Large Intestine.

DECOCTION AND ADMINISTRATION: To achieve a mild purgative effect, cook Rhei Radix et Rhizoma *(dà huáng)* and honey-toasted Glycyrrhizae Radix preparata *(zhì gān cǎo)* for 15 minutes. This is because laboratory research and clinical experience have shown that the longer Rhei Radix et Rhizoma *(dà huáng)* is cooked, the weaker its purgative action. In this formula, filter the other herbs from the decoction and then add Natrii Sulfas *(máng xiāo)*. Cook the decoction over a slow fire until it boils, and then take warm.

Differentiation and Treatment of Wind-Warmth in the Nutritive Level

BURNING OF YIN IN THE NUTRITIVE LEVEL BY HEAT

Manifestations. There are three concurrent aspects to this pattern:

1. *Disturbance of the Heart spirit by heat* with irritability, restlessness, or delirium.

2. *Injury to the yin by heat* with fever that worsens at night, dry lips and mouth (with no desire to drink), deep-red tongue with thin or no coating, and a thin, rapid pulse.

3. *Failure of the collaterals to control blood due to invasion of heat* with faint eruptions and rashes. The skin manifestations are faint here because the heat is merely in the nutritive level and no toxin is present. Because the heat is not so intense, little blood is forced out of the vessels.

NOTE: Among the signs and symptoms, fever that worsens at night, irritability, restlessness, and a deep-red tongue without coating are the key identifiers for this pattern. If heat has only recently progressed from the qi to the nutritive level, there may also be a yellow coating over part of the tongue. Insomnia is commonly seen in this pattern.

Irritability and restlessness can be caused by:

- Heat from excess in the Stomach
- Heat from constraint in the chest and diaphragm
- Burning of yin in the nutritive level by heat (also known as disturbance of the Heart spirit due to invasion of heat)

Table 7.7 shows how the practitioner can differentiate among these three patterns.

Table 7.7	Comparison of Three Types of Restlessness
Pathology	**Signs and symptoms**
HEAT FROM EXCESS IN STOMACH	
Disturbance of the Heart spirit by excess qi-level heat in the Stomach through its collateral	Vigorous fever, profuse sweating, thirst with a preference for large amounts of cold beverages, red tongue with yellow coating
HEAT FROM CONSTRAINT IN CHEST AND DIAPHRAGM	
Disturbance of the Heart spirit by heat in the chest and diaphragm at the qi level	Irritability, insomnia, slightly yellow tongue coating
BURNING OF YIN IN NUTRITIVE LEVEL BY HEAT	
Disturbance of the Heart spirit by heat in the nutritive level	Fever that worsens at night, faint eruptions and rashes, deep-red tongue, thin and rapid pulse

Delirium is one aspect of the pattern of clumping of dry stool and heat in the Large Intestine, as well as of the present pattern. If there is constipation, distending pain in the abdomen, and a thick tongue coating, the delirium is caused by clumping of dry stool and heat in the Large Intestine. Otherwise, particularly if the presentation includes fever that worsens at night and a deep-red tongue, the delirium is due to the burning of yin in the nutritive level by heat.

Pathology. Disturbed Heart spirit, injury to the yin at the nutritive level, and failure of the collaterals to control blood due to invasion of heat.

Treatment principles. Dispel heat from the nutritive level to the qi level by cooling the blood, enriching the yin, and clearing heat from the Heart.

Formula:

CLEAR THE NUTRITIVE LEVEL DECOCTION *(qīng yíng tāng)*

SOURCE: *Systematic Differentiation of Warm Pathogen Diseases*

Bubali Cornu *(shuǐ niú jiǎo)*[32] 30-120g

Scrophulariae Radix *(xuán shēn)* 9g

Rehmanniae Radix *(shēng dì huáng)* 15g

Ophiopogonis Radix *(mài mén dōng)* 9g

Lonicerae Flos *(jīn yín huā)* 9g

Forsythiae Fructus *(lián qiào)* 6g

Coptidis Rhizoma *(huáng lián)* 4.5g

Lophatheri Herba *(dàn zhú yè)* [33] 3g

Salviae miltiorrhizae Radix *(dān shēn)* 6g

ANALYSIS OF FORMULA: Bubali Cornu *(shuǐ niú jiǎo)* is combined here with Coptidis Rhizoma *(huáng lián)* to clear heat and resolve toxicity from the Heart. Rehmanniae Radix *(shēng dì huáng)*, Scrophulariae Radix *(xuán shēn)*, and Ophiopogonis Radix *(mài mén dōng)* clear heat and enrich yin. Lonicerae Flos *(jīn yín huā)*, Forsythiae Fructus *(lián qiào)*, and Lophatheri Herba *(dàn zhú yè)* are mostly used to cope with the heat in the upper burner and qi level. They are cool, acrid, and light herbs that promote qi circulation and dispel the heat from the nutritive to the qi level. Salviae miltiorrhizae Radix *(dān shēn)* removes blood stasis and calms the spirit to relieve restlessness. In sum, because it promotes qi circulation, this formula is able to clear heat from the nutritive level and enrich the yin without trapping the warm-heat pathogen inside the body. According to Zhao Shao-Qin in *Length and Breadth of Warm Pathogen Disease [Differentiation]*,[34] promoting the circulation of qi is a very important principle of treatment when dealing with nutritive level patterns because there are many other factors besides the warm-heat pathogen that can cause the qi to stagnate, including phlegm, dampness, food retention, blood stasis, and dry, hard stool. Once it becomes stagnant, qi is unable to battle with the warm-heat pathogen, which then remains in the nutritive level. Thus, any method that can restore qi circulation, especially when combined with clearing heat from the nutritive level and enriching the yin, should be helpful in moving the warm-heat pathogen to the qi level. Such methods include eliminating food retention, removing blood stasis, and transforming phlegm and dampness.

MODIFICATIONS: The basic formula can be modified as follows:

- For residual protective level signs and symptoms, add Sojae Semen preparatum *(dàn dòu chǐ)*, Arctii Fructus *(niú bàng zǐ)*, and Menthae haplocalycis Herba *(bò hé)*.

- For severe coma, combine with Calm the Palace Pill with Cattle Gallstone *(ān gōng niú huáng wán)*. [35]

- For convulsions due to stirring of Liver wind, add Saigae tataricae Cornu *(líng yáng jiǎo)*, Uncariae Ramulus cum Uncis *(gōu téng)*, Bombyx batryticatus *(bái jiāng cán)*, and Chrysanthemi Flos *(jú huā)*.

- Once heat and toxins enter the blood level and the tongue body becomes very deep red, remove the herbs that dispel heat from the nutritive to the qi level, such as Forsythiae Fructus *(lián qiào)* and Lophatheri Herba *(dàn zhú yè)*. Add others, such as Paeoniae Radix rubra *(chì sháo)* and Moutan Cortex *(mǔ dān pí)*, that cool the blood.

- For heat that has combined with dampness (greasy tongue coating), add herbs with an aromatic nature, such as Curcumae Radix *(yù jīn)* and Acori tatarinowii Rhizoma *(shí chāng pǔ)*, to resolve the dampness.

DECOCTION AND ADMINISTRATION: Bubali Cornu *(shuǐ niú jiǎo)* should be powdered and cooked separately for 30 minutes before adding the other herbs.

ONSET OF RASH DUE TO HEAT IN THE LUNG

Manifestations. There are two concurrent aspects to this pattern:

1. *Accumulation of heat in the Lung* with cough, chest distention, red tongue with a thin, yellow coating, and a rapid pulse.
2. *Invasion of the blood level by heat in the Lung and heat forcing blood out of the collaterals* with rashes.

Pathology. Heat in the Lung invading the blood level and forcing blood out of the collaterals.

NOTE: This pattern is actually a combination of a qi-level disturbance, especially of the Lung, and a blood-level disturbance marked by a rash from heat forcing blood out of the collaterals.

Treatment principles. Clear and vent heat by promoting the Lung's disseminating function, cool the blood level, and promote the expression of rashes.

Formula:

MODIFIED HONEYSUCKLE AND FORSYTHIA POWDER
(jiā jiǎn yín qiáo sǎn)

SOURCE: *Systematic Differentiation of Warm Pathogen Diseases*

Lonicerae Flos *(jīn yín huā)* 30g

Forsythiae Fructus *(lián qiào)* 30g

Platycodi Radix *(jié gěng)* 18g

Menthae haplocalycis Herba *(bò hé)* 18g

Lophatheri Herba *(dàn zhú yè)* 12g

Glycyrrhizae Radix *(gān cǎo)* 15g

Schizonepetae Herba *(jīng jiè)* 12g

Arctii Fructus *(niú bàng zǐ)* 18g

Rehmanniae Radix *(shēng dì huáng)* 12g

Isatidis Folium *(dà qīng yè)* 9g

Moutan Cortex *(mǔ dān pí)* 9g

Scrophulariae Radix *(xuán shēn)* 30g

ANALYSIS OF FORMULA: Honeysuckle and Forsythia Powder *(yín qiào sǎn)* consists of acrid and cool herbs and is used to disperse wind-heat. Sojae Semen preparatum *(dàn dòu chǐ),* if prepared by soaking in Ephedrae Herba *(má huáng),* is acrid and warm. However, since there are no exterior signs and symptoms, Sojae Semen preparatum *(dàn dòu chǐ)* is not used in this modified formula. Schizonepetae Herba *(jīng jiè)* is used to ease itching and express skin eruptions, as well as to counteract the possible congealing effects of the many cold herbs in the formula. To cool the blood, clear heat, and resolve toxicity, Rehmanniae Radix *(shēng dì huáng),* Moutan Cortex *(mǔ dān pí),* Isatidis Folium *(dà qīng yè),* and Scrophulariae Radix *(xuán shēn)* are added. This formula serves to vent heat from the nutritive to the protective level, promote qi and blood circulation, and cool the blood.

MODIFICATIONS: Add Arnebiae Radix/Lithospermi Radix *(zǐ cǎo)* if the skin eruptions are severe.

Invasion of the Pericardium or Heart by Heat

VEILING OF THE PERICARDIUM BY TRANSMISSION OF HEAT AND PHLEGM

Manifestations. There are four concurrent aspects to this pattern:

1. *Attack on the nutritive level by heat* with a deep-red tongue body.

2. *Disturbance of the Heart spirit* with a muddled consciousness and delirium.

231

3. *Blockage of yang qi in the Pericardium by heat* with cold extremities and a hot chest.

4. *Obstruction of the Heart channel by phlegm-heat* with stiffness of the tongue and difficulty speaking.

NOTE: Delirium is a symptom of both the burning of yin in the nutritive level by heat and of the present pattern. However, the former pattern often begins in the protective level, then progresses to the qi level, and finally to the nutritive level, and *sometimes* presents with delirium. By contrast, the present pattern often progresses directly from the protective to the nutritive level, and delirium and muddled consciousness are *always* present. (See Table 7.8 for a comparison of the two patterns.)

Table 7.8	Comparison of Two Types of Delirium
Pathology	**Signs and Symptoms**
BURNING OF YIN IN NUTRITIVE LEVEL BY HEAT	
Heat often progresses from the qi to the nutritive level	Condition is milder, although there is sometimes delirium
VEILING OF THE PERICARDIUM BY TRANSMISSION OF HEAT AND PHLEGM	
Heat often progresses from the protective level directly to the nutritive level	Condition is severe: muddled consciousness and delirium

In this pattern, the blockage of qi in the Pericardium causing the extremities to become cold is a more serious sign than the delirium, because blockage of qi is more severe than stagnation of qi. The phlegm in this pattern is either derived from heat causing the fluids to congeal or was present prior to the onset of the warm pathogen disease.

Pathology. Veiling of the Pericardium by transmission of heat and phlegm.

Treatment principles. Clear heat from the Pericardium, resolve the phlegm, and open the orifices.

Formula No. 1:

CALM THE PALACE PILL WITH CATTLE GALLSTONE *(ān gōng niú huáng wán)*

SOURCE: *Systematic Differentiation of Warm Pathogen Diseases*

Bovis Calculus *(niú huáng)* 30g

Rhinocerotis Cornu *(xī jiǎo)* 30g
Moschus *(shè xiāng)* 7.5g
Coptidis Rhizoma *(huáng lián)* 30g
Scutellariae Radix *(huáng qín)* 30g
Gardeniae Fructus *(zhī zǐ)* 30g
Arnebiae Radix/Lithospermi Radix Realgar *(xióng huáng)* 30g
Borneolum *(bīng piàn)* 7.5g
Cinnabaris *(zhū shā)* 30g
Curcumae Radix *(yù jīn)* 30g
Margarita *(zhēn zhū)* 15g
Auri Lamina *(jīn bó)*[36] 30g

ANALYSIS OF FORMULA: One of the chief ingredients, Bovis Calculus *(niú huáng)*, which is bitter, cool, and aromatic, is very effective in clearing heat from both the Heart and Liver channels. Its aromatic properties vent heat to the exterior by way of the collaterals of the Pericardium. Additionally, this ingredient resolves toxicity and dislodges phlegm to open the sensory orifices, extinguishes wind, and stops spasms, tremors, and convulsions. It thereby addresses all of the major aspects of this condition.

The second chief ingredient, Rhinocerotis Cornu *(xī jiǎo)*, which is salty and cold, enters the nutritive and blood levels and plays an important role in clearing fire and heat from the Heart, Liver, and Stomach. It clears heat from the Heart, calms the spirit, cools the blood, and resolves toxicity. Its cool, aromatic properties quickly vent pathogenic heat from the Pericardium. The third chief ingredient, Moschus *(shè xiāng)*, which is aromatic, opens the orifices and revives the spirit as it penetrates all twelve channels of the body. Its strong, aromatic nature is essential in treating a disorder in which the sensory orifices are veiled by phlegm.

The three major deputies—Scutellariae Radix *(huáng qín)*, Coptidis Rhizoma *(huáng lián)*, and Gardeniae Fructus *(zhī zǐ)*—con-duct the heat downward, helping Bovis Calculus *(niú huáng)* and Rhinocerotis Cornu *(xī jiǎo)* clear and drain the heat and toxin from the Pericardium. Another ingredient, Arnebiae Radix/Lithospermi Radix Realgar *(xióng huáng)*, dislodges phlegm and resolves toxicity, thus helping to open the orifices by draining the turbid phlegm. The remaining ingredients, Borneolum *(bīng piàn)* and Curcumae Radix *(yù jīn)*, aromatically open the orifices and disperse constrained heat, thereby helping the chief ingredients to vent heat through the channel of the Pericardium. The three assistants—Cinnabaris *(zhū shā)*, Auri Lamina *(jīn bó)*, and Margarita *(zhēn zhū)*—sedate the Heart and calm the spirit while clearing heat from the Heart and Liver.

Formula No. 2:

GREATEST TREASURE SPECIAL PILL *(zhì bǎo dān)*

SOURCE: *Formulary of the Bureau of Medicines of the Taiping Era*[37]

Bovis Calculus *(niú huáng)* 15g
Rhinocerotis Cornu *(xī jiǎo)* 30g
Moschus *(shè xiāng)* 0.3g
Arnebiae Radix/Lithospermi Radix Realgar *(xióng huáng)* 30g
Borneolum *(bīng piàn)* 0.3g
Argenti Lamina *(yín bó)* . . . . 10 pieces
Cinnabaris *(zhū shā)* 30g
Eretmochelydis Carapax *(dài mào)*[38] 30g
Benzoinum *(ān xī xiāng)* 45g
Succinum *(hǔ pò)* 30g
Auri Lamina *(jīn bó)*[39] . . . . 25 pieces
Cinnabaris *(zhū shā)* 30g

ANALYSIS OF FORMULA: The chief ingredient, Rhinocerotis Cornu *(xī jiǎo)*, clears heat from the nutritive level and cools the blood. Its cool, aromatic properties make it useful for treating heat that affects the collateral of the Pericardium. Phlegm and heat interact: unless the turbid phlegm is eliminated, it will be difficult to clear the heat. Bovis Calculus *(niú huáng)*, which clears heat, resolves toxicity, clears away phlegm, and opens the orifices, is therefore used to eliminate the phlegm-heat that veils the Pericardium.

Eretmochelydis Carapax *(dài mào)*, which is sweet and cold, enters both the Heart and Liver channels, sedates the Heart, calms the Liver, clears heat, and resolves toxicity. It is particularly useful in cooling the Liver, extinguishing wind, and stopping spasms and convulsions. The Heart stores the spirit and the Liver stores the ethereal soul. Clearing heat from these two organs serves to calm the spirit and the ethereal soul.

Borneolum *(bīng piàn)* and Benzoinum *(ān xī xiāng)* are very aromatic substances that break up turbid phlegm and open the orifices, thus eliminating internal obstruction. Cinnabaris *(zhū shā)*, Succinum *(hǔ pò)*, Auri Lamina *(jīn bó)*, and Argenti Lamina *(yín bó)* sedate the Heart and calm the spirit, resolving the irritability and impairment of speech and consciousness. Arnebiae Radix/Lithospermi Radix Realgar *(xióng huáng)* eliminates phlegm and resolves toxicity. It strengthens the actions of Bovis Calculus *(niú huáng)* in breaking up phlegm and opening the orifices.

Formula No. 3:

> **PURPLE SNOW SPECIAL PILL** *(zǐ xuě dān)*[40]
>
> SOURCE: *Supplement to Important Formulas Worth a Thousand Gold Pieces*

Gypsum fibrosum *(shí gāo)* 1500g
Glauberitum *(hán shuǐ shí)* 1500g

Talcum *(huá shí)* 1500g

Rhinocerotis Cornu *(xī jiǎo)* 150g

Saigae tataricae Cornu *(líng yáng jiǎo)* 150g

Moschus *(shè xiāng)* 37.5g

Scrophulariae Radix *(xuán shēn)* 500g

Magnetitum *(cí shí)* 1500g

Aquilariae Lignum resinatum *(chén xiāng)* 150g

Cimicifugae Rhizoma *(shēng má)* 500g

Honey-toasted Glycyrrhizae Radix preparata *(zhì gān cǎo)* 240g

Aristolochiae Radix (*qīng mù xiāng)*[41] 150g

Caryophylli Flos *(dīng xiāng)* 30g

Cinnabaris *(zhū shā)* 90g

Natrii Sulfas *(máng xiāo)* 5000g

Nitrum *(xiāo shí)* 96g

Gold *(huáng jīn)* . . . . 3000g[42]

ANALYSIS OF FORMULA: There are two groups of chief ingredients. The first consists of Gypsum fibrosum *(shí gāo)*, Glauberitum *(hán shuǐ shí)*, and Talcum *(huá shí)*. Gypsum fibrosum *(shí gāo)* is an important substance for clearing fire and heat from the qi level, causing the heat to recede and encouraging the generation of fluids. It thereby eliminates irritability. Glauberitum *(hán shuǐ shí)* likewise clears heat and drains fire to eliminate irritability. The slippery quality of Talcum *(huá shí)* enables it to conduct heat downward so that it can be eliminated through the urine.

The second group of chief ingredients consists of Rhinocerotis Cornu *(xī jiǎo)*, Saigae tataricae Cornu *(líng yáng jiǎo)*, and Moschus *(shè xiāng)*. Rhinocerotis Cornu *(xī jiǎo)*, which is cool and aromatic, both rises and disperses. It enters the nutritive and blood levels, and is an important substance for clearing fire and heat from the Heart and Liver. It clears heat from the nutritive level, cools the blood, and resolves toxicity. Due to its active nature, it can be cold without retarding movement; this quality makes it useful for venting heat through the collaterals of the Pericardium. Saigae tataricae Cornu *(líng yáng jiǎo)* is particularly helpful in draining Liver fire and is an important substance for cooling the Liver and fire, and extinguishing wind. Together, these three animal products treat the heat in the Heart and Liver, and effectively resolve spasms, convulsions, and impaired consciousness. The aromatic properties of Moschus *(shè xiāng)* enable it to open the orifices of the Heart and restore consciousness.

Among the deputies and assistant ingredients, Scrophulariae Radix *(xuán shēn)* conducts fire downward, enriches yin, and eliminates irritability. It is combined with Cimicifugae Rhizoma *(shēng má)* to strengthen its ability to clear heat and resolve toxicity. Aristolochiae Radix *(qīng mù xiāng)*, Caryophylli Flos *(dīng xiāng)*, and

Aquilariae Lignum resinatum *(chén xiāng)* promote the movement of qi and assist Moschus *(shè xiāng)* in opening the orifices. Cinnabaris *(zhū shā)* and Magnetitum *(cí shí)* sedate the Heart and calm the spirit, which strengthens the formula's action in eliminating irritability. Natrii Sulfas *(máng xiāo)* and Nitrum *(xiāo shí)* also drain heat and dissipate clumps, especially when combined with Scrophulariae Radix *(xuán shēn)*. This strong, heat-clearing action is called 'removing the firewood from under the cauldron' (釜抵抽薪 *fǔ dǐ chōu xīn)*.

Formula No. 4:

CLEAR THE PALACE DECOCTION *(qīng gōng tāng)*

SOURCE: *Systematic Differentiation of Warm Pathogen Diseases*

Core Scrophulariae Radix *(xuán shēn)* 9g
Nelumbinis Plumula *(lián zǐ xīn)* 1.5g
Lophatheri Folium immaturus *(zhú yè juǎn xīn)* . . . . .6g[43]
Forsythiae Semen *(lián qiào xīn)*[44] 6g
Ophiopogonis Radix *(mài mén dōng)* 9g
Rhinocerotis Cornu *(xī jiǎo)* 6g

ANALYSIS OF FORMULA: Clear the Palace Decoction *(qīng gōng tāng)* is a special formula for clearing heat from the Pericardium. In Chinese medicine, the Pericardium is like the wall around a palace *(gōng qiáng* 宮牆) that protects the sovereign (that is, the Heart) who lives inside. Hence the name of the formula, which means to clear heat specifically from the Pericardium. In this formula, Rhinocerotis Cornu *(xī jiǎo)* clears heat from the Pericardium. Core Scrophulariae Radix *(xuán shēn)*, Nelumbinis Plumula *(lián zǐ xīn)*, and Ophiopogonis Radix *(mài mén dōng)* nourish the fluids of the Heart and the Pericardium. Lophatheri Folium immaturus *(zhú yè juǎn xīn)* and Forsythiae Fructus *(lián qiào)* are chosen to clear and disperse heat from the Pericardium. According to Wu Tang, the kernel of a seed, the core of a root, and an unfolded leaf from the bamboo are needed in this formula, because these parts of the plants represent the center *(xīn* 心) and thus correspond to the Heart *(xīn* 心). As a result of this correspondence, it is believed that they can specifically reach to the Heart and Pericardium. However, it is generally used without the special parts of the plants specified here. Clinically, Clear the Palace Decoction *(qīng gōng tāng)* only serves to clear heat from the Pericardium and enrich the yin of the Heart; it cannot resolve the phlegm and open the orifices. Therefore, Calm the Palace Pill with Cattle Gallstone *(ān gōng niú huáng wán)*, Purple Snow Special Pill *(zǐ xuě dān)*, or Greatest Treasure Special Pill *(zhì bǎo dān)* must be added for these purposes. (See 'Administration' below for a discussion of combining these formulas.)

MODIFICATIONS

- For high fever and muddled consciousness, use Calm the Palace Pill with Cattle Gallstone *(ān gōng niú huáng wán)*. If there are many red spots over the tip of the tongue, add Coptidis Rhizoma *(huáng lián)*, Isatidis Folium *(dà qīng yè)*, and Isatidis/Baphicacanthis Radix *(bǎn lán gēn)* to enhance the function of the other herbs in clearing heat from the Pericardium.

- For much phlegm that manifests as gurgling of phlegm in the throat and bronchi, and a bright red tongue with a thick, greasy coating, add Bambusae Succus *(zhú lì)*, Bambusae Concretio silicea *(tiān zhú huáng)*, and Trichosanthis Pericarpium *(guā lóu pí)* to clear heat and resolve the phlegm.

- For convulsions due to heat from excess in the nutritive level leading to stirring of internal wind, combine Purple Snow Special Pill *(zǐ xuě dān)* with Uncariae Ramulus cum Uncis *(gōu téng)* to extinguish the internal wind.

- For a pattern that is associated with clumping of dry stool and heat in the Large Intestine, add Rhei Radix et Rhizoma *(dà huáng)* and Natrii Sulfas *(máng xiāo)* to purge heat and dry stool.

- For obstruction of the orifices and channel of the Heart (purple lips, nails, and tongue), add Rhinoceros Horn and Succinum Greatest Treasure Special Pill *(xī pò zhì bǎo dān)*[45] to enhance the formula's ability to remove blood stasis and open the orifices. The formula will clear heat, resolve phlegm, promote blood circu-lation, and remove blood stasis. However, due to concerns of toxicity and the endangered status of the rhinoceros, Bubali Cornu *(shuǐ niú jiǎo)* should be substituted for Rhinocerotis Cornu *(xī jiǎo)*. Also, Coptidis Rhizoma *(huáng lián)* is used in place of Cinnabaris *(zhū shā)*, and Margaritiferae Concha usta *(zhēn zhū mǔ)* is substituted for Eretmochelydis Carapax *(dài mào)*.

In addition, acupuncture should be used to deal with these conditions. Recommended points include GV-26 *(rén zhōng)*, LI-11 *(qū chí)*, and LU-11 *(shào shāng)*.

ADMINISTRATION: The first three formulas, which, when used to treat a warm patho-gen disease, are referred to collectively as the 'three treasures,' are available as pat-ent medicines, and are selected according to different conditions. They are similar to each other, but also quite different (see Table 7.9). Any of the three can be swallowed with a decoction of Clear the Palace Decoction *(qīng gōng tāng)*. However, the com-bination of Clear the Palace Decoction *(qīng gōng tāng)* and Calm the Palace Pill with Cattle Gallstone *(ān gōng niú huáng wán)* is best for this pattern. Clinically, these formulas can be melted in boiled water and given to the patient drop by drop through the mouth. The dosage suggested is 5-10 drops every hour. Nowadays a nasogastric tube is used, but the decoction must still be administered slowly, a small amount at a time.

Table 7.9	Comparison of Calm the Palace Pill with Cattle Gallstone, Greatest Treasure Special Pill, and Purple Snow Special Pill	
Indications	**Focus of Treatment**	
CALM THE PALACE PILL WITH CATTLE GALLSTONE *(ān gōng niú huáng wán)*		
High fever, muddled consciousness	Clear heat, resolve toxicity, resolve phlegm	
GREATEST TREASURE SPECIAL PILL *(zhì bǎo dān)*		
Severe coma, fever that is not as high as in the other patterns	Open the orifices	
PURPLE SNOW SPECIAL PILL *(zǐ xuě dān)*		
High fever and convulsions	Clear heat and extinguish internal wind	

If none of the three formulas is available, add Bovis Calculus *(niú huáng)* (0.3g) or Bubali Cornu *(shuǐ niú jiǎo)* (15g), Bambusae Succus *(zhú lì)* (30g), Arisaema cum Bile *(dǎn nán xīng)* (9g), Acori tatarinowii Rhizoma *(shí chāng pǔ)* (6g), and Curcumae Radix *(yù jīn)* (6g) to Clear the Palace Decoction *(qīng gōng tāng)* to resolve the phlegm and open the orifices. If there are convulsions, add Saigae tataricae Cornu *(líng yáng jiǎo)* (0.3g) and Uncariae Ramulus cum Uncis *(gōu téng)* (15g) to extinguish the Liver wind.

Blockage of the Heart by Transmission of Heat Coupled with Clumping of Dry Stool and Heat in the Large Intestine

Manifestations. There are two concurrent aspects to this pattern:

1. *Blockage of the Heart by transmission of heat* with fever, coma, stiff tongue with difficulty speaking, cold extremities, and a deep-red tongue.
2. *Clumping of dry stool and heat in the Large Intestine* with an intense, distending pain in the abdomen, constipation, a dry and yellow tongue coating, and a deep, forceful, rapid pulse.

NOTE: Fever, coma, and cold extremities may appear in the pattern of clumping of dry stool and heat in the Large Intestine. However, stiff tongue with difficulty speaking is absent from that pattern. This is a key identifier for distinguishing the combined pattern here from just the clumping of dry stool and heat in the Large Intestine. It is significant because the tongue is the mirror of the Heart. When heat blocks the Heart, movement of the tongue will be affected; the tongue will be stiff, and speech will be impaired.

Pathology. Blockage of the Heart by heat combined with clumping of dry stool and heat in the Large Intestine.

Treatment principles. Clear heat from the Heart, open the orifices, and remove dry stool and heat from the Large Intestine by purging.

Formula:

> **CATTLE GALLSTONE DECOCTION TO ORDER THE QI**
> *(niú huáng chéng qì tāng)*

SOURCE: *Systematic Differentiation of Warm Pathogen Diseases*

ANALYSIS OF FORMULA: Cattle Gallstone Decoction to Order the Qi *(niú huáng chéng qì tāng)* consists of two Calm the Palace Pills with Cattle Gallstone *(ān gōng niú huáng wán)* and powdered Rhei Radix et Rhizoma *(dà huáng)* (3g). Calm the Palace Pill with Cattle Gallstone *(ān gōng niú huáng wán)* is used to clear heat and open the orifices, and Rhei Radix et Rhizoma *(dà huáng)* purges heat through bowel movements. Purging heat through bowel movements is an example of a famous treatment strategy: 'removing firewood from under the cauldron.' As in this situation, a strong purgative effect is desired. Untreated Rhei Radix et Rhizoma *(dà huáng)* is used for this purpose.

MODIFICATIONS: The basic formula can be modified as follows:

- When Rhei Radix et Rhizoma *(dà huáng)* is not strong enough by itself to clear extreme heat from the Heart and remove dry stool from the Large Intestine, add Natrii Sulfas *(máng xiāo)* and Scrophulariae Radix *(xuán shēn)* to soften dry stool and to generate fluids for the discharge of dry stool as well as heat.

- For severe damage to the fluids, add Ophiopogonis Radix *(mài mén dōng)*, Rehmanniae Radix *(shēng dì huáng)*, and Scrophulariae Radix *(xuán shēn)*.

DECOCTION AND ADMINISTRATION: First, dissolve two Calm the Palace Pills with Cattle Gallstone in warm boiled water. Then mix with 3g powdered Rhei Radix et Rhizoma *(dà huáng)*. Begin by giving just one half of this mixture by nasogastric tube. If there is no movement of the bowels and the patient remains unconscious, give the rest of the mixture to the patient.

INTERIOR BLOCKAGE AND EXTERIOR COLLAPSE

Manifestations. There are two concurrent aspects to this pattern:

1. *Interior blockage of phlegm and heat* with fever, coma, and a very deep-red and dry tongue.
2. *Exterior collapse of yang qi* with either:
   • Shortness of breath, profuse sweating, thin and weak pulse; or
   • Pale face with profuse sweating, cold sensation in the extremities, and a feeble pulse.

Pathology. Interiorly, a blockage of the Heart by phlegm and heat combined with an exterior collapse of yang qi.

Treatment principles. Clear heat, resolve phlegm, open the orifices, and arrest collapse.

Formulas. Calm the Palace Pill with Cattle Gallstone *(ān gōng niú huáng wán)*, Greatest Treasure Special Pill *(zhì bǎo dān)*, or Purple Snow Special Pill *(zǐ xuě dān)* combined with Generate the Pulse Powder *(shēng mài sǎn)* or Ginseng and Aconite Accessory Root Decoction *(shēn fù tāng)*.

Formula No. 1:

GENERATE THE PULSE POWDER *(shēng mài sǎn)*

SOURCE: *Origins of Medicine* [46]

Ginseng Radix *(rén shēn)* 9g
Ophiopogonis Radix *(mài mén dōng)* 6g
Schisandrae Fructus *(wǔ wèi zǐ)* 3g

ANALYSIS OF FORMULA: Ginseng Radix *(rén shēn)*, the chief herb in this formula, strongly tonifies the source qi (which also generates fluids) and calms the spirit. When the source qi is strong, the qi of the Lung is replete and is properly able to regulate the interstices and pores; as a consequence, the fluids are no longer lost through the superficial levels of the body.

The deputy herb is Ophiopogonis Radix *(mài mén dōng)*, which enriches the yin and moistens the Lung. It also benefits the Stomach, generates fluids, and clears heat from the Heart to eliminate the irritability that may occur with this condition. The chief herb acts on the qi and the fluids, while the deputy herb acts directly on the fluids, a combination that gives the formula a very strong fluid-generating effect.

The assistant herb, Schisandrae Fructus *(wǔ wèi zǐ)*, restrains the leakage of Lung qi and sweat, generates fluids, and calms the spirit. In concert with the deputy, it forms a powerful combination for generating fluids. With the chief herb, this enables the formula to rescue the injured qi and yin. This formula is simple, yet well-balanced. The chief herb tonifies, the deputy clears, and the assistant restrains leakage.

Formula No. 2:

GINSENG AND ACONITE ACCESSORY ROOT DECOCTION *(shēn fù tāng)*

SOURCE: *Great Collection of Fine Formulas for Women* [47]

Ginseng Radix *(rén shēn)* 30g
Aconiti Radix lateralis preparata *(zhì fù zǐ)* 15g

ANALYSIS OF FORMULA: Very warm and strong tonifying herbs must be used to restore the exhausted yang and rescue the qi from collapse. The Spleen is the foundation of the postnatal qi and the source of blood. The Lung governs the body's qi. The chief ingredient, sweet and warm Ginseng Radix *(rén shēn)*, strongly tonifies the Spleen and Lung qi as well as the source qi in the Kidney. Its actions of nourishing, tonifying, and strengthening enable it to stabilize a condition of imminent collapse.

The deputy herb, Aconiti Radix lateralis preparata *(zhì fù zǐ)*, warms and tonifies the yang of the Kidney. Together these herbs restore the yang and rescue it from collapse. Although the formula is composed of only two herbs, the relatively large dosage has a quick effect on the body. It is therefore suitable for the condition of acute collapse of yang qi.

NOTE: Generate the Pulse Powder *(shēng mài sǎn)* is used for treating collapse of qi and yin. Ginseng and Aconite Accessory Root Decoction *(shēn fù tāng)* is used for collapse of yang qi.

DECOCTION AND ADMINISTRATION: The source text advises to decoct in water in which Zingiberis Rhizoma recens *(shēng jiāng)* and Jujubae Fructus *(dà zǎo)* have been boiled. Ginseng Radix *(rén shēn)* may be separately prepared by cooking it for 30 minutes in a double boiler and adding the resulting liquid to a strained decoction of Aconiti Radix lateralis preparata *(zhì fù zǐ)*.[48]

Summary

Wind-warmth is the disease caused by an attack of wind-heat, which usually occurs in the spring or winter. There are two avenues of progression in the development of wind-warmth, normal and abnormal. Generally speaking, in the early stage there is involvement of the Lung and/or the protective level. In the middle stage when heat has invaded the qi level, the Lung, diaphragm, Stomach, and Large Intestine are mostly involved. And at a later stage, injury to the yin of the Lung and Stomach is most commonly seen. The principles and methods of treatment for wind-warmth are summarized in Table 7.10.

Table 7.10	Differentiation and Treatment of Wind-Warmth	
Patterns	**Treatment Principles**	**Formulas**
PROTECTIVE LEVEL		
Attack on protective level by wind-heat, slightly affecting the Lung	Release the exterior and disseminate the Lung qi	Honeysuckle and Forsythia Powder (*yín qiào sǎn*)
Attack on the Lung by wind- heat	Disseminate the Lung qi and induce it to descend, release the exterior	Mulberry Leaf and Chrysanthemum Drink (*sāng jú yǐn*)
QI LEVEL		
Accumulation of heat in the Lung and Stomach	Clear heat from the Lung and Stomach, disseminate and induce the Lung qi to descend	Ephedra, Apricot Kernel, Gypsum, and Licorice Decoction (*má xìng shí gān tāng*)
Heat from constraint in the chest and diaphragm	Clear and disperse heat from the chest and diaphragm with light herbs	Gardenia and Prepared Soybean Decoction (*zhì zǐ chǐ tāng*)
Stagnation of phlegm and heat in the chest and epigastrium	Clear heat, resolve phlegm, and disperse phlegm and heat	Minor Sinking into the Chest Decoction plus Unripe Bitter Orange (*xiǎo xiàn xiōng jiā zhǐ shí tāng*)
Remnants of heat with injury to the Lung and Stomach yin	Enrich the Lung and Stomach yin	Glehnia/Adenophora and Ophiopogon Decoction (*shā shēn mài mén dōng tāng*)
Blockage of the Lung by phlegm and heat coupled with clumping of stool and heat in the Large Intestine	Induce the Lung qi to descend, resolve phlegm, clear heat by purging	Disseminate the White and Order the Qi Decoction (*xuān bái chéng qì tāng*)
Transmission of heat to the Large Intestine from the Lung	Clear heat from the Large Intestine and stop diarrhea	Kudzu, Scutellaria, and Coptis Decoction (*gé gēn huáng qín huáng lián tāng*)
Heat from excess in the Stomach injuring the fluids	Clear heat from the Stomach and generate fluids	White Tiger Decoction (*bái hǔ tāng*)

Table 7.10, cont.		
Clumping of dry stool and heat in the Large Intestine	Soften the dry stool and clear heat by purging	Regulate the Stomach and Order the Qi Decoction (*tiáo wèi chéng qì tāng*)
NUTRITIVE AND BLOOD LEVEL		
Burning of yin in the nutritive level by heat, which also affects the collaterals	Dispel heat from the nutritive level to the qi level by cooling blood, enriching yin, and clearing heat from the Heart	Clear the Nutritive Level Decoction (*qīng yíng tāng*)
Onset of rash due to heat in the Lung	Clear and vent heat by promoting the Lung's disseminating function, cool the blood level, promote the expression of rashes	Modified Honeysuckle and Forsythia Powder (*jiā jiǎn yín qiáo sǎn*)
INVASION OF THE PERICARDIUM BY HEAT		
Veiling of the Pericardium by transmission of heat with phlegm	Clear heat from the Pericardium, resolve phlegm, and open the orifices	Calm the Palace Pill with Cattle Gallstone (*ān gōng niú huáng wán*), Greatest Treasure Special Pill (*zhì bǎo dān*), or Purple Snow Special Pill (*zǐ xuě dān*) taken with Clear the Palace Decoction (*qīng gōng tāng*)
Blockage of the Heart by transmission of heat coupled with clumping of dry stool and heat in the Large Intestine	Clear heat from the Heart, open the orifices, and remove dry stool and heat from the Large Intestine by purgation	Cattle Gallstone Decoction to Order the Qi (*niú huáng chéng qì tāng*)
Interior blockage of the Heart by phlegm and heat with exterior collapse of yang qi	Clear heat, resolve phlegm, open the orifices, and arrest collapse	Calm the Palace Pill with Cattle Gallstone (*ān gōng niú huáng wán*), Greatest Treasure Special Pill (*zhì bǎo dān*), or Purple Snow Special Pill (*zǐ xuě dān*) combined with Generate the Pulse Powder (*shēng mài sǎn*) or Ginseng and Aconite Accessory Root Decoction (*shēn fù tāng*)

Endnotes

1. While most textbooks in China state that wind-warmth only occurs during spring or winter, patterns associated with wind-warmth, such as those for which Mulberry Leaf and Chrysanthemum Drink *(sāng jú yǐn)* or Honeysuckle and Forsythia Powder *(yín qiào sǎn)* are indicated, are also often seen during the summer or fall.

2. Tang Da-Lie (Tang Li-San), *Collections of Discourses by Wu [Area] Physicians (Wú yī huì jiǎng)*. Shanghai: Shanghai Science and Technology Publishing House, 1983: 7

3. The term 'remnants of heat' refers to a situation where heat from excess has been fighting with the body's yin. In the process both sides are injured and the heat thus becomes less forceful due to the yin's moderating influence, while the yin becomes damaged.

4. The combination of sweet-flavored and cold-natured herbs serves to produce fluids.

5. Each pattern described in this book has several coexisting aspects that are described to assist in the differentiation of the patterns.

6. Wu Tang, *Systematic Differentiation of Warm Pathogen Diseases (Wēn bìng tiáo biàn)*. Beijing: People's Health Publishing House, 1963: 16.

7. He Lian-Chen, *Revised and Expanded Discussion of Warm-Heat Pathogen Diseases (Chóng dìng guǎng wēn rè lùn)*. Beijing: People's Health Publishing House, 1960: 35.

8. Anonymous, *Yellow Emperor's Inner Classic: Basic Questions (Huáng Dì nèi jīng sù wèn)*. Beijing: People's Health Publishing House, 1963: 510

9. Alternatives to decocting: For convenience, many of the formulas described in this book are available in prepared form as tablets or powders. They are very easy to take, particularly for patients who travel or who do not have time to cook raw herbs. While it is a good idea to follow the manufacturer's directions, for this formula to be effective in prepared form it should be taken every two hours, at least six times a day.

10. For more information about the proper method for preparing Chinese medicine, see the preface to this book.

11. Anonymous, *Yellow Emperor's Inner Classic: Basic Questions,* 4-5. In my opinion, we should not be too rigid in adhering to this concept.

12. Throughout this book are case studies that illustrate the use of particular formulas. These cases focus on specific pathologies and not necessarily unique manifestations of an individual pattern. It is important to note this emphasis on pathology, because manifestations can differ from person to person due to differences in constitution, diet, lifestyle, and environment. Always remember that the formulas are designed to treat the pathology, not necessarily a specific manifestation.

13. Meng Shu-Jiang et al., *Warm Pathogen Diseases (Wēn bìng xué)*. Shanghai: Shanghai Science and Technology Publishing House, 1985: 50. This case was submitted by the doctors in the Internal Medicine Department at the First Teaching Hospital of the Jiangsu College of New Medicine.

14. We have reproduced this case as set forth in the original work and have not edited out some of its odder aspects, such as a diagnosis of a viral disease followed by treatment with multiple antibiotics.

15. Meng Shu-Jiang et al., *Warm Pathogen Diseases*, 50. This case study was reported by Pu Fu-Zhou.

16. The ingredients in this formula are identical to those in a formula with a similar but longer name, Ephedra, Apricot Kernel, Licorice and Gypsum Decoction *(má huáng xìng rén gān cǎo shí gaō tāng)* from the *Discussion of Cold Damage* by Zhang Ji. Unfortunately, the English translation is the same. The difference is that in Zhang's formula, the dosage of the main herbs is much greater. Wu uses a smaller dosage because he saw this as heat in the upper and middle burners, that is, the Lung and Stomach, necessitating herbs that are light in weight. This way they will disperse heat in the upper burner and open the pores to vent heat, for which relatively small doses are more effective. In particular, he reduced the dosage of Gypsum fibrosum *(shí gāo)* from 48g to 9g to avoid the possibility of its heavy and cold qualities congealing the heat. In my opinion, 9g of Gypsum fibrosum *(shí gāo)* is sometimes insufficient for severe heat in the Lung and Stomach, and 18g is often used in the clinic.

17. When combined with Cinnamomi Ramulus *(guì zhī)*, which can warm the channels, Ephedrae Herba *(má huáng)* can induce a great deal of sweating because blood in the channels is the source of sweat. When combined with Gypsum fibrosum *(shí gāo)*, which is acrid and cold and counteracts the warming effects of Ephedrae Herba *(má huáng)*, the use of Ephedrae Herba *(má huáng)* will only induce very mild sweating, and will merely open the pores on the skin. In this way Gypsum fibrosum *(shí gāo)* modulates the effects of Ephedrae Herba *(má huáng)*, whereas Cinnamomi Ramulus *(guì zhī)* works synergistically with it.

18. In *Discussion of Cold Damage*, Zhang Ji recommends cooking Ephedrae Herba *(má huáng)* first and skimming off the froth before adding other herbs to the decoction. The sixth-century writer Tao Hong-Jing noted that this froth can make a patient feel restless. *Collection of Commentaries on the Classic of the Materia Medica (Běn cǎo jīng jí zhù)*. Beijing: People's Health Publishing House, 1994: 271. In the early twentieth century, Zhang Xi-Chun wrote that the froth actually has a very strong sweat-inducing effect and should be skimmed off if intense sweating is not indicated. *Essays on Medicine Esteeming the Chinese and Respecting the Western (Yī xué zhōng zhōng cān xī lù)*. Shijiazhuang: Hebei People's Publishing House, 1957: 506. In my own experience, however, there is neither excessive sweating nor restlessness when Ephedrae Herba *(má huáng)* is combined with Gypsum fibrosum *(shí gāo)*, regardless of whether Ephedrae Herba *(má huáng)* is decocted first or the froth is skimmed off.

19. Dong Jian-Hua, *Selected Case Studies from Famous Modern Chinese Doctors (Zhōng guó xiàn dài míng zhōng yī yī àn jīng huá)*. Beijing: Beijing Publishing House, 1990: 1655. This case study was reported by Zhao Xi-Wu.

20. Anonymous, *Yellow Emperor's Inner Classic: Basic Questions*, 501.

21. Chen Ming and Zhang Yin-Sheng, *Selected Case Studies from Famous Doctors who Specialize in Cold Damage (Shāng hán míng yī yàn àn jīng xuǎn)*. Beijing: Learning Garden Publishing House, 1998: 79. This case study was reported by Wei Peng-Chun.

22. This is a modification of Minor Sinking into the Chest Decoction *(xiǎo xiàn xiōng tāng)* from *Discussion of Cold Damage*.

23. Zhao Xu-Chu et al., *Compendium of Modern Chinese Medicine Applications and Research: Warm Pathogen Diseases (Xiàn dài zhōng yī yào yìng yòng yǔ yán jiù dà xì: wēn bìng)*. Shanghai: Shanghai University of Chinese Medicine Publishing House, 1995: 251.

24. The manifestations of the pattern for which Major Order the Qi Decoction *(dà chéng qì tāng)* is indicated are tidal fever, constipation with hard and dry stool in the Large Intestine or diarrhea with a discharge of foul-smelling liquid, strong and distending pain in the abdomen, and a submerged, forceful pulse.

25. Wang Shi-Xiong, *Cases Studies of Wang Meng-Ying (Wáng Mèng-Yīng yī àn)*. Beijing: Chinese Medicine and Pharmacology Publishing House, 1999: 27.

26. Meng Shu-Jiang et al., *Warm Pathogen Diseases*, 46.

27. This formula is taken from *Systematic Differentiation of Warm Pathogen Diseases.*

28. In the source text Wu Tang states that sugar cane juice can be substituted for lotus node juice.

29. See Appendix C.

30. Both of these formulas were first recorded in *Discussion of Cold Damage.* Major Order the Qi Decoction *(dà chéng qì tāng)* contains the following herbs: Rhei Radix et Rhizoma *(dà huáng)* (12g), Natrii Sulfas *(máng xiāo)* (9-12g), Aurantii Fructus immaturus *(zhǐ shí)* (12-15g), and Magnoliae officinalis Cortex *(hòu pò)* (24g). Minor Order the Qi Decoction *(xiǎo chéng qì tāng)* is discussed in Chapter 11.

31. Wu Tang, *Systematic Differentiation of Warm Pathogen Diseases*, 65.

32. The source text calls for Rhinocerotis Cornu *(xī jiǎo)*. Because this is taken from an endangered species, Bubali Cornu *(shuǐ niú jiǎo)* is used as a substitute, with a dosage of 30–120g.

33. The source text uses Lophatheri Folium immaturus *(zhú yè juǎn xīn)*, which is difficult to find outside of East Asia. I recommend substituting Lophatheri Herba *(dàn zhú yè)*.

34. Zhao Shao-Qin, Hu Ding-Bang, and Liu Jing-Yuan, *Length and Breadth of Warm Pathogen Disease [Differentiation] (Wēn bìng zòng héng)*. Beijing: Beijing College of Traditional Chinese Medicine, 1979: 97.

35. For an extensive discussion of this formula, see below under the blockage of the Heart by transmission of heat and phlegm.

36. According to the source text, Auri Lamina *(jīn bó)*, which is a thin layer of gold made by striking gold, has been used to sedate the Heart and calm the spirit, and comprises the outer layer of the pill. Because of its expense, it is now impossible to obtain. Fortunately, Calm the Palace Pill with Cattle Gallstone *(ān gōng niú huáng wán)* can be obtained from many herbal companies or Chinese groceries, and we do not have to make the pill ourselves. However, if you choose to do so, it is my opinion that Succinum *(hǔ pò)* can be substituted for Auri Lamina *(jīn bó)*.

37. Chen Shi-Wen et al., *Formulary of the Bureau of Medicines of the Taiping Era (Tàipíng huì mín hé jì jú fāng)*. Beijing: People's Health Publishing House, 1959: 1.

38. This is a hawksbill turtle shell. It is sweet, salty, and cold and enters the Heart and Liver channels. It calms the Liver and settles convulsions, and also clears heat and resolves toxicity. The normal dosage is 3-6g. It is rarely used in decoctions.

39. See n. 36 above.

40. In the source text, the formula was simply called Purple Snow *(zǐ xuě)*. This formula is available in prepared powder form. The normal dosage is 1-3g taken once or twice a day. In my own experience, it is also effective for reducing fever due to wind-heat attacking the protective level.

41. Recently there has been some question as to whether the small amount of the known nephrotoxin aristolochic acid in this herb could lead to renal damage in some patients. In May, 2000 the U.S. Federal Drug Administration issued a warning in this regard. Although there has been discussion about the clinical implications of this matter and whether the harm from this herb is more theoretical than real, at the present time I would suggest that, in an effort to ensure patient safety, this herb not be used until the matter is resolved.

42. Gold is not discussed in this formula due to its expense. Clinically, Succinum *(hǔ pò)* can be substituted to sedate the Heart and calm the spirit.

43. This is the immature leaves of Lophatheri Herba *(dàn zhú yè)* which are difficult to find outside of East Asia. I recommend substituting Lophatheri Herba *(dàn zhú yè)*.

44. This is the seed of Forsythiae Fructus *(lián qiào)*. It is bitter and slightly cold and enters the Heart and Gallbladder channels. It clears heat from the Heart and calms the spirit. Commonly used for fever, irritability, restlessness, and insomnia. The normal dosage is 3-9g.

45. He Lian-Chen, *Revised and Expanded Discussion of Warm-Heat Pathogen Diseases.* Beijing: People's Health Publishing House, 1961: 102. This formula is composed of Rhinocerotis Cornu *(xī jiǎo)*, Saigae tataricae Cornu *(líng yáng jiǎo)*, Curcumae Radix *(yù jīn)*, Succinum *(hǔ pò)*, Manitis Squama *(chuān shān jiǎ)* which is no longer used because of its endangered species status—Forsythiae Semen *(lián qiào xīn)*, Acori tatarinowii Rhizoma *(shí chāng pǔ)*, Bufonis Venenum *(chán sū)*, Cinnabaris *(zhū shā)*, Eretmochelydis Carapax *(dài mào)*, Moschus *(shè xiāng)*, Daemonoropis Resina *(xuè jié)*, *Carthami Flos (hóng huā)*, Cinnamomi Ramulus *(guì zhī)*, Moutan Cortex *(mǔ dān pí)*, and blood from a pig's heart.

46. Zhang Yuan-Su, *Origins of Medicine (Yī xué qǐ yuán)*, annotated by Ren Ying-Qiu. Beijing: People's Health Publishing House, 1978: 198.

47. Written by Chen Zi-Ming in 1237.

48. There are many different ideas about the best way to decoct Aconiti Radix lateralis preparata *(zhì fù zǐ)*. One common way is to differentiate the cooking time based on where the herb is grown. For example, 15 to 25 minutes of cooking will be enough to reduce the toxicity of Aconiti Radix lateralis preparata *(zhì fù zǐ)* grown in Sichuan province, while it might take 20 to 25 minutes for that grown in Yunnan province. However, I believe the safest course is that advocated by my teacher, Dr. Ran Ping-Zhen. He told his patients to cook the Aconiti Radix lateralis preparata *(zhì fù zǐ)* for two hours, regardless of the dosage, and then asked them to taste the decoction. If this did not result in any numbness on the tongue within a few minutes, the decoction was considered safe to drink.

8 Spring-Warmth

S PRING-WARMTH (春溫 *chūn wēn*) was first discussed in the twelfth-century *Supplement to What Has Been Lost from [Discussion of] Cold Damage (Shāng hán bǔ wàng lùn)* by Guo Yong (Guo Zi-He, 1165–1173). If external cold attacks a person with constitutional deficiency of Kidney yin and essence during the winter, the pathogen may lurk within the body and transform into heat. Then, during the spring, two distinct triggers can cause the lurking pathogen to emerge. The first is an attack by another external pathogen, either wind-cold or wind-heat. The second is some irregularity in life-style—irregular food intake, stress, overstrain, emotional imbalance—which has the effect of weakening the antipathogenic qi and further compromising the yin. Should either trigger injure the antipathogenic qi, the lurking pathogen can be reactivated.

The significance of these events occurring in the spring is that this is the time of year when the energy of the Liver and Gallbladder rises, causing the lurking pathogen to rise as well. Thus, spring-warmth initially occurs primarily at the qi level and/or nutritive level. If the initial signs and symptoms are those of the *shao yang*, it is the Gallbladder that will be chiefly involved. And since the pathogen is attacking a person with constitutional yin deficiency, even the initial stages of the disease will further injure the yin, more so than in other warm pathogen diseases, and then progress rather quickly to severe yin deficiency.

Yet although this disease initially results from underlying yin deficiency, it will manifest in patterns of heat from excess. Spring-warmth is characterized by acute onset, interior heat, a multitude of changes, and severe signs and symptoms. In its early

249

stage, the symptoms include high fever, irritability, and thirst; there can even be loss of consciousness and convulsions.

The initial *external* cause of spring-warmth is cold, not heat. The secondary external trigger can be either wind-cold or wind-heat. Nevertheless, spring-warmth is traditionally included in discussions of warm pathogen diseases because:

- Lurking cold transforms into heat.

- Wind-heat can be the secondary trigger.

- Its etiology, pathology, and treatment principles are similar to those described for other warm pathogen diseases.

- Historically, it was the first type of warm pathogen disease to be described.

Biomedical diseases such as epidemic cerebrospinal meningitis, viral encephalitis, and severe influenza that occur in the spring have some overlap with the Chinese medical diagnosis of spring-warmth and can be treated using the methods described below for spring-warmth.

Etiology and Pathology

Spring-warmth occurs as a result of the confluence of two disharmonies, one external and one internal. The external factor is cold that attacks during the winter and lurks within the body, gradually transforming into heat. The internal factor is constitutional deficiency of Kidney yin and essence. Clinically, the internal factor is of greater concern.

There are two types of early stage spring-warmth, differentiated by the symptoms:

1. *Heat from excess arises spontaneously from lurking cold stagnating in the interior.* It appears because the antipathogenic qi has been injured by an irregular aspect in one's lifestyle (irregular food intake, stress, emotional imbalance). As Wu You-Xing observed in *Discussion of Warm Epidemics (Wēn yì lùn):*

   > If an external pathogen is not strong enough to fight against antipathogenic qi, it just lurks and does not make trouble for the body. However, it will make trouble for the body when the antipathogenic qi is weakened by irregular food intake, overwork, anxiety, anger, and pensiveness.[1]

It is the pathology of interior heat from excess that presents with high fever, irritability, and thirst. This is the type most frequently seen in the clinic.

NOTE: Since this type does not result from an attack by a secondary external patho-gen, the exterior symptom of aversion to cold is not present.

The basis for the onset of this type of spring-warmth is lurking cold in the body, which stagnates and constrains the qi and gradually produces interior heat from ex-cess. However, depending on the strength of the anti-pathogenic qi and the severity of the heat, this type of spring-warmth can be further differentiated:

- If the antipathogenic qi is strong enough to resist the heat from constraint that is caused by the lurking cold, the heat will be controlled and manifest in the qi level. Although the fact that there is a lurking pathogen at all reflects a problem with the antipathogenic qi, if that qi is strong enough to resist the pathogen, heat from constraint will appear in the qi level.

- If on the other hand the antipathogenic qi is too weak to resist the heat from constraint due to lurking cold, the heat will appear in the nutritive level.

2. *A secondary external pathogen induces the appearance of the heat from excess.* The secondary pathogen may be wind-cold or wind-heat, but *most* patients present with signs and symptoms related to a secondary attack by wind-heat. In fact, however, what appears to be wind-heat may actually be wind-cold that has rapidly transformed into heat due to the pre-existence of interior heat. This type manifests with signs and symptoms of both interior heat (high fever, irritabil-ity, thirst) and an exterior condition (aversion to cold, chills, headache, nasal congestion). While this type is rare in China, it has been my experience that it is quite common in the United States. The exterior presentation will last for two to three days. As it disappears, the warm-heat pathogen penetrates deeper into the body, and the interior heat can progress rapidly.

Table 8.1	Types of Early Stage Spring-Warmth
Type	**Pathology and Symptoms**
Heat arises from lurking cold stagnating internally; irregular lifestyle habits are the trigger	Interior heat from excess: high fever, restlessness, thirst, no aversion to cold and chills
Lurking cold constrains the qi and generates internal heat; a secondary external pathogen is the trigger	Interior heat from excess and an exterior condition: high fever, restlessness, thirst, aversion to cold, headache, nasal congestion

Identifying Spring-Warmth

Key indicators. There are two important indicators that help in the identification of spring-warmth:

1. *The disease is acute and appears in the spring.*[2] It presents with a particular series of interior heat signs and symptoms, including high fever that is unchanged by sweating, irritability, thirst, and dark-yellow urine. The dark-yellow urine results from heat injuring the fluids, and causing the urine to be concentrated.

2. *Maculopapular rashes, loss of consciousness, and convulsions are apt to be present in the development of spring-warmth.* At a later stage, exhaustion of yin of the Liver and Kidney may lead to stirring of Liver wind.

Location of signs and symptoms. If the disease occurs in the qi level there will be signs and symptoms that are typical of the qi level such as high fever, sweating, irritability, thirst, bitter taste, nausea, dark-yellow urine, red tongue with a yellow coating, and a flooding, rapid pulse. If it occurs in the nutritive level the signs and symptoms will be fever that worsens at night, irritability, dry mouth with no desire to drink, perhaps delirium, deep-red tongue, and a thin, rapid pulse. If the patient does not present with these typical symptoms, or if the history is unclear, the diagnosis of spring-warmth cannot be made.[3] The only way this diagnosis can be made at the beginning of an illness is if there are significant interior heat signs and symptoms from the very onset.

NOTE: A high fever can result from either external or internal pathogenic factors. The way to distinguish between them is to determine if there are also exterior signs and symptoms and if the high fever declines after sweating. Generally speaking, the cause is external if the high fever is associated with exterior signs and symptoms (aversion to cold and chills) and if it declines, even slightly, subsequent to sweating.[4] Otherwise, the cause is internal. At some point, the external pathogen that causes the exterior presentation will transform into interior heat, and the condition will rapidly evolve into an interior presentation. For this reason it is important to gauge the relative strength of the exterior and interior conditions.

Comparison to wind-warmth. A comparison between the description of spring-warmth above and that of wind-warmth in Chapter 7 highlights the differences between the two. Specifically, wind-warmth:

- May occur during winter or spring
- Is caused by an attack of wind-heat with immediate manifestations in the protective level
- Blocks the protective qi and Lung qi leading to a failure of the Lung to disseminate

- Causes only slight injury to the fluids in its early stages, with a slight increase in thirst
- In its early stages may present with a number of exterior symptoms—severe aversion to cold, chills, body aches, sweating, headache, sore throat, runny nose, plugged ears, cough—but no signs or symptoms of interior heat—irri-tability, thirst, dark-yellow urine.

Table 8.2	Distinguishing Spring-Warmth from Wind-Warmth		
Seasonal Onset	**Etiology**	**Pathology**	**Early Stage Symptoms**
▶ SPRING-WARMTH			
Only in the spring	Attack during winter in one with constitutional deficiency of Kidney yin and essence by external cold, which lurks inside body and gradually transforms into heat	Lurking cold transforms into interior heat from excess, first attacking the qi or nutritive level, then exhausting the yin of the Kidney and Liver, stirring up internal wind	Interior heat in the qi or nutritive level: high fever, thirst, restlessness, dark-yellow urine or fever that worsens at night, restlessness, dry mouth with no desire to drink, possible delirium, deep-red tongue, thin, rapid pulse; mild and usually transient exterior signs and symptoms
▶ WIND-WARMTH			
In the spring or winter	Attack by external wind-heat	Wind-heat blocks the protective qi and Lung qi, leading to failure of Lung to disseminate; first attacks protective level and the Lung, then the Stomach or Pericardium	Exterior wind-heat in the protective level: fever, aversion to cold, body aches, sweating, sore throat, plugged ears, headache, cough, slight thirst

Progression of Spring-Warmth

Spring-warmth can progress in three ways:

1. Heat from constraint in the qi level may progress to the nutritive or blood level if the antipathogenic qi fails to eliminate it. If the antipathogenic qi is strong enough, the heat can be cleared.

2. Heat from constraint in the nutritive level can progress in two ways. If the antipathogenic qi is strong enough to dispel the interior heat, improvement may occur as the heat reverses direction and moves from the nutritive to the qi level. If the antipathogenic qi is too weak to dispel the interior heat, this heat from constraint may invade the blood level. This will lead to bleeding problems or injury to the Liver and Kidney yin in the lower burner during a later stage of the disease, resulting in low-grade fever in the evening and insomnia. Alternatively, it may lead to stirring of Liver wind due to interior heat from excess, resulting in dizziness, loss of balance, and trembling of the limbs.

3. If the interior heat is too extreme, the heat may progress to the Pericardium.

Treatment principles. The treatment principles are to clear interior heat directly, to protect and enrich the yin, and to provide an avenue for the interior heat to exit the body. If there is heat in the qi level, it is cleared from the body with bitter and cold herbs. If it is in the nutritive level, the heat is vented back to the qi level.[5] The question arises, why not clear heat when it is in the nutritive or blood level? Heat by itself is a pathogen without form. However, when it enters the nutritive or blood level, it combines with the nutritive qi or blood, which are thought to have form, and transforms into a relatively substantial complex with form. As a result, trying to clear heat from this complex in the nutritive or blood level can injure the nutritive qi or blood. By venting the heat it can be separated from the nutritive qi or blood, dispersed to the qi level, and then cleared from the body. In later stages of spring-warmth, attention should be paid to enriching the yin, especially the Liver and Kidney yin.

Treatment strategies for secondary signs and symptoms are as follows:

- Releasing the exterior should be used if there are exterior signs and symptoms. However, those herbs that strongly relieve exterior signs and symptoms and promote sweating should not be used as they readily injure the yin.

- Cooling blood and clearing heat should be used for bleeding problems when heat invades the blood level.

- Cooling the Liver and extinguishing Liver wind should be used for the stirring of Liver wind.

Differentiation and Treatment of Combined Protective and Qi Level Patterns

Secondary Attack by Wind-Cold

Manifestations. There are two concurrent aspects to this pattern:

1. *Exogenous cold attacking the exterior* with aversion to cold, chills, absence of sweating, fever, headache, and a floating pulse.
2. *Interior heat* with thirst, irritability, dark-yellow urine, red tongue, and a rapid pulse.

NOTE: This pattern results from a secondary attack by wind-cold, as described above. Although this does occur, it is relatively rare. The pattern is also somewhat similar to the *tai yang* stage of cold damage (wind-cold) described in *Discussion of Cold Damage (Shāng hán lùn)* as both patterns share the symptoms of aversion to cold, chills, fever, headache, and the absence of sweating. However, spring-warmth will also present with interior heat and signs and symptoms of the qi level such as thirst, irritability, dark-yellow urine, red tongue, and a rapid pulse.

Table 8.3	Combined Protective and Qi Level Pattern vs. *Tai Yang* Stage Cold Damage
Pathology	**Signs and Symptoms***
▶ COMBINED PROTECTIVE AND QI LEVEL PATTERN	
Associated with interior heat	Thirst, dark-yellow urine, floating and rapid pulse, red tongue
▶ TAI YANG STAGE COLD DAMAGE	
Absence of interior heat	Absence of thirst, clear urine, floating and tight pulse, slightly red tongue

*Common points: attack on the exterior by cold resulting in fever, aversion to cold, headache, and absence of sweating.

Pathology. Wind-cold, acting as a secondary external pathogen, triggers the manifestation of lurking interior heat.

Treatment principles. Eliminate exterior signs and symptoms with acrid and slightly warm herbs, and clear interior heat with bitter and cold herbs.

Formula:

> SCALLION, PREPARED SOYBEAN, AND PLATYCODON DECOCTION
> (*cōng chǐ jié gěng tāng*)
>
> SOURCE: *Revised Popular Guide to the Discussion of Cold Damage*

Allii fistulosi Bulbus *(cōng bái)* .... 3–5 pieces (9–12g)

Platycodi Radix *(jié gěng)* 3–4.5g

Gardeniae Fructus *(zhī zǐ)* 6–9g

Sojae Semen preparatum *(dàn dòu chǐ)* 9–15g

Menthae haplocalycis Herba *(bò hé)* 3–4.5g

Forsythiae Fructus *(lián qiào)* 4.5–6g

Glycyrrhizae Radix *(gān cǎo)* 1.8–2.4g

Lophatheri Herba *(dàn zhú yè)* .... 30 leaves (1.5–3g)

ANALYSIS OF FORMULA: This is a common formula, but is especially used for lurking cold that has caused the qi to stagnate, become constrained, and produced heat, and which itself has been induced to emerge following a new attack of external cold. Because of their acrid flavor, Allii fistulosi Bulbus *(cōng bái)*, Sojae Semen preparatum *(dàn dòu chǐ)*, Platycodi Radix *(jié gěng)*, and Menthae haplocalycis Herba *(bò hé)* eliminate the exterior signs and symptoms by dispersing external wind-cold. The first three substances are mild and will therefore not cause further damage to the yin or increase the heat. Clinically, with its acrid flavor and cool nature, Menthae haplocalycis Herba *(bò hé)* has a slight effect in inducing sweating. With Allii fistulosi Bulbus *(cōng bái)* it induces slight sweating to remove the wind-cold from the body; it also serves to buffer the warm nature of Allii fistulosi Bulbus *(cōng bái)*, which might otherwise increase the interior heat. It is common for practitioners specializing in four-level theory to prescribe Menthae haplocalycis Herba *(bò hé)* for exterior conditions. With its function of disseminating Lung qi, Platycodi Radix *(jié gěng)* enhances the cold-dispersing actions of Sojae Semen preparatum *(dàn dòu chǐ)* and Allii fistulosi Bulbus *(cōng bái)*. With their bitter flavor and cold nature, Forsythiae Fructus *(lián qiào)*, Gardeniae Fructus *(zhī zǐ)*, and Lophatheri Herba *(dàn zhú yè)* clear interior heat. Glycyrrhizae Radix *(gān cǎo)* harmonizes the effects of the other herbs.

MODIFICATIONS: The basic formula can be modified as follows:

• For significant interior heat with a bitter taste, add Scutellariae Radix *(huáng qín)* to increase the heat-clearing action.

• For severe heat in the *yang ming* with pronounced thirst and irritability, disperse the heat with Cold Resolving Decoction *(hán jiě tāng)*:[6]

Gypsum fibrosum *(shí gāo)* 30g

Anemarrhenae Rhizoma *(zhī mǔ)* 24g

Forsythiae Fructus *(lián qiào)* 4.5g

Cicadae Periostracum *(chán tuì)* 4.5g

While this formula focuses on heat in the *yang ming*, it also relieves external heat. Gypsum fibrosum *(shí gāo)* and Anemarrhenae Rhizoma *(zhī mǔ)*, which comprise half the ingredients of White Tiger Decoction *(bái hǔ tāng),*[7] are combined to disperse heat from the *yang ming.* A small dosage of Forsythiae Fructus *(lián qiào)* and Cicadae Periostracum *(chán tuì)*, which are acrid and light, mildly releases exterior disorders and allows heat in the Stomach to reach the surface where it is discharged. According to Zhang Xi-Chun, who designed this formula, sweating may accompany its ingestion. If there are marked exterior signs and symptoms, increase the dosage of Forsythiae Fructus *(lián qiào)* and Cicadae Periostracum *(chán tuì)* to 15g each.

Differentiation and Treatment of Qi Level Patterns

HEAT FROM CONSTRAINT IN THE GALLBLADDER

Manifestations. There are two concurrent aspects to this pattern:

1. *Heat from constraint in the Gallbladder* with fever, bitter taste, irritability, nausea, belching or dry heaving, and a wiry, rapid pulse.
2. *Injury to the fluids* with thirst and scanty, dark-yellow urine.

Pathology. Heat from constraint in the Gallbladder. While both this pattern and those treated by White Tiger Decoction *(bái hǔ tāng)* are characterized by interior heat in the qi level, this pattern is situated in the Gallbladder where the heat is stagnating, unable to reach the exterior. Thus, although the heat in this pattern is quite severe, the patient only presents with fever and internal symptoms, such as a bitter taste, nausea, and irritability. Conversely, for the patterns treated by White Tiger Decoction *(bái hǔ tāng)*, the heat stagnates only in the Stomach from which it can move out toward the surface, leading to high fever, profuse sweating, strong thirst, and a flooding pulse. White Tiger Decoction *(bái hǔ tāng)* reinforces the natural movement of the heat upward and outward, where it is dispersed.

Treatment principles. Clear the heat with bitter and cold herbs, coupled with acrid and cool herbs to disperse heat from constraint.

Formula:

> SCUTELLARIA DECOCTION PLUS PREPARED SOYBEAN AND SCROPHULARIA
> *(huáng qín tāng jiā dàn dòu chǐ hé xuán shēn)*

SOURCE: *Encountering the Sources of Warm-Heat Pathogen Diseases*[8]

Scutellariae Radix *(huáng qín)* 9g

Paeoniae Radix alba *(bái sháo)* 6g

Honey-toasted Glycyrrhizae Radix preparata *(zhì gān cǎo)* 6g

Jujubae Fructus *(dà zǎo)* . . . . 12 pieces

Scrophulariae Radix *(xuán shēn)* 9g

Sojae Semen preparatum *(dàn dòu chǐ)*. 12g

ANALYSIS OF FORMULA: As the principal herb, Scutellariae Radix *(huáng qín)* clears heat from the Gallbladder directly. With their sour and sweet flavors, respectively, the combination of Paeoniae Radix alba *(bái sháo)* and honey-toasted Glycyrrhizae Radix preparata *(zhì gān cǎo)* produces yin and fluids. It is better to substitute Glycyrrhizae Radix *(gān cǎo)* for honey-toasted Glycyrrhizae Radix preparata *(zhì gān cǎo)* because the former can clear heat and resolve toxicity as well as harmonize the functions of the other herbs. Scrophulariae Radix *(xuán shēn)* clears heat, resolves toxicity, enriches yin, and produces fluids. Jujubae Fructus *(dà zǎo)* prevents the bitter and cold herbs from injuring the qi of the Spleen and Stomach. Sojae Semen preparatum *(dàn dòu chǐ)* disperses heat from constraint with its acrid flavor.

The use of Scutellaria Decoction *(huáng qín tāng)* was first recorded in *Discussion of Cold Damage (Shāng hán lùn)* where it is prescribed for treating dysenteric diarrhea resulting from heat in the Gallbladder attacking the Large Intestine. According to Ye Gui:

> Cold that attacks the body in the winter lurks in the Kidney, transforms into heat, and manifests in the Gallbladder in the spring. The treatment for this situation is to take Scutellaria Decoction *(huáng qín tāng)* as the main formula to clear heat with bitter and cold herbs.[9]

However, as the focus of this formula is only on clearing heat with bitter and cold herbs, it cannot disperse heat from constraint. In its unmodified form, the practitioner risks congealing the heat from constraint. In addition, the astringent quality of Paeoniae Radix alba *(bái sháo)* is not helpful for dealing with heat from constraint, especially when combined with bitter and cold herbs. Based on his own experience, Liu Bao-Yi added Sojae Semen preparatum *(dàn dòu chǐ)* and Scrophulariae Radix *(xuán shēn)* to this formula. In *Encountering the Sources of Warm-Heat Pathogen Diseases*, Liu explained that "Sojae Semen preparatum *(dàn dòu chǐ)* is made with black soybeans that reach the Kidney. It can ventilate lurking heat in the Kidney. Scrophulariae Radix *(xuán shēn)* can enrich the Kidney yin."[10] By adding these two herbs to Scutellaria Decoction *(huáng qín tāng)*, the formula works in two ways:

1. The acrid flavor and light nature of Sojae Semen preparatum *(dàn dòu chǐ)*, and the bitter flavor and cold nature of Scrophulariae Radix *(xuán shēn)*, serve to disperse and clear the heat.

2. The acrid flavor of Sojae Semen preparatum *(dàn dòu chǐ)* buffers the astringent properties of Paeoniae Radix alba *(bái sháo)*, and its warm nature balances the cold nature of Scutellariae Radix *(huáng qín)* and reduces its heat-congealing properties.

In *Systematic Differentiation of Warm Pathogen Diseases (Wēn bìng tiáo biàn)*, Wu Tang indicated that he preferred using Scutellaria and Coptis Decoction *(huáng qín huáng lián tāng)*.[11] This formula includes Scutellariae Radix *(huáng qín)* (6g), Coptidis Rhizoma *(huáng lián)* (6g), Curcumae Radix *(yù jīn)* (4.5g), and Sojae Semen preparatum *(dàn dòu chǐ)* (6g). Scutellaria and Coptis Decoction *(huáng qín huáng lián tāng)* would seem to be more appropriate for treating this condition than Scutellaria Decoction *(huáng qín tāng)*, as it clears and disperses heat, and promotes the movement of Gallbladder qi. However, it is less capable of enriching the yin than Scutellaria Decoction plus Prepared Soybean and Scrophularia *(huáng qín tāng jiā dàn dòu chǐ hé xuán shēn)*. Since yin deficiency is part of the background of spring-warmth, the latter formula is preferred in this case.

MODIFICATIONS: The basic formula can be modified as follows:

- For exterior wind-heat that triggers the emergence of heat from constraint caused by lurking cold, with headache, stiffness of the neck, and aversion to cold, add Puerariae Radix *(gé gēn)*, Menthae haplocalycis Herba *(bò hé)*, and Cicadae Periostracum *(chán tuì)* to disperse wind-heat.

- For heat from constraint in both the *shao yang* channel and organ (Gallbladder) with alternating chills and fever, distention in the hypochondriac and costal regions, and pronounced irritability and restlessness, add Bupleuri Radix *(chái hú)* and Gardeniae Fructus *(zhī zǐ)* to clear and disperse heat in the Gallbladder.

- For an attack on the Stomach by Gallbladder heat with severe vomiting, add Bambusae Caulis in taeniam *(zhú rú)* and Coptidis Rhizoma *(huáng lián)* to drain the Stomach heat and direct its qi downward.

HEAT FROM CONSTRAINT IN THE CHEST AND DIAPHRAGM

Manifestations. There are two concurrent aspects to this pattern:

1. *Initial invasion of the qi level and disappearance of exterior signs and symptoms* with slight fever, no aversion to cold, thirst, and a slightly yellow tongue coating.
2. *Disturbance of the spirit due to heat from constraint in the chest and the diaphragm* with restlessness, irritability, and insomnia with tossing and turning in bed.

NOTE: Restlessness, irritability, and insomnia with tossing and turning in bed, and a slightly yellow tongue coating are the key identifiers for this pattern. The restlessness in this pattern, and that associated with heat progressing to the nutritive level, are quite different. In this pattern the restlessness is not accompanied by a deep-red tongue or a fever that worsens at night, which would reflect a nutritive level pattern.

Pathology. Initial invasion of the qi level by heat, leading to heat from constraint in the chest and diaphragm.

Treatment principle. Clear heat from the chest and diaphragm with light herbs.

Formula:

GARDENIA AND PREPARED SOYBEAN DECOCTION *(zhī zǐ chǐ tāng)*

SOURCE: *Discussion of Cold Damage*

Gardeniae Fructus *(zhī zǐ)* 12g

Sojae Semen preparatum *(dàn dòu chǐ)* 9g

ANALYSIS OF FORMULA: Since there is interior heat situated in the upper burner, the treatment method of dispersing and venting heat is selected. Sojae Semen preparatum *(dàn dòu chǐ)* disperses heat from constraint in the chest and diaphragm, while Gardeniae Fructus *(zhī zǐ)* clears interior heat directly.

MODIFICATIONS: The basic formula can be modified as follows:

- For injury to the fluids with thirst, add Trichosanthis Radix *(tiān huā fěn)* to generate fluids.

- When this pattern occurs simultaneously with a protective level pattern with chills, aversion to cold, fever, and sore throat, add herbs such as Menthae haplocalycis Herba *(bò hé)*, Arctii Fructus *(niú bàng zǐ)*, and Cicadae Periostracum *(chán tuì)* to release the exterior and improve the condition of the throat.

- For vomiting, add Bambusae Caulis in taeniam *(zhú rú)* and Zingiberis Rhizoma recens *(shēng jiāng)* to clear heat and direct Stomach qi downward.

DECOCTION AND ADMINISTRATION: Refer to the method for decocting this formula discussed in Chapter 7.

HEAT BURNING THE CHEST AND DIAPHRAGM WITH LACK OF PASSAGE THROUGH THE INTESTINES

Manifestations.

There are three concurrent aspects to this pattern:

1. *Heat burning the chest and diaphragm* with persistent fever, hot sensation in the area of the chest and diaphragm, irritability, restlessness, red tongue with a yellow coating, and a slippery, rapid pulse.

2. *Injury to the fluids by heat from excess* with thirst, and dry lips and throat.

3. *Severe heat in the upper burner affecting the lower burner* with constipation and dark-yellow urine.

NOTE: In some cases the constipation, thirst, and yellow tongue coating could mislead the practitioner into concluding that the constipation is *only* a result of dry stool and heat in the Large Intestine, which corresponds to the *yang ming* organ syndrome in *Discussion of Cold Damage*. In fact, it is *mainly* caused by the failure of the Lung qi to descend, leading in turn to a failure of the Large Intestine's qi to descend, resulting in some dryness and heat. This conclusion is reinforced by the absence of a hard and distended sensation in the abdomen, a submerged and forceful pulse, or a dry, yellow tongue coating.

This pattern is situated primarily in the chest and diaphragm. As a part of the pattern, the Lung is unable to direct its qi downward to the Large Intestine. Since qi circulation in the Large Intestine is abnormal, the stool does not move smoothly, resulting in a reduction in the frequency of bowel movements. Depending on the degree of heat in the Large Intestine, there may or may not be hard, dry stools. However, the constipation will exacerbate the qi stagnation and heat in the upper burner because there is no way for the heat to exit the body. Consequently, treatment must address the constipation since the heat must be given an avenue for exiting the body as soon as possible.

Pathology. Heat from excess burns in the chest and diaphragm, and there is a lack of passage through the Intestines. The pattern here and that of heat from constraint in the chest and diaphragm share the symptom of heat in the chest and diaphragm. In the latter pattern, however, there are no Large Intestine problems. By contrast, in this pattern the heat in the upper burner is so severe that it acts like fire burning the chest and diaphragm, affecting the Lung's ability to direct it's qi downward to the Large Intestine, thus leading to constipation.

Treatment principles. Clear heat, disperse heat from the upper burner, and drain heat from the Large Intestine by purging.

Table 8.4	Heat From Constraint in the Chest and Diaphragm vs. Heat Burning the Chest and Diaphragm with Lack of Intestinal Passage
Pathology	**Signs and Symptoms***
▶ HEAT FROM CONSTRAINT IN THE CHEST AND DIAPHRAGM	
Heat from constraint without form in the chest and diaphragm	Insomnia with tossing and turning in bed
▶ BURNING OF THE CHEST AND DIAPHRAGM BY HEAT FROM EXCESS WITH SLIGHT CONSTIPATION	
Heat from constraint without form in the chest and diaphragm, coupled with mild dryness and heat in Large Intestine	Hot sensation in the chest and diaphragm, thirst, dry lips and mouth, constipation

*Both are qi level patterns situated in the upper burner. Common points include heat in the chest and diaphragm, along with restlessness.

Formula:

COOL THE DIAPHRAGM POWDER *(liáng gé sǎn)*

SOURCE: *Formulary of the Bureau of Medicines of the Taiping Era*[12]

Rhei Radix et Rhizoma *(dà huáng)* 60g
Natrii Sulfas *(máng xiāo)* 30g
Glycyrrhizae Radix *(gān cǎo)* 18g
Scutellariae Radix *(huáng qín)* 30g
Gardeniae Fructus *(zhī zǐ)* 24g
Menthae haplocalycis Herba *(bò hé)* 21g
Forsythiae Fructus *(lián qiào)* 30g
Lophatheri Herba *(dàn zhú yè)* 3g

ANALYSIS OF FORMULA: In this formula, Gardeniae Fructus *(zhī zǐ)* and Scutellariae Radix *(huáng qín)* clear heat directly from the upper burner. Rhei Radix et Rhizoma *(dà huáng)* and Natrii Sulfas *(máng xiāo)* drain the heat via the lower burner by purging it from the Large Intestine. While these herbs are typically used in patterns that include severe constipation with dry stools and heat in the Large Intestine, they are nevertheless used here because the heat must be given an avenue to exit the body. Finally, Lophatheri Herba *(dàn zhú yè)* also drains heat via the lower burner through the urine, which is another avenue for removing heat from the body. Menthae haplocalycis Herba *(bò hé)* and Forsythiae Fructus *(lián qiào)* disperse heat. Glycyrrhizae Radix *(gān cǎo)* coordinates and harmonizes the functions of the other herbs in the formula.

Why should purging and promoting urination be used in this case? Ordinarily, interior heat located in the upper burner is treated by dispersing the heat and venting it with light herbs such as Menthae haplocalycis Herba *(bò hé)*, Lonicerae Flos *(jīn yín huā)*, and Forsythiae Fructus *(lián qiào)*. However, if the interior heat is too severe, or if it has influenced the lower burner, this method will not be strong enough. It will then be necessary to find alternative methods to get rid of the interior heat, like purging and promoting urination. As previously noted, purging and promoting urination are usually used to discharge interior heat, but here they are used to drain interior heat without form and provide an avenue for the heat to exit the body.

Clinically, the interior heat in this pattern is so severe that the symptoms will include irritability, restlessness, thirst, a hot sensation in the chest and diaphragm, persistent fever, and dry lips and throat. Using just one or two methods to deal with such severe interior heat will not suffice. The practitioner must also attempt to immediately drain the interior heat with a combination of dispersing, clearing, purging, and promoting urination. Otherwise, the interior heat will soon exhaust the fluids and yin. In addition, a relatively large dosage of herbs should be used. The dosage shown in the formula above reflects the ratio of herbs to be used. The amount of Rhei Radix et Rhizoma *(dà huáng)* and Natrii Sulfas *(máng xiāo)* can be reduced to 12g and 9g, respectively.[13]

MODIFICATIONS: The basic formula can be modified as follows:

- To generate fluids and relieve irritability, add Trichosanthis Radix *(tiān huā fěn)* and Phragmitis Rhizoma *(lú gēn)*.

- If there is no constipation, remove Natrii Sulfas *(máng xiāo)*.

HEAT FROM EXCESS IN THE STOMACH

Manifestations. Vigorous fever, profuse sweating, thirst with a preference for cold beverages, and a flooding pulse.

Pathology. Heat from excess in the Stomach injuring the Stomach fluids.

Treatment principles. Clear heat with acrid and cold herbs, and produce fluids with sweet and cold herbs.

Formula:

WHITE TIGER DECOCTION *(bái hǔ tāng)*

For further details, see the pattern of heat from excess in the Stomach described in Chapter 7.

Differentiation and Treatment of Qi Level Patterns Involving Constipation with Dry Stool and Heat in the Large Intestine

SEVERE CONSTIPATION WITH DRY STOOL AND HEAT IN THE LARGE INTESTINE COMBINED WITH EXHAUSTION OF THE YIN AND FLUIDS

Manifestations. There are two concurrent aspects to this pattern:

1. *Severe constipation with dry stool and heat in the Large Intestine* with fever, constipation (consisting of dry and hard stools), and distending pain in the abdomen.
2. *Exhaustion of yin and fluids* with dry lips and mouth, dry tongue coating, and a submerged and thin pulse.

Pathology. Severely dry stools (consisting of dry and hard stools) and heat in the Large Intestine, combined with exhaustion of the yin and fluids.

Treatment principles. Eliminate heat by purging, enrich the yin, and generate fluids.

Formula:

INCREASE THE FLUIDS AND ORDER THE QI DECOCTION
(zēng yè chéng qì tāng)

SOURCE: *Systematic Differentiation of Warm Pathogen Diseases*

Scrophulariae Radix *(xuán shēn)* 30g
Ophiopogonis Radix *(mài mén dōng)* 24g
Rehmanniae Radix *(shēng dì huáng)* 24g
Rhei Radix et Rhizoma *(dà huáng)* 9g
Natrii Sulfas *(máng xiāo)* 4.5g

ANALYSIS OF FORMULA: Increase the Fluids Decoction *(zēng yè tāng)*, first described in *Systematic Differentiation of Warm Pathogen Diseases*, consists of Rehmanniae Radix *(shēng dì huáng)*, Ophiopogonis Radix *(mài mén dōng)*, and Scrophulariae Radix *(xuán shēn)*, all sweet and cold herbs. They serve to enrich the yin, moisten dryness, add fluids to the Large Intestine to improve bowel movement, and prevent further damage to the yin and fluids. Rhei Radix et Rhizoma *(dà huáng)* and Natrii Sulfas *(máng xiāo)* purge heat via bowel movement. According to Wu Tang:

The wonderful thing about this formula is that it includes purging herbs among those that enrich the yin, while the herbs that enrich the yin add more fluids to the Large Intestine and moisten it, which can help the purging herbs to discharge heat. Overall, this formula can eliminate heat from excess and dry stool while preventing further injury to the yin and fluids from the purging herbs.[14]

The dosage of Rhei Radix et Rhizoma *(dà huáng)* and Natrii Sulfas *(máng xiāo)* is reduced significantly since the use of too large a dose of these substances will further injure the yin and fluids. Conversely, large amounts of Rehmanniae Radix *(shēng dì huáng)*, Ophiopogonis Radix *(mài mén dōng)*, and Scrophulariae Radix *(xuán shēn)* are used to enrich the yin and generate fluids.

MODIFICATIONS: According to Wu Tang there are four basic formulas that deal with severe constipation with dry stool and heat in the Large Intestine, which can be differentiated based upon the degree of heat and injury to the yin and fluids:

1. For heat from excess in the Large Intestine that is actively injuring the yin and fluids, use Major Order the Qi Decoction *(dà chéng qì tāng)*[15] to purge the heat and dry stool in order to prevent serious injury to the yin and fluids. If one were to try to purge heat and enrich the yin and fluids simultaneously in this context, it would be ineffective, as the yin tonics would adversely affect the strength of the purging herbs. As a result, it would take longer to discharge the heat. Therefore, the heat must first be purged before tackling the development of the disease, which is the heat that is injuring the yin and fluids. After the heat has been drained, the yin and fluids can be enriched.

2. For severe constipation (or dry stools and the discharge of foul-smelling water) and heat in the Large Intestine, but no injury to the yin and fluids, use Regulate the Stomach and Order the Qi Decoction *(tiáo wèi chéng qì tāng)*[16] to clear the heat by purging and softening the dry stools.

3. Exhaustion of yin and fluids may be coupled with slight constipation with dry stool and heat in the Large Intestine. The exhaustion of the yin and fluids can result in constipation due to the lack of fluids in the Large Intestine. In such cases, use Increase the Fluids Decoction *(zēng yè tāng)*[17] to avoid further injury to the yin and fluids.

4. For dry and hard stools (but without distending abdominal pain), dry mouth, dry lips, and a thin pulse due to yin deficiency, use Increase the Fluids Decoction *(zēng yè tāng)* first; that is, do not use Rhei Radix et Rhizoma *(dà huáng)* and Natrii Sulfas *(máng xiāo)*. If the patient still has not had a bowel movement twenty-four hours after taking the formula, then combine this with Regulate the Stomach and Order the Qi Decoction *(tiáo wèi chéng qì tāng)* to purge the stools.

Case study: Increase the Fluids and Order the Qi Decoction
(*zēng yè chéng qì tāng*)

Ms. Song, female, 65 years old

First visit: Since the beginning of spring the patient had been sick for more than 20 days with a fever. Her temperature was 38.5°C. She was emaciated and had a dark face that lacked luster. Her tongue was deep red with cracks and a lack of saliva, and her lips were dry. The coating was dry, thick, and yellow. She had a poor appetite, thirst for cold beverages, and constipation. Her epigastrium and abdomen were distended and felt worse with pressure. Her throat was red, dry, and sore. Her pulse was deep, thin, small, and slippery, but forceful. The patient had suffered from pulmonary tuberculosis for more than ten years, with frequent night sweats and a low-grade fever at times.

Recently, the patient was treated by another physician who had mistakenly diagnosed her condition as wind-cold, for which acrid and warm herbs were prescribed to induce sweating. Therefore, her yin and fluids were badly damaged, and heat had accumulated in the Large Intestine, leading to constipation. This led to a vicious cycle where the more deficient the yin became, the more heat was generated, leading to more dryness, which in turn further aggravated the injury to the yin. The appropriate treatment was to purge heat from the Large Intestine, and enrich the yin and fluids to moisten dryness. Increase the Fluids and Order the Qi Decoction (*zēng yè chéng qì tāng*) was prescribed: Scrophulariae Radix (*xuán shēn*) (45g), Rehmanniae Radix (*shēng dì huáng*) (30g), Ophiopogonis Radix (*mài mén dōng*) (25g), Paeoniae Radix alba (*bái sháo*) (30g), Dendrobii Herba (*shí hú*) (25g), Natrii Sulfas (*máng xiāo*) (1.5g, taken with the strained decoction), Rhei Radix et Rhizoma (*dà huáng*) powder (1.2g, taken with the strained decoction). One packet of the herbs was given to the patient.

Second visit: Last night after finishing the herbs the patient had a bowel movement. At first, it was as hard as goat feces, but became softer. The hard stool caused some bleeding per rectum. Her temperature was 37.5°C. She still had a deep-red tongue with cracks and insufficient saliva. Her appetite increased while the epigastric and abdominal distention was reduced. Her throat was still red, but less dry and sore than previously. Her pulse was also less forceful. The patient had underlying yin deficiency that was further injured by the combination of wind-heat and the mistaken treatment. This led to constipation. The situation was like that of a boat being unable to move because there was too little water in the river.

The initial treatment was to enrich the yin, moisten the Large Intestine, and purge heat. Now that her stool was moving and the heat had been drained, it was inappropriate to continue purging with substances such as Natrii Sulfas (*máng xiāo*) and Rhei Radix et Rhizoma (*dà huáng*). The proper course was to use sweet and cold herbs to enrich the yin and moisten the dryness: Glehniae/Adenophorae Radix *(shā shēn)* (30g), Rehmanniae Radix *(shēng dì huáng)* (25g), Paeoniae Radix alba *(bái sháo)* (25g), Asini Corii Colla *(ē jiāo)* (15g, divided into two portions and melted into the strained decoction), Auricularia *(hēi mù ěr)*[18] (12g), Trionycis Carapax *(biē jiǎ)* (15g, cooked first), and Ophiopogonis Radix *(mài mén dōng)* (15g). Two packets of the herbs were given to the patient.

Third visit: The patient's fever was gone and her temperature was now 37°C. Her thick, dry, yellow tongue coating was back to normal. The tongue body was still deep red with cracks and less than normal saliva. Her appetite was normal. Her bowel movements had become normal in frequency and consistency. There was no distention in her abdomen or epigastrium. The red, dryness, and pain in her throat were gone. Her pulse was thin, wiry, and small. The treatment to enrich the yin with sweet, cold herbs continued: Rehmanniae Radix *(shēng dì huáng)* (25g), Glehniae/Adenophorae Radix *(shā shēn)* (25g), Paeoniae Radix alba *(bái sháo)* (25g), Coicis Semen *(yì yǐ rén)* (15g), Lablab Semen album *(bái biǎn dòu)* (25g), Asini Corii Colla *(ē jiāo)* (12g, divided into two portions and melted into the strained decoction), Ophiopogonis Radix *(mài mén dōng)* (10g), Asparagi Radix *(tiān mén dōng)* (10g), and Gigeriae galli Endothelium corneum *(jī nèi jīn)* (10g). Five packets of the herbs were given to the patient. After finishing the herbs, all signs and symptoms were gone. The patient had a good appetite and slept well. She was told to avoid spicy and greasy foods, and to eat lightly.[19]

Comparison. The dosage of Natrii Sulfas *(máng xiāo)* in this formula is much lower than in Cool the Diaphragm Powder *(liáng gé sǎn)*. This is because the key pathology in the pattern of burning of the chest and diaphragm by heat from excess with lack of passage in the Intestines, discussed above, is heat in the chest and diaphragm. By contrast, the key pathology in the pattern here is exhaustion of both the yin and fluids, as well as severe constipation with dry stool and heat. The heat in the pattern here is not as severe, but the injury to the fluids and yin is much more severe. Therefore, much more attention is placed here on enriching the yin and generating fluids.

SEVERE CONSTIPATION WITH DRY STOOL AND HEAT IN THE LARGE INTESTINE COMBINED WITH QI AND YIN DEFICIENCY

Manifestations. There are three concurrent aspects to this pattern:

1. *Severe constipation with dry stool and heat in the Large Intestine* with fever, abdominal distention, constipation, and a dry tongue coating that is either yellow or black.

2. *Exhaustion of yin* with dry lips, throat, and mouth.
3. *Deficiency of qi* with listlessness, shortness of breath, and a submerged, weak or a submerged, thin pulse.

Pathology. Severe constipation with dry stool and heat in the Large Intestine, accompanied by deficiency of yin and qi. This pattern commonly occurs as a result of waiting too long to purge severe constipation with dry stool and heat in the Large Intestine. The heat can injure the yin. In addition, as noted in Chapter 5 of *Basic Questions*,[20] extreme heat can exhaust the qi. Therefore, if there is severe constipation with dry stool and heat in the Large Intestine, the purging method with Rhei Radix et Rhizoma *(dà huáng)* and Natrii Sulfas *(máng xiāo)* should be used *immediately* in order to protect the qi and fluids from the extreme heat. Otherwise, both the qi and yin will be damaged and severe constipation with dry stool and heat will persist in the Large Intestine. This condition can be so severe that the patient may develop twitching of the hands from stirring up of Liver wind.

Treatment principles. Purge heat and dry stools, tonify the qi, and enrich the yin.

Formula:

NEWLY AUGMENTED YELLOW DRAGON DECOCTION *(xīn jiā huáng lóng tāng)*

SOURCE: *Systematic Differentiation of Warm Pathogen Diseases*

Scrophulariae Radix *(xuán shēn)*. 15g
Ophiopogonis Radix *(mài mén dōng)* 15g
Rehmanniae Radix *(shēng dì huáng)* 15g
Natrii Sulfas *(máng xiāo)* 3g
Glycyrrhizae Radix *(gān cǎo)* 6g
Ginseng Radix *(rén shēn)* 4.5g
Angelicae sinensis Radix *(dāng guī)* .4.5g
Stichopus *(hǎi shēn)*. . . . . 2 pieces
Zingiberis Rhizomatis Succus *(jiāng zhī)* . . . . 6 spoonfuls
Rhei Radix et Rhizoma *(dà huáng)*[21] .9g

ANALYSIS OF FORMULA: This represents a modification of two formulas:

1. Regulate the Stomach and Order the Qi Decoction *(tiáo wèi chéng qì tāng)*[22] and
2. Increase the Fluids Decoction *(zēng yè tāng)*

The former is used to purge heat as well as dry stool from the Large Intestine. The latter, discussed above, enriches the yin and generates fluids.

Stichopus *(hǎi shēn)* and Angelicae sinensis Radix *(dāng guī)* enrich the yin and improve bowel movement. Ginseng Radix *(rén shēn)* tonifies the qi. Zingiberis Rhizomatis Succus *(jiāng zhī)* harmonizes the Stomach qi. Angelicae sinensis Radix *(dāng guī)* invigorates the blood to improve the movement of qi and blood in the Large Intestine.

DECOCTION AND ADMINISTRATION: According to Wu Tang, Ginseng Radix *(rén shēn)* should be cooked separately, and the other herbs cooked later. The decoction of Ginseng Radix *(rén shēn)* and Zingiberis Rhizomatis Succus *(jiāng zhī)* is then added into the strained decoction made from the other herbs. Take one cup of the decoction. If there is no bowel movement within one to two hours after taking the formula, take a second cup. If there is a bowel movement, the patient should stop taking this formula and begin taking Benefit the Stomach Decoction *(yì wèi tāng)*, which is composed of Glehniae/Adenophorae Radix *(shā shēn)* (9g), Ophiopogonis Radix *(mài mén dōng)* (15g), Rehmanniae Radix *(shēng dì huáng)* (15g), rock sugar *(bīng táng)* (3g), and Polygonati odorati Rhizoma *(yù zhú)* (4.5g). This formula should continue to be taken until the mouth, lips, and throat are no longer dry.[23]

Case study: Newly Augmented Yellow Dragon Decoction
(xīn jiā huáng lóng tāng)

Ms. Pang, female, 80 years old

First visit: The patient had a history of opium smoking for over thirty years and was often constipated with a bowel movement every seven to eight days. In late April she contracted wind-warmth with fever, cough, and a red, swollen, painful throat. She had been treated with both Western and Chinese medicine for ten days, but to no avail.

The patient had a fever (38.3°C) and a rapid, thin, wiry, small, and slippery pulse. She was dizzy, restless, feverish, and had abdominal distention. Her lips and mouth were dry, and her throat at this time was mildly sore. Her tongue coating was dry, thick, yellow, and black with cracks. She was listless and fatigued. Opium smoking gave her constitutional yin deficiency that led to fire from deficiency and injured the fluids. Her recent warm pathogen disease further injured the yin. The diagnosis was qi and yin deficiency with accumulation of heat and dry stool in the Large Intestine. The treatment principle was to purge heat and tonify qi to ward off qi collapse. A modified version of Newly Augmented Yellow Dragon Decoction *(xīn jiā huáng lóng tāng)* was prescribed: fresh Rehmanniae Radix recens *(xiān dì huáng)* (60g), Glycyrrhizae Radix *(gān cǎo)* (10g), Scrophulariae Radix *(xuán shēn)* (25g), Ophiopogonis Radix *(mài mén dōng)* (15g), Paeoniae Radix rubra *(chì sháo)* (25g), Paeoniae Radix alba *(bái sháo)* (25g), Angelicae sinensis Radix *(dāng guī)* (10g), and Rhei Radix et Rhizoma *(dà huáng)* and Natrii Sulfas *(máng xiāo)* powder (1.2g each, both taken with the strained decoction). A packet of the herbs was given to the patient. She was also told that two hours after taking these herbs she would feel movement or gas in her intestines that would tell her she was about to have a bowel movement. She was instructed that, to prevent the exertion from the bowel movement leading to qi collapse, she should take Panacis quinquefolii Radix *(xī yáng shēn)* powder (4.5g) with a decoction made from Ginseng Radix *(rén shēn)* (25g).

As predicted, two hours after taking the herbs she felt some abdominal pain and had an urge to defecate. She swallowed 4.5g of Panacis quinquefolii Radix *(xī yáng shēn)* powder with the decoction cooked from Ginseng Radix *(rén shēn)* before going to the bathroom. A few minutes later she passed a fair amount of stool and then felt some shortness of breath. She then drank some more of the Ginseng Radix *(rén shēn)* decoction without the Panacis quinquefolii Radix *(xī yáng shēn)* and went to sleep.

Second visit: After taking the herbs, the patient had another bowel movement yesterday without any signs of qi collapse. She slept through the night. Her pulse was thin and frail and her temperature was now 36.7°C. The abdominal distention, dizziness, and restlessness were reduced. Her tongue coating was no longer dry or black and showed no cracks; however, it was still thick and yellow. She was extremely fatigued. The yin had been so badly damaged that it could not recover quickly. She was given a formula with sweet, cold herbs to enrich the yin and clear heat from deficiency along with sweet and slightly warm herbs to tonify qi: Stichopus *(hǎi shēn)* (15g, cooked first), Glehniae/Adenophorae Radix *(shā shēn)* (30g), Scrophulariae Radix *(xuán shēn)* (30g), Ophiopogonis Radix *(mài mén dōng)* (25g), Polygonati Rhizoma *(huáng jīng)* (25g), fresh Dendrobii Herba *(xiān shí hú)* (30g), Paeoniae Radix alba *(bái sháo)* (30g), Rehmanniae Radix *(shēng dì huáng)* (25g), Rehmanniae Radix preparata *(shú dì huáng)* (25g), and Panacis quinquefolii Radix *(xī yáng shēn)* powder (10g, divided into three portions and swallowed with the strained decoction). She was given two packets and told to be careful about her diet and to avoid drafts.

Third visit: She returned feeling better without any fever and with some appetite. The thick tongue coating had gradually diminished until it was only present on the root of the tongue. She was sleeping well and had an increase in urination.[24] She was given a formula to enrich the yin and blood while tonifying the Spleen and Stomach: Panacis quinquefolii Radix *(xī yáng shēn)* powder (10g, divided into three portions and swallowed with the decoction), Glehniae/Adenophorae Radix *(shā shēn)* (30g), Adenophorae Radix *(nán shā shēn)* (30g), Paeoniae Radix alba *(bái sháo)* (30g), Scrophulariae Radix *(xuán shēn)* (30g), Ophiopogonis Radix *(mài mén dōng)* (25g), Nelumbinis Semen *(lián zǐ)* (25g), Rehmanniae Radix *(shēng dì huáng)* (30g), Lilii

Bulbus *(băi hé)* (25g), Dioscoreae Rhizoma *(shān yào)* (30g), fried Coicis Semen *(yì yǐ rén)* (30g), and Armeniacae Semen *(xìng rén)*(10g). Three packets were given to the patient.

Fourth visit: The patient's energy and appetite continued to improve. She had a bowel movement yesterday with stool that was dry at first and then of normal consistency. Only a slightly thick coating at the root of the tongue remained. She had a thin, frail, small, and slippery pulse. She was given three packets of the same formula.

Fifth visit: The patient stated that her energy was almost normal this week and that she was able to walk a bit. Her appetite was continually improving and she was sleeping well. Her face has a rosy glow with luster and her tongue coating is almost normal. She was told to eat rice porridge with Coicis Semen *(yì yǐ rén)* and Lilii Bulbus *(băi hé)* every day, take porridge made from rice and Dioscoreae Rhizoma *(shān yào)* at noon, and drink the soup made from Longan Arillus *(lóng yǎn ròu)* with pork meat. Two weeks later the patient had recovered.[25]

Severe Constipation with Dry Stool and Heat in the Large Intestine Combined with Heat from Excess in the Small Intestine

Manifestations. There are two concurrent aspects to this pattern:

1. *Severe constipation with dry stool and heat in the Large Intestine* with fever and constipation.

2. *Heat from excess in the Small Intestine* with dribbling, painful, scanty, dark-yellow or reddish urine.[26]

Pathology. Severe constipation with dry stool and heat in the Large Intestine, combined with heat from excess in the Small Intestine.

Treatment principles. Drain heat from the Large Intestine by purging, and clear heat from the Small Intestine.

Formula:

> **GUIDE OUT THE RED AND ORDER THE QI DECOCTION**
> *(dǎo chì chéng qì tāng)*

SOURCE: *Systematic Differentiation of Warm Pathogen Diseases*

Rehmanniae Radix *(shēng dì huáng)* 15g
Rhei Radix et Rhizoma *(dà huáng)* 9g
Natrii Sulfas *(máng xiāo)* 3g
Paeoniae Radix rubra *(chì sháo)* 9g
Coptidis Rhizoma *(huáng lián)* 6g
Phellodendri Cortex *(huáng bǎi)* 6g

ANALYSIS OF FORMULA: When both the Large and Small Intestines are involved, heat will exit the body through both the urine and stool. The treatment principle should promote this process by conducting the heat downward to discharge it. The name of the formula reflects this strategy. Guide out the red (導赤 *dǎo chì*) means to conduct heat out of the Small Intestine; the word red (赤 *chì*) refers to the color, which corresponds to the Heart and Small Intestine. Order the qi (承氣 *chéng qì*) refers to getting the qi to follow the natural direction of the Large Intestine, which is downward.

In this formula, Rhei Radix et Rhizoma *(dà huáng)* and Natrii Sulfas *(máng xiāo)* drain heat and discharge dry stool from the Large Intestine. Coptidis Rhizoma *(huáng lián)* and Phellodendri Cortex *(huáng bǎi)* clear heat from the Small Intestine. Rehmanniae Radix *(shēng dì huáng)* and Paeoniae Radix rubra *(chì sháo)* enrich the yin and cool the blood.

MODIFICATIONS: The basic formula can be modified as follows:

- To increase its ability to drain heat from the Small Intestine via the urine, add Lophatheri Herba *(dàn zhú yè)*, Akebiae Caulis *(mù tōng)*,[27] and Glycyrrhizae Radix *(gān cǎo)*.
- For intensely painful urination, which indicates that the heat has transformed into toxin and is obstructing the blood in the Bladder, add Succinum *(hǔ pò)* and Patriniae Herba *(bài jiàng cǎo)* to clear heat, resolve toxicity, and invigorate the blood.
- For reddish urine, add Imperatae Rhizoma *(bái máo gēn)*, Gardeniae Fructus *(zhī zǐ)*, and Cirsii Herba *(xiǎo jì)*.
- For severe restlessness and thirst, add Trichosanthis Radix *(tiān huā fěn)*, Ophiopogonis Radix *(mài mén dōng)*, and Phragmitis Rhizoma *(lú gēn)*.

REVIEW OF THE EIGHT PATTERNS INVOLVING CONSTIPATION WITH DRY STOOL AND HEAT IN THE LARGE INTESTINE

So far in this book, a total of seven patterns involving constipation with heat and/or dry stool in the Large Intestine have been discussed. An eighth pattern, combined heat and blood stasis, is discussed below in the context of nutritive and blood level patterns of spring-warmth. Table 8.5 summarizes these eight patterns and their associated formulas.

Table 8.5	Eight Patterns with Severe Constipation, Dry Stools, and Heat in the Large Intestine		
Patterns	**Signs and Symptoms**	**Treatment Principles**	**Formulas**
► WIND-WARMTH			
Blockage of Lung by phlegm and heat with clumping of stool and heat in Large Intestine	Cough, persistent labored breathing, profuse sputum, tidal fever, constipation, yellow, greasy tongue coating	Disseminate and induce Lung qi to descend, transform phlegm, purge heat	Disseminate the White and Order the Qi Decoction (*xuān bái chéng qì tāng*)
Blockage of Heart spirit by transmission of heat coupled with clumping of dry stool and heat in Large Intestine	Deep-red tongue, loss of consciousness, stiff tongue with difficult speech, cold extremities, hard, distending pain in abdomen, constipation, dry, yellow tongue coating, submerged, forceful, rapid pulse	Clear heat from Pericardium, open orifices, purge dry stools and heat from Large Intestine	Cattle Gallstone Decoction to Order the Qi (*niú huáng chéng qì tāng*)
Clumping of dry stool and heat in Large Intestine	Tidal fever, constipation with hard and dry stool or diarrhea with discharge of foul-smelling liquid, hard and distending pain in abdomen, dry, yellow tongue coating, submerged, forceful pulse	Soften dry stools, purge heat	Regulate the Stomach and Order the Qi Decoction (*tiáo wèi chéng qì tāng*)
Heat burning chest and diaphragm with lack of passage through Intestines	Persistent fever, hot sensation in chest and diaphragm, restlessness, constipation; thirst, dry lips and throat, red tongue with yellow coating, slippery and rapid pulse	Clear heat, disperse heat, and drain heat by purging	Cool the Diaphragm Powder (*liáng gé sǎn*)

Table 8.5, cont.			
Severe constipation with dry stools and heat in Large Intestine combined with exhaustion of yin and fluids	Fever, constipation (dry and hard stools), distending pain in abdomen, dry lips and mouth, dry tongue coating, submerged and thin pulse	Purge heat, enrich the yin, and generate fluids	Increase the Fluids and Order the Qi Decoction (*zēng yè chéng qì tāng*)
Severe constipation with dry stools and heat in Large Intestine combined with qi and yin deficiency	Fever, abdominal distention, constipation, dry lips, throat, and mouth, listlessness, shortness of breath, dry, yellow tongue coating or dry, black tongue coating, submerged pulse that is weak or thin	Purge heat and dry stools, tonify the qi, and enrich the yin	Newly Augmented Yellow Dragon Decoction (*xīn jiā huáng lóng tāng*)
Severe constipation with dry stools and heat in Large Intestine combined with heat from excess in Small Intestine	Fever, constipation, dribbling, painful, scanty, and dark-yellow or reddish urine	Purge heat from Large Intestine and clear heat from Small Intestine	Guide Out the Red and Order the Qi Decoction (*dǎo chì chéng qì tāng*)
Clumping of heat and blood stasis	Constipation with dry, black stools, hardness, distention, and pain in lower abdomen, dry mouth, mania, purplish tongue or purplish spots over tongue, submerged and forceful or hesitant pulse	Purge heat, invigorate the blood, and dispel blood stasis	Peach Kernel Decoction to Order the Qi (*táo rén chéng qì tāng*)

Differentiation and Treatment of Nutritive and Blood Level Patterns

INTENSE HEAT IN BOTH THE QI AND NUTRITIVE LEVELS

Manifestations. There are two concurrent aspects to this pattern:

1. *Heat from excess in the Stomach in the qi level* with vigorous fever, sweating, thirst, and a yellow tongue coating.
2. *Heat from excess in the nutritive level* with restlessness and a deep-red tongue.

Pathology. Intense heat in both the qi and nutritive levels.

Treatment principles. Clear heat from the qi and nutritive levels.

Formula:

> **MODIFIED JADE WOMAN DECOCTION**
> *(jiā jiǎn yù nǚ jiān)*
>
> SOURCE: *Systematic Differentiation of Warm Pathogen Diseases*
>
> Gypsum fibrosum *(shí gāo)* 30g
> Anemarrhenae Rhizoma *(zhī mǔ)* 12g
> Scrophulariae Radix *(xuán shēn)* 12g
> Ophiopogonis Radix *(mài mén dōng)* 18g
> Rehmanniae Radix *(shēng dì huáng)* 18g

ANALYSIS OF FORMULA: This formula is often used for intense heat in both the qi and nutritive levels. Gypsum fibrosum *(shí gāo)* and Anemarrhenae Rhizoma *(zhī mǔ)*, two of the main herbs in White Tiger Decoction *(bái hǔ tāng)*,[28] clear heat from the qi level, while the other three herbs, Rehmanniae Radix *(shēng dì huáng)*, Scrophulariae Radix *(xuán shēn)*, and Ophiopogonis Radix *(mài mén dōng)*, cool the blood and enrich the yin.

HEAT FLARING IN BOTH THE QI AND BLOOD LEVELS

Manifestations. There are two concurrent aspects to this pattern:

1. *Heat from excess in the Stomach in the qi level* with vigorous fever, sweating, thirst, and a yellow tongue coating.
2. *Heat from excess in the blood level* with maculopapular rash, hematemesis (vomiting of blood), and/or epistaxis.

275

Pathology. Intense heat in both the qi and blood levels.

Treatment principles. Clear heat from the qi and blood levels.

Formula No. 1:

> ### TRANSFORM MACULAS DECOCTION *(huà bān tāng)*
>
> SOURCE: *Systematic Differentiation of Warm Pathogen Diseases*
>
> Gypsum fibrosum *(shí gāo)* 30g
>
> Anemarrhenae Rhizoma *(zhī mǔ)* 12g
>
> Glycyrrhizae Radix *(gān cǎo)* 9g
>
> Scrophulariae Radix *(xuán shēn)* 9g
>
> Rhinocerotis Cornu *(xī jiǎo)* 6g
>
> Nonglutinous rice *(gěng mǐ)* 9g

ANALYSIS OF FORMULA: Transform Maculas Decoction *(huà bān tāng)* consists of White Tiger Decoction *(bái hǔ tāng)*[29] plus Scrophulariae Radix *(xuán shēn)* and Rhinocerotis Cornu *(xī jiǎo)* to clear heat from the Stomach and blood level, and resolve toxicity. It is mostly used for treating maculas that result from heat in the Stomach and blood level. While the formula as originally designed effectively clears heat from the qi and blood levels, it cannot invigorate the blood for blood stasis. This is important because blood stasis is commonly seen after bleeding and can block the vessels and thereby induce further bleeding. In addition, the cold herbs themselves can cause the blood to congeal. Since Moutan Cortex *(mǔ dān pí)* and Paeoniae Radix rubra *(chì sháo)* cool and invigorate the blood and remove blood stasis, while Rehmanniae Radix *(shēng dì huáng)* cools the blood, 15g of each herb should be added to the formula to improve its efficacy. In addition, since Rhinocerotis Cornu *(xī jiǎo)* is from an endangered species, Bubali Cornu *(shuǐ niú jiǎo)* should be substituted, and its dosage doubled.[30]

Formula No. 2:

> ### CLEAR EPIDEMICS AND OVERCOME TOXIN DRINK *(qīng wēn bài dú yǐn)*
>
> SOURCE: *Achievements Regarding Epidemic Rashes*

Herbs (Dosage)	Large	Medium	Small
Gypsum fibrosum *(shí gāo)* 180–240g	60–120g	24–36g	
Rehmanniae Radix *(shēng dì huáng)* 18–30g	9–15g	6–12g	
Rhinocerotis Cornu *(xī jiǎo)* 18–24g	9–15g	6–12g	
Coptidis Rhizoma *(huáng lián)* 12–18g	6–12g	3–4.5g	

This formula was originally designed to treat the warm pathogen diseases caused by epidemic qi and warm toxin. According to its originator, Yu Lin, it can drain fire from all twelve channels and can be used for treating heat and fire and such associated problems as restlessness, mania, dry mouth, sore throat, dry heaves, delirium, insomnia, vomiting of blood, nose bleeds, and maculopapular rashes. As Yu noted in *Achievements Regarding Epidemic Rashes:*

> A large dosage of the ingredients in the formula should be used when a submerged, thin, rapid pulse accompanies the symptoms noted above. The medium dosage should be used when a submerged, rapid pulse accompanies the symptoms noted above. A small dosage should be used when a floating, big, rapid pulse accompanies the symptoms noted above.[31]

This formula also includes Gardeniae Fructus *(zhī zǐ)*, Platycodi Radix *(jié gěng)*, Scutellariae Radix *(huáng qín)*, Anemarrhenae Rhizoma *(zhī mǔ)*, Paeoniae Radix rubra *(chì sháo)*, Scrophulariae Radix *(xuán shēn)*, Forsythiae Fructus *(lián qiào)*, fresh Lophatheri Herba *(xiān dàn zhú yè)*, Glycyrrhizae Radix *(gān cǎo)*, and Moutan Cortex *(mǔ dān pí)*. The source text does not specify the dosage for these ingredients; usually, 9-15g of each herb is recommended. According to one respected modern source, the dosage should be: Gardeniae Fructus *(zhī zǐ)* (9g), Platycodi Radix *(jié gěng)* (3g), Scutellariae Radix *(huáng qín)* (9g), Anemarrhenae Rhizoma *(zhī mǔ)* (12g), Paeoniae Radix rubra *(chì sháo)* (12g), Scrophulariae Radix *(xuán shēn)* (24g), Forsythiae Fructus *(lián qiào)* (15g), Glycyrrhizae Radix *(gān cǎo)* (6g), Moutan Cortex *(mǔ dān pí)* (9g), and fresh Lophatheri Herba *(dàn zhú yè)* (9g).[32]

ANALYSIS OF FORMULA: The formula Clear Epidemics and Overcome Toxin Drink *(qīng wēn bài dú yǐn)* should be used when the heat from excess in the Stomach is transforming into fire and toxin and invading the nutritive and blood levels. This formula includes important ingredients from four other formulas:

1. Gypsum fibrosum *(shí gāo)*, from White Tiger Decoction *(bái hǔ tāng)*,[33] is used to clear heat from the Stomach.

2. Gardeniae Fructus *(zhī zǐ)*, Scutellariae Radix *(huáng qín)*, and Forsythiae Fructus *(lián qiào)*, from Cool the Diaphragm Powder *(liáng gé sǎn)*,[34] are used to clear heat.

3. Coptidis Rhizoma *(huáng lián)* and Scutellariae Radix *(huáng qín)*, from Coptis Decoction to Resolve Toxicity *(huáng lián jiě dú tāng)*,[35] are used to clear heat and resolve toxicity.

4. Rhinocerotis Cornu *(xī jiǎo)*, Anemarrhenae Rhizoma *(zhī mǔ)*, Moutan Cortex *(mǔ dān pí)*, and Rehmanniae Radix *(shēng dì huáng)*, from Rhinoceros Horn

and Rehmannia Decoction *(xī jiǎo dì huáng tāng)*,[36] are used to cool blood and resolve toxicity.

According to Yu Lin, the reason for using such a large dosage of Gypsum fibrosum *(shí gāo)* is to eliminate the extreme heat in the qi level. This heat exists prior to its invasion of the nutritive and blood levels, and prior to its transformation into toxin. Once the extreme heat in the qi level has been cleared, the heat in the other levels can be easily cleared because its primary source is gone.

MODIFICATIONS: The basic formula can be modified as follows:

- For maculopapular rashes that are purplish in color, indicating blood stasis, add Arnebiae Radix/Lithospermi Radix *(zǐ cǎo)*, Persicae Semen *(táo rén)*, and *Carthami Flos (hóng huā)* to cool and invigorate the blood.

- For epistaxis, add Imperatae Rhizoma *(bái máo gēn)* and Agrimoniae Herba *(xiān hè cǎo)* to cool the blood and stop the bleeding.

- For loss of consciousness, immediately administer Calm the Palace Pill with Cattle Gallstone *(ān gōng niú huáng wán)* or Purple Snow Special Pill *(zǐ xuě dān)*.[37]

- For convulsions due to stirring of Liver wind, add Saigae tataricae Cornu *(líng yáng jiǎo)*, Uncariae Ramulus cum Uncis *(gōu téng)*, and Chrysanthemi Flos *(jú huā)* to cool the Liver and extinguish Liver wind.

- For abdominal distention and constipation, add Rhei Radix et Rhizoma *(dà huáng)* and Natrii Sulfas *(máng xiāo)* to eliminate heat from the body through bowel movement.

Case study: Transform Maculas Decoction *(huà bān tāng)*

First visit: An adult female developed aversion to cold, chills, fever, and headache a day after giving birth. She was treated with warm, acrid herbs that release the exterior, but without effect. Another doctor treated her for an attack of wind-cold with underlying blood deficiency, but again there was no improvement. The patient presented with a vigorous fever, restlessness, thirst, and a painful and swollen throat. She had bright maculas over her body. Her pulse was flooding and rapid. She had a deep-red tongue with a yellow coating. In addition, her white blood cell count was elevated to 18,000/mm³. The diagnosis was intense heat in both the qi and blood levels. A modified form of Transform Maculas Decoction *(huà bān tāng)* was prescribed: Gypsum fibrosum *(shí gāo)* (30g), Anemarrhenae Rhizoma *(zhī mǔ)* (15g), Glycyrrhizae Radix *(gān cǎo)* (6g), Scrophulariae Radix *(xuán shēn)* (24g), Rhinocerotis Cornu *(xī jiǎo)* (10g, cooked before the other herbs), Lonicerae Flos *(jīn yín huā)* (15g), Forsythiae Fructus *(lián qiào)* (30g), Scutellariae Radix *(huáng qín)* (25g), Moutan Cortex *(mǔ dān pí)* (12g), and Paeoniae Radix rubra *(chì sháo)* (15g). The patient was told to take the medicine six times a day (every four hours) using two packets a day.

Second visit: The day after finishing two packets of the herbs, the signs and symptoms of heat were significantly reduced. The formula was modified slightly and continued for two more days. By that time all signs and symptoms had disappeared.[38]

Case study: Clear Epidemics and Overcome Toxin Drink

(qīng wēn bài dú yǐn)

Ms. Yao, 44 years old, complained of abdominal pain, fever, and chills for three days. She had also developed yellowing of the skin and sclera. She was hospitalized and diagnosed with an acute attack of chronic cholecystitis, chronic cholelithiasis, necrotic cholecystitis, and toxic shock. She was treated with antibiotics, but to no avail. It was then suggested that she try Chinese medicine.

First visit: She looked acutely ill and in significant distress. She had muddled consciousness, delirium, restlessness, a green and yellow complexion, purple lips, yellow sclera and skin, some skin eruptions, and she looked as if she had bruises under her eyes. There was persistent distending abdominal pain that waxed and waned, chills, shivers, high fever, profuse sweating, nausea and vomiting, grayish stool that came twice a day, and scanty, dark-yellow urine. Her tongue was extremely red with a thick, dry coating, and her pulse was deep and weak. There were areas of tenderness along with a hard lump in the upper abdomen. Temperature was 39.5°C; blood pressure was 80-60/50-30mmHg; WBC 15100/mm³ with 95% neutrophils; urinalysis protein ++ with 5-10 RBC and slight WBC; BUN was 53.1mg%. The Chinese diagnosis was severe heat and toxin blocking the Gallbladder and Pericardium and forcing blood out of the vessels. The treatment principles were to clear the heat and resolve the toxicity, cool the blood and promote the function of the Gallbladder. The formula prescribed was a modified version of Clear Epidemics and Overcome Toxin Drink (qīng wēn bài dú yǐn): Rehmanniae Radix (shēng dì huáng) (30g), Moutan Cortex (mǔ dān pí) (15g), Paeoniae Radix alba (bái sháo) (15g), Rhinocerotis Cornu (xī jiǎo) (9g), Anemarrhenae Rhizoma (zhī mǔ) (9g), Gypsum fibrosum (shí gāo) (60g), nonglutinous rice (gěng mǐ) (15g), honey-toasted Glycyrrhizae Radix preparata (zhì gān cǎo) (9g), fried Coptidis Rhizoma (chǎo huáng lián) (9g), fried Scutellariae Radix (chǎo huáng qín) (6g), Phellodendri Cortex (huáng bǎi) (9g), fried Gardeniae Fructus (chǎo zhī zǐ) (12g), fried Aurantii Fructus immaturus (chǎo zhǐ shí) (9g), and Rhei Radix et Rhizoma (dà huáng) (9g). She was told to take one packet each day, and continued to be closely observed.

Second visit: The patient improved after taking one packet, and continued to take the formula for seven days. At this time her temperature and blood pressure had returned to normal, and the quantity of stool and urine had increased and were yellow. The skin eruptions and the look of bruising under her eyes were fading, as was the yellowing of her skin and sclera. There was slight edema of the lower legs. Her tongue was red with a yellow coating, and her pulse was thin and rapid. The same basic formula was used: Rehmanniae Radix *(shēng dì huáng)* (30g), Moutan Cortex *(mǔ dān pí)* (15g), Paeoniae Radix alba *(bái sháo)* (9g), Saigae tataricae Cornu *(líng yáng jiǎo)* (3g), Anemarrhenae Rhizoma *(zhī mǔ)* (24g), Gypsum fibrosum *(shí gāo)* (30g), nonglutinous rice *(gěng mǐ)* (15g), honey-toasted Glycyrrhizae Radix preparata *(zhì gān cǎo)* (9g), Coptidis Rhizoma *(huáng lián)* (9g), dry-fried Scutellariae Radix *(chǎo huáng qín)* (9g), Phellodendri Cortex *(huáng bǎi)* (9g), fried Gardeniae Fructus *(chǎo zhī zǐ)* (9g), and Artemisiae scopariae Herba *(yīn chén)* (15g).

Third visit: After taking two packets of the herbs the sclera and skin were only slightly yellow and the bruise spots under the eyes had faded even more. There was no change in the edema, tongue, or pulse. Her temperature and blood pressure remained normal. The diagnosis at this point was remnants of damp-heat along with injured Liver and Kidney yin. The treatment principles were to enrich the Liver and Kidney yin while continuing to clear the heat and drain the dampness. The formula was a modified version of Anemarrhena, Phellodendron, and Rehmannia Pill *(zhī bái dì huáng wán):*[39] Rehmanniae Radix *(shēng dì huáng)* (24g), Dioscoreae Rhizoma *(shān yào)* (12g), *Corni Fructus (shān zhū yú)* (12g), Moutan Cortex *(mǔ dān pí)* (9g), Poria *(fú líng)* (9g), Alismatis Rhizoma *(zé xiè)* (9g), Anemarrhenae Rhizoma *(zhī mǔ)* (12g), Phellodendri Cortex *(huáng bǎi)* (9g), and Artemisiae scopariae Herba *(yīn chén)* (15g).

Fourth visit: After taking three packets of the formula, it was modified by removing Poria *(fú líng)*, Alismatis Rhizoma *(zé xiè)*, and *Corni Fructus (shān zhū yú)*, and adding Akebiae Caulis *(mù tōng)* (9g), Polyporus *(zhū líng)* (9g), Ophiopogonis Radix *(mài mén dōng)* (15g), and Glehniae/Adenophorae Radix *(shā shēn)* (9g).

Fifth visit: After taking two packets of the modified formula, the bruise spots had almost completely disappeared and the skin and sclera were only slightly yellow. Her urination and bowel movements were normal. She had a red tongue with a white coating and a thin pulse. At this time she was given Six-Ingredient Pill with Rehmannia *(liù wèi dì huáng wán)*[40] with the addition of Artemisiae scopariae Herba *(yīn chén)*.

Sixth visit: After taking nine packets of the modified formula, the sclera and skin were no longer yellow, the bruise spots had disappeared, and so had the edema of the lower legs. Her appetite was fair and her blood pressure normal. She was discharged from the hospital.[41]

BURNING OF THE YIN IN THE NUTRITIVE LEVEL

Manifestations. There are three concurrent aspects to this pattern:

1. *Heat disturbing the spirit* with restlessness, irritability, or sometimes delirium.

2. *Injury to the yin in the nutritive level by heat* with fever that worsens at night, dry lips and mouth but with little desire to drink, a deep-red tongue with little or no coating, and a thin, rapid pulse.

3. *Failure of the collaterals to control the blood due to invasion of heat* with faint maculopapular rashes.

NOTE: Among these signs and symptoms, the deep-red tongue with no coating, fever that worsens at night, and restlessness are the key identifiers for this pattern. If the heat has just progressed from the qi to the nutritive level, there may be a yellow coating over part of the tongue.

Restlessness, a symptom of disturbance of the spirit, can be caused by heat from excess in the Stomach, heat from constraint in the chest and diaphragm, and invasion of the Pericardium by heat. Distinguishing among them is a common problem in the clinic, and was addressed in Chapter 7 (see Table 7.7).

Delirium can be seen in both this pattern and in severe constipation with dry stool and heat in the Large Intestine. The way to distinguish between them is to observe if there is constipation and distending pain in the abdomen, and if the tongue coating is thick. If so, the delirium is caused by severe constipation with dry stool and heat in the Large Intestine. If not, the delirium is due to burning of yin in the nutritive level by heat. Delirium can also be seen in invasion of the Pericardium by heat. However, the delirium in that pattern is constant with severe muddled consciousness, rather than being intermittent and without muddled consciousness, as seen here.

Pathology. Disturbance of the spirit, injury to the yin in the nutritive level, and failure of the collaterals to control blood due to invasion of heat.

Treatment principles. Dispel heat from the nutritive to the qi level by cooling the blood, enriching the yin, and clearing heat from the Heart.

Formula:

CLEAR THE NUTRITIVE LEVEL DECOCTION *(qīng yíng tāng)*

For a discussion of this formula, see the pattern of burning of yin in the nutritive level by heat in Chapter 7.

MODIFICATIONS: The basic formula can be modified as follows:

- For protective level involvement (aversion to cold, headache), add Sojae Semen preparatum *(dàn dòu chǐ)*, Arctii Fructus *(niú bàng zǐ)*, and Menthae haplocalycis Herba *(bò hé)* to disperse the heat in the protective level.

- Once heat and toxin progress to the blood level and the tongue body becomes very deep red, remove the herbs that dispel heat from the nutritive to the qi level—Forsythiae Fructus *(lián qiào)* and Lophatheri Herba *(dàn zhú yè)* — and add herbs that cool the blood, e.g., Paeoniae Radix rubra *(chì sháo)*.

- For stirring of Liver wind leading to convulsions, add Chrysanthemi Flos *(jú huā)*, Uncariae Ramulus cum Uncis *(gōu téng)*, and Saigae tataricae Cornu *(líng yáng jiǎo)*.

- For heat that has combined with dampness (greasy tongue coating), add herbs that are aromatic in nature, such as Curcumae Radix *(yù jīn)*, to transform the dampness.

BLEEDING DUE TO HEAT FROM EXCESS AND TOXIN IN THE BLOOD LEVEL

Manifestations. There are three concurrent aspects to this pattern:

1. *Bleeding due to heat from excess and toxin in the blood level* with various kinds of acute bleeding, usually of several types. This bleeding may take the form of large maculas, or it may appear in the stools or urine, or come from the nose or throat.

2. *Blood stasis* with purplish nails, face, and lips, and a very deep-red tongue.

3. *Blockage of the Heart's spirit* with loss of consciousness or sustained delirium.

NOTE: Compared with the pattern of burning of yin in the nutritive level by heat, this pattern is more severe because many large maculas appear, coupled with bleeding over the entire body and loss of consciousness or sustained delirium. By contrast, in the former pattern there are only faint maculopapular rashes without other signs of bleeding, and the patient only sometimes has delirium. Bleeding is mostly seen in warm pathogen diseases and internal diseases, and it is necessary to distinguish between them (see Table 8.6).

Pathology. Heat from excess and toxin in the blood level forcing the blood out of the vessels and leading to blood stasis.

Treatment Principles. Cool and invigorate the blood, clear heat, and resolve toxicity in the blood level.

Table 8.6	Distinguishing Bleeding in Warm Pathogen Diseases from Bleeding in Internal Diseases	
Pathology	**Signs and Symptoms**	**Treatment Principles**
▶ WARM PATHOGEN DISEASES		
Heat forces blood out of the vessels	Acute bleeding over several areas at once associated with blood stasis and fever	Cool the blood, clear heat from the nutritive and blood levels, invigorate the blood, enrich the yin
▶ INTERNAL DISEASES		
Injury to vessels by internal heat or failure of Spleen to control blood	Chronic and limited bleeding, no fever or low grade fever	Stop the bleeding, dispel blood stasis, eliminate internal heat, or tonify the Spleen qi

Formula:

RHINOCEROS HORN AND REHMANNIA DECOCTION *(xī jiǎo dì huáng tāng)*

SOURCE: *Important Formulas Worth a Thousand Gold Pieces*

Rhinocerotis Cornu *(xī jiǎo)* . . . . 30g[42]
Rehmanniae Radix *(shēng dì huáng)* 24g
Moutan Cortex *(mǔ dān pí)* 6g
Paeoniae Radix alba *(bái sháo)* 9g

ANALYSIS OF FORMULA: Rhinocerotis Cornu *(xī jiǎo)* is the chief herb in this formula. When combined with Rehmanniae Radix *(shēng dì huáng)*, Rhinocerotis Cornu *(xī jiǎo)* cools the blood and resolves toxicity to stop the bleeding. Moutan Cortex *(mǔ dān pí)* and Paeoniae Radix alba *(bái sháo)* cool and invigorate the blood (respectively) to stop the bleeding. It is strongly recommended that Paeoniae Radix rubra *(chì sháo)* be substituted for Paeoniae Radix alba *(bái sháo)* since Paeoniae Radix rubra *(chì sháo)* can both cool and invigorate the blood. In this formula much attention has been paid to selecting herbs that cool the blood because the cause of the bleeding here is heat in the blood. Without clearing the heat and cooling the blood, the bleeding will not stop. However, a large dosage of herbs to clear the heat and cool the blood may cause the blood to congeal, leading to blood stasis, which could give rise to further bleeding. Thus, Paeoniae Radix rubra *(chì sháo)* and Moutan Cortex *(mǔ dān pí)* play important multipurpose roles in clearing heat, cooling blood, invigorating the blood, and removing blood stasis.[43]

MODIFICATIONS: The basic formula can be modified as follows:

- For a high fever, add Isatidis Folium *(dà qīng yè)* and Anemarrhenae Rhizoma *(zhī mǔ)* to increase the actions of clearing heat and resolving toxicity.

- For a patient in a coma, use Calm the Palace Pill with Cattle Gallstone *(ān gōng niú huáng wán)*[44] to clear heat from the Heart and open the orifice.

- For severe blood stasis and purplish maculas, add Arnebiae Radix/Lithospermi Radix *(zǐ cǎo)* and Manitis Squama *(chuān shān jiǎ)*[45] to remove the blood stasis.

- Different herbs affect bleeding in different areas of the body. Add Scutellariae Radix *(huáng qín)*, Coptidis Rhizoma *(huáng lián)*, and Bambusae Caulis in taeniam *(zhú rú)* for hematemesis. Add Scutellariae Radix *(huáng qín)* and Imperatae Rhizoma *(bái máo gēn)* for hemoptysis. Add Sanguisorbae Radix *(dì yú)* and Sophorae Flos immaturus *(huái mǐ)* for hematochezia. Add Knoxiae Radix/Euphorbiae pekinensis Radix *(dà jǐ)*, Cirsii Herba *(xiǎo jì)*, Scutellariae Radix *(huáng qín)*, and Imperatae Rhizoma *(bái máo gēn)* for hematuria.

Case study: Rhinoceros Horn and Rehmannia Decoction *(xī jiǎo dì huáng tāng)*

The patient, a 23-year-old female, had purple maculas over her body for three days and required hospitalization. The maculas worsened during those three days. In addition, she suffered dizziness, palpitations, poor appetite, fatigue, loose stools, and bleeding from the nose. Prior to this, she had missed her menstrual period for three months. A blood test revealed a platelet count of only 20,000/mm³.[46] She had a red tongue with purple blisters and a slippery, rapid pulse. The biomedical diagnosis was acute thrombocytopenic purpura.

First visit: The traditional Chinese doctor diagnosed the condition as heat attacking the blood level, forcing blood out of the vessels. The treatment principle was to clear the heat, cool the blood, enrich the yin, and drain the fire. A modified form of Rhinoceros Horn and Rehmannia Decoction *(xī jiǎo dì huáng tāng)* was prescribed for this purpose: Bubali Cornu *(shuǐ niú jiǎo)* (30g), Rehmanniae Radix *(shēng dì huáng)* (30g), Scrophulariae Radix *(xuán shēn)* (30g), Paeoniae Radix alba *(bái sháo)* (15g), Testudinis Plastrum *(guī bǎn)* (20g), Ligustri lucidi Fructus *(nǚ zhēn zi)* (15g), Ecliptae Herba *(mò hàn lián)* (15g), Anemarrhenae Rhizoma *(zhī mǔ)* (10g), charred Platycladi Cacumen *(cè bǎi tàn)* (10g), Agrimoniae Herba *(xiān hè cǎo)* (10g), and Asini Corii Colla *(ē jiāo)* (10g). Since the patient's condition was severe, she also received 200cc of blood by transfusion to prevent her condition from deteriorating.

Second visit: After taking three packets of the formula, the patient's energy improved, her nosebleeds stopped, and her maculas were reduced. Moutan Cortex *(mǔ dān pí)* (6g) and Rumicis Radix *(yáng tí)*[47] (15g) were added to the formula.

Third visit: After taking four packets of the modified formula, all of the signs and symptoms continued to improve. The patient still had a red face and a red and tender tongue, showing that heat remained. She continued taking the same formula.

Fourth visit: After taking an additional seven packets of the modified formula, all of her signs and symptoms were gone, except for occasional palpitations, red tongue, and a thin pulse that showed yin deficiency. The formula was modified to Bubali Cornu *(shuǐ niú jiǎo)* (30g), Moutan Cortex *(mǔ dān pí)* (6g), Asini Corii Colla *(ē jiāo)* (10g), Paeoniae Radix alba *(bái sháo)* (10g), Dendrobii Herba *(shí hú)* (10g), and Ecliptae Herba *(mò hàn lián)* (10g). The patient was hospitalized for a total of twenty days, after which the signs and symptoms were fully resolved. Her platelet count also improved, rising from 20,000 to 67,000/mm³. Following these results, the patient was discharged from the hospital.[48]

CLUMPING OF HEAT AND BLOOD STASIS

Manifestations. There are two concurrent aspects to this pattern:

1. *Combination of heat and blood stasis in the lower burner* with constipation and dry, black stools, hardness, distention, and pain in the lower abdomen, dry mouth, and normal urination.
2. *Disturbance of the spirit of the Heart by heat and blood stasis* with mania, a purplish tongue or purplish spots over the tongue, and a submerged and forceful or hesitant pulse.

NOTE: The key identifiers for this pattern are hardness, distention, and pain in the lower abdomen, black stools, normal urination, purplish tongue or purplish spots over the tongue, and a submerged and forceful or hesitant pulse.

Pathology. A combination of heat and blood stasis in the lower burner.

Treatment principles. Drain heat by purging, invigorate the blood, and remove blood stasis.

Formula:

PEACH KERNEL DECOCTION TO ORDER THE QI *(táo rén chéng qì tāng)*

SOURCE: *Systematic Differentiation of Warm Pathogen Diseases*

Rhei Radix et Rhizoma *(dà huáng)* 15g

Natrii Sulfas *(máng xiāo)* 6g

Paeoniae Radix alba *(bái sháo)* 6g

Persicae Semen *(táo rén)* 9g

Moutan Cortex *(mǔ dān pí)* 9g

Angelicae sinensis Radix *(dāng guī)* 9g

ANALYSIS OF FORMULA: Paeoniae Radix alba *(bái sháo)*, Persicae Semen *(táo rén)*, Moutan Cortex *(mǔ dān pí)*, and Angelicae sinensis Radix *(dāng guī)* clear heat, cool the blood, invigorate the blood, and remove blood stasis. Rhei Radix et Rhizoma *(dà huáng)* and Natrii Sulfas *(máng xiāo)* drain heat by purging and provide an avenue for the heat and blood stasis to exit the body. It is better to use Paeoniae Radix rubra *(chì sháo)* than Paeoniae Radix alba *(bái sháo)* because Paeoniae Radix rubra *(chì sháo)* can clear heat and invigorate the blood. Angelicae sinensis Radix *(dāng guī)* invigorates the blood as well as induces bowel movements, both of which are beneficial for this pattern.

Wu You-Xing (Wu You-Ke, c. 1582–1652) first introduced this formula in *Discussion of Warm Epidemics.* It is a modification of Peach Pit Decoction to Order the Qi *(táo hé chéng qì tāng)* from which Cinnamomi Ramulus *(guì zhī)* and Glycyrrhizae Radix *(gān cǎo)* have been removed, and Angelicae sinensis Radix *(dāng guī)*, Paeoniae Radix alba *(bái sháo)*, and Moutan Cortex *(mǔ dān pí)* added. These modifications reflect the strategy of providing an avenue for the pathogenic factors to exit the body. Here, in addition to the heat, the blood stasis too can exit via bowel movements.

Another formula by the same name was introduced by Yu Gen-Chu in *Revised Popular Guide to the Discussion of Cold Damage.* [49] This formula contains Persicae Semen *(táo rén)* (9g), Trogopterori Faeces *(wǔ líng zhī)* (6g), Typhae Pollen *(pú huáng)* (4.5g), Rehmanniae Radix *(shēng dì huáng)* (24g), Rhei Radix et Rhizoma *(dà huáng)* (6g), Natrii Sulfas *(máng xiāo)* (3g), Glycyrrhizae Radix *(gān cǎo)* (1.8g), and ground Rhinocerotis Cornu *(xī jiǎo)* (4 spoonfuls).[50] Relative to the formula above, it is more effective at cooling and invigorating the blood, and at relieving pain, but is less effective at purging heat and blood stasis. It is therefore indicated when the blood stasis aspects of the condition predominate.

If the patient shows intense mania and has a strong physical constitution, the treatment of choice is Dead-on Decoction *(dǐ dǎng tāng)*, which was first recorded in *Discussion of Cold Damage.* It is composed of Hirudo *(shuǐ zhì)* (30g), Tabanus *(méng chóng)* (30g), Persicae Semen *(táo rén)* (20 pieces), and Rhei Radix et Rhizoma *(dà huáng)* (9g). For these patients, the dosage of Hirudo *(shuǐ zhì)* and Tabanus *(méng chóng)* should be reduced, and that of Rhei Radix et Rhizoma *(dà huáng)* and Persicae Semen *(táo rén)* should be increased: Rhei Radix et Rhizoma *(dà huáng)* (15g), Tabanus *(méng chóng)* (20 pieces), Persicae Semen *(táo rén)* (15g), and Hirudo *(shuǐ zhì)* (1.5g).[51] Relative to the formula above, it is more effective at cooling and invigorating the blood, and at relieving pain, but is less effective at purging heat. It is therefore indicated when the blood stasis aspects of the condition predominate.

MODIFICATIONS: For severe low abdomen and low back pain, add Sudden Smile Powder *(shī xiào sǎn)*,[52] which consists of Trogopterori Faeces *(wǔ líng zhī)* and Typhae Pollen *(pú huáng)*, to increase the actions of removing blood stasis and relieving lower abdominal pain.

Differentiation and Treatment of Invasion of the Pericardium by Heat

VEILING OF THE PERICARDIUM BY HEAT AND PHLEGM

The differentiation and treatment of this pattern is identical to that of wind-warmth related veiling of the Pericardium by transmission of heat and phlegm (see Chapter 7). Also, note that delirium is present both in this pattern and in that of burning of yin in the nutritive level by heat. The delirium due to veiling of the Pericardium by heat and phlegm is more severe (see Table 8.7).

INTERIOR BLOCKAGE AND EXTERIOR COLLAPSE

The differentiation and treatment of this pattern and the wind-warmth related pattern of interior blockage and exterior collapse (see Chapter 7) are identical.

Table 8.7	Delirium Associated with Burning of Yin by Heat in Nutritive Level vs. Veiling of Pericardium by Heat and Phlegm
Pathology	**Signs and Symptoms**
▶ BURNING OF YIN BY HEAT IN NUTRITIVE LEVEL	
Invasion of heat leading to disturbance of the Heart spirit, injury of yin in the nutritive level, failure of collaterals to control the blood	Mild delirium, intermittent wakefulness, and possible speech difficulty (but w/o stiffness of tongue or coldness in extremities)
▶ VEILING OF THE PERICARDIUM BY HEAT AND PHLEGM	
Veiling of Pericardium by heat associated with phlegm	Severe delirium, coma, stiffness of tongue with speech difficulty, cold extremities

287

STIRRING OF INTERNAL WIND DUE TO HEAT FROM EXCESS IN THE LIVER

Manifestations. There are three concurrent aspects to this pattern:

1. *Stirring of internal wind due to heat from excess in the Liver* with involuntary movements of the limbs, spasms of the sinews, convulsions (or even rigidity of the neck and trunk), high fever, dizziness, headache with a sense of pressure, and a wiry, rapid pulse.

2. *Blockage or disturbance of the spirit of the Heart by heat* with loss of consciousness or mania.

3. *Blockage of yang by accumulation of extreme interior heat and obstruction of qi activity* with cold extremities.

NOTE: Involuntary movements of the limbs, spasms of the sinews, convulsions (or even rigidity of the neck and trunk), and a high fever are the key identifiers for this condition. It is important to note that the internal wind is a result of excess rather than deficiency. While heat from excess in the Liver usually leads to a mild, temporary injury of the Liver yin, the internal wind is due to heat from excess causing the sinews to move violently, and not from the mild, temporary injury to the yin. If the heat is drained quickly, the Liver yin will recover very soon. There are other instances of internal wind due to excess, apart from this one (see Table 8.8). Note that the principal sign of stirring of internal wind is the involuntary movements of the limbs and opisthotonos.

Pathology. Heat from excess invading the Liver, leading to stirring of Liver wind.

Treatment principles. Cool the Liver and extinguish Liver wind.

NOTE: Since this is due to heat from excess in the Liver, treatment should clear heat from the Liver as well as extinguish the internal wind.

Formula:

ANTELOPE HORN AND UNCARIA DECOCTION *(líng jiǎo gōu téng tāng)*

SOURCE: *Revised Popular Guide to the Discussion of Cold Damage*

Saigae tataricae Cornu *(líng yáng jiǎo)* 4.5g
Mori Folium *(sāng yè)* 6g
Fritillariae cirrhosae Bulbus *(chuān bèi mǔ)* 12g
Rehmanniae Radix *(shēng dì huáng)* 15g
Uncariae Ramulus cum Uncis *(gōu téng)* 9g
Chrysanthemi Flos *(jú huā)* 9g

Table 8.8	Comparison of Four Types of Internal Wind Due to Heat from Excess*		
Manifestations	**Treatment Principles**	**Formulas**

▶ INVASION OF PERICARDIUM BY HEAT FROM EXCESS IN PROTECTIVE LEVEL LEADING TO STIRRING OF INTERNAL WIND

Coma, fever, convulsions, cold extremities, stiff and deep-red tongue with speech difficulty	Clear heat from the Pericardium, open the orifices, cool the Liver, extinguish internal wind	Clear the Palace Decoction (*qīng gōng tāng*) plus Antelope Horn and Uncaria Decoction (*líng jiǎo gōu téng yǐn*); or Calm the Palace Pill with Cattle Gallstone (*ān gōng niú huáng wán*), Purple Snow Special Pill (*zǐ xuě dān*), or Greatest Treasure Special Pill (*zhì bǎo dān*)

▶ STIRRING OF INTERNAL WIND DUE TO HEAT FROM EXCESS IN STOMACH

Vigorous fever, strong thirst, profuse sweating, convulsions, flooding pulse	Clear and vent heat, cool the Liver, and extinguish internal wind	White Tiger Decoction (*bái hǔ tāng*) plus herbs that clear heat and extinguish wind

▶ STIRRING OF INTERNAL WIND DUE TO SEVERE CONSTIPATION WITH DRY STOOL AND HEAT IN LARGE INTESTINE

Tidal fever, convulsions, hard and dry stool or diarrhea with discharge of foul water, hard and distending pain in abdomen, red tongue with dry, yellow coating, submerged and forceful pulse	Drain heat from the Large Intestine by purging, extinguish internal wind	Regulate the Stomach and Order the Qi Decoction (*tiáo wèi chéng qì tāng*) plus herbs that clear heat and extinguish wind

▶ STIRRING OF INTERNAL WIND DUE TO HEAT FROM EXCESS IN THE LIVER

Spasm of sinews, convulsions, or even rigidity of neck and trunk, high fever, dizziness, distending headache, wiry and rapid pulse	Cool the Liver and extinguish internal wind	Antelope Horn and Uncaria Decoction (*líng jiǎo gōu téng yǐn*)

*See Chapter 7 for discussion of the first and second types. The third type is rarely seen as the heat in this pattern is usually not intense enough to stir up internal wind, and is often eliminated via foul-smelling diarrhea before it reaches that point.

Poriae Sclerotium pararadicis *(fú shén)* 9g

Paeoniae Radix alba *(bái sháo)* 9g

Glycyrrhizae Radix *(gān cǎo)* 2.4g

Bambusae Caulis in taeniam *(zhú rú)* 15g

ANALYSIS OF FORMULA: As the chief herbs, Saigae tataricae Cornu *(líng yáng jiǎo)* and Uncariae Ramulus cum Uncis *(gōu téng)* work together to cool the Liver and extinguish Liver wind. Chrysanthemi Flos *(jú huā)* and Mori Folium *(sāng yè)* disperse heat and enhance the effect of Saigae tataricae Cornu *(líng yáng jiǎo)* and Uncariae Ramulus cum Uncis *(gōu téng)*. Clinically, extreme heat in the Liver can injure the Liver yin, reducing nourishment to the sinews and aggravating the convulsions. The sweet and sour flavor of Rehmanniae Radix *(shēng dì huáng)*, Paeoniae Radix alba *(bái sháo)*, and Glycyrrhizae Radix *(gān cǎo)* enrich the Liver yin, which then nourishes and relaxes the sinews. The other herbs clear heat from constraint in the Liver and Gallbladder and transform phlegm, which results from heat congealing the fluids.

MODIFICATIONS: The basic formula can be modified as follows:

- For significant rigidity of the neck, add Puerariae Radix *(gé gēn)*.

- To extinguish Liver wind and to relieve convulsions with rigidity of the trunk, add Bombyx batryticatus *(bái jiāng cán)* and Pheretima *(dì lóng)*.

- For severe conditions with loss of consciousness, use Calm the Palace Pill with Cattle Gallstone *(ān gōng niú huáng wán)* or Purple Snow Special Pill *(zǐ xuě dān)*.[53]

- For heat from excess in the nutritive level with maculopapular rash and a deep-red tongue, add Rhinocerotis Cornu *(xī jiǎo)*, Moutan Cortex *(mǔ dān pí)*, and Arnebiae Radix/Lithospermi Radix *(zǐ cǎo)* to cool the blood and resolve toxicity.

- For heat in the Large Intestine with constipation, add Bubali Cornu *(shuǐ niú jiǎo)*, Coptidis Rhizoma *(huáng lián)*, Rhei Radix et Rhizoma *(dà huáng)*, and Natrii Sulfas *(máng xiāo)*.

Case study: Antelope Horn and Uncaria Decoction *(líng jiǎo gōu téng tāng)*

Xie XX, male, 5 years old

In mid-June the patient came down with a fever and began coughing up thick, yellow sputum. He went to the outpatient department of a hospital for treatment. That night he developed projectile vomiting, vigorous fever, and stiffness of the neck, and became comatose. He was diagnosed with purulent encephalitis, hospitalized, and treated with a wide spectrum of antibiotics for more than forty days, with no significant improvement. He was then transferred to the provincial children's hospital for a week. The signs and symptoms showed slight improvement, and he was discharged.

The second day after returning home (August 1) he developed a vigorous fever and again became lethargic and comatose. He was taken to the emergency room and then hospitalized at the Linggang County Traditional Chinese Medical Hospital (in Jiangxi province).

At this time the patient had a vigorous fever, headache, muddled consciousness, and was lethargic. He also had projectile vomiting and was coughing up thick, yellow sputum. He was very thirsty, his neck was stiff, and he suffered violent spasms of the limbs. He was constipated and incontinent of urine. His tongue was red with a greasy, yellow coating. The pulse was wiry and slippery. The biomedical exam revealed a temperature of 41.1°C; a lump behind his right ear; moist rales in his lungs; blood pressure of 92/60mmHg; WBC 22400/mm^3 with 92% neutrophils. His cerebrospinal fluid was turbid and contained *Strep. pneumococcus*.

As soon as he was hospitalized, the patient was treated with a continuous infusion of penicillin, which was the only Western medicine used. In addition, he was immediately given five Cattle Gallstone Pills to Calm the Brain *(ān nǎo niú huáng piàn)*.[54] Also, a combination of a modified version of Antelope Horn and Uncaria Decoction *(líng jiǎo gōu téng tāng)* along with Five-Ingredient Decoction to Eliminate Toxin *(wǔ wèi xiāo dú yǐn)*[55] were prepared and given to the patient frequently throughout the day and night. The prescription was: Saigae tataricae Cornu *(líng yáng jiǎo)* powder (two small bottles, taken with the strained decoction), Uncariae Ramulus cum Uncis *(gōu téng)* (10g, added near the end of the decocting), Arisaema cum Bile *(dǎn nán xīng)* (5g), Bambusae Caulis in taeniam *(zhú rú)* (5g), Chrysanthemi Flos *(jú huā)* (30g), Mori Folium *(sāng yè)* (6g), Rehmanniae Radix *(shēng dì huáng)* (7g), Fritillariae cirrhosae Bulbus *(chuān bèi mǔ)* (7g), Paeoniae Radix alba *(bái sháo)* (6g), Poria *(fú líng)* (6g), Puerariae Radix *(gé gēn)* (10g), Scolopendra *(wú gōng)* (1 piece), Rhei Radix et Rhizoma *(dà huáng)* (6g, added near the end of the decocting), Lonicerae Flos *(jīn yín huā)* (15g), Violae Herba *(zǐ huā dì dīng)* (20g), and Taraxaci Herba *(pú gōng yīng)* (20g).

By 4 A.M. the following morning his temperature began to gradually decrease, until it reached 38.5°C at 8 A.M. He had a bowel movement of loose, strong-smelling stool. His mind became clear. His head and violent spasms were reduced. But he still had a stiff neck, looked sleepy, and was coughing. His tongue was still red with a thick, yellow, greasy coating, and his pulse was slippery and rapid. At this time the infusion of penicillin was stopped and the same formula, with the addition of Trichosanthis Semen *(guā lóu rén)* (9g), was continued at a dosage of one packet per day. He was also given five Cattle Gallstone Pills to Calm the Brain *(ān nǎo niú huáng piàn)* twice a day.

By August 6 (five days after admission) the fever, vomiting, and spasms were gone and this treatment was stopped. The next day he was started on one packet a day of the following formula: Taraxaci Herba *(pú gōng yīng)* (20g), Violae Herba *(zǐ huā dì dīng)* (20g), Lonicerae Flos *(jīn yín huā)* (15g), Chrysanthemi Flos *(jú huā)* (20g),

Uncariae Ramulus cum Uncis *(gōu téng)* (10g, added near the end of the decocting), Arisaema cum Bile *(dǎn nán xīng)* (5g), Bambusae Caulis in taeniam *(zhú rú)* (5g), Mori Folium *(sāng yè)* (6g), Rehmanniae Radix *(shēng dì huáng)* (7g), Fritillariae cirrhosae Bulbus *(chuān bèi mǔ)* (7g), Paeoniae Radix alba *(bái sháo)* (6g), Poria *(fú líng)* (6g), and Trichosanthis Fructus *(guā lóu)* (3g). He was also given one pill a day of Cattle Gallstone Pill to Resolve Toxicity *(niú huáng jiě dú wán)*.[56] He was discharged from the hospital a week later, and was instructed to take Five-Ingredient Decoction to Eliminate Toxin *(wǔ wèi xiāo dú yǐn)* with sugar as a tea for two weeks to dispel the residual heat and toxin. The follow-up visit showed that the boy was normal both physically and mentally.[57]

Differentiation and Treatment of Patterns Involving Injury to the Kidney Yin by Heat (Nutritive Level)

BLAZING FIRE DUE TO KIDNEY YIN DEFICIENCY

Manifestations. Fever, difficulty falling asleep, red tongue with yellow coating or thin, black, and dry coating, and a thin, rapid pulse.

NOTE: Clinically, less tongue coating than normal or a mirror-like tongue is an important sign for identifying yin deficiency.

Pathology. Blazing Heart fire due to heat injuring Kidney yin. This is also called disharmony between the Heart and Kidney due to failure of the Kidney to enrich the Heart with its yin.

Treatment principles. Enrich the Kidney yin and drain fire from the Heart.

Formula:

COPTIS AND ASS-HIDE GELATIN DECOCTION *(huáng lián ē jiāo tāng)*
SOURCE: *Systematic Differentiation of Warm Pathogen Diseases*

Coptidis Rhizoma *(huáng lián)* 12g

Scutellariae Radix *(huáng qín)* 3g

Asini Corii Colla *(ē jiāo)* 9g

Paeoniae Radix alba *(bái sháo)* 3g

egg yolks *(jī zǐ huáng)* . . . . 2 yolks

ANALYSIS OF FORMULA: Coptis and Ass-Hide Gelatin Decoction *(huáng lián ē jiāo tāng)* was first described by Zhang Ji in *Discussion of Cold Damage*. Wu Tang modified this by reducing the dosage of Paeoniae Radix alba *(bái sháo)* and Scutellariae Radix *(huáng qín)* from 6g to 3g. According to Wu Tang, Coptidis Rhizoma *(huáng lián)* and Scutellariae Radix *(huáng qín)* drain Heart fire to prevent further injury to the yin. Asini Corii Colla *(ē jiāo)* and Paeoniae Radix alba *(bái sháo)* enrich the yin of the Kidney and Liver to control blazing fire. Egg yolks *(jī zǐ huáng)* enrich the yin of the Kidney and Heart and promote Kidney and Heart communication.

DECOCTION AND ADMINISTRATION: Once the decoction has been prepared, dissolve Asini Corii Colla *(ē jiāo)* in the strained decoction. Then stir the egg yolks *(jī zǐ huáng)* into the resulting liquid.

Case study: Coptis and Ass-Hide Gelatin Decoction *(huáng lián ē jiāo tāng)*

First visit: A three-year-old male presented in mid-July. He had suffered a ten-day course of measles in May, and since early June had a fever (38.5°C – 39.0°C) with thirst, no sweating, and profuse urine. The blood tests and x-ray imaging tests were negative. He had been treated by Western medical doctors without noticeable improvement.

The patient had dry lips and tongue. His stool was dry and hard. The tongue was red with little coating, and his pulse was thin and rapid. He was diagnosed with injury to the Kidney yin by summerheat. The treatment principle was to clear the heat and enrich the yin for which he was given a modified version of Coptis and Ass-Hide Gelatin Decoction *(huáng lián ē jiāo tāng)*: Coptidis Rhizoma *(huáng lián)* (3g), Asini Corii Colla *(ē jiāo)* (6g, melted in the strained decoction), egg yolks *(jī zǐ huáng)* (one yolk), Paeoniae Radix alba *(bái sháo)* (10g), and Panacis quinquefolii Radix *(xī yáng shēn)* (3g, cooked separately and mixed with the strained decoction).

Second visit: After taking five packets of the herbs, the patient's temperature was reduced to 37.6°C. His dry lips, tongue, and thirst had improved. A thin coating grew on the tongue. The patient was cured after continuing to take herbs to enrich the yin and tonify the qi for two more weeks.[58]

EXHAUSTION OF THE KIDNEY AND LIVER YIN

Manifestations. There are two concurrent aspects to this pattern:

1. *Exhaustion of the Kidney and Liver yin by the remnants of heat* with dry throat, dry teeth (lack of luster), diminished hearing or deafness, listlessness, and a dry, deep-red tongue.

2. *Deficiency of yin leading to hyperactivity of yang* with a hotter sensation on the soles and palms than on the back of the hands and top of the feet, and slight but persistent fever.

NOTE: Compared with blazing fire due to Kidney yin deficiency, there are no significant signs or symptoms of fire or heat in this pattern. However, there are many more signs and symptoms of exhaustion of Kidney yin. Dry throat and teeth, slight but persistent fever, a hotter sensation in the soles and palms than on the back of the hands and top of the feet, and deafness are the key identifiers for this pattern.

In this pattern, both the Kidney and Liver yin are badly damaged. Since the Pericardium is associated with the Liver (they are both *jue yin* channels), heat from deficiency begins to manifest at PC-8 *(láo gōng)* and KI-1 *(yōng quán)*, which are located in the center of the palm of the hand and sole of the foot, respectively. Therefore, when there is Kidney and Liver yin deficiency, coupled with heat from deficiency, the patient will feel a hot sensation in the soles and palms that is greater than on the back of the hands and top of the feet.

Deafness or diminished hearing is a key feature of this pattern. They can also be seen in an attack on the Gallbladder by heat, but in those cases it is always accompanied by a plugged sensation in the ears coupled with signs and symptoms of Gallbladder heat.

Pathology. Exhaustion of Kidney yin by the remnants of heat, leading to hyperactive yang.

Treatment principles. Enrich the yin of the Kidney and the Liver.

Formula:

MODIFIED RESTORE THE PULSE DECOCTION *(jiā jiǎn fù mài tāng)*

SOURCE: *Systematic Differentiation of Warm Pathogen Diseases*

Honey-toasted Glycyrrhizae Radix preparata *(zhì gān cǎo)* 18g

Rehmanniae Radix *(shēng dì huáng)* 18g

Cannabis Semen *(huǒ má rén)* 9g

Ophiopogonis Radix *(mài mén dōng)* 15g

Asini Corii Colla *(ē jiāo)* 9g

Paeoniae Radix alba *(bái sháo)* 18g

---

ANALYSIS OF FORMULA: This formula is based on Restore the Pulse Decoction *(fù mài tāng)*, also called Honey-Fried Licorice Decoction *(zhi gan cao tang)* from *Discussion of Cold Damage*. Restore the Pulse Decoction *(fù mài tāng)* contains honey-toasted Glycyrrhizae Radix preparata *(zhì gān cǎo)* (12g), Zingiberis Rhizoma recens *(shēng jiāng)* (9g), Ginseng Radix *(rén shēn)* (6g), Rehmanniae Radix *(shēng dì huáng)* (48g),

Cinnamomi Ramulus *(guì zhī)* (9g), Asini Corii Colla *(ē jiāo)* (6g), Ophiopogonis Radix *(mài mén dōng)* (9g), Cannabis Semen *(huǒ má rén)* (9g), Jujubae Fructus *(dà zǎo)* (30 pieces), and wine (10ml). Wu Tang removed Ginseng Radix *(rén shēn)*, Cinnamomi Ramulus *(guì zhī)*, Zingiberis Rhizoma recens *(shēng jiāng)*, Jujubae Fructus *(dà zǎo)*, and wine because they are warm in nature and would aggravate the injured yin. He added Paeoniae Radix alba *(bái sháo)*. This formula reflects the idea of enriching the yin with sweet and sour herbs. In the formula, honey-toasted Glycyrrhizae Radix preparata *(zhì gān cǎo)* tonifies the Spleen, which is the source of qi and blood. Rehmanniae Radix *(shēng dì huáng)*, Paeoniae Radix alba *(bái sháo)*, Ophiopogonis Radix *(mài mén dōng)*, Cannabis Semen *(huǒ má rén)*, and Asini Corii Colla *(ē jiāo)* enrich the Kidney and Liver yin.

MODIFICATIONS: According to Wu Tang, if there is diarrhea, one should remove Cannabis Semen *(huǒ má rén)* and add Ostreae Concha *(mǔ lì)* (30g). He also suggested that if the condition were severe, the dosage of the following herbs should be increased: honey-toasted Glycyrrhizae Radix preparata *(zhì gān cǎo)* (30g), Rehmanniae Radix *(shēng dì huáng)* (24g), Paeoniae Radix alba *(bái sháo)* (24g), and Ophiopogonis Radix *(mài mén dōng)* (21g).

STIRRING OF LIVER WIND DUE TO KIDNEY YIN DEFICIENCY

Manifestations. There are three concurrent aspects to this pattern:

1. *Stirring of Liver wind due to Kidney yin deficiency* with trembling of the fingers or limbs or convulsions of the feet and hands.
2. *Exhaustion of the Kidney yin* with cracked lips, "black" teeth,[59] extreme mental and physical fatigue, a dry and deep-red tongue without coating or with cracks, and a deficient pulse.
3. *Malnutrition of the Heart spirit due to Kidney yin deficiency* with violent palpitations or even chest pain.

Pathology. Kidney yin deficiency leading to stirring of Liver wind and malnourishment of the Heart spirit.

Treatment principles. Enrich the Kidney yin, extinguish the Liver wind, and calm the spirit.

Formula No. 1:

TWO-SHELL DECOCTION TO RESTORE THE PULSE *(èr jiǎ fù mài tāng)*
SOURCE: *Systematic Differentiation of Warm Pathogen Diseases*

Honey-toasted Glycyrrhizae Radix preparata *(zhì gān cǎo)* 18g
Rehmanniae Radix *(shēng dì huáng)* 18g
Paeoniae Radix alba *(bái sháo)* 18g
Ostreae Concha *(mǔ lì)* 15g
Ophiopogonis Radix *(mài mén dōng)* 15g
Asini Corii Colla *(ē jiāo)* 9g
Cannabis Semen *(huǒ má rén)* 9g
Trionycis Carapax *(biē jiǎ)* 24g

ANALYSIS OF FORMULA: This formula is based on Modified Restore the Pulse Decoction *(jiā jiǎn fù mài tāng)* with Ostreae Concha *(mǔ lì)* and Trionycis Carapax *(biē jiǎ)* added to enrich the Kidney yin, clear the heat, subdue the rising Liver yang, and extinguish the Liver wind. It is suitable for treating a slight stirring of Liver wind with mild trembling of the fingers.

Formula No. 2:

THREE-SHELL DECOCTION TO RESTORE THE PULSE *(sān jiǎ fù mài tāng)*

SOURCE: *Systematic Differentiation of Warm Pathogen Diseases*

Honey-toasted Glycyrrhizae Radix preparata *(zhì gān cǎo)* 18g
Rehmanniae Radix *(shēng dì huáng)* 18g
Paeoniae Radix alba *(bái sháo)* 18g
Ostreae Concha *(mǔ lì)* 15g
Testudinis Plastrum *(guī bǎn)* 30g
Ophiopogonis Radix *(mài mén dōng)* 15g
Asini Corii Colla *(ē jiāo)* 9g
Cannabis Semen *(huǒ má rén)* 9g
Trionycis Carapax *(biē jiǎ)* 24g

ANALYSIS OF FORMULA: This formula is based on Two-Shell Decoction to Restore the Pulse *(èr jiǎ fù mài tāng)*, with Testudinis Plastrum *(guī bǎn)* added to enrich the Kidney yin, subdue the ascendant Liver yang, and calm the spirit. It is suitable for relatively severe disturbances of the Heart spirit due to Kidney yin deficiency, with such symptoms as violent palpitations (often accompanied by a sensation of emptiness in the chest) or even chest pain.

Formula No. 3:

MAJOR ARREST THE WIND PEARL *(dà dìng fēng zhū)*

SOURCE: *Systematic Differentiation of Warm Pathogen Diseases*

Honey-toasted Glycyrrhizae Radix preparata *(zhì gān cǎo)* 18g
Rehmanniae Radix *(shēng dì huáng)* 18g

Paeoniae Radix alba *(bái sháo)* 18g

Ostreae Concha *(mŭ lì)* 15g

Testudinis Plastrum *(guī băn)* 30g

egg yolks *(jī zĭ huáng)* . . . . 2 pieces

Ophiopogonis Radix *(mài mén dōng)* 15g

Asini Corii Colla *(ē jiāo)* 9g

Cannabis Semen *(huŏ má rén)* 9g

Trionycis Carapax *(biē jiă)* 24g

Schisandrae Fructus *(wŭ wèi zĭ)* 6g

ANALYSIS OF FORMULA: This formula is based on Three-Shell Decoction to Restore the Pulse *(sān jiă fù mài tāng)*, with Schisandrae Fructus *(wŭ wèi zĭ)* and egg yolks *(jī zĭ huáng)* added to enrich the Kidney yin, extinguish the Liver wind, preserve the yin, and anchor the yang. It is suitable for severe Liver wind with marked trembling of the fingers or limbs (or clonic convulsions of the feet and hands), extreme mental and physical fatigue, deep-red tongue without coating, very weak pulse, and symptoms of yin and yang beginning to separate.[60] The formula contains many cloying and astringent ingredients that can possibly trap the warm-heat pathogen, so it should only be used when there is pure deficiency of the Kidney yin *without* heat.

note: We have discussed two kinds of interior wind, one caused by heat from excess, the other by yin deficiency of the Liver and Kidney. In the clinic, it is very important to distinguish between them (see Table 8.9). While both manifest with convulsions, the movement associated with yin deficiency of the Liver and Kidney is small and relatively mild.

Table 8.9	Internal Wind Due to Heat From Excess vs. Internal Wind Due to Yin Deficiency	
Pathology	**Signs and Symptoms**
► INTERIOR WIND DUE TO HEAT FROM EXCESS	
Heat from excess in Liver forces sinews to move violently, resulting in stirring of Liver wind	Convulsions accompanied by high fever, cold extremities, loss of consciousness, thirst, and wiry, rapid pulse
► INTERIOR WIND DUE TO KIDNEY YIN DEFICIENCY	
Deficiency of Liver and Kidney yin with malnourishment of sinews, resulting in spasms and stirring of Liver wind	Trembling of fingers or clonic convulsions of feet and hands, listlessness, emaciation, dry lips, 'black'teeth, dry and deep-red tongue or one w/o coating, deficient pulse

MODIFICATIONS: Major Arrest Wind Pearl can be modified as follows:[61]

- For shortness of breath, add Ginseng Radix *(rén shēn)*.

- For spontaneous sweating, add Fossilia Ossis Mastodi *(lóng gǔ)*, Tritici Fructus *(xiǎo mài)*,[62] and Ginseng Radix *(rén shēn)*.

- For palpitations, add Poria *(fú líng)*, Ginseng Radix *(rén shēn)*, and Tritici Fructus *(xiǎo mài)*.

REMNANTS OF HEAT IN THE LIVER AND KIDNEY

Manifestations. There are two concurrent aspects to this pattern:[63]

1. *Exhaustion of the Liver and Kidney yin due to a prolonged warm pathogen disease* with emaciation, a red tongue with little coating, and a submerged, thin, and slightly rapid pulse.

2. *Remnants of heat in the Liver and Kidney* with fever in the evening that disappears in the morning, with absence of sweating after the fever subsides. The temperature is usually not elevated.

NOTE: Why is there fever in the evening that disappears in the morning, and an absence of sweating after the fever has subsided? According to Chapter 28 of *Divine Pivot (Líng shū)*, the protective qi moves through the exterior during the day and into the interior at night.[64] The protective qi pertains to yang; it increases the yang in the interior when it begins to flow inside the body. In a patient with this pattern, the yin and yang are already out of balance, which is aggravated by the additional yang. This leads to more heat from deficiency with fever in the evening, which is not necessarily accompanied by an increase in temperature. The patient is unable to produce sweat due to the injury to the fluids. As day dawns the protective qi returns to the exterior; this reduces the imbalance between yin and yang, and, even though there is no sweating, the fever declines.

Pathology. Remnants of heat in the Liver and Kidney combine with yin deficiency of the Liver and Kidney.

NOTE: Why does the heat remain? The Kidney and Liver yin are not strong enough to eliminate the heat, and Kidney and Liver yin deficiency results in heat from deficiency. The root is the Kidney and Liver yin deficiency, and the remnants of heat should be regarded as heat from both excess and deficiency.

Treatment principles. Disperse the remnants of heat and enrich the Liver and Kidney yin.

Formula:

Sweet Wormwood and Soft-Shelled Turtle Shell Decoction	
(qīng hào biē jiǎ tāng)	

SOURCE: *Systematic Differentiation of Warm Pathogen Diseases*

Artemisiae annuae Herba *(qīng hāo)* 6g

Trionycis Carapax *(biē jiǎ)* 15g

Rehmanniae Radix *(shēng dì huáng)* 12g

Anemarrhenae Rhizoma *(zhī mǔ)* 6g

Moutan Cortex *(mǔ dān pí)*................................9g

ANALYSIS OF FORMULA: As the chief herbs, Artemisiae annuae Herba *(qīng hāo)* (with its aromatic flavor) and Trionycis Carapax *(biē jiǎ)* (with its salty flavor and moist nature) enter the Liver and Kidney to eliminate the remnants of heat and enrich the yin of both organs. Careful attention should be paid to the dosage of these two herbs. Artemisiae annuae Herba *(qīng hāo)* readily induces sweating. Since in this case there is heat from deficiency resulting from Kidney and Liver yin deficiency, only small amounts of Artemisiae annuae Herba *(qīng hāo)* are required in this formula; the practitioner thus avoids inducing profuse sweating, which would aggravate the injury to the Kidney and Liver yin. By contrast, a large dosage of Trionycis Carapax *(biē jiǎ)* is needed to strongly enrich the yin. Moutan Cortex *(mǔ dān pí)* is used to clear heat from deficiency and cool the blood, and to help Artemisiae annuae Herba *(qīng hāo)* disperse the remnants of heat in the nutritive level. Rehmanniae Radix *(shēng dì huáng)* and Anemarrhenae Rhizoma *(zhī mǔ)* clear the remnants of heat from the Liver and the Kidney and enrich the yin of the Liver and Kidney to support the ability of Trionycis Carapax *(biē jiǎ)* to enrich the yin.

DECOCTION AND ADMINISTRATION: Add Artemisiae annuae Herba *(qīng hāo)* near the end of the decocting process; otherwise its aromatic flavor will evaporate, and the effect of the formula will not be optimal.

Summary

Cold can attack a person with constitutional deficiency of Kidney yin and essence during the winter and lurk within the body, where it can lead to qi constraint and subsequent heat. If attacked during the spring by a secondary external pathogen, such as wind-cold or wind-heat, this will induce the lurking heat to manifest. Alternatively, lifestyle habits that compromise the antipathogenic qi can also induce the lurking heat to manifest during the spring. Spring-warmth is characterized by an acute onset, the presence of interior heat at the very beginning of the condition, a multitude of changes, and severe signs and symptoms. In the early stage, clinical features include a high fever, restlessness, and thirst, or even loss of consciousness and convulsions.

Generally speaking, there are two types of pathologies at the early stage of spring-warmth, which differ based on the strength of the antipathogenic qi and the severity of the heat from constraint due to the lurking cold. First, even though the heat is intense, if the antipathogenic qi is strong enough to resist it, the pathology will be one of heat from constraint in the qi level. But if the antipathogenic qi is not strong enough to resist, the pathology will be one of heat from constraint in the nutritive level.

Apart from its seasonality, the key variable used in identifying spring-warmth is the presence of an interior heat pattern at an early stage. It is very important to distinguish between spring-warmth and wind-warmth because both may occur in the spring and present with exterior signs and symptoms.

Since spring-warmth is caused by a constitutional deficiency of yin combined with lurking cold that produces interior heat, a pattern of interior heat from excess often appears in the early stage of the disease, with immediate injury to the yin and fluids. It is therefore necessary to apply the treatment principles of clearing and draining the heat directly, combined with protecting the yin and fluids. Table 8.10 summarizes the varieties of spring-warmth and their associated treatments.

Table 8.10	Differentiation and Treatment of Spring-Warmth	
Patterns (Pathology)	**Treatment Principles**	**Formulas**
▶ PROTECTIVE AND QI LEVELS		
Combined protective and qi level due to wind-cold, a secondary external pathogen that brings out stagnant interior heat	Eliminate exterior signs and symptoms with acrid and slightly warm herbs, and clear interior heat with bitter and cold herbs	Scallion, Prepared Soybean and Platycodon Decoction (*cōng chǐ jié gěng tāng*)
▶ QI LEVEL		
Heat from constraint in Gallbladder	Clear heat with bitter and cold herbs and disperse heat from constraint with acrid and cool herbs	Scutellaria Decoction plus Prepared Soybean and Scrophularia (*huáng qín tāng jiā dàn dòu chǐ hé xuán shēn*)
Heat from constraint in chest and diaphragm due to initial invasion of qi level	Clear heat from chest and diaphragm with light herbs	Gardenia and Prepared Soybean Decoction (*zhì zǐ chǐ tāng*)

Table 8.10, cont.		
Heat burning chest and diaphragm with lack of passage through Intestines	Clear heat, disperse heat, and drain heat by purging	Cool the Diaphragm Powder (*liáng gé săn*)
Heat from excess in Stomach leading to injury of fluids in Stomach	Clear heat from Stomach with acrid and cold herbs, and supply Stomach with fluids with sweet and cold herbs	White Tiger Decoction (*bái hǔ tāng*)
Severe constipation with dry stool and heat in Large Intestine combined with exhaustion of yin and fluids	Eliminate heat by purging, enrich the yin, and generate fluids	Increase the Fluids and Order the Qi Decoction (*zēng yè chéng qì tāng*)
Severe constipation with dry stool and heat in Large Intestine combined with qi and yin deficiency	Purge heat and dry stools, tonify qi, and enrich the yin	Newly Augmented Yellow Dragon Decoction (*xīn jiā huáng lóng tāng*)
Severe constipation with dry stool and heat in Large Intestine combined with heat from excess in Small Intestine	Drain heat from Large Intestine by purging, and clear heat from Small Intestine	Guide Out the Red and Order the Qi Decoction (*dǎo chì chéng qì tāng*)
▶ NUTRITIVE AND BLOOD LEVELS		
Intense heat in both qi and nutritive levels	Clear heat from qi and nutritive levels	Modified Jade Woman Decoction (*jiā jiǎn yù nǔ jiān*)
Intense heat in both qi and blood levels	Clear heat from qi and blood levels	Transform Maculas Decoction (*huà bān tāng*) or Clear Epidemics and Overcome Toxins Decoction (*qīng wēn bài dú yǐn*)
Burning of yin in nutritive level by heat (invasion of heat leads to disturbance of Heart, injury to yin in nutritive level, and failure of collaterals to control blood)	Dispel heat from nutritive to qi level by cooling the blood, enriching the yin, and clearing heat from Heart	Clear the Nutritive Level Decoction (*qīng yíng tāng*)
Bleeding due to heat from excess and toxin in blood level (leading to blood stasis)	Cool and invigorate the blood, clear heat, and resolve toxicity from blood level	Rhinoceros Horn and Rehmannia Decoction (*xī jiǎo dì huáng tāng*)

301

Table 8.10, cont.		
Combination of heat and blood stasis in the lower burner	Drain heat by purging, invigorate the blood, and remove blood stasis	Peach Kernel Decoction to Order the Qi (*táo rén chéng qì tāng*)
Veiling of Pericardium by heat and phlegm	Clear heat and resolve phlegm in Pericardium, and open the orifices	Calm the Palace Pill with Cattle Gallstone (*ān gōng niú huáng wán*), Purple Snow Special Pill (*zǐ xuě dān*), or Greatest Treasure Special Pill (*zhì bǎo dān*) in combination with Clear the Palace Decoction (*qīng gōng tāng*)
Interior blockage and exterior collapse (of yang qi)	Clear heat, resolve phlegm, open the orifices, and arrest collapse	Calm the Palace Pill with Cattle Gallstone (*ān gōng niú huáng wán*), Greatest Treasure Special Pill (*zhì bǎo dān*) or Purple Snow Special Pill (*zǐ xuě dān*) combined with Generate the Pulse Powder (*shēng mài sǎn*) or Ginseng and Aconite Accessory Root Decoction (*shēn fù tāng*)
Stirring of internal wind due to heat from excess in the Liver	Cool the Liver and extinguish the Liver wind	Antelope Horn and Uncaria Decoction (*líng jiǎo gōu téng yǐn*)
▶ INJURY TO KIDNEY YIN BY HEAT (NUTRITIVE LEVEL)		
Blazing fire due to Kidney yin deficiency	Enrich Kidney yin and drain Heart fire	Coptis and Ass-Hide Gelatin Decoction (*huáng lián ē jiāo tāng*)
Exhaustion of Kidney and Liver yin (exhaustion of yin by remnants of heat, leading to hyperactive yang)	Enrich Kidney and Liver yin	Modified Restore the Pulse Decoction (*jiā jiǎn fù mài tāng*)
Stirring of Liver wind due to Kidney yin deficiency (leading to malnutrition of Heart spirit)	Enrich Kidney yin, extinguish Liver wind, and calm the spirit	Two-Shell Decoction to Restore the Pulse (*èr jiǎ fù mài tāng*), Three-Shell Decoction to Restore the Pulse (*sān jiǎ fù mài tāng*), or Major Arrest Wind Pearl (*dà dìng fēng zhū*)
Remnants of heat in Liver and Kidney (combined with Liver and Kidney yin deficiency)	Disperse remnants of heat and enrich the Liver and Kidney yin	Sweet Wormwood and Soft-Shelled Turtle Shell Decoction (*qīng hào biē jiǎ tāng*)

Endnotes

1. Wu You-Xing, *Discussion of Warm Epidemics (Wēn yì lùn)*. Shenyang: Liaoning Science and Technology Publishing House, 1997: 1.

2. While theoretically spring-warmth should occur only during the spring, if the pathology and presentation are the same, the differentiations and treatments described in this chapter are applicable regardless of the season.

3. When this occurs, we should just approach the diagnosis based on an appropriate diagnostic method, such as four levels, three burners, or organ pathology, and treat accordingly. The difference is that if we make the diagnosis of spring-warmth, we are then aware of the underlying Kidney yin deficiency and will avoid herbs that might deplete the yin. Whenever you believe there is a possibility of spring-warmth, pay close attention to the status of the yin as the disease progresses.

4. This is because an external pathogen can exit the exterior via sweating, and there is no severe qi blockage or struggle between the external pathogen and the antipathogenic qi. It should be noted that sometimes the exterior signs and symptoms are minor, for example, the patient may present with an acute headache without any sweating.

5. Clearing heat implies moving it out of the body in a downward direction, while venting heat means that heat is moved out of the body in a transverse direction.

6. Zhang Xi-Chun (Zhang Shou-Fu), *Essays on Medicine Esteeming the Chinese and Respecting the Western (Yī xúe zhōng zhōng cān xī lù)*. Shijiazhuang: Hebei People's Publishing House, 1957: 191.

7. Zhang Ji, *Discussion of Cold Damage (Shāng hán lùn)*. Beijing: People's Health Publishing House, 1983: 50. This formula is composed of Gypsum fibrosum *(shí gāo)* (30g), Anemarrhenae Rhizoma *(zhī mǔ)* (9g), nonglutinous rice *(gěng mǐ)* (9-15g), and honey-toasted Glycyrrhizae Radix preparata *(zhì gān cǎo)* (3g). See Chapter 7 for further details.

8. Liu Bao-Yi, *Encountering the Sources of Warm-Heat Pathogen Diseases (Wēn rè féng yuán)*. Beijing: People's Health Publishing House, 1959: 65. Note that the source text provides no dosages. Those shown here are from Meng Shu-Jiang et al., *Warm Pathogen Diseases (Wēn bìng xué)*. Shanghai: Shanghai Science and Technology Publishing House, 1985: 53.

9. Ye Gui, *Differentiating Lurking Pathogens and Externally-Contracted Diseases during Three Seasons (Sān shí fú xié wài gǎn piàn)*. This book does not exist as a stand-alone volume but is included in the book by Ye Gui, *Case Records as a Guide to Clinical Practice (Lín zhèng zhǐ nán yī àn)*. Shanghai: Shanghai Science and Technology Publishing House, 1959: 734.

10. Liu Bao-Yi, *Encountering the Sources of Warm-Heat Pathogen Diseases*, 65

11. Wu Tang, *Systematic Differentiation of Warm Pathogen Diseases (Wēn bìng tiáo biàn)*. Beijing: People's Health Publishing House, 1963: 71.

12. Originally the dosages were as follows: Rhei Radix et Rhizoma *(dà huáng)* (600g), Natrii Sulfas *(máng xiāo)* (600g), Glycyrrhizae Radix *(gān cǎo)* (600g), Gardeniae Fructus *(zhī zǐ)* (300g), Menthae haplocalycis Herba *(bò hé)* (300g), Scutellariae Radix *(huáng qín)* (600g), Forsythiae Fructus *(lián qiào)* (1200g), Lophatheri Herba *(dàn zhú yè)* (7 pieces). The ingredients were ground into powder and the normal dose was 6g decocted with a small

amount of honey and seven pieces of Lophatheri Herba *(dàn zhú yè)*. Administration of the formula was terminated after the patient reported loose stools. The dosages shown here are from Meng Shu-Jiang et al., *Warm Pathogen Diseases,* 54.

13. Cool the Diaphragm Powder *(liáng gé sǎn)* was originally used to treat accumulation of heat in the yin and yang organs, leading to irritability, restlessness, thirst, flushed face, dizziness, dry lips and throat, swollen tongue, hoarse voice, constipation, red eyes, nosebleeds, and canker sores of the mouth or tongue. We can say the original problem for which this formula is designed includes not only heat, but also upward-flaring of fire. The large dosage of Rhei Radix et Rhizoma *(dà huáng)* and Natrii Sulfas *(máng xiāo)* was intended to strongly purge this severe heat and fire via the Large Intestine. However, the pattern of heat burning the chest and diaphragm with slight constipation is different, as there is underlying yin deficiency along with spring-warmth. In addition, the heat from excess has damaged the fluids. In order to prevent overly intense purging, which would further injure the fluids, a smaller dosage is highly recommended. Moreover, once there have been smooth bowel movements and a reduction in the heat signs, this formula should be discontinued and the patient given something to mildly clear heat and generate fluids.

14. Wu Tang, *Systematic Differentiation of Warm Pathogen Diseases*, 64.

15. This formula was first recorded in *Discussion of Cold Damage* by Zhang Ji in the early third century. It contains Rhei Radix et Rhizoma *(dà huáng)* (12g), Natrii Sulfas *(máng xiāo)* (912g), Aurantii Fructus immaturus *(zhǐ shí)* (5 pieces, or 9-12g), and Magnoliae officinalis Cortex *(hòu pò)* (24g).

16. This formula was first recorded in *Discussion of Cold Damage*. It is discussed in Chapter 7 of the present volume.

17. Increase the Fluids Decoction *(zēng yè tāng)* was first recorded in Wu Tang's *Systematic Differentiation of Warm Pathogen Diseases*. It consists of Scrophulariae Radix *(xuán shēn)* (30g), Ophiopogonis Radix *(mài mén dōng)* (24g), and Rehmanniae Radix *(shēng dì huáng)* (24g). See Chapter 7 for further details.

18. This is a kind of "wood ear" fungus that is sweet and neutral and enters the Stomach and Large Intestine channels. It cools blood and stops bleeding and is used for bloody stools, dysenteric disorder, abnormal menstrual bleeding, and hemorrhoids.

19. Peng Jian-Zhong and Yang Lian-Zhu, *Selected Case Studies from Zhao Shao-Qin (Zhào Shào-Qín lín zhèng yàn àn jīng xuǎn)*. Beijing: Learning Garden Publishing House, 1996: 11.

20. Anonymous, *Yellow Emperor's Inner Classic: Basic Questions (Huáng Dì nèi jīng sù wèn)*. Beijing: People's Health Publishing House, 1963: 33.

21. According to the source text, Rhei Radix et Rhizoma *(dà huáng)* in this formula is not prepared but cooked with the other herbs at the same time. This serves to weaken its purgative effect, which is appropriate for this condition.

22. See Chapter 7.

23. Wu Tang, *Systematic Differentiation of Warm Pathogen Diseases*, 67.

24. Although not previously mentioned in the case report, this patient must originally have had scanty urination due to her qi and yin deficiency.

25. Peng Jian-Zhong and Yang Lian-Zhu, *Selected Case Studies from Zhao Shao-Qin*, 13.

26. In general, it is rare to see red-colored urine with this condition. Note that it is different from bloody painful urinary difficulty, which is also characterized by frequent, urgent urination.

27. As of May, 2000 the U.S. Federal Drug Administration had put Akebiae Caulis *(mù tōng)* on a warning list as some plants that are used as this herb may theoretically contain aristolochic acid, a known nephrotoxin. Although there is some controversy about the clinical implications of this matter and whether there is any possible real harm from this herb, until the matter is resolved, prudence would suggest that the herb not be used. Clinically, Tetrapanacis Medulla *(tōng cǎo)* can be substituted.

28. This formula is discussed in Chapter 7.

29. See Chapter 7.

30. Often, when Bubali Cornu *(shuǐ niú jiǎo)* is substituted for Rhinocerotis Cornu *(xī jiǎo)*, the dosage is increased many times. Here the condition involves both the qi and blood levels, so it is better to use a relatively small dosage to avoid congealing the blood.

31. Lu Zhen, ed., *Collected Rare Recent Books on Chinese Medicine: Warm Pathogen Disease Section (Jìn dài zhōng yī zhēn běn jí: wēn bìng fēn cè)*. Hangzhou: Zhejiang Science and Technology Publishing House, 1987: 189.

32. Zhao Shao-Qin, Hu Ding-Bang, Liu Jing-Yuan, *Length and Breadth of Warm Pathogen Disease [Differentiation]*. Beijing: Beijing College of Traditional Chinese Medicine, 1979: 97.

33. See Chapter 7.

34. See text above.

35. Wang Tao, *Arcane Essentials from the Imperial Library (Wài tái mì yào)*. Shanghai: Shanghai Publishing House of Ancient Literature, 1991: 65. This text was first published in 752. This formula contains Coptidis Rhizoma *(huáng lián)* (9g), Scutellariae Radix *(huáng qín)* (6g), Phellodendri Cortex *(huáng bǎi)* (6g), and Gardeniae Fructus *(zhī zǐ)* (14 pieces).

36. See text below.

37. See Chapter 7.

38. Dong Jian-Hua et al., *Selected Case Studies from Famous Modern Chinese Doctors (Zhōng guó xiàn dài míng zhōng yī yī àn jīng huá)*. Beijing: Beijing Publishing House, 1990: 1304. This case study was reported by Xu You-Ling.

39. This formula was first recorded in *Golden Mirror of the Medical Tradition (Yī zōng jīn jiàn)*. Beijing: People's Health Publishing House, 1973: 753. It contains Rehmanniae Radix preparata *(shú dì huáng)* (240g), *Corni Fructus (shān zhū yú)* (120g), Poria *(fú líng)* (90g), Dioscoreae Rhizoma *(shān yào)* (120g), Moutan Cortex *(mǔ dān pí)* (90g), and Alismatis Rhizoma *(zé xiè)* (90g).

40. This formula was first recorded in *Craft of Medicines and Patterns for Children (Xiǎo ér yào zhèng zhēn jué)*. Shenyang: Liaoning Science and Technology Publishing House, 1997: 14. The book was written by Qian Yi in 1093. There the formula was called Rehmannia Pill

(dì huáng wán) and contained Rehmanniae Radix preparata *(shú dì huáng)* (24g), *Corni Fructus (shān zhū yú)* (12g), Dioscoreae Rhizoma *(shān yào)* (12g), Alismatis Rhizoma *(zé xiè)* (9g), Moutan Cortex *(mǔ dān pí)* (9g), and Poria *(fú líng)* (9g).

41. Dong Jian-Hua et al., *Selected Case Studies from Famous Modern Chinese Doctors,* 1507. This case study was reported by Mi Bo-Rang.

42. These dosages are based on the seventh-century work by Sun Si-Miao, *Important Formulas Worth a Thousand Gold Pieces (Qiān jīn yào fāng).* Beijing: People's Health Publishing House, 1982: 222. This dosage of Rhinocerotis Cornu *(xī jiǎo)* is much higher than any used clinically nowadays. Because Rhinocerotis Cornu *(xī jiǎo)* is from an endangered species, it should not be used. Today most people follow the dosage set forth in Wu Tang's *Systematic Differentiation of Warm Pathogen Diseases:* Rehmanniae Radix *(shēng dì huáng)* (30g), Paeoniae Radix alba *(bái sháo)* (9g), Moutan Cortex *(mǔ dān pí)* (9g), and Rhinocerotis Cornu *(xī jiǎo)* (9g). In my opinion, Paeoniae Radix rubra *(chì sháo)* (in a dosage of 12-15g), which cools the blood and removes blood stasis, is more appropriate here than Paeoniae Radix alba *(bái sháo).*

43. Based on this idea, charred herbs with an astringent property are usually contraindicated for these conditions: not only can they lead to blood stasis, they can also stop up heat inside the body.

44. See Chapter 7.

45. The source text calls for this substance, which is from an endangered species. Today, Eupolyphaga/Stelophaga *(tǔ biē chóng)* is substituted, with a dosage of 9-15g.

46. A normal count runs between 100,000 and 300,000/mm^3.

47. This is bitter, astringent, and cold and enters the Heart, Liver, and Large Intestine channels. It cools the blood and stops bleeding, kills parasites and treats tinea-like rashes, and also serves as a mild laxative. The normal dosage is 10-15g.

48. Dong Jian-Hua, *Selected Case Studies from Famous Modern Chinese Doctors,* 307. This case study was reported by Xie Chang-Ren.

49. Yu Gen-Chu, *Revised Popular Guide to the Discussion of Cold Damage (Chóng dìng tōng sú shāng hán lùn).* Hangzhou: New Medicine Press, 1956: 65.

50. Today, powdered Bubali Cornu *(shuǐ niú jiǎo)* (15g) is substituted.

51. Wu Tang, *Systematic Differentiation of Warm Pathogen Diseases,* 129.

52. Chen Shi-Wen et al., *Formulary of the Bureau of Medicines of the Taiping Era (Tàipíng huì mín hé jì jú fāng).* Beijing: People's Health Publishing House, 1959: 182. Originally, equal amounts of the herbs were ground into a powder, and 2g of the powder were mixed with vinegar and made into a paste. The paste was then decocted with water. Today, usually 15g of each herb is used and taken as a decoction.

53. All of these formulas are discussed in Chapter 7.

54. This is similar to Calm the Palace Pill with Cattle Gallstone *(ān gōng niú huáng wán).*

55. This formula was first recorded in *Golden Mirror of the Medical Tradition,* 1911. It contains Lonicerae Flos *(jīn yín huā)* (9g), Taraxaci Herba *(pú gōng yīng)* (3.6g), Chrysanthemi indici Flos *(yě jú huā)* (3.6g), Violae Herba *(zǐ huā dì dīng)* (3.6g), and Begoniae fimbristipulatae Herba *(hóng tiān kuí)* (3.6g).

56. This is a prepared medicine recorded in the *Formula Section of Encyclopedia of Traditional Chinese Medicine (Zhōng yī dà cí diǎn fāng jì fèn cè)*. Beijing: People's Health Publishing House, 1983: 105. It contains Saposhnikoviae Radix *(fáng fēng)* (9g), Ophiopogonis Radix *(mài mén dōng)* (9g), Glycyrrhizae Radix *(gān cǎo)* (9g), Paeoniae Radix rubra *(chì sháo)* (15g), Coptidis Rhizoma *(huáng lián)* (15g), Scutellariae Radix *(huáng qín)* (15g), Uncariae Ramulus cum Uncis *(gōu téng)* (15g), Phellodendri Cortex *(huáng bǎi)* (15g), Gardeniae Fructus *(zhī zǐ)* (15g), Angelicae sinensis Radix *(dāng guī)* (15g), Rhei Radix et Rhizoma *(dà huáng)* (30g), Gypsum fibrosum *(shí gāo)* (30g), Forsythiae Fructus *(lián qiào)* (30g), Lonicerae Flos *(jīn yín huā)* (30g), and Platycodi Radix *(jié gěng)* (12g). Grind these herbs into powder. Mix 26.4g of the powder with Bovis Calculus *(niú huáng)* (3g), decoction of Menthae haplocalycis Herba *(bò hé)* (3g), Borneolum *(bīng piàn)* (3g), Arnebiae Radix/ Lithospermi Radix Realgar *(xióng huáng)* (15g), Cinnabaris *(zhū shā)* (30g), and Moschus *(shè xiāng)* (1.5g). Grind all the herbs and mix them with honey to make pills.

57. Chongqing Traditional Chinese Medicine Research Institute, *Traditional Chinese Medicine and Acute Conditions Report (Zhōng yī jí zhèng tōng xùn)*. Chongqing: Chongqing Traditional Chinese Medicine Research Institute, 1985(6): 13. This case study was reported by Xie Bing-Guo.

58. Meng Yong-Li, Shen Guo-Nan, Li Xiao-Lu, *Modern Research and Clinical Application of the Discussion of Cold Damage (Shāng hán lùn xiàn dài yán jiù yǔ lín chuáng yìng yòng)*. Beijing: Learning Garden Publishing House, 1998: 671. This case study was reported by Cao Shi-Bao.

59. This refers to a darkening of the teeth, which can appear black. When observed in patients with dry tongues, it is an important sign of Kidney yin deficiency.

60. Patients with this pattern usually present with dry lips, dry skin, thin muscles, malar flush, blurred vision, dry teeth, vomiting, weak voice, and cold extremities.

61. Wu Tang, *Systematic Differentiation of Warm Pathogen Diseases*, 127.

62. This is wheat. It is sweet, cool, and enters the Heart, Spleen, and Kidney channels. It nourishes the Heart, tonifies the Kidney, and clears heat to ease thirst. Used for melancholy, irritability, restlessness, thirst, diarrhea, carbuncles, burns, and bleeding secondary to trauma.

63. There is some disagreement as to the level of this pattern. Some theorists in the Ming and Qing periods describe it as a late stage of spring-warmth, and not necessarily a nutritive level pattern. Others suggest that if there is damage to the yin of the Liver and Kidney, it must be considered a nutritive level pattern. I agree with the latter position.

64. Anonymous, *Yellow Emperor's Inner Classic: Divine Pivot (Huáng Dì nèi jīng líng shū)*. Beijing: People's Health Publishing House, 1963: 66.

9 Autumn-Dryness

AUTUMN-DRYNESS (秋燥 *qiū zào)* is, as might be expected, caused by an attack of dryness during the autumn season. In its early stage it is characterized by injury to the fluids, with typical symptoms of a dry throat and nose, cough with little sputum, and dry skin. Generally speaking, autumn-dryness does not progress as readily as other warm pathogen diseases; it remains at one place in the body for some time and does not quickly penetrate to deeper levels. Thus, it is more easily cured. Geographically, autumn-dryness occurs most frequently in areas that are dry and of high altitude, such as northwest China, Tibet, or the Colorado Plateau in the United States. However, neither seasonality nor geographical location is the only cause for dry conditions. For example, dryness and its associated illnesses are common throughout the developed world where many people live and work in air-conditioned or centrally-heated environments, which can be quite dry.

Other warm pathogen diseases can injure the fluids and produce *internal* dryness in their early stages, especially those caused by warm-heat pathogens unaccompanied by dampness, such as wind-warmth and spring-warmth. However, the internal dryness and injury to the yin or fluids are very mild during the early stages of these other warm pathogen diseases; the main signs and symptoms are those of heat from excess with slight thirst, or dry throat and/or dry nose. By contrast, autumn-dryness is an exogenous disorder that presents early on (even the first day) with clear signs and symptoms of fluid or yin damage and dryness. Furthermore, any signs or symptoms of heat associated with autumn-dryness mainly result from injury to the yin or fluids from attack by the dry pathogen, rather than directly from heat. Biomedical diseases such as upper respiratory tract infections and acute bronchitis overlap somewhat with the Chinese medical diagnosis of autumn-dryness, and can be treated with the same methods outlined in this chapter.

Autumn-dryness can be divided into two subcategories. The first is warm-dryness (溫燥 *wēn zào*), which is caused by the dry-heat (燥熱 *zào rè*[1]) aspect of the dry pathogen. Dry-heat appears in early autumn when the weather is just beginning to shift from summer, and some warmth still remains. The second subcategory is cool-dryness (涼燥 *liáng zào*), which is caused by the cool-dry aspect of the dry pathogen. Cool-dryness appears in late autumn when the weather is dry and cooler, and cold winter weather is approaching. These seasonal differences are worth considering, but should not be followed too rigidly. Cool-dryness and dry-heat are two different aspects of the same dry pathogen.

Etiology and Pathology

Regardless of whether autumn-dryness manifests as warm-dryness or cool-dryness, it occurs in the autumn and results from a common exogenous pathogenic factor: dryness. However, the manner of its appearance may differ. Warm-dryness occurs in early autumn and is similar in nature to an attack by wind-warmth, although it more readily injures the fluids. The basic pathology of warm-dryness is an attack on the Lung and exterior by dry-heat, leading to injury of the fluids. By contrast, cool-dryness occurs in late autumn. The basic pathology of cool-dryness is an attack on the exterior by cool-dryness, which impairs the Lung's ability to disseminate and disperse fluids throughout the body, slightly injuring the fluids. While it is somewhat similar to the *tai yang* stage of wind-cold described in *Discussion of Cold Damage (Shāng hán lùn)*, there are significant differences, the principal one being that it slightly damages the Lung fluids early in the process.[2]

Dryness may occur in other seasons than autumn, especially for those who live and work in an air-conditioned environment, which can be quite dry. In that environment, individuals may manifest either warm-dryness or cool-dryness, primarily depending on their physical constitution. That is, those with underlying yin or blood deficiency will tend to develop warm-dryness, while those with yang or qi deficiency will usually present with cool-dryness.

Factors for Identifying Autumn-Dryness

There are two important factors for identifying autumn-dryness:

1. The disease must occur during the autumn or the patient must have spent a significant amount of time in a dry environment.

2. Apart from signs and symptoms of the Lung and protective level (aversion to cold, chills, fever, cough) there must also be signs and symptoms of injury to the Lung yin in the early stage of the disease, such as dry mouth, skin, throat, and nose.

The Lung is the pathological center of an attack by either wind-warmth or autumn-dryness, and the symptoms are fever, aversion to cold, chills, and cough. However, wind-warmth, unlike autumn-dryness, usually appears in the spring or winter instead of autumn. In addition, the signs and symptoms of injury to Lung yin in the early stages of the illness—dry nose, throat, skin, or mouth, and a dry cough—are not as remarkable in wind-warmth as they are in autumn-dryness. While these differences should not be followed too rigidly, it is important to remember that wind-warmth can progress more rapidly to a severe stage, particularly a direct transmission to the Pericardium.

Lurking summerheat can also occur in the autumn, presenting with exterior signs and symptoms that are often confused with autumn-dryness.[3] The two types of warm pathogen disease are easily distinguished: there will be manifestations of dampness in the early stage of lurking summerheat which, of course, are absent from autumn-dryness.

The practitioner must also distinguish between the early stages of warm-dryness and cool-dryness. Table 9.1 lists the differences between these two forms of dryness. It should be noted that while there are two subcategories for autumn-dry-ness, once either of them has progressed and transformed into heat at the qi level, the treatment is the same regardless of etiology.

Table 9.1	Comparison of Early Stages of Cool-Dryness and Warm-Dryness	
Basis of Difference	**Cool-Dryness**	**Warm-Dryness**
Pathology	Cool-dryness slightly injures fluids of the Lung and constrains protective qi	Dry-heat injures Lung fluids, and heat attacks Lung and protective qi
Fever	Slight fever and severe aversion to cold	Intense fever and slight aversion to cold
Mouth and nose	Dry mouth but only slight or no thirst; dry nose with congestion	Intense thirst and drinking copious amounts of fluids; dry nose
Nature of cough	Small amount of frothy sputum	Small amount of viscous sputum
Tongue signs	Tongue body color normal; white, thin, dry coating	Tongue body and tip red; white, thin, dry coating

Progression of Autumn-Dryness

In the case of warm-dryness, dry-heat injures the yin of the Lung. Dryness in the body can transform into heat and progress to the Large Intestine, the paired organ of the Lung. Once dry-heat has progressed to the Large Intestine, it can injure its fluids, leading to the pattern of severe constipation with dry stool and heat in the Large Intestine combined with injury to the yin. If dry-heat persists for a long time it will exhaust the yin and fluids, especially the yin of the Liver and Kidney. In terms of five-phase theory, this will lead to stirring of Liver wind due to the failure of water to enrich wood.

By contrast, cool-dryness is unlikely to progress unless it is a severe case that results in injury to the body's yin. This type of progression is rare, and in such cases its progress will be slow.

Generally speaking, the pathological center of an attack by autumn-dryness is the Lung, and autumn-dryness is less likely to progress than are other warm pathogen diseases. Injury to the fluids of the Lung and Stomach by dry-heat is the most commonly seen pattern. Progression of dry-heat to the lower burner is seldom seen unless the patient has constitutional Kidney yin deficiency or was improperly treated by inducing profuse sweating or strong purging.

Treatment Principles

According to Chapter 74 of *Basic Questions (Sù wèn)*, dryness should be treated by moistening.[4] Thus, the treatment principle for autumn-dryness is to moisten and enrich the yin and generate fluids. However, the practitioner must also focus on eliminating autumn-dryness, a warm-heat pathogen. Different treatment principles must be applied for the different stages and locations of the disease. For example, in the early stage the treatment protocol depends on the nature of the pathogen, that is, whether it is warm-dryness or cool-dryness.

Table 9.2	General Treatment Principles for Cool-Dryness and Warm-Dryness	
Type	**Herb Qualities**	**Comments**
Cool-dryness	Slightly warm, acrid, and moistening	Avoid very warm and acrid herbs
Warm-dryness	Acrid, cool, sweet, and moistening	Focus on clearing heat and protecting the fluids

As previously mentioned, autumn-dryness can attack different organs and thereby give rise to different patterns. The treatment principle is chosen accordingly. In *Case Records as a Guide to Clinical Patterns (Lín zhèng zhǐ nán yī àn)*,[5] Ye Gui pointed out that patterns of dryness in the upper burner must be treated by promoting qi circulation, and those in the lower burner by enriching the blood.[6] According to Yu Gen-Chu in *Revised Popular Guide to the Discussion of Cold Damage (Chóng dìng tōng sú shāng hán lùn)*, autumn-dryness first injures the fluids of the Lung, then those of the Stomach, and finally Liver blood and Kidney yin.[7] Based on the experience of these physicians, the treatment of autumn-dryness will vary depending on whether it is located in the upper, middle, or lower burner.

Table 9.3	Treatment Principles for Warm-Dryness Patterns Based on Location
Location	**Treatment Principle**
Upper burner	Disseminate Lung qi with acrid, sweet, cool, and moistening herbs
Middle burner	Support the fluids of the Stomach with sweet and cold herbs
Lower burner	Enrich the blood and yin of the Liver and Kidney with sweet, salty, and moistening herbs

NOTE: Dry-heat is comprised of two yang pathogenic factors and progresses more rapidly than cool-dryness, which is comprised of a yang and a yin pathogenic factor. Thus, the pathological center of a cool-dryness pattern generally remains in the upper burner.

In general, once an exogenous pathogenic factor transforms into heat or fire, heat must be cleared with bitter and cold herbs. However, since autumn-dryness is characterized by injury to the fluids, bitter, cold herbs cannot be used in isolation, as they are drying and damage the yin. Instead, moistening herbs that are sweet and cold must be combined with the bitter, cold herbs to enrich the yin and fluids.

Differentiation and Treatment of Autumn-Dryness in the Protective Level

DRY-HEAT ATTACKING THE LUNG AND EXTERIOR

Manifestations. There are three concurrent aspects to this pattern:

1. *Dry-heat attacking the protective level* with fever, slight aversion to cold or chills, headache, slight sweating, and a white tongue coating.
2. *Dry-heat attacking the Lung and injuring its fluids* with a dry throat and nose, thirst with a desire to drink a lot of water, and a red tongue with a white, thin, and dry coating.
3. *Failure of the Lung qi to disseminate and descend due to an attack by dry-heat* with cough with scanty, viscous sputum.

Pathology. Dry-heat attacks the Lung and protective level, leading to injury of the Lung fluids.

Treatment principles. Gently disperse dry-heat from the Lung and protective level with acrid, cool, sweet, and moistening herbs.

Formula:

MULBERRY LEAF AND APRICOT KERNEL DECOCTION *(sāng xìng tāng)*

SOURCE: *Systematic Differentiation of Warm Pathogen Diseases*

Mori Folium *(sāng yè)* 3g
Armeniacae Semen *(xìng rén)* 4.5g
Gardeniae Epicarpium *(shān zhī pí)*[8] 3g
Glehniae/Adenophorae Radix *(shā shēn)* 6g
Sojae Semen preparatum *(dàn dòu chǐ)* 3g
Fritillariae Bulbus *(bèi mǔ)*[9] 3g
Pyri Exocarpium *(lí pí)* 3g

ANALYSIS OF FORMULA: This formula is based on the notion that heat patterns are treated with cool herbs, and dryness is treated with moistening herbs. In this formula, Mori Folium *(sāng yè)* and Sojae Semen preparatum *(dàn dòu chǐ)* expel exogenous dry-heat. Armeniacae Semen *(xìng rén)* and Fritillariae cirrhosae Bulbus *(chuān bèi mǔ)* direct the Lung qi downward, transform phlegm, and stop the coughing. Gardeniae Fructus *(zhī zǐ)* clears heat. Glehniae/Adenophorae Radix *(shā shēn)* and Pyri Exocarpium *(lí pí)* enrich the yin and moisten the Lung. The formula reflects the concern of dispersing dry-heat without injuring the fluids, and moistening the Lung without trapping the dry-heat.

MODIFICATIONS: The basic formula can be modified as follows:

- For severe thirst, add Trichosanthis Radix *(tiān huā fěn)* to supplement the fluids.
- For severe cough and pain in the chest, add Trichosanthis Pericarpium *(guā lóu pí)* and Citri reticulatae Vascular *(jú luò)*[10] to transform phlegm and ease the chest.

- For labored breathing due to accumulation of phlegm-heat secondary to dry-heat, add Lepidii/ Descurainiae Semen *(tíng lì zǐ)* and Mori Cortex *(sāng bái pí)* to direct the Lung qi downward.

- For bloody sputum, add Imperatae Rhizoma *(bái máo gēn)* and Nelumbinis Nodus rhizomatis *(ǒu jié)* to enhance the effect of the other herbs in clearing heat from the Lung and stopping bleeding.

- For dizziness, add Chrysanthemi Flos *(jú huā)* and Prunellae Spica *(xià kū cǎo)* to eliminate exogenous wind and clear heat from the Liver channel.

Case study: Mulberry Leaf and Apricot Kernel Decoction *(sāng xìng tāng)*

First visit. When autumn began, the weather was very dry, and this 31-year-old male patient developed a slight fever with chills. He coughed frequently, expectorating blood-tinged sputum. His pulse was wiry and thin, and the tongue coating was yellow in the center and white around the edges. He was diagnosed with a combination of:

1. An internal pattern of Liver yang excess due to Liver fire, which was attacking the Lung and injuring the yin; and

2. An external pattern of autumn-dryness attacking the Lung and exterior.

The initial treatment focused on dispersing autumn-dryness with acrid and cool herbs. The formula Mulberry Leaf and Apricot Kernel Decoction *(sāng xìng tāng)* was selected for this purpose: Mori Folium *(sāng yè)* (5g), Armeniacae Semen *(xìng rén)*(12g), Sojae Semen germinatum *(dà dòu juǎn)* (6g), fried Gardeniae Fructus *(zhī zǐ)* (5g), Bambusae Caulis in taeniam *(zhú rú)* (6g), Benincasae Semen *(dōng guā zǐ)* (12g), Adenophorae Radix *(nán shā shēn)* (9g), Fritillariae thunbergii Bulbus *(zhè bèi mǔ)* (9g), Polygonati odorati Rhizoma *(yù zhú)* (12g), Trichosanthis Radix *(tiān huā fěn)* (9g), Ecliptae Herba *(mò hàn lián)* (12g), and one pear.

Second visit. The fever and chills were gone. However, the cough was worse in the morning and evening, and he was still expectorating bloody sputum. His pulse was still wiry and thin, and he had a red tongue with a thin coating. The diagnosis therefore changed to Liver and Kidney yin deficiency, and dry-heat attacking the Lung, leading to injury of the vessels. Treatment was now focused on subduing the Liver yang, moistening the Lung, and clearing heat from the Lung. The following herbs were chosen: Chrysanthemi Flos *(jú huā)* (6g), Armeniacae Semen *(xìng rén)*(9g), Fritillariae cirrhosae Bulbus *(chuān bèi mǔ)* (9g), Polygonati odorati Rhizoma *(yù zhú)* (9g), Trichosanthis Radix *(tiān huā fěn)* (12g), Quartz album *(bái shí yīng)*[11] (24g), Moutan Cortex *(mǔ dān pí)* (5g), Paeoniae Radix alba *(bái sháo)* (5g), Ligustri lucidi Fructus *(nǚ zhēn zǐ)* (15g), Ecliptae Herba *(mò hàn lián)* (12g), Benincasae Semen *(dōng guā zǐ)* (12g), and fried Eriobotryae Folium *(chǎo pí pá yè)* (12g). After finishing the formula, all of the patient's signs and symptoms were gone.[12]

COOL-DRYNESS ATTACKING THE LUNG AND EXTERIOR

Manifestations. There are three concurrent aspects to this pattern:

1. *Cool-dryness attacking the Lung and protective level* with fever, chills, aversion to cold, headache, and the absence of sweating.
2. *Failure of the Lung to disseminate fluids throughout the body, with slight injury to the Lung fluids,* with dry nose and nose congestion, dry mouth but little thirst, dry throat and lips.
3. *Production of phlegm due to failure of the Lung to distribute fluids throughout the body* with nasal congestion and a cough with white and frothy sputum.

NOTE: As previously mentioned, this pattern is similar in appearance to an attack by wind-cold. However, cool-dryness exhibits significant signs and symptoms of injury to the fluids, while wind-cold does not. This raises a question: Why is there a lack of fluids together with frothy, white sputum in an attack by cool-dryness? This is because the cold in cool-dryness is a yin pathogenic factor that obstructs the Lung and thereby impairs its ability to distribute the fluids. This leads to a general lack of fluids, along with stagnation of fluids in the Lung, which turn into frothy, white sputum. Cool-dryness must also be differentiated from warm-dryness, as described in Table 9.2 above.

Pathology. Failure of the Lung to disseminate fluids due to an attack on the Lung and protective level by cool-dryness, with slight injury to the fluids.

Treatment principles. Disseminate the Lung qi, dispel the exterior condition, and transform the phlegm.

Formula No. 1:

APRICOT KERNEL AND PERILLA LEAF POWDER *(xìng sū sǎn)*[13]

SOURCE: *Systematic Differentiation of Warm Pathogen Diseases*

Armeniacae Semen *(xìng rén)* 6g
Perillae Folium *(zǐ sū yè)* 9g
Peucedani Radix *(qián hú)* 9g
Platycodi Radix *(jié gěng)* 6g
Aurantii Fructus *(zhǐ ké)* 6g
Citri reticulatae Pericarpium *(chén pí)* 6g

Poria *(fú líng)* 6g

Pinelliae Rhizoma preparatum *(zhì bàn xià)* 6g

Zingiberis Rhizoma recens *(shēng jiāng)* .6g

Jujubae Fructus *(dà zǎo)*. . . . . 2 pieces

Glycyrrhizae Radix *(gān cǎo)* 3g

ANALYSIS OF FORMULA: In this formula, Perillae Folium *(zǐ sū yè)* and Peucedani Radix *(qián hú)* expel exogenous cool-dryness. Platycodi Radix *(jié gěng)*, Armeniacae Semen *(xìng rén)*, and Glycyrrhizae Radix *(gān cǎo)* disseminate and direct the Lung qi downward to stop the coughing. Pinelliae Rhizoma preparatum *(zhì bàn xià)*, Citri reticulatae Pericarpium *(chén pí)*, Poria *(fú líng)*, and Aurantii Fructus *(zhǐ ké)* transform phlegm. Zingiberis Rhizoma recens *(shēng jiāng)*, Jujubae Fructus *(dà zǎo)*, and Glycyrrhizae Radix *(gān cǎo)* support the Spleen and Stomach in producing fluids for the Lung. If the patient coughs up a large amount of white and frothy sputum, or has had phlegm in the Lung before attack of cool-dryness (e.g., chronic bronchitis or allergic asthma), this formula is a good choice because it contains Two Cured Decoction *(èr chén tāng)*,[14] which transforms phlegm. However, Two Cured Decoction *(èr chén tāng)* focuses more on middle burner patterns and contains Poria *(fú líng)*, which drains dampness via urination. Therefore, by itself, it is not recommended for dryness-related diseases. If the patient does not cough up a large amount of white and frothy sputum and there is no tightness in the chest or chest pain, Modified Cyperus, Perilla Leaf, Scallion, and Prepared Soybean Decoction *(jiā jiǎn xiāng sū cóng chǐ tāng)*[15] is a better choice because this formula effectively disseminates the Lung qi and eliminates cool-dryness.

MODIFICATIONS: According to Wu Tang,[16] the basic formula can be modified as follows:

- For absence of sweating, a wiry or tight pulse, add Notopterygii Rhizoma seu Radix *(qiāng huó)* to slightly induce sweating.

- For continuous coughing after sweating, remove Perillae Folium *(zǐ sū yè)* and add Perillae Caulis *(zǐ sū gěng)*.

- For diarrhea with abdominal bloating, add Atractylodis Rhizoma *(cāng zhú)* and Magnoliae officinalis Cortex *(hòu pò)*.

- For headache with pain over the superior orbit, add Angelicae dahuricae Radix *(bái zhǐ)*.

Case study: Apricot Kernel and Perilla Leaf Powder *(xìng sū sǎn)*

First visit. The patient, a 48-year-old male, suffered from a distending pain on the top of his head, aversion to cold, cough with frothy and white sputum, nasal congestion, dry throat, floating and wiry pulse, and a white and thin tongue coating. He was diagnosed with cool-dryness attacking the exterior and Lung. The treatment strategy chosen was to eliminate cool-dryness with bitter and warm herbs, plus others to transform the phlegm and disseminate the Lung qi. Specifically, Apricot Kernel and Perilla Leaf Powder *(xìng sū sǎn)* was modified, using Armeniacae Semen *(xìng rén)*(12g), Perillae Folium *(zǐ sū yè)* (5g), Peucedani Radix *(qián hú)* (12g), Platycodi Radix *(jié gěng)* (5g), Glycyrrhizae Radix *(gān cǎo)* (5g), Menthae haplocalycis Herba *(bò hé)* (2g), Poria *(fú líng)* (12g), Aurantii Fructus *(zhǐ ké)* (6g), Pinelliae Rhizoma preparatum *(zhì bàn xià)* (5g), Citri reticulatae Exocarpium rubrum *(jú hóng)* (3g), Tribuli Fructus *(cì jí lí)* (12g), and Farfarae Flos *(kuǎn dōng huā)* (9g).

Second visit. The headache was considerably diminished, although he still had a cough with frothy and white sputum, dry lips and throat, white and greasy tongue coating, and a wiry and slippery pulse. He continued taking the same formula with the following modifications: Peucedani Radix *(qián hú)* (12g), Perillae Folium *(zǐ sū yè)* (3g), Armeniacae Semen *(xìng rén)*(12g), Platycodi Radix *(jié gěng)* (5g), Poria *(fú líng)* (12g), Aurantii Fructus *(zhǐ ké)* (5g), Pinelliae Rhizoma preparatum *(zhì bàn xià)* (5g), Citri reticulatae Exocarpium rubrum *(jú hóng)* (3g), Farfarae Flos *(kuǎn dōng huā)* (9g), Polygonati odorati Rhizoma *(yù zhú)* (12g), and fried Eriobotryae Folium *(pí pá yè)* (12g). After finishing the formula, all of the patient's signs and symptoms were gone.[17]

Formula No. 2:

> **MODIFIED CYPERUS, PERILLA LEAF, SCALLION, AND PREPARED**
> Soybean Decoction *(jiā jiǎn xiāng sū cóng chǐ tāng)*

SOURCE: *Revised Popular Guide to the Discussion of Cold Damage*

Armeniacae Semen *(xìng rén)* 9g

Asteris Radix *(zǐ wǎn)* 9g

Perillae Folium *(zǐ sū yè)* 9g

Allii fistulosi Bulbus *(cōng bái)* . . . . 2 pieces

Honey-toasted Glycyrrhizae Radix preparata *(zhì gān cǎo)* 6g

Stemonae Radix *(bǎi bù)* 6g

Cynanchi stauntonii Rhizoma *(bái qián)* 6g

Citri reticulatae Pericarpium *(chén pí)* 6g

Sojae Semen preparatum *(dàn dòu chǐ)* 12g

ANALYSIS OF FORMULA: In this formula, Sojae Semen preparatum *(dàn dòu chǐ)*, Perillae Folium *(zǐ sū yè)*, and Allii fistulosi Bulbus *(cōng bái)* are used to eliminate cool-dryness in the exterior. Asteris Radix *(zǐ wǎn)*, Stemonae Radix *(bǎi bù)*, Armeniacae Semen *(xìng rén)*, and Cynanchi stauntonii Rhizoma *(bái qián)*, which are warm and moistening in nature, are used to warm and moisten the Lung and aid in the recovery of the Lung's disseminating and descending functions. Citri reticulatae Pericarpium *(chén pí)* and honey-toasted Glycyrrhizae Radix preparata *(zhì gān cǎo)* are used to harmonize the middle burner.

Differentiation and Treatment of Autumn-Dryness in the Qi Level

DYSFUNCTION OF THE UPPER ORIFICES DUE TO AN ATTACK BY DRY-HEAT

Manifestations. There are two concurrent aspects to this pattern:

1. *Fire attacking the upper orifices of the body* with tinnitus and red eyes. In this pattern, the dry-heat has transformed into fire.

2. *Dry-heat attacking the orifices of the Lung and the Stomach* with a red and sore throat, dryness and burning pain in the nose, and swollen gums.

NOTE: A red tongue with a dry, thin, and yellow coating and a rapid pulse are commonly seen with this pattern.

Pathology. Dry-heat in the Lung transforming into fire and attacking the upper orifices of the body.

Treatment principles. Drain the fire and disperse the dry-heat from the upper burner.

Formula:

FORSYTHIA AND MENTHA DECOCTION *(qiào hé tāng)*

SOURCE: *Systematic Differentiation of Warm Pathogen Diseases*

Menthae haplocalycis Herba *(bò hé)* 4.5g

Forsythiae Fructus *(lián qiào)* .4.5g

Gardeniae Epicarpium *(shān zhī pí)* 4.5g

Platycodi Radix *(jié gěng)*. 6g

Glycinis Testa *(lǜ dòu yī)*[18] 6g

Glycyrrhizae Radix *(gān cǎo)* 3g

ANALYSIS OF FORMULA: It is unnecessary to wait for all the signs and symptoms mentioned above to manifest before using this formula. Once the patient presents with two or three of them, the development of the problem (which can be very rapid) becomes clear and the formula should be used. In this formula, Menthae haplocalycis Herba *(bò hé)*, with its acrid flavor and cool nature, improves the condition of the head and eyes. Forsythiae Fructus *(lián qiào)*, Gardeniae Epicarpium *(shān zhī pí)* and Glycinis Testa *(lǔ dòu yī)* drain fire and clear dry-heat from the upper burner. Platycodi Radix *(jié gěng)* and Glycyrrhizae Radix *(gān cǎo)* are used in many classic formulas to treat sore throat. All the herbs in this formula are light, reflecting the idea of treating upper burner problems with herbs that are as light as the feathers of a bird. It is usually difficult to obtain Gardeniae Epicarpium *(shān zhī pí)* (the peel of Gardeniae Fructus *[zhī zǐ]*), and Glycinis Testa *(lǔ dòu yī)* (the skin of Phaseoli radiati Semen *[lù dòu)]*). Gardeniae Fructus *(zhī zǐ)* and Phaseoli radiati Semen *(lù dòu)* can be substituted, but their dosage should be cut in half.[19]

MODIFICATIONS: The basic formula can be modified as follows:

- To enhance the heat-dispersing properties of this formula, add Mori Folium *(sāng yè)* and Cicadae Periostracum *(chán tuì)*.

- For tinnitus, add Saigae tataricae Cornu *(líng yáng jiǎo)*, Ilicis latifoliae Folium *(kǔ dīng chá)*,[20] and Prunellae Spica *(xià kū cǎo)* to drain the heat from the Liver that has descended from the Lung (source text).[21]

- For red eyes, add Chrysanthemi Flos *(jú huā)*, Ilicis latifoliae Folium *(kǔ dīng chá)*,[22] and Prunellae Spica *(xià kū cǎo)* to disperse the heat in the Liver and Gallbladder (source text).

- For a sore throat, add Arctii Fructus *(niú bàng zǐ)*, Belamcandae Rhizoma *(shè gān)*, Scrophulariae Radix *(xuán shēn)*, and Scutellariae Radix *(huáng qín)* to clear heat from the Lung and ease the throat (source text).

- For swollen gums, add Gypsum fibrosum *(shí gāo)* and Lycii Cortex *(dì gǔ pí)* to clear heat from the Stomach.

Comparisons. This pattern and that treated by Mulberry Leaf and Apricot Kernel Decoction *(sāng xìng tāng)* attack on the Lung and exterior by dry-heat—both fall into the category of warm-dryness. However, the pattern treated by Mulberry Leaf and Apricot Kernel Decoction *(sāng xìng tāng)* is marked by injury to the fluids, and the goal of treatment is therefore to disperse dry-heat gently from the Lung and protective level with acrid, cool, sweet, and moistening herbs. By contrast, in the pattern here, the dry-heat has transformed into fire and affects the upper orifices of the body. The goal of treatment is therefore somewhat different: to drain fire and disperse dry-heat from the upper burner with herbs that are more acrid than bitter. Of course, there may be slight injury to the fluids from the dry-heat and fire, as evidenced in the red tongue and dry, thin, and yellow coating. However, the dry-heat and fire are so severe in this pattern that they must be dealt with first. It is true that enriching the yin and supporting the fluids will also have the effect of draining fire and clearing heat, but these methods work indirectly, and, in the context of this case, would be too slow in taking effect.

Injury to the Lung Yin and Fluids by Dry-Heat

Manifestations. There are two concurrent aspects to this pattern:

1. *Failure of the Lung qi to descend due to transformation of dryness into heat* with fever, irritability, labored breathing, wheezing, distending pain in the chest, and a red tongue tip and edges.
2. *Injury to the Lung yin and fluids by fire* with a dry cough, dry nose and throat, thirst, and a thin and dry tongue coating.

Pathology. Dryness transforming into heat and injuring the yin and fluids of the Lung, impairing the descent of the Lung qi.

Treatment principles. Clear and disperse dry-heat from the Lung, moisten dryness, enrich Lung yin, and direct the Lung qi downward.

Formula:

> ### Eliminate Dryness and Rescue the Lung Decoction
> *(qīng zào jiù fèi tāng)*
>
> SOURCE: *Precepts for Physicians*
>
> Gypsum fibrosum *(shí gāo)* 7.5g
> Mori Folium *(sāng yè)* 7.5g
> Glycyrrhizae Radix *(gān cǎo)* 3g
> Ginseng Radix *(rén shēn)* 2.1g
> Sesami Semen nigrum *(hēi zhī má)* 3g
> Asini Corii Colla *(ē jiāo)* 2.4g
> Ophiopogonis Radix *(mài mén dōng)* 3.6g
> Armeniacae Semen *(xìng rén)* 2.1g
> Eriobotryae Folium *(pí pá yè)* . . . . 1 piece

ANALYSIS OF FORMULA: According Ye Gui in *Differentiating Lurking Pathogens and Externally-Contracted [Diseases] During Three Seasons (Sān shí fú xié wài gǎn piàn)*, dry-heat should be treated with acrid, cool, sweet, and moistening herbs.[23] In this formula, Gypsum fibrosum *(shí gāo)*, which is acrid and cold, and Mori Folium *(sāng yè)*, which is sweet and cold, disperse and clear heat from the Lung. Armeniacae Semen *(xìng rén)* and Eriobotryae Folium *(pí pá yè)* direct the Lung qi downward to stop the coughing. Asini Corii Colla *(ē jiāo)*, Ophiopogonis Radix *(mài mén dōng)*, and Sesami Semen nigrum *(hēi zhī má)* enrich the yin and moisten the dryness.

But why did Yu Chang, the author of the *Precepts for Physicians*, recommend the use of Ginseng Radix *(rén shēn)* and Glycyrrhizae Radix *(gān cǎo)*, which are warm and sweet in nature, in this formula? In this pattern, prolonged coughing due to dry-heat will injure both the Lung and Stomach qi, resulting in such symptoms as shortness of breath and poor appetite. According to Yu, Ginseng Radix *(rén shēn)* and Glycyrrhizae Radix *(gān cǎo)* generate fluids and tonify the Lung qi. In addition, he said that the formula should focus on the Stomach and Spleen qi because they correspond to earth, which is the mother of metal, the Lung. Here is his explanation for choosing these herbs instead of more obvious ones:

Asparagi Radix *(tiān mén dōng)* can enrich the yin of the Lung, but it has a bitter flavor and cold nature that can damage the qi and cause it to stagnate in the Stomach and Spleen, leading to production of phlegm. Anemarrhenae Rhizoma *(zhī mǔ)* can enrich both the Lung and Kidney yin, but it is bitter, and herbs that are too cold cannot be used here. In conclusion, the use of bitter and cold herbs is forbidden for this pattern in which the Lung yin and qi are badly damaged. Otherwise, how would the patient have a chance to live?[24]

NOTE: It is recommended that the patient eat pears or water chestnuts to help build up the Lung yin to fight the dry-heat.

MODIFICATIONS: The basic formula can be modified as follows:

- For severe injury to the yin due to heat from excess, substitute Panacis quinquefolii Radix *(xī yáng shēn)* for Ginseng Radix *(rén shēn)* and add Glehniae/Adenophorae Radix *(shā shēn)* and Phragmitis Rhizoma *(lú gēn)* to enhance the formula's ability to enrich the yin.

- For profuse yellow sputum that is difficult to expectorate (indicating that there is accumulation of phlegm-heat in the Lung), add Fritillariae cirrhosae Bulbus *(chuān bèi mǔ)*, Trichosanthis Pericarpium *(guā lóu pí)*, and Bambusae Caulis in taeniam *(zhú rú)*.

- For sputum tinged with blood, add Scutellariae Radix *(huáng qín)*, Imperatae Rhizoma *(bái máo gēn)*, and Rehmanniae Radix *(shēng dì huáng)* to cool the blood, clear heat, and stop bleeding.

- For constipation consisting of either dry and hard stools or bowel movements that occur only once every two or three days (commonly seen with this pattern due to insufficient qi and fluids descending from the Lung to the Large Intestine), add Trichosanthis Semen *(guā lóu rén)* and Cannabis Semen *(huǒ má rén)*, and increase the dosage of Armeniacae Semen *(xìng rén)*.

DECOCTION AND ADMINISTRATION: Dissolve Asini Corii Colla *(ē jiāo)* in the strained decoction before drinking it.

Comparisons. Both this pattern and that for which Mulberry Leaf and Apricot Kernel Decoction *(sāng xìng tāng)* is indicated (attack on the Lung and exterior by dry-heat) are due to an attack on the Lung by warm-dryness. Both patterns also include the symptom of dry cough. However, the protective level is involved in the pattern for which Mulberry Leaf and Apricot Kernel Decoction *(sāng xìng tāng)* is indicated, as evidenced by the aversion to cold and recent onset. These factors are absent here, and there is greater damage to the yin, since this pattern is located in the Lung and in the qi level.

Both this pattern and that for which Forsythia and Mentha Decoction *(qiào hé tāng)* is indicated are located in the qi level. However, the pattern here is located in the Lung with injury to Lung yin, as evidenced by the dry cough, labored breathing, wheezing, and dry nose and throat. The latter pattern is located in the orifices of the head, without significant injury to the Lung yin.

INJURY TO THE FLUIDS OF THE LUNG AND STOMACH BY DRY-HEAT

Manifestations. There are three concurrent aspects to this pattern:

1. *Remnants of dry-heat* with slight fever.
2. *Injury to the Lung fluids* with severe dry cough.
3. *Injury to the Stomach fluids* with a dry mouth and tongue, and thirst.

Pathology. Transmission of dry-heat to the interior of the body, leading to injury of the fluids of the Lung and Stomach.

Treatment principles. Enrich the yin and support the fluids of the Lung and Stomach.

Formula No. 1:

GLEHNIA/ADENOPHORA AND OPHIOPOGON DECOCTION
(shā shēn mài mén dōng tāng).

See Chapter 7 for a discussion of this formula.

Formula No. 2:

FIVE JUICE DRINK *(wǔ zhī yǐn)*

SOURCE: *Systematic Differentiation of Warm Pathogen Diseases*

ANALYSIS OF FORMULA: Five Juice Drink consists of the juices of the following five herbs: Ophiopogonis Radix *(mài mén dōng)*, Phragmitis Rhizoma *(lú gēn)*, Pyri Fructus *(lí)* [pears], Eleocharitis Rhizoma *(bí qì)*,[25] and Nelumbinis Nodus rhizomatis *(ǒu jié)*. All five of these juices are sweet in flavor and cold in nature and have the function of moistening dryness and supporting the fluids.

The herbs in these two formulas enrich the yin and support the fluids. They are suitable for treating injury to the yin and fluids of the Lung and Stomach. However, many of the herbs in these two formulas are cloying, so it is forbidden to use them when there are still exterior signs and symptoms, or when there is heat from excess, because they will block the qi and trap exogenous pathogenic factors in the body. Outside of East Asia it is very difficult to obtain all of the fresh herbs above, much less their juices. As a substitute, a patient can make a juice by pressing edible fungi such as white wood ears, as well as radishes, oranges, or grapefruit.

DRY-HEAT INJURING THE LUNG COLLATERALS AND BEING TRANSMITTED TO THE LARGE INTESTINE

Manifestations. There are two concurrent aspects to this pattern:

1. *Injury of the collaterals of the Lung by fire that has transformed from dry-heat* with an itchy throat, dry cough, blood-tinged viscous sputum, and pain in the chest.

2. *Transmission of heat from the Lung to the Large Intestine* with a hot sensation in the abdomen and diarrhea, red tongue with yellow, dry, and thin coating, and a rapid pulse.

NOTE: The consistency of the diarrhea in this pattern may be either watery with burning pain in the rectum, or a small amount of loose stool that is hard to discharge, coupled with abdominal pain. The diarrhea is caused by too much heat from the Lung forcing out the fluids from the Large Intestine. This kind of diarrhea is similar to that found in the pattern of transmission of heat to the Large Intestine from the Lung, a wind-warmth pattern discussed in Chapter 7. However, the two patterns differ in the quality of their cough. The pattern here displays a cough with blood-tinged sputum, indicating that the collaterals of the Lung have been injured by dry-heat.

Pathology. Injury to the collaterals of the Lung by dry-heat and a transmission of the heat from the Lung to the Large Intestine. This transmission can occur when heat in the Lung becomes intense.

Treatment principles. Enrich the yin and moisten dryness, clear heat, and drain heat to stop the bleeding.

Formula:

Ass-Hide Gelatin and Scutellaria Decoction *(ē jiāo huáng qín tāng)*

SOURCE: *Revised Popular Guide to the Discussion of Cold Damage*

Asini Corii Colla *(ē jiāo)*	9g
Scutellariae Radix *(huáng qín)*	9g
Armeniacae Semen *(xìng rén)*	6g
Mori Cortex *(sāng bái pí)*	6g
Paeoniae Radix alba *(bái sháo)*	3g
Plantaginis Herba *(chē qián cǎo)*	15g
Glycyrrhizae Radix *(gān cǎo)*	2.4g
Sacchari Caulis tenuis *(gān zhe shāo)*[26]	15g

ANALYSIS OF FORMULA: In this formula, Armeniacae Semen *(xìng rén)* and Mori Cortex *(sāng bái pí)* are combined with Sacchari Caulis tenuis *(gān zhe shao)* to moisten the Lung, support the fluids, and stop the coughing. Asini Corii Colla *(ē jiāo)* enriches the blood and stops bleeding. Scutellariae Radix *(huáng qín)* clears heat from the Lung. Paeoniae Radix alba *(bái sháo)* and Glycyrrhizae Radix *(gān cǎo)*, with their sweet and sour flavors, enrich yin and relax muscle spasms to relieve pain. Plantaginis Herba *(chē qián cǎo)* drains and discharges heat via the urine.

The inclusion of an herb in this formula to drain damp-heat via urination may seem odd, especially since this pattern is characterized by dry-heat and injury to the fluids. Why then did Yu Gen-Chu choose Plantaginis Herba *(chē qián cǎo)*? Among herbs that drain damp-heat, this is the only one that can leach out dampness and clear heat without injuring the yin; its function in promoting urination is very mild. Since there is so much heat being transmitted from the Lung to the Large Intestine, which is located in the lower burner, and there is a hot sensation in the abdomen, using this herb will allow the heat to exit without injuring the yin.

NOTE: It is forbidden to purge in this case because the dryness has injured the fluids, which would be exacerbated by inducing diarrhea.

MODIFICATIONS: The basic formula can be modified as follows:

- For cough with profuse sputum, add Eriobotryae Folium *(pí pá yè)*, Fritillariae cirrhosae Bulbus *(chuān bèi mǔ)*, and Bambusae Succus *(zhú lì)*.
- For a significant amount of hemoptysis, add Imperatae Rhizoma *(bái máo gēn)* and Agrimoniae Herba *(xiān hè cǎo)*.
- For severe pain in the chest and hypochondriac region, add Curcumae Radix *(yù jīn)* and Luffae Fructus Retinervus *(sī guā luò)*.

Comparisions. Both this formula and Kudzu, Scutellaria, and Coptis Decoction *(gé gēn huáng qín huáng lián tāng)* treat diarrhea and cough caused by a transmission of a warm-heat pathogen from the Lung to the Large Intestine. However, the condition here is due to dry-heat and must be treated with sweet and sour as well as bitter and cold herbs. This is because dryness and heat have injured the fluids. By contrast, as the latter formula is designed to treat heat alone, bitter and cold herbs will suffice.

Case study: Ass-Hide Gelatin and Scutellaria Decoction *(ē jiāo huáng qín tāng)*

Male, 30 years old. During the autumn this patient suffered from diarrhea more than ten times a day. He was feverish and had a slight cough. Herbs to disperse the exterior were prescribed, but to no effect. He was then treated with herbs to direct the Lung qi downward and disperse wind, again without any apparent change in his condition. The same physician then gave him herbs to warm, tonify, and ascend, which made everything worse. By now the patient had no luster in his face and looked very anxious. His tongue was pale with a thin coating and red dots. His pulse was floating and deficient. A modified version of Ass-Hide Gelatin and Scutellaria Decoction *(ē jiāo huáng qín tāng)* was prescribed: Asini Corii Colla *(ē jiāo)* (9g), Scutellariae Radix *(huáng qín)* (6g), Glycyrrhizae Radix *(gān cǎo)* (3g), Lycii Cortex *(dì gǔ pí)* (15g), Platycodi Radix *(jié gěng)* (4.5g), and Mori Cortex *(sāng bái pí)* (15g). After finishing seven packets of these herbs, all signs and symptoms of the disorder were gone.[27]

DRYNESS OF THE LUNG AND BLOCKAGE OF THE LARGE INTESTINE

Manifestations. There are three concurrent aspects to this pattern:

1. *Failure of the Lung to disseminate qi due to attack of dry-heat* with cough and chest distention.
2. *Accumulation of phlegm in the Lung from failure of the Lung to disseminate fluids* with profuse sputum.
3. *Lack of moisture and retention of stool in the Large Intestine due to failure of the Lung to disseminate fluids* with distention in the abdomen and chest, constipation, and a white, dry tongue coating.

NOTE: The pattern here and that of severe constipation with dry stool and heat in the Large Intestine (discussed in Chapter 7) both display the symptoms of abdominal distention and constipation. However, in this case, there is no abdominal pain, yellow tongue coating, or tidal fever. Instead, there is a productive cough.

Pathology. Insufficient fluids in the Large Intestine due to failure of the Lung to disseminate the fluids, leading to phlegm.

Treatment principles. Disseminate and direct the Lung qi downward, transform the phlegm, moisten the Large Intestine, and unblock the bowels.

NOTE: Constipation in this case means hard and dry stools and is a result of a lack of fluids in the Large Intestine due to failure of the Lung to disseminate the fluids. It is not a consequence of the complex of dry stool and heat in the Large Intestine. The formula should therefore be directed at promoting the Lung's function of disseminating the qi downward, moistening the Large Intestine, and promoting the circulation of qi in the Large Intestine—not purging.

Formula:

FIVE SEED AND CITRUS PEEL DECOCTION (*wǔ rén jú pí tāng*)

SOURCE: *Revised Popular Guide to the Discussion of Cold Damage*

Armeniacae Semen (*xìng rén*) 9g
Pini Semen (*sōng zǐ rén*)[28] 9g
Pruni Semen (*yù lǐ rén*) 12g
Persicae Semen (*táo rén*) 6g
Platycladi Semen (*bǎi zǐ rén*) 6g
Citri reticulatae Pericarpium (*chén pí*) 4.5g

ANALYSIS OF FORMULA: According to Yu Gen-Chu, dryness in the upper burner presents with cough, dryness in the middle burner presents with thirst, and dryness in the lower burner presents with constipation.[29] In his book *Comprehensive Medicine According to Master Zhang (Zhāng shì yī tōng)*, Zhang Lu (Zhang Shi-Wan) noted that when dryness progresses from the upper to the lower burner, it will affect the Large Intestine.[30] This pattern shows dryness in both of the paired metal organs. Therefore, cough and constipation present simultaneously. The constipation here is due to dryness in the Lung, impairing its ability to direct qi downward, which further obstructs the qi in the Large Intestine. Conversely, the obstruction of qi in the Large Intestine aggravates the Lung's inability to direct its qi downward.

Getting the qi in the Large Intestine to move properly, and moistening that organ, will help move the bowels. This in turn will help restore the Lung's function of directing its qi downward and disseminating the fluids. Since the constipation is not caused primarily by heat, the use of bitter and cold herbs to purge would be inappropriate. In this formula, Pini Semen *(sōng zǐ rén)*, Armeniacae Semen *(xìng rén)*, Pruni Semen *(yù lǐ rén)*, Persicae Semen *(táo rén)*, and Platycladi Semen *(bǎi zǐ rén)* contain rich oils that will moisten the Large Intestine and promote bowel movements without injuring the fluids. Citri reticulatae Pericarpium *(chén pí)* promotes the circulation of qi in the Large Intestine, and Armeniacae Semen *(xìng rén)* moistens the Lung, directs the Lung qi downward, and promotes bowel movements.

SEVERE CONSTIPATION AND DRY-HEAT IN THE LARGE INTESTINE COMBINED WITH INJURY OF THE YIN

Manifestations. There are two concurrent aspects to this pattern:

1. *Severe constipation with dry stools and heat in the Large Intestine* with fever, distention in the abdomen, and constipation (hard and dry stools).

2. *Dry-heat exhausting the fluids and yin* with a black, dry tongue coating, and a submerged, thin pulse.

NOTE: It is necessary to distinguish between this pattern and dryness of the Lung and blockage of the Large Intestine, since they both involve constipation (see Table 9.4).

Table 9.4	Comparison of Dryness of Lung and Blockage of Large Intestine vs. Dry-Heat in Large Intestine Combined with Injury to Yin	
Pathology	**Signs and Symptoms***	**Treatment**
▶ DRYNESS OF LUNG AND BLOCKAGE OF LARGE INTESTINE		
Located in Large Intestine and Lung; lack of fluids in Large Intestine due to failure of Lung to disseminate fluids	Profusely productive cough, distention in chest	Disseminate and direct Lung qi downward, transform phlegm, moisten Large Intestine, promote bowel movements
▶ SEVERE CONSTIPATION WITH DRY-HEAT IN LARGE INTESTINE COMBINED WITH INJURY TO YIN		
Severe constipation with dry- heat in Large Intestine combined with injury to the fluids and yin	Black and dry tongue coating	Purge the Large Intestine, enrich the yin, and support the fluids

*Both are qi-level patterns situated primarily in the Large Intestine. Common symptoms include constipation and abdominal distention.

Pathology. Severe constipation with dry-heat in the Large Intestine combined with injury to the fluids and yin.

Treatment principles. Purge the Large Intestine, enrich the yin, and support the fluids.

Formula:

> ### Augmented Regulate the Stomach and Order the Qi Decoction
> *(jiā wèi tiáo wèi chéng qì tāng)*

This formula is comprised of Regulate the Stomach and Order the Qi Decoction *(tiáo wèi chéng qì tāng)*, discussed in Chapter 7, plus fresh Polygoni multiflori Radix *(xiān hé shǒu wū)* (15g), fresh Rehmanniae Radix recens *(xiān dì huáng)* (12g), and fresh Dendrobii Herba *(xiān shí hú)* (12g).[31] It is better to use fresh herbs as they contain more juice than dry ones and are more effective at enriching the yin. But since it is almost impossible, outside of East Asia, to obtain these herbs in their fresh form, the dried herbs—at double the dosage indicated above—can still be used to effectively enrich the yin.

Intense Dry-Heat in Both the Qi and Nutritive Levels

Although this pattern and that of intense heat in both the qi and nutritive levels (see Chapter 8) are associated with entirely different pathogens, they have the same pathology. The practitioner can therefore use the same treatment strategy and formula discussed in Chapter 8 for resolving this pattern.

Injury to the Liver and Kidney Yin

This pattern bears a striking resemblance to another discussed in Chapter 8: exhaustion of the Kidney yin and Liver yin. The practitioner can therefore use the same treatment strategy and formula discussed in that chapter for resolving this pattern.

Summary

Autumn-dryness is a type of warm pathogen disease that results from an attack of cool-dry-ness or dry-heat during the autumn. It is characterized by injury to the fluids in the early stage of the disease, with symptoms of a dry throat and nose, cough with little sputum, and dry skin. Generally speaking, autumn-dryness does not progress as quickly as other types of warm pathogen disease, and is easily cured. Since exogenous dryness is likely to injure the fluids, the treatment principles for autumn-dryness are to moisten dryness, support the fluids, and enrich the yin.

Table 9.5	Differentiation and Treatment of Autumn-Dryness Diseases	
Patterns	**Treatment Principles**	**Formulas**
▶ PROTECTIVE LEVEL		
Dry-heat attacking Lung and exterior leading to injury of Lung fluids	Gently disperse dry-heat from Lung and protective level with acrid, cool, sweet, and moistening herbs	Mulberry Leaf and Apricot Kernel Decoction (*sang jú yĭn*)
Failure of Lung to disseminate fluids due to attack on the Lung and protective level by cool-dryness, slightly injuring the fluids	Disseminate the Lung qi, dispel the exterior condition, and transform phlegm	Apricot Kernel and Perilla Leaf Powder (*xìng sū săn*)
▶ QI LEVEL		
Dysfunction of the upper orifices due to attack by dry- heat which has transformed into fire and attacked the upper orifices	Drain fire and disperse dry-heat in the upper burner	Forsythia and Mentha Decoction (*qiào hé tāng*)
Injury to Lung yin and fluids by dry-heat	Clear and disperse dry-heat in Lung, moisten dryness, enrich Lung yin, and direct Lung qi downward	Eliminate Dryness and Rescue the Lung Decoction (*qīng zào jiù fèi tāng*)
Injury to fluids of Lung and Stomach by dry-heat	Enrich the yin and support the fluids of the Lung and Stomach	Glehnia/Adenophora and Ophiopogonis Decoction (*shā shēn mài mén dōng tāng*) plus Five Juice Drink (*wǔ zhī yǐn*)
Injury to Lung collaterals by dry-heat, shifting to the Large Intestine	Enrich the yin and moisten dryness, clear dry-heat, and drain heat to stop the bleeding	Ass-Hide Gelatin and Scutellaria Decoction (*ē jiāo huáng qín tāng*)
Dryness of Lung and blockage of Large Intestine due to failure of Lung to disseminate fluids	Disseminate and direct the Lung qi downward, transform phlegm, moisten the Large Intestine, and unblock the bowels	Five-Seed and Citrus Peel Decoction (*wǔ rén jú pí tāng*)
Severe constipation with dry-heat in Large Intestine combined with injury to yin and fluids	Purge the Large Intestine, enrich the yin, and support the fluids	Augmented Regulate the Stomach and Order the Qi Decoction (*jiā wèi tiáo wèi chéng qì tāng*)

Endnotes

1. This is a combination of dryness and heat in the same way that wind-cold is a combination of wind and cold. It should not be misconstrued as a dry type of heat.

2. Strictly speaking, cool-dryness is not a real warm pathogen disease at all, as cool-dryness is not due to a warm-heat pathogen. It is discussed in this chapter in part because of its relationship to dryness, which is a warm-heat pathogen, and in part because of its close connection in diagnosis and treatment to warm-dryness.

3. Lurking summerheat is discussed in Chapter 13.

4. Anonymous, *Yellow Emperor's Inner Classic: Basic Questions (Huáng Dì nèi jīng sù wèn).* Beijing: People's Health Publishing House, 1963: 541.

5. Ye Gui, *Case Records as a Guide to Clinical Patterns (Lín zhèng zhǐ nán yī àn).* Shanghai: Shanghai Science and Technology Publishing House, 1959: 363.

6. My interpretation of this sentence is that it means that as the Lung is an organ that focuses on qi, sweet, cool, and moistening herbs should be used to preserve the yin and fluids in the Lung from dryness in the upper burner. Treatment of dryness in the lower burner should focus on nourishing blood and bolstering the essence with sweet, salty, and moistening herbs as fluids in this area depend on the Liver, which stores the blood, and the Kidney, which stores the essence.

7. Yu Gen-Chu, *Revised Popular Guide to the Discussion of Cold Damage (Chóng ding tōng sú shāng hán lùn).* Hangzhou: New Medicine Press, 1956: 32.

8. This is bitter and cold and enters the Heart, Liver, Lung, Stomach, and Triple Burner channels. Those who distinguish it from Gardeniae Fructus *(zhī zǐ)* believe that it has a more superficial effect and eliminates heat from the skin and muscle layer.

9. The source text does not specify the exact variety of this herb. It is generally agreed that sweet, cold Fritillariae cirrhosae Bulbus *(chuān bèi mǔ)* is the appropriate variety as it resolves phlegm, stops cough, moistens the Lung, and clears heat.

10. This is the pith of the mandarin orange or tangerine peel. It is sweet, bitter, and neutral and enters the Liver and Spleen channels. It unblocks the channels and collaterals, promotes the movement of qi, and transforms phlegm. Often used for phlegm stagnating in the chest with coughing and pain in the chest and hypochondria. The normal dosage is 3-6g.

11. This is white quartz. It is sweet and slightly warm, and enters the Lung, Kidney, and Heart channels. It warms and moistens the Lung, warms the Kidney, calms the spirit, and promotes urination.

12. Dong Jian-Hua et al., *Selected Case Studies from Famous Modern Chinese Doctors (Zhōng guó xiàn dài míng zhōng yī yī àn jīng huá).* Beijing: Beijing Publishing House, 1990: 763. This is a case study of the physician Yan Er-Ling.

13. The source text does not list the dosage for each herb. Those shown here are the recommendation of the author.

14. This formula was first recorded in *Formulary of the Bureau of Medicines of the Taiping Era (Tàipíng huì mín hé jì jú fāng)* written by Chen Shi-Wen et al. Beijing: People's Health Publishing House, 1959: 77. It contains Pinelliae Rhizoma preparatum *(zhì bàn xià)* (15g),

Citri reticulatae Exocarpium rubrum *(jú hóng)* (15g), Poria *(fú líng)* (9g), Honey-toasted Glycyrrhizae Radix preparata *(zhì gān cǎo)* (4.5g), Zingiberis Rhizoma recens *(shēng jiāng)* (7 pieces), and Mume Fructus *(wū méi)* (1 piece).

15. Yu Gen-Chu, *Revised Popular Guide to the Discussion of Cold Damage*, 259. This formula is discussed below.

16. Wu Tang, *Systematic Differentiation of Warm Pathogen Diseases (Wēn bìng tiáo biàn).* Beijing: People's Health Publishing House, 1963: 51.

17. Dong Jian-Hua, *Selected Case Studies from Famous Modern Chinese Doctors*, 764. This case study was reported by the physician Yan Er-Ling.

18. This is the skin of the mung bean. It is sweet and cold and enters the Heart and Stomach channels. It can disperse wind, clear heat, resolve toxicity, transform maculas, and reduce superficial visual obstructions.

19. While Ye Gui says that the peel or skin of these two substances should be used, he does not provide a rationale, nor are they discussed in the materia medica. While there may be a theoretical justification for using the peels, which are thought to be related to the Lung, good results are obtained from using the whole fruit or beans.

20. This is bitter and very cold and enters the Liver, Stomach, and Gallbladder channels. It disperses wind-heat, clears the head and eyes, and eliminates thirst and irritability. The normal dosage is 3-9g.

21. This is an example of excessive metal (Lung) attacking wood (Liver), leading to rising Liver yang and tinnitus. One example of this phenomenon is a patient with an allergy attack presenting with watery and burning eyes in addition to sneezing, nasal congestion, and nasal discharge.

22. See n. 20 above.

23. Ye Gui, *Differentiating Lurking Pathogens and Externally-Contracted [Diseases] During Three Seasons (Sān shí fú xié wài gǎn piàn).* This book does not exist as a stand-alone volume, but is included in Ye Gui, *Case Records as a Guide to Clinical Practice (Lín zhèng zhǐ nán yī àn).* Shanghai: Shanghai Science and Technology Publishing House, 1959: 744.

24. Yu Chang (Yu Jia-Yan), *Precepts for Physicians (Yī mén fǎ lǜ).* Shanghai: Shanghai Science and Technology Publishing House, 1983: 163.

25. See Appendix C.

26. This is the tip of the sugar cane. It clears heat, generates fluids, directs qi downward, and moistens what is dry. It is used for injury to the fluids, irritability, thirst, and vomiting in febrile diseases, as well as cough and dry and hard stools due to Lung dryness. Sometimes the juice is substituted, with a dosage of 60-120g.

27. He Lian-Chen, *Revised Classified Case Studies from Nationally Famous Doctors (Chóng dìng quán guó míng yī yàn àn lèi biān).* Shanghai: Shanghai Science and Technology Publishing House, 1959: 195.

28. This is the seed of the Korean pin. It is sweet and warm and enters the Lung, Liver, Spleen, Heart, and Large Intestine channels. It enriches the yin, moistens the Lung, and stops coughs while also dispelling wind and unblocking the collaterals and tonifying the blood. It is commonly used for dry coughs, dizziness, constipation, and wind-predominant painful obstruction.

29. Yu Gen-Chu, *Revised Popular Guide to the Discussion of Cold Damage*, 32.

30. Zhang Lu, *Comprehensive Medicine According to Master Zhang (Zhāng shì yī tōng)*. Beijing: Chinese Medicine Publishing House, 1995: 22.

31. The use of this modification of Regulate the Stomach and Order the Qi Decoction *(jiā wèi tiáo wèi chéng qì tāng)* for treating this condition was first noted by Lu Ting-Zheng in *Systematic Differentiation of the Six Etiologies (Liù yīn tiáo biàn)*, which can be found in *Collection of Rare Chinese Medical Books (Zhēn běn yī shū jí chéng)*. Beijing: Chinese Medicine and Pharmacology Publishing House, 1996: 713. I have given the resulting formula its name and provided the dosages.

10 Warm-Toxin

W ARM-TOXIN (溫毒 *wēn dú*) is caused by an attack of the warm-toxin pathogen. Among its characteristics are:

- Rapid progression from the protective level to the qi, nutritive, and blood levels

- Acute onset with local redness and swelling that progresses to either ulcerations in the throat or eruptions over the entire body.

Previous commentators, from the seventeenth-century writer Chen Shi-Gong[1] to the early twentieth-century physician Ding Gan-Ren,[2] have noted that the warm-toxin pathogen attacks the body during either winter or spring when the weather is abnormal, such as a warm spell in the winter or a cold spell in the spring. This may be true to some extent, but there are many, many exceptions to this rule, and warm-toxin can in fact manifest during any season. One clear example of this is mumps.

In winter the warm-toxin pathogen will appear if the weather is relatively warm, and in spring it will appear if it is very hot. Both of these abnormal weather patterns will produce warm-toxin pathogen, which readily attacks the upper part of the body, such as the head and throat.[3] Warm-toxin can also appear at other times depending on the constitution of the patient and the extent to which the weather varies from normal. If the warm-toxin pathogen reaches the blood vessels and forces blood out of them, a maculopapular rash will occur. There are many types of warm-toxin, whose names are based on their clinical manifestations. Biomedical diseases such as infections of the head, scarlet fever, and mumps overlap somewhat with the diagnosis of warm-toxin in traditional Chinese medicine, and can likewise be treated with the methods presented in this chapter.

Three types of warm-toxin disease are mentioned in the seminal texts on warm pathogen diseases:

1. Massive head febrile disorder (大頭溫 *dà tóu wēn*) is described in *Collected Treatises of [Zhang] Jing-Yue (Jǐng-Yuè quán shū)*, written by Zhang Jie-Bing about 1637, and in *Systematic Differentiation of Warm Pathogen Diseases (Wēn bìng tiáo biàn)*, written by Wu Tang in 1798. Massive head febrile disorders are characterized by an attack of warm-toxin on the head and face in which they become red, hot, and swollen. A subcategory of this pattern is mumps (痄腮 *zhà sāi*), which is characterized by fever and swollen and painful cheeks.

2. Putrefying throat granular disorder (爛喉痧 *làn hóu shā*) is described in *Case Records as a Guide to Clinical Practice (Lín zhèng zhǐ nán yī àn)*, written by Ye Gui in 1746, and in *Summary of Putrefying Throat Red Granular Disorder (Làn hóu dān shā jí yào)*, written by Jin De-Jian in 1867. Putrefying throat granular disorder presents with a red, swollen, painful, and ulcerous throat and with eruptions over the body. There is some overlap between this disorder and the biomedical diagnosis of scarlet fever.

3. Entangling throat wind disorder (纏喉風 *chán hóu fēng*) is mentioned in relatively early works, such as the twelfth-century *Comprehensive Recording of Sage-like Benefit from the Zhenghe Era (Zhènghé shèng jì zǒng lù)*,[4] but is not described in detail. This disorder appears to be similar to the biomedical diseases of acute laryngeal infection as well as diphtheria. Owing to the dearth of information about this disease in pre-modern texts, it will not be discussed in much detail here.

In general, warm-toxin diseases require a more aggressive approach than do other warm pathogen diseases. For example, treatment of these diseases include bitter and cold herbs during their early stages. However, even for warm-toxin diseases, one must still rely on the dispersing effects of acrid, cool herbs at this stage.

Massive Head Febrile Disorder

Massive head febrile disorder usually occurs in the winter or spring and is caused by an attack on the head and face by a combination of warm-toxin pathogen and wind. This attack leads to a red, hot, and swollen head and face, fever, and aversion to cold and chills (in the early stage) or to heat (later stage). The identifying signs are the red, hot, and swollen face and head. As previously noted, there is some overlap between this disorder and mumps.

ETIOLOGY AND PATHOLOGY

This disease initially attacks the protective level and presents for a brief time with aversion to cold and chills coupled with fever. The warm-toxin pathogen then attacks the qi level, particularly the Lung and Stomach, leading to symptoms such as vigorous fever with aversion to heat rather than aversion to cold, thirst for cold beverages, and sore throat. Concurrently, the warm-toxin pathogen attacks the exterior and upper part of the body, resulting in a red and swollen or even ulcerated face and head.

The qi level is the pathological focus of this disorder, that is, it seldom invades the nutritive and blood levels. However, if the warm-toxin pathogen is severe, it can invade the lower burner leading to red, hot, swollen, and painful testicles in men. Should this occur, the patient might suffer from sterility. This is called warm-toxin pathogen attacking the essence chamber (精室 *jīng shì*). In traditional Chinese medicine, sterility results from badly injured Kidney essence.

FACTORS FOR IDENTIFYING MASSIVE HEAD FEBRILE DISEASE

There are two important factors for identifying massive head febrile disorder:

1. The onset of the disease is acute and usually occurs either in winter or spring.
2. Besides aversion to cold, chills, and fever for a brief time, the patient quickly presents with a red, hot, and swollen face and head.

TREATMENT PRINCIPLES

Treatment of massive head febrile disease combines both oral and topical approaches. For those medicines taken orally, the main treatment principles are to disperse wind, clear heat, resolve toxicity, and reduce swelling. Topical herbs usually focus on draining fire, resolving toxicity, dispelling blood stasis and reducing swelling. Treatment must be aggressive with this disease. Especially in men it is very important that progression of the warm toxin from the upper burner to the lower burner be prevented, as this can damage the essence and lead to sterility.

ATTACK ON THE UPPER PART OF THE BODY BY WARM-TOXIN PATHOGEN AND WIND

Manifestations. There are three concurrent aspects to this pattern:

1. *Dysfunction of the protective qi as a result of warm-toxin pathogen and wind attacking the exterior* with aversion to cold, chills, and high fever.
2. *Attack on the upper body by warm-toxin pathogen* with a red, hot, and swollen head and face.

3. *Extreme heat in the Lung and Stomach* with thirst for cold beverages, irritability, restlessness, sore throat, red tongue with a dry, yellow coating, and a rapid, forceful pulse.

Pathology. A combination of warm-toxin pathogen and wind attacking the protective and qi levels, especially affecting the Lung and the Stomach.

Treatment principles. Internally disperse wind and clear heat, resolve toxicity, and reduce swelling. Topically drain fire and resolve toxicity, dissipate blood stasis, and reduce swelling.

Formula No. 1:

UNIVERSAL BENEFIT DRINK TO ELIMINATE TOXIN *(pǔ jì xiāo dú yǐn)*

SOURCE: *Ten Books from Dong Yuan*[5]

Coptidis Rhizoma *(huáng lián)*	2.4g
Scutellariae Radix *(huáng qín)*	6g
Arctii Fructus *(niú bàng zǐ)*	9g
Menthae haplocalycis Herba *(bò hé)*	3g
Forsythiae Fructus *(lián qiào)*	9g
Bombyx batryticatus *(bái jiāng cán)*	6g
Scrophulariae Radix *(xuán shēn)*	9g
Lasiosphaera/Calvatia *(mǎ bó)*	4.5g
Platycodi Radix *(jié gěng)*	3g
Glycyrrhizae Radix *(gān cǎo)*	3g
Citri reticulatae Pericarpium *(chén pí)*	4.5g
Isatidis/Baphicacanthis Radix *(bǎn lán gēn)*	9g
Bupleuri Radix *(chái hú)*	3g
Cimicifugae Rhizoma *(shēng má)*	2.4g

ANALYSIS OF FORMULA: This formula treats warm-toxin pathogen that has combined with wind and is attacking the upper regions of the body. It includes acrid, cool, and light herbs, such as Menthae haplocalycis Herba *(bò hé)*, Bombyx batryticatus *(bái jiāng cán)*, Arctii Fructus *(niú bàng zǐ)*, and Bupleuri Radix *(chái hú)*, to disperse the wind and heat and provide an avenue for them to exit the body, instead of allowing them to stagnate in the body where they will exacerbate future conditions. Scutellariae Radix *(huáng qín)* and Coptidis Rhizoma *(huáng lián)*, bitter and cold herbs, are effective in clearing and resolving the warm-toxin pathogen in the Lung and Stomach. Forsythiae Fructus *(lián qiào)*, Cimicifugae Rhizoma *(shēng má)*, Lasiosphaera/Calvatia *(mǎ bó)*, Isatidis/Baphicacanthis Radix *(bǎn lán gēn)*, Platycodi

Radix *(jié gěng)*, and Glycyrrhizae Radix *(gān cǎo)* drain fire and toxin, reduce swelling, and improve the condition of the throat. Scrophulariae Radix *(xuán shēn)* enriches the yin, which helps control the fire, and Citri reticulatae Pericarpium *(chén pí)* moves the qi and protects the Stomach, which might otherwise be injured by the cold nature of Coptidis Rhizoma *(huáng lián)* and Scutellariae Radix *(huáng qín)*.

Platycodi Radix *(jié gěng)* is known for its ability to conduct other herbs to the upper part of the body. Bupleuri Radix *(chái hú)* conducts herbs to the *shao yang* channel, while Cimicifugae Rhizoma *(shēng má)* conducts herbs to the *yang ming* channel. Together these three herbs guide the effects of the other ingredients to the head.

Based on his own clinical experience, Wu Tang thought it best to modify this formula by removing Cimicifugae Rhizoma *(shēng má)* and Bupleuri Radix *(chái hú)*.[6] He did this because, in this disorder, the warm-toxin pathogen has already attacked the upper part of the body. As a result, herbs that disperse and clear heat and resolve toxicity should be used, rather than those that lift the yang and might thereby exacerbate the heat, fire, and toxin. Wu Tang also observed that if the Stomach is not involved, Coptidis Rhizoma *(huáng lián)* and Scutellariae Radix *(huáng qín)*, which are bitter in flavor and cold in nature, and which clear heat from the Stomach, should also be discarded because they can congeal and trap the warm-toxin pathogen in the exterior.[7] In my own experience as well, if the warm-toxin pathogen is so severe that the patient presents with a very red, hot, and swollen head and face, it is better to remove Bupleuri Radix *(chái hú)* and Cimicifugae Rhizoma *(shēng má)* so as not to exacerbate the warm-toxin pathogen. However, if the patient presents with swollen and hard cheeks, Bupleuri Radix *(chái hú)* and Cimicifugae Rhizoma *(shēng má)* are needed to conduct the other herbs to the *shao yang* and *yang ming* channels, and to resolve toxicity.

MODIFICATIONS: The basic formula can be modified as follows:

- For occipital pain and stiffness, which reflects involvement of the *tai yang* channel, add Puerariae Radix *(gé gēn)* and Notopterygii Rhizoma seu Radix *(qiāng huó)*.
- For involvement of the Gallbladder channel (alternating chills and fever, bitter taste, dry throat, swelling and pain around the ear), add Gentianae Radix *(lóng dǎn cǎo)*, Prunellae Spica *(xià kū cǎo)*, and Bambusae Caulis in taeniam *(zhú rú)*.
- For involvement of the Stomach channel (red and swollen face, frontal headache, vigorous fever, thirst), add Gypsum fibrosum *(shí gāo)* and Anemarrhenae Rhizoma *(zhī mǔ)*.
- For constipation, add Rhei Radix et Rhizoma *(dà huáng)*.
- For swelling that does not decrease, add Paeoniae Radix rubra *(chì sháo)*,

Moutan Cortex *(mǔ dān pí)*, and Rhei Radix et Rhizoma *(dà huáng)* to cool and invigorate the blood.

- For pain in the testicles, add Taraxaci Herba *(pú gōng yīng)*, Smilacis glabrae Rhizoma *(tǔ fú líng)*, and Patriniae Herba *(bài jiàng cǎo)*.

Formula No. 2:

THREE YELLOW AND TWO FRAGRANT POWDER *(sān huáng èr xiāng sǎn)*

SOURCE: *Systematic Differentiation of Warm Pathogen Diseases*

Coptidis Rhizoma *(huáng lián)* 30g
Phellodendri Cortex *(huáng bǎi)* 30g
Rhei Radix et Rhizoma *(dà huáng)* 30g
Olibanum *(rǔ xiāng)* 5g
Myrrha *(mò yào)* 5g

ANALYSIS OF FORMULA: This formula is indicated for external use. It drains fire, resolves toxicity, and reduces swelling and pain. Coptidis Rhizoma *(huáng lián)*, Phellodendri Cortex *(huáng bǎi)*, and Rhei Radix et Rhizoma *(dà huáng)* drain fire and resolve toxicity. Olibanum *(rǔ xiāng)* and Myrrha *(mò yào)* invigorate the blood and remove blood stasis. Mixing the herbs with warm green tea can enhance their action in draining fire because green tea is bitter and cold. Also, because sesame oil can protect the skin, it is helpful to mix it with the powder when the skin has been broken.

DECOCTION AND ADMINISTRATION: Grind the herbs into a powder, mix with green tea to make a paste, and apply locally. Once the paste on the skin has become dry, repeat the application with a fresh dose every two hours. However, if the skin is broken, mix the paste with sesame oil instead of green tea.

Case study: Universal Benefit Drink to Eliminate Toxin *(pǔ jì xiāo dú yǐn)*

Male, 28 years old. In the spring of 1962, the patient suddenly developed swelling in his face and head that was so severe that he could not open his eyes. He also experienced slight aversion to cold, vigorous fever (39°C), wheezing and rough breathing, dry mouth, sore throat, scanty, yellow urine, and constipation. The tongue coating was yellow and greasy and his pulse was wiry and rapid. His tonsils and cheeks were also swollen. His WBC was 18,000mm³. The Western medical diagnosis was facial erysipelas. The Chinese medical diagnosis was wind-heat and toxin attacking the *tai yang, shao yang,* and *yang ming.* The treatment principles were to use primarily acrid and cool herbs to disperse and clear heat, resolve toxicity, and reduce the swelling. The formula chosen for this purpose was a modified version of Universal Benefit

Drink to Eliminate Toxin *(pǔ jì xiāo dú yǐn)*:Scutellariae Radix *(huáng qín)* (9g), Coptidis Rhizoma *(huáng lián)* (6g), Isatidis/Baphicacanthis Radix *(bǎn lán gēn)* (15g), Arctii Fructus *(niú bàng zǐ)* (9g), Platycodi Radix *(jié gěng)* (15g), Forsythiae Fructus *(lián qiào)* (21g), Bupleuri Radix *(chái hú)* (6g), Schizonepetae Herba *(jīng jiè)* (6g), Saposhnikoviae Radix *(fáng fēng)* (9g), and Rhei Radix et Rhizoma *(dà huáng)* (9g).

After finishing three packets of the formula, the fever was gone and his bowel movements were normal. All other signs and symptoms were diminished. The patient was cured after taking another three packets of the same formula.[8]

LUNG AND STOMACH FIRE TOXIN CONSTRAINING AND OBSTRUCTING

Manifestations. There are four concurrent aspects to this pattern:

1. *Slight injury to the yin by heat from excess in the qi level* with fever, thirst, and a thin and rapid pulse.

2. *Obstruction of the channels by heat* with head and body aches.

3. *Flare-up of fire and toxin* with a red, hot, and swollen head, ulcers on the tongue and in the mouth, and a feeling of obstruction in the throat.

4. *Skin eruptions* may appear, which are due to invasion of the blood by the warm-toxin pathogen.

Pathology. Slight injury to the yin by stagnant fire and toxin in the Lung and Stomach.

Treatment principles. Clear heat, enrich the yin, resolve toxicity, and drain the fire.

Formula:

> **FRAGRANT DRINK** *(fāng xiāng yǐn)*
>
> SOURCE: *Systematic Differentiation of Cold Damage and Warm Epidemics*[9]
>
> Scrophulariae Radix *(xuán shēn)* 30g
> Gypsum fibrosum *(shí gāo)* 15g
> Bombyx batryticatus *(bái jiāng cán)* 9g
> Trichosanthis Radix *(tiān huā fěn)* 9g
> Sophorae flavescentis Radix *(kǔ shēn)* 9g
> Citri reticulatae Pericarpium *(chén pí)* 3g
> Poria *(fú líng)* 15g

Cicadae Periostracum *(chán tuì)* 6g

Schizonepetae Herba *(jīng jiè)* 9g

Massa medicata fermentata *(shén qū)* 9g

Scutellariae Radix *(huáng qín)* 6g

Glycyrrhizae Radix *(gān cǎo)* 3g

ANALYSIS OF FORMULA: This formula focuses on both eliminating warm-toxin pathogens while also enriching the yin. The large dosage of Scrophulariae Radix *(xuán shēn)* enriches the yin as well as resolves toxicity. Gypsum fibrosum *(shí gāo)* and Trichosanthis Radix *(tiān huā fěn)* clear heat from the Lung and Stomach and generate fluids. Bombyx batryticatus *(bái jiāng cán)*, Schizonepetae Herba *(jīng jiè)*, and Cicadae Periostracum *(chán tuì)* are good for resolving and dissipating stagnating toxin. Scutellariae Radix *(huáng qín)* and Sophorae flavescentis Radix *(kǔ shēn)* clear heat, drain fire, and resolve toxicity. Poria *(fú líng)*, Citri reticulatae Pericarpium *(chén pí)*, Massa medicata fermentata *(shén qū)*, and Glycyrrhizae Radix *(gān cǎo)* prevent injury to the Spleen and Stomach from the bitter, cold herbs in the formula.

MODIFICATIONS: For eruptions, add Rehmanniae Radix *(shēng dì huáng)* and Moutan Cortex *(mǔ dān pí)* to clear heat and cool the blood.

Putrefying Throat Granular Disorder

Putrefying throat granular disorder is also caused by a combined attack of warm-toxin pathogen and wind. It presents with fever, swollen and ulcerous throat, and eruptions over the body. Putrefying throat granular disorder also mostly occurs in the spring or winter. Since it can be transmitted from one person to another, some ancient texts refer to it as both epidemic throat granular disorder (疫喉痧 *yì hóu shā*) and seasonal throat granular disorder (時喉痧 *shí hóu shā*). Many patients with this disorder are diagnosed in biomedicine with scarlet fever.

ETIOLOGY AND PATHOLOGY

Putrefying throat granular disorder occurs when a warm-toxin pathogen attacks the body and the antipathogenic qi is weak. Warm-toxin pathogen first attacks the Lung and Stomach through the nose, mouth, and throat. The nose is the gate of the Lung and the mouth is the gate of the Stomach. Some consider the throat to be a gate for both the Lung *and* the Stomach. In traditional Chinese medical theory, the Lung governs the skin and the Stomach governs the muscles. After an attack on the Lung and Stomach by warm-toxin pathogen, the following occurs:

- *Fever, chills, and aversion to cold* as a result of the attack on the protective level.
- *A red, swollen, and ulcerated throat* as a result of the attack by the warm-toxin pathogen on the throat, the gate of the Lung and Stomach.
- *Skin eruptions* as a result of the warm-toxin pathogen invading the vessels of the skin and the muscles.

The presence of a red, swollen, and ulcerated throat, in addition to maculas, are the principal features of putrefying throat granular disorder. In the early stages, the warm-toxin pathogen attacks the Lung and Stomach, affecting the protective, qi, and blood levels. In the middle stages, the warm-toxin pathogen is found predominantly in both the qi and blood levels. It may invade the Pericardium or even lead to collapse of the qi externally, and blockage of the Heart spirit internally. During the later stages, there are remnants of warm-toxin pathogen and symptoms of severe injury to the yin and essence.

The practitioner can reach a prognosis by examining the condition of the skin eruptions and of the throat, and the overall mental and physical state of the patient. The latter is done by observing the spirit and feeling the pulse. The prognosis is good if:

- The maculas are sparse, shining, and red.
- The ulcerations in the throat are shallow.
- The mind is clear.
- The pulse is rapid.

By contrast, the prognosis is poor if:

- The maculas are dense and dull in color.
- The ulcers in the throat are deep.
- The patient's mind is not clear.
- The pulse is submerged, thin, and weak.

In general, if the warm-toxin pathogen is mild, it will remain in the Lung and Stomach, and can be easily cleared through treatment. However, if the warm-toxin pathogen is severe, it will move on to invade the Pericardium, a pattern discussed in both Chapters 7 and 8. This pattern presents with a high fever, muddled consciousness, delirium, deep-red tongue, and dark-red maculas, or even blockage of the spirit of the Heart and external collapse of the qi. Collapse of the qi manifests with cold extremities, profuse sweating, pale face, and a feeble pulse. This can be terminal.

Factors for Identifying Putrefying Throat Granular Disorder

There are three important characteristics that help in the identification of putrefying throat granular disorder:

1. The disease usually occurs in the winter or spring.
2. The patient will have been in contact with another person who has had putrefying throat granular disorder.
3. The onset of the disease is acute, with a fever, swollen and ulcerated throat, maculas over the body, and a deep-red tongue body with pronounced thorns, making it look like a strawberry.

TREATMENT PRINCIPLES

Since an attack on the Lung and Stomach by warm-toxin pathogen leads to heat and toxin from excess in the qi, nutritive, or blood level, the general treatment principles are to clear and disperse heat and resolve toxicity. However, the treatment methods vary, depending on the stage of the disease. In the early stage, the warm-toxin pathogen only attacks the protective level and the Lung with slight involvement of the blood level. One can therefore open the pores of the skin and disperse the warm-toxin pathogen with acrid and cool herbs such as Cicadae Periostracum *(chán tuì)*, Arctii Fructus *(niú bàng zǐ)*, Mori Folium *(sāng yè)*, Chrysanthemi Flos *(jú huā)*, Lonicerae Flos *(jīn yín huā)*, Schizonepetae Herba *(jīng jiè)*, and Belamcandae Rhizoma *(shè gān)*. In *Revised Classified Case Studies from Famous Doctors throughout the Country (Chóng dìng quán guó míng yī yàn àn lèi biān)*, the early twentieth-century physician He Lian-Chen noted that "Treatment at the early stage should disperse warm-toxin pathogen as soon as possible: Use Cicadae Periostracum *(chán tuì)* and Arctii Fructus *(niú bàng zǐ)* for mild cases, and Ephedrae Herba *(má huáng)* and Allii fistulosi Bulbus *(cōng bái)* for severe cases."[10]

Why should Ephedrae Herba *(má huáng)* be used here, and what role does it play in treating this condition? Another early twentieth-century physician, Ding Gan-Ren, noted that "The key way of treating putrefying throat granular disorder is to induce unimpeded sweating."[11] This is because unimpeded sweating indicates that there is harmony between the protective and nutritive qi, and that the body can focus its energy to fight the warm-toxin pathogen. Furthermore, sweating can carry the warm-toxin pathogen out of the body. As would be expected, only slight sweating is appropriate here, which is what Ephedrae Herba *(má huáng)* does if it is used by itself and not with Cinnamomi Ramulus *(guì zhī)*. If a large amount of bitter and cold herbs are used to clear heat and resolve toxicity without simultaneously dispersing the warm-toxin pathogen through sweating, the pathogen will congeal and stagnate inside the body. This may lead to invasion of the blood and Pericardium, and injure the yin and essence. The best strategy is therefore to combine dispersing methods with those that clear and resolve the warm-toxin pathogen.

In the middle stages, the warm-toxin pathogen has penetrated deeply, and the patient's condition has become severe, since both the qi and nutritive or blood levels are involved. The practitioner must therefore drain the fire, resolve the toxicity, and cool the blood with herbs such as Rehmanniae Radix *(shēng dì huáng)*, Moutan Cortex *(mǔ dān pí)*, Bubali Cornu *(shuǐ niú jiǎo)*, and Coptidis Rhizoma *(huáng lián)*. Sometimes the purging method is necessary to encourage the heat and toxin to exit the body via the stool. In these cases, herbs such as Natrii Sulfas *(máng xiāo)* and Rhei Radix et Rhizoma *(dà huáng)* should be used. According to He Lian-Chen in *Revised Classified Case Studies From Famous Doctors throughout the Country*:

> Two or three days after an attack by warm-toxin pathogen leading to putrefying throat granular disorder, if the exterior symptoms are gone and heat and fire flare up, herbs that cool blood and clear or purge heat and toxin, like Rhinocerotis Cornu *(xī jiǎo)*, Rehmanniae Radix *(shēng dì huáng)*, Coptidis Rhizoma *(huáng lián)*, Rhei Radix et Rhizoma *(dà huáng)*, and Natrii Sulfas *(máng xiāo)*, must be used immediately. This method is called 'removing the firewood from under the caldron' (釜抵加薪 *fǔ dǐ jiā xīn)*. Once the qi in the Large Intestine, which is closely related to the Lung and Stomach, descends normally, the flaring fire and toxin will be extinguished and the disease will be cured.[12]

There is another important point to consider. Is the warm-toxin pathogen predominantly in the qi level or in the nutritive and blood levels? For the former, the heat in the qi level must be cleared. For the latter, the blood must be both cooled and invigorated. However, regardless of its location, acrid, warm herbs should not be used at this stage. They will exacerbate the flaring-up of fire and toxin because they are quite yang in nature and have a tendency to lift the yang.

By the time the disease has entered its later stages, the yin has been injured and there are persistent remnants of the warm-toxin pathogen still in the body. The practitioner must enrich the yin, support the fluids, clear the remnants of heat, and resolve toxicity with such herbs as Rehmanniae Radix *(shēng dì huáng)*, Scrophulariae Radix *(xuán shēn)*, Ophiopogonis Radix *(mài mén dōng)*, and Anemarrhenae Rhizoma *(zhī mǔ)*.

Attack on the Protective Level and Lung by Warm-Toxin Pathogen

Manifestations. There are two concurrent aspects to this pattern:

1. *Dysfunction of protective qi* with aversion to cold, chills, and fever.

2. *Warm-toxin pathogen attacking the Lung* with slight thirst, a red, swollen, and painful or even ulcerated throat, faint maculas over the body, red tongue with a thin yellow and white coating, and a rapid pulse. The faint maculas are indicative of slight involvement of the blood level in this pattern.

Pathology. Warm-toxin pathogen attacking the protective level and the Lung.

Treatment principles. Disperse and clear the heat, resolve the toxicity, and improve the condition of the throat.

Formula No. 1 (internal):

DECOCTION TO CLEAR THE THROAT WTIH PREPARED SOYBEAN AND GARDENIA *(qīng yān zhī chǐ tāng)*

SOURCE: *Initial Discussion on Putrefying Throat Granular Disorder*[13]

Sojae Semen preparatum *(dàn dòu chǐ)* 9g

Lonicerae Flos *(jīn yín huā)* 9g

Menthae haplocalycis Herba *(bò hé)* 3g

Arctii Fructus *(niú bàng zǐ)* 9g

Gardeniae Fructus *(zhī zǐ)* 9g

Bombyx batryticatus *(bái jiāng cán)* 6g

Rhinocerotis Cornu *(xī jiǎo)* 2.4g

Phragmitis Rhizoma *(lú gēn)* 30g

Forsythiae Fructus *(lián qiào)*.........................9g

Platycodi Radix *(jié gěng)* 4.5g

Lasiosphaera/Calvatia *(mǎ bó)* 4.5g

Junci Medulla *(dēng xīn cǎo)* 3g

Lophatheri Herba *(dàn zhú yè)* 3g

Glycyrrhizae Radix *(gān cǎo)* 9g

Cicadae Periostracum *(chán tuì)* 2.4g

ANALYSIS OF FORMULA: This pattern represents an early stage of the disease. It presents with stagnation of warm-toxin pathogen in the exterior, as evidenced by the aversion to cold, chills, and fever, as well as symptoms of interior heat. As Xiao Chun-Long observed in the source text, it is best to disperse the warm-toxin pathogen under these conditions through the pores of the skin by inducing unimpeded sweating.[14] Sojae Semen preparatum *(dàn dòu chǐ)*, Menthae haplocalycis Herba *(bò hé)*, Cicadae Periostracum *(chán tuì)*, and Platycodi Radix *(jié gěng)* are thus used to disperse the warm-toxin pathogen from the Lung. In addition, Lonicerae Flos *(jīn yín huā)*, Forsythiae Fructus *(lián qiào)*, Gardeniae Fructus *(zhī zǐ)*, Junci Medulla *(dēng xīn cǎo)*, Phragmitis Rhizoma *(lú gēn)*, and Lophatheri Herba *(dàn zhú yè)* clear and discharge heat through the urine, while Rhinocerotis Cornu *(xī jiǎo)*, Lasiosphaera/

Calvatia *(mǎ bó)*, Arctii Fructus *(niú bàng zǐ)*, Bombyx batryticatus *(bái jiāng cán)*, and Glycyrrhizae Radix *(gān cǎo)* resolve toxicity and improve the condition of the throat. Since Rhinocerotis Cornu *(xī jiǎo)* is derived from an endangered species, the practitioner should substitute three pieces of Canarii albii Fructus *(gǎn lǎn)*[15] or 60g of Bubali Cornu *(shuǐ niú jiǎo)* in this formula.

MODIFICATIONS: The basic formula can be modified as follows:

- For severe stagnation of qi in the exterior with significant body aches, add Saposhnikoviae Radix *(fáng fēng)* and Schizonepetae Herba *(jīng jiè)*. These herbs enhance the formula's ability to disperse the warm-toxin pathogen from the exterior. However, their dosage should be limited to 6g because they will otherwise increase the heat in the body.

- For profuse sputum and vomiting, add Citri reticulatae Exocarpium rubrum *(jú hóng)* and Curcumae Radix *(yù jīn)*, and remove Glycyrrhizae Radix *(gān cǎo)*.

Formula No. 2 (topical):

JADE KEY *(yù yào shi)*

SOURCE: *Discussion of Illnesses, Patterns, and Formulas Related to the Unification of the Three Etiologies*[16]

Natrii Sulfas *(máng xiāo)* 4.5g

Borax *(péng shā)* 15g

Borneolum *(bīng piàn)* 0.3g

Bombyx batryticatus *(bái jiāng cán)* 7.5g

ANALYSIS OF FORMULA: Jade Key *(yù yào shi)* is a topical formula that clears heat, resolves toxicity, and improves the condition of the throat. It is indicated for putrefying throat granular disorder when there are *no* ulcerations in the throat. In this formula, Natrii Sulfas *(máng xiāo)* softens masses and dissipates the mixture of heat and toxin. Borax *(péng shā)* clears heat, transforms phlegm, and resolves toxicity. Borneolum *(bīng piàn)* disperses stagnant warm-toxin pathogen, and Bombyx batryticatus *(bái jiāng cán)* transforms phlegm and dissipates the mixture of heat and phlegm.

ADMINISTRATION: Grind the herbs into a fine powder and use a thin bamboo pipe to blow 1.5g of the powder into the throat. The powder should only be applied to the red, swollen area once or twice a day. A plastic or steel pipe can be substituted for the bamboo pipe.

STAGNATION OF WARM-TOXIN PATHOGEN IN THE QI LEVEL

Manifestations. There are three concurrent aspects to this pattern:

1. *Heat from excess in the qi level* with vigorous fever without aversion to cold, irritability, and thirst for cold beverages. There may be aversion to heat.
2. *Stagnation of the warm-toxin pathogen* with a red, swollen, painful, and ulcerated throat.
3. *Blood moving out of the vessels due to the warm-toxin pathogen* with maculas over the entire body.

Pathology. Stagnation of warm-toxin pathogen in the qi level with slight invasion of the blood level. The latter leads to blood being forced out of the vessels.

Treatment principles. Clear and disperse heat, resolve toxicity in the qi level, and cool the blood.

Formula No. 1 (internal):

YU'S CLEAR THE HEART AND COOL THE DIAPHRAGM POWDER
(Yú shì qīng xīn liáng gé sǎn)

SOURCE: *Achievements Regarding Epidemic Rashes*[17]

Forsythiae Fructus *(lián qiào)* . . . . .9g[18]
Scutellariae Radix *(huáng qín)* 9g
Gardeniae Fructus *(zhī zǐ)* 9g
Menthae haplocalycis Herba *(bò hé)* 3g
Gypsum fibrosum *(shí gāo)* . . . . 18g[18]
Platycodi Radix *(jié gěng)* 3g
Glycyrrhizae Radix *(gān cǎo)* 3g
Lophatheri Herba *(dàn zhú yè)* 3g

ANALYSIS OF FORMULA: Although there is blood level involvement in this pattern, the pathogen is located primarily in the qi level. The formula therefore serves to clear heat and resolve toxicity in the qi level. Since the disease is situated in the upper part of the body, it is still useful to disperse and clear heat.

This formula is a modified version of Cool the Diaphragm Powder *(liáng gé sǎn)*, discussed in Chapter 8. The modification involves removing Natrii Sulfas *(máng xiāo)* and Rhei Radix et Rhizoma *(dà huáng)* and adding Platycodi Radix *(jié gěng)* and Gypsum fibrosum *(shí gāo)*. The purpose of the modification is to focus on clearing and dispersing heat and toxin in the upper burner, instead of purging heat and toxin in the lower burner. In this formula, Gypsum fibrosum *(shí gāo)* is the chief herb for clearing heat from the qi level. Forsythiae Fructus *(lián qiào)*, Scutellariae

Radix *(huáng qín)*, Lophatheri Herba *(dàn zhú yè)*, and Gardeniae Fructus *(zhī zǐ)* clear and disperse heat and toxin. Menthae haplocalycis Herba *(bò hé)*, Platycodi Radix *(jié gěng)*, and Glycyrrhizae Radix *(gān cǎo)* disperse the Lung to help the qi move through the upper burner and ease the throat.

MODIFICATIONS: The basic formula can be modified as follows:

- Based on the experience of Zhao Shao-Qin, described in *Length and Breadth of Warm Pathogen Disease [Differentiation] (Wēn bìng zòng héng)*, it is best to add Lonicerae Flos *(jīn yín huā)* (9g), Violae Herba *(zǐ huā dì dīng)* (9g), Arnebiae Radix/Lithospermi Radix *(zǐ cǎo)* (9g), Moutan Cortex *(mǔ dān pí)* (9g), Paeoniae Radix rubra *(chì sháo)* (9g), Rehmanniae Radix *(shēng dì huáng)* (9g), fresh Phragmitis Rhizoma recens *(xiān lú gēn)* (30g), and fresh Imperatae Rhizoma *(xiān bái máo gēn)* (30g) to enhance the formula's action in clearing heat, resolving toxicity, cooling the blood, invigorating the blood, and enriching the yin.[19] Personally, in place of these additions, I often add Arnebiae Radix/Lithospermi Radix *(zǐ cǎo)* (24g), Cicadae Periostracum *(chán tuì)* (9g), and Patriniae Herba *(bài jiàng cǎo)* (9g) to cool the blood and enhance the formula's ability to disperse heat and toxin.

- For constipation, add Rhei Radix et Rhizoma *(dà huáng)* and Natrii Sulfas *(máng xiāo)* to purge the heat.

- For widespread skin maculas, add Moutan Cortex *(mǔ dān pí)*, Rehmanniae Radix *(shēng dì huáng)*, and Arnebiae Radix/Lithospermi Radix *(zǐ cǎo)*.

Formula No. 2 (topical):

MEDICINE FOR REMOVING ROT FROM A PUTREFYING THROAT *(làn hóu qù fǔ yào)*

SOURCE: *Revised and Expanded Discussion of Warm-Heat Pathogen Diseases*[20]

Cyathulae Radix *(chuān niú xī)*	30g
Menthae haplocalycis Herba *(bò hé)*	1.5g
Indigo naturalis *(qīng dài)*	1.5g
Borneolum *(bīng piàn)*	0.9g

ANALYSIS OF FORMULA: Indigo naturalis *(qīng dài)* clears heat and resolves toxicity. The combination of Menthae haplocalycis Herba *(bò hé)* and Borneolum *(bīng piàn)* is used to disperse heat and relieve pain in the throat. Cyathulae Radix *(chuān niú xī)* promotes blood circulation and removes blood stasis, which results from heat and toxin.

ADMINISTRATION: Grind all the herbs into a fine powder and place in a small glass bottle with a tight lid. Store the bottle in a refrigerator or in another cool and dry place. Use a thin bamboo pipe (or other tube) to blow 0.5g of powder into the throat onto the red, swollen, ulcerated areas twice a day.

BURNING OF WARM-TOXIN PATHOGEN IN THE QI, NUTRITIVE, AND BLOOD LEVELS

Manifestations. There are two concurrent aspects to this pattern:

1. *Heat from excess in the qi level* with vigorous fever, profuse sweating, thirst for cold beverages, irritability, and restlessness.

2. *Heat from excess and toxin in the nutritive and blood levels* with a severe red, swollen, painful, and ulcerated throat that may lead to partial blockage of the respiratory tract. This, in turn, can lead to shortness of breath or even labored breathing. There may also be a deep-red tongue with thorns, making the tongue look like a strawberry, and dense patches of maculas over the entire body.

NOTE: This is the most severe and critical pattern of putrefying throat granular disorder. The warm-toxin pathogen has transformed into fire and is burning the qi, nutritive, and blood levels. If left untreated, the patient will suffer from blockage of the Heart spirit internally, and collapse of the yang qi externally, and will consequently die.

Pathology. Warm-toxin transforming into fire and burning and injuring the qi and blood.

Treatment principles. Clear heat from the qi level, and cool the blood and resolve toxicity in the nutritive and blood levels.

Formula:

COOL THE NUTRITIVE AND CLEAR THE QI DECOCTION *(liáng yíng qīng qì tāng)*

SOURCE: *Collected Clinical Writings of Ding Gan-Ren*

Rhinocerotis Cornu *(xī jiǎo)* 1.5g
fresh Dendrobii Herba *(xiān shí hú)* 24g
Gardeniae Fructus *(zhī zǐ)* 6g
Moutan Cortex *(mǔ dān pí)* 6g
fresh Rehmanniae Radix recens *(xiān dì huáng)* 24g

Menthae haplocalycis Folium *(bò hé yè)* [21] 2.4g

Coptidis Rhizoma *(huáng lián)* 1.5g

Paeoniae Radix rubra *(chì sháo)* 6g

Scrophulariae Radix *(xuán shēn)* 9g

Gypsum fibrosum *(shí gāo)* 24g

Glycyrrhizae Radix *(gān cǎo)* 2.4g

Forsythiae Fructus *(lián qiào)* 9g

Lophatheri Herba *(dàn zhú yè)* . . . . 30 pieces

Phragmitis Rhizoma *(lú gēn)* 30g

Imperatae Rhizoma *(bái máo gēn)* 30g

Succus Faecalis Aureus *(jīn zhī)* 30g

ANALYSIS OF FORMULA: This formula is a modification of White Tiger Decoction *(bái hǔ tāng)* and Clear the Nutritive Level Decoction *(qīng yíng tāng)*, both of which are discussed in Chapter 7. Both formulas were modified and combined to clear heat and cool the blood. In this formula, Gypsum fibrosum *(shí gāo)*, Gardeniae Fructus *(zhī zǐ)*, Forsythiae Fructus *(lián qiào)*, Menthae haplocalycis Folium *(bò hé yè)*, Lophatheri Herba *(dàn zhú yè)*, and Coptidis Rhizoma *(huáng lián)* clear heat and resolve toxicity in the qi level. Rhinocerotis Cornu *(xī jiǎo)*, Rehmanniae Radix *(shēng dì huáng)*, Moutan Cortex *(mǔ dān pí)*, Paeoniae Radix rubra *(chì sháo)*, Glycyrrhizae Radix *(gān cǎo)*, and Succus Faecalis Aureus *(jīn zhī)* cool the blood and resolve toxicity in the nutritive and blood levels. Dendrobii Herba *(shí hú)*, Phragmitis Rhizoma *(lú gēn)*, Imperatae Rhizoma *(bái máo gēn)*, and Scrophulariae Radix *(xuán shēn)* enrich the yin and prevent further injury to the yin from the heat and toxin. In addition, since Rhinocerotis Cornu *(xī jiǎo)* is derived from an endangered species, Bubali Cornu *(shuǐ niú jiǎo)* should be substituted, but its dosage should be at least 30g in this formula.

MODIFICATIONS: The basic formula can be modified as follows:

- For blockage of the Heart by warm-toxin pathogen with muddled consciousness, delirium, cold extremities, and a deep pulse, use Calm the Palace Pill with Cattle Gallstone *(ān gōng niú huáng wán)* to clear heat from the Heart and open the orifices.[22]

- For collapse of yang qi with shallow breathing, cold body, and profuse sweating, use Ginseng, Aconite Accessory Root, Dragon Bone and Oyster Shell Decoction *(shēn fù lóng mù tāng)*[23] to quickly restore the yang. Such patients should be sent immediately to the emergency room, as it is impossible to adequately care for them as outpatients. In China such patients are sometimes treated with these herbs taken via a nasogastric tube. You may also apply some salt on the skin at CV4 *(guān yuán)* and CV-8 *(shén jué)* and burn three moxa cones over each point.

Case study: Cool the Nutritive and Clear the Qi Decoction
(liáng yíng qīng qì tāng)

Male, 25 years old

First visit. After suffering from a fever for two or three days, the patient developed faint maculas on his face, chest, abdomen, and extremities along with a swollen and painful throat the morning of his first visit. His tonsils were swollen with pustules, and his temperature was 39.5°C. The area around his mouth was pale. The tip of his tongue had many red thorns and looked like a strawberry, and the tongue body was deep red and dry, with a yellow and thick coating at the root. He was dizzy, restless, irritable, and had insomnia. His lips were cracked with bleeding. The patient had not had a bowel movement for two days. His urine was scanty and dark red. He was diagnosed with severe putrefying throat granular disorder due to burning from the warm pathogen and collection of heat in the qi and nutritive levels.

The treatment principles were to clear heat from the qi level and in the nutritive level, while promoting the eruption of the rash. A modified version of Cool the Nutritive and Clear the Qi Decoction *(liáng yíng qīng qì tāng)*[24] was prescribed: Rhinocerotis Cornu *(xī jiǎo)* powder (0.6g, swallow with the strained decoction), fresh Imperatae Rhizoma *(xiān bái máo gēn)* (45g), fresh Phragmitis Rhizoma recens *(xiān lú gēn)* (45g), Gypsum fibrosum *(shí gāo)* (24g), Scrophulariae Radix *(xuán shēn)* (45g), Forsythiae Fructus *(lián qiào)* (15g), Lonicerae Flos *(jīn yín huā)* (3g), Arnebiae Radix/Lithospermi Radix *(zǐ cǎo)* (9g), Glycyrrhizae Radix *(gān cǎo)* (10g), Violae Herba *(zǐ huā dì dīng)* (9g), Trichosanthis Radix *(tiān huā fěn)* (9g), Patriniae Herba *(bài jiàng cǎo)* (9g), and Armeniacae Semen *(xìng rén)*(9g). The patient was given two packets of these herbs and instructed to avoid greasy and sweet foods.

Second visit. After these herbs were finished, maculas clearly developed all over the patient's face, chest, abdomen, and extremities. He felt calmer and less restless, and his throat was less swollen and painful. His temperature had come down to 38°C. His tonsils, while less swollen, still had pustules. The tongue was unchanged. The patient had slept well for the previous two nights, and had experienced less restlessness, but his lips were still cracked. He had had a bowel movement, but with little stool, and his urine was scanty and red. There had been some improvement, but the heat and toxicity were still intense. In order to prevent them from invading the Pericardium, it was decided to add some herbs to vent the heat. The new formula was composed of: Rhinocerotis Cornu *(xī jiǎo)* powder (0.3g, swallow with the strained decoction), Gardeniae Fructus *(zhī zǐ)* (6g), Forsythiae Fructus *(lián qiào)* (30g), Moutan Cortex *(mǔ dān pí)* (9g), Gypsum fibrosum *(shí gāo)* (24g), Scrophulariae Radix *(xuán shēn)*

(45g), Lophatheri Herba *(dàn zhú yè)* (6g), fresh Imperatae Rhizoma *(xiān bái máo gēn)* (45g), fresh Phragmitis Rhizoma recens *(xiān lú gēn)* (45g), Scutellariae Radix *(huáng qín)* (9g), and Lonicerae Flos *(jīn yín huā)* (30g). The patient was given two packets of this prescription.

Third visit: The fever had gradually diminished and on this day was 37.4°C. His sore and swollen throat and restlessness had disappeared, and he was sleeping well. He had a bowel movement once a day. His urine was scanty and yellow. His tongue coating was less yellow and there were no more deep red thorns over the tip of his tongue. However, his lips were deep purple. There were remnants of heat and injury to the yin. At this time it was important to begin enriching the yin, and the following herbs were given to the patient: Rehmanniae Radix *(shēng dì huáng)* (30g), Anemarrhenae Rhizoma *(zhī mǔ)* (9g), Lophatheri Herba *(dàn zhú yè)* (3g), Forsythiae Fructus *(lián qiào)* (24g), Lonicerae Flos *(jīn yín huā)* (24g), Moutan Cortex *(mǔ dān pí)* (9g), Scrophulariae Radix *(xuán shēn)* (30g), Paeoniae Radix rubra *(chì sháo)* (9g), Glehniae/Adenophorae Radix *(shā shēn)* (30g), and Benincasae Exocarpium *(dōng guā pí)* (30g). The patient was given three packets of this prescription.

Fourth visit. The patient no longer had a fever. The skin was gradually peeling off where there had been maculas. His energy was good and his appetite, urination, and bowel movements were all normal. The yellow tongue coating was gone and the tongue body was just slightly red. His pulse was thin and frail. The putrefying throat granular disorder had been cured, and it was now time to adjust the function of the Spleen and Stomach. Four packets of the following herbs were given to the patient: Glehniae/Adenophorae Radix *(shā shēn)* (24g), Rehmanniae Radix *(shēng dì huáng)* (24g), Paeoniae Radix rubra *(chì sháo)* (9g), Paeoniae Radix alba *(bái sháo)* (9g), Benincasae Exocarpium *(dōng guā pí)* (30g), Poriae Cutis *(fú líng pí)* (24g), Hordei Fructus germinatus *(mài yá)* (9g), and Gigeriae galli Endothelium corneum *(jī nèi jīn)* (9g).

Fifth visit. At this point all the problems related to putrefying throat granular disorder were gone, except for the flakes on the skin. His appetite was good and he was sleeping well. The following powdered herbs were given to the patient to harmonize the Stomach and promote digestion: fried Massa medicata fermentata *(shén qū)* (150g), fried Crataegi Fructus *(shān zhā)* (150g), fried Hordei Fructus germinatus *(mài yá)* (150g), Gigeriae galli Endothelium corneum *(jī nèi jīn)* (150g), and Amomi Fructus *(shā rén)* (3g). Nine grams of this powder mixed with an equal amount of sugar were taken with boiled water in the morning and evening.[25]

Injury to Yin by the Remnants of Warm-Toxin Pathogen

Manifestations. There are two concurrent aspects to this pattern:

1. *The remnants of warm-toxin pathogen* with a swollen and slightly ulcerated throat (but one that is *not* red or painful) coupled with maculas over the entire body.

2. *Injured yin* with slight fever in the afternoon, hot sensation in the palms and soles, red and dry tongue with little saliva, and a thin and rapid pulse.

Pathology. Injured yin with the remnants of warm-toxin pathogen, with the injured yin being the predominant feature.

Treatment principles. Enrich the yin, support the fluids, and clear the remnants of warm-toxin pathogen.

Formula:

Clear the Throat and Enrich the Nutritive Qi Decoction
(qīng yān yǎng yíng tāng)

SOURCE: *Initial Discussion on Putrefying Throat Granular Disorder*[26]

Panacis quinquefolii Radix *(xī yáng shēn)*	9g
Rehmanniae Radix *(shēng dì huáng)*	9g
Poriae Sclerotium pararadicis *(fú shén)*	9g
Ophiopogonis Radix *(mài mén dōng)*	9g
Paeoniae Radix alba *(bái sháo)*	6g
Trichosanthis Radix *(tiān huā fěn)*	12g
Asparagi Radix *(tiān mén dōng)*	6g
Scrophulariae Radix *(xuán shēn)*	12g
Anemarrhenae Rhizoma *(zhī mǔ)*	9g
Honey-toasted Glycyrrhizae Radix preparata *(zhì gān cǎo)*	3g

ANALYSIS OF FORMULA: This formula is used to treat the later stage of putrefying throat granular disorder. Since the predominant feature is injury to the yin, enrichment of the yin comes first. Otherwise, it will be very difficult to clear the remnants of warm-toxin pathogen. In this formula, Scrophulariae Radix *(xuán shēn)*, Ophiopogonis Radix *(mài mén dōng)*, and Rehmanniae Radix *(shēng dì huáng)* are combined with Asparagi Radix *(tiān mén dōng)*, Paeoniae Radix alba *(bái sháo)*, and honey-toasted Glycyrrhizae Radix preparata *(zhì gān cǎo)* to enrich yin with the combination of sweet and sour flavors. Panacis quinquefolii Radix *(xī yáng shēn)* can tonify both the qi and yin. If the injury to the qi is mild, Glehniae Radix *(běi shā shēn)* can be used instead. Anemarrhenae Rhizoma *(zhī mǔ)* and Trichosanthis Radix *(tiān huā fěn)*, which are bitter, sweet, and moist, clear heat without injuring the yin, especially compared to Scutellariae Radix *(huáng qín)* and Coptidis Rhizoma *(huáng lián)*, which are bitter and cold and readily injure the yin. Poriae Sclerotium pararadicis *(fú shén)* is simply used to calm the spirit of the Heart, since the spirit may be disturbed by the remnants of the warm-toxin pathogen.

Summary

Warm-toxin is caused by warm-toxin pathogens. These pathogens result in heat from excess or fire, and the ensuing illnesses are characterized by local areas of redness and swelling that either progress to ulcerations that affect the head and throat, or to maculas that cover the entire body. In all cases, the main goals of treatment are to clear heat and resolve toxicity. In this chapter, we have only discussed two types of warm-toxin—massive head febrile disorder and putrefying throat granular dis-order—because there is simply not enough information about the other types in our sources.

The term massive head febrile disorder is derived from the disorder's primary characteristic, a red and swollen head. In the early stage, there is an attack on the protective level, Lung, and Stomach by the warm-toxin pathogen and wind, leading to the accumulation of wind, heat, and toxin in the head. In a later stage, there is injury to the yin by stagnant fire and toxin in the Lung and Stomach. The principles of treatment, and the specific formulas chosen, vary depending on the stage of the disease.

The term putrefying throat granular disorder is derived from the disorder's primary characteristics: redness, swelling, pain, and ulcerations in the throat, as well as eruptions over the entire body. In the early stage of this disorder, the warm-toxin pathogen and wind attack the exterior, protective level, and Lung. Later stages are characterized by stagnation of warm-toxin pathogen in the qi level (and slight invasion of the blood level, forcing blood out of the vessels) or by burning of the warm-toxin pathogen in the qi, nutritive, and blood levels. Finally, remnants of warm-toxin pathogen can injure the yin. Again, the principles of treatment, and the particular formulas, will vary depending upon the stage of the disease.

Table 10.1	Differentiation and Treatment of Warm-Toxin	
Patterns	**Treatment Principles**	**Formulas**
▶ MASSIVE HEAD FEBRILE DISORDER		
Attack on upper part of body by warm-toxin pathogen and wind	Disperse and clear heat, resolve toxicity, and reduce swelling	Universal Benefit Drink to Eliminate Toxin (*pǔ jì xiāo dú yǐn*), or Three Yellow and Two Fragrant Powder (*sān huáng èr xiāng sǎn*)
Lung and Stomach fire toxin constraining and obstructing and injuring the yin	Clear heat, enrich the yin, resolve toxicity, and drain fire	Fragrant Drink (*fāng xiāng yǐn*)
▶ PUTREFYING THROAT GRANULAR DISORDER		
Attack on protective level and Lung by warm-toxin	Disperse and clear heat, resolve toxicity and benefit the throat	Decoction to Clear the Throat with Prepared Soybean and Gardenia (*qīng yān zhī chǐ tāng*) and Jade Key (*yù yào shí*)
Stagnation of warm-toxin pathogen in qi level with minor invasion of blood level forcing blood out of the vessels	Clear and disperse heat, resolve toxicity in qi level, and cool the blood	Yu's Clear the Heart and Cool the Diaphragm Powder (*Yú shì qīng xīn liáng gé sǎn*), and Medicine for Removing Rot from a Putrefying Throat (*làn hóu qù fǔ yào*)
Burning of warm-toxin pathogen in qi, nutritive, and blood levels	Clear heat from qi level, cool blood and resolve toxicity in nutritive and blood levels	Cool the Nutritive and Clear the Qi Decoction (*liáng yíng qīng qì tāng*)
Injury to yin by the remnants of warm-toxin pathogen	Enrich the yin, support the fluids, and clear remnants of warm-toxin pathogen	Clear the Throat and Enrich the Nutritive Decoction (*qīng yān yǎng yíng tāng*)

Endnotes

1. Chen Shi-Gong, *Orthodox Lineage of External Medicine (Wài kē zhèng zōng)*. Tianjin: Tianjin Science and Technology Publishing House, 1999: 130.

2. Ding Gan-Ren, *Outline of the Presentation and Treatment of Throat Granular Disorder (Hóu shā zhèng zhì gài yào)*. This book was published in 1927 and is contained in Lu Zhen, *Collected Rare Recent Books on Chinese Medicine, Five Sensory Organ Section (Jīn dài zhōng yī zhēn běn jí: wēn bìng fèn cè)*. Hangzhou: Zhejiang Science and Technology Publishing House, 1987: 567.

3. See Chapters 2 and 3 for a review of the general traits of the warm-toxin pathogen.

4. Zhao Ji, *Comprehensive Recording of Sage-like Benefit from the Zhenghe Era (Zhènghé shèng jì zǒng lù)*. Beijing: People's Health Publishing House, 1962: 2069. This book was written by order of the Hui Zong emperor of the Song dynasty during the Zhenghe era (1111–1117).

5. Meng Shu-Jiang et al., *Warm Pathogen Diseases (Wēn bìng xué)*. Shanghai: Shanghai Science and Technology Publishing House, 1985: 103. We have been unable to find a copy of the source text itself.

6. Wu Tang, *Systematic Differentiation of Warm Pathogen Diseases (Wēn bìng tiáo biàn)*. Beijing: People's Health Publishing House, 1963: 29

7. Ibid.

8. Gansu People's Publishing House, *A Selection of Chinese Case Studies and Medical Discussions (Zhōng yī yī àn yī huà jí jǐn)*. Lanzhou: Gansu People's Publishing House, 1980: 453. This case study was reported by the physician Zhang Zhong-Xuan.

9. This was written by Yang Xuan in 1784.

10. He Lian-Chen, *Revised Case Studies of Famous Doctors throughout the Country Organized by Category (Chóng dìng quán guó míng yī yàn àn lèi biān)*. Shanghai: Shanghai Science and Technology Publishing House, 1959: 302. He Lian-Chen, also known as He Bing-Yuan, lived from 1860-1929.

11. Shen Zhong-Li et al., *Collected Clinical Writings of Ding Gan-Ren (Dīng Gān-Rén lín zhèng yī jí)*. Shanghai: Shanghai University of Traditional Chinese Medicine Publishing House, 2000: 342. Ding Gan-Ren was also known as Ding Ze-Zhou. This statement was originally written in 1927.

12. He Lian-Chen, *Revised Case Studies of Famous Doctors Throughout the Country*, 302.

13. This book was written by Xia Chun-Long (Xia Yun) and published in the late nineteenth century.

14. Meng Shu-Jiang, *Warm Pathogen Diseases*, 108.

15. This is the Chinese olive. It is sweet, sour, and neutral and enters the Lung channel. It clears heat, resolves toxicity, improves the condition of the throat, and transforms phlegm. Often used for a swollen, painful throat and cough due to Lung heat. The normal dosage is 6-15g.

16. Written by Chen Yan in 1174.

17. Written by Yu Lin (Yu Shi-Yu) in 1794.

18. In the source text, no dosage is provided. These come from Meng Shu-Jiang, *Warm Pathogen Diseases*, 108.

19. Zhao Shao-Qin, Hu Ding-Bang, Liu Jing-Yuan, *Length and Breadth of Warm Pathogen Disease [Differentiation]*. Beijing: Beijing College of Traditional Chinese Medicine, 1979: 90.

20. He Lian-Chen, *Revised and Expanded Discussion of Warm-Heat Pathogen Diseases (Chóng dìng guǎng wēn rè lùn.)* Beijing: People's Health Publishing House, 1960: 38-39.

21. This is acrid and cool and enters the Lung and Liver channels. It has the same functions as Menthae haplocalycis Herba *(bò hé)*, but is stronger at inducing sweating.

22. See Chapter 7 for further details.

23. This is Ginseng and Aconite Accessory Root Decoction *(shēn fù tāng)*, discussed in Chapter 7, with the addition of Fossilia Ossis Mastodi *(lóng gǔ)* (10-20g) and Ostreae Concha *(mǔ lì)* (10-20g).

24. The source text provides no name for this formula. The name was devised by myself based on the ingredients.

25. Peng Jian-Zhong and Yang Lian-Zhu, *Selected Case Studies from Zhao Shao-Qin (Zhào Shào-Qín lín zhèng yàn àn jīng xuǎn)*. Beijing: Learning Garden Publishing House, 1996: 57.

26. Meng Shu-Jiang, *Warm Pathogen Diseases*, 108. The source text is unavailable.

Differentiation and Treatment of Warm Pathogen Diseases

Section B – Damp-Heat Pathogen Diseases

WARM PATHOGEN DISEASES caused by a combination of warm-heat pathogen and dampness include summerheat-warmth, damp-warmth, and lurking summerheat. On the face of it, treatment of these disorders may appear to be simple, that is, clear the heat and eliminate the dampness. However, the focus should always be on eliminating dampness, regardless of whether dampness or heat predominates. This is because dampness is a viscous yin pathogen that has form. It can readily lead to stagnation and constraint of qi, which in turn will generate more heat. It can also serve as a foundation to which heat attaches and becomes trapped. Therefore, the elimination of dampness should be the priority in treatment and no effort should be spared in dealing with it. Methods for treating dampness alone are discussed in Chapter 6. But when it appears in combination with heat, there are five treatment methods:

1. *Disperse damp-heat with acrid and warm herbs, or acrid and cool herbs, and transform dampness using aromatic herbs.* This method is used when dampness predominates and attacks the exterior, leading to a slight fever, severe chills, aversion to cold, heaviness or stiffness throughout the body, absence of sweating, and a white, yellow, and slightly greasy tongue coating. Among the herbs used for this treatment method are Pogostemonis/Agastaches Herba (*huò xiāng*), Angelicae dahuricae Radix (*bái zhǐ*), Perillae Folium (*zǐ sū yè*), Moslae Herba (*xiāng rú*), Eupatorii Herba (*pèi lán*), Menthae haplocalycis Herba (*bò hé*), Arctii Fructus (*niú bàng zǐ*), and Notopterygii Rhizoma seu Radix (*qiāng huó*). These herbs serve to disperse dampness and heat by opening the pores in the skin and inducing a slight sweat.

2. *Disperse damp-heat with acrid and cool herbs, leach out dampness with bland herbs, and transform dampness with aromatic herbs.* This method is used when heat predominates and attacks the exterior, leading to contained fever, chills, heaviness in the body, joint pain, thirst, sweating, chest distention, and a yellow and slightly greasy tongue coating. The herbs used in connection with this method include Menthae haplocalycis Herba *(bò hé)*, Atractylodis Rhizoma *(cāng zhú)*, Tetrapanacis Medulla *(tōng cǎo)*, Talcum *(huá shí)*, Poria *(fú líng)*, Sojae Semen germinatum *(dà dòu juǎn)*, Pogostemonis/Agastaches Herba *(huò xiāng)*, Nelumbinis Folium *(hé yè)*, and Platycodi Radix *(jié gěng)*. Not only does this method disperse dampness and heat from the body through the skin, it also promotes urination and provides an avenue for both dampness and heat to exit the body through the urine.

3. *Regulate qi circulation with acrid and warm herbs, and dry dampness with bitter and warm herbs.* This method is used for damp-heat in the middle burner, especially when dampness predominates, leading to chest and epigastric distention, abdominal bloating, loose stools or an incomplete feeling after finishing a bowel movement, fatigue, a fuzzy-headed feeling, and a white, yellow, and greasy tongue coating. The herbs used for this method include Pinelliae Rhizoma preparatum *(zhì bàn xià)*, Atractylodis Rhizoma *(cāng zhú)*, Magnoliae officinalis Cortex *(hòu pò)*, Tsaoko Fructus *(cǎo guǒ)*, Amomi Fructus rotundus *(bái dòu kòu)*, Alpiniae katsumadai Semen *(cǎo dòu kòu)*, Arecae Pericarpium *(dà fù pí)*, and Citri reticulatae Pericarpium *(chén pí)*. Those herbs with an acrid flavor and warm nature serve to lift the Spleen qi and eliminate dampness, and those with a bitter flavor and warm nature dry dampness and direct the Stomach qi downward.

4. *Clear heat and dry dampness with bitter and cold herbs.* Like the third method, this one is also used for damp-heat in the middle burner, but in situations where the dampness and heat are present in roughly equal amounts. This condition can lead to a low-grade fever, loose stools with a strong odor and a burning sensation around the anus, dry mouth and thirst, abdominal bloating, and a yellow and greasy tongue coating. The herbs used for this method include Coptidis Rhizoma *(huáng lián)*, Scutellariae Radix *(huáng qín)*, Phellodendri Cortex *(huáng bǎi)*, and Gardeniae Fructus *(zhī zǐ)*.

5. *Leach out dampness with bland herbs.* This method is primarily used for treating damp-heat in the lower burner, and serves to drain the damp-heat from the body through urination. However, regardless of where it is situated in the body, when treating dampness it is always a good idea to use one or two herbs to leach out dampness through urination, which provides an avenue for damp-heat to exit the body. For damp-heat in the lower burner leading to cloudy urine, an incomplete feeling after urination, slow urination, lower abdominal distention,

and a yellow and greasy tongue coating, use Talcum *(huá shí)*, Tetrapanacis Medulla *(tōng cǎo)*, Poria *(fú líng)*, Coicis Semen *(yì yǐ rén)*, Alismatis Rhizoma *(zé xiè)*, Polyporus *(zhū líng)*, and Plantaginis Semen *(chē qián zǐ)*. If heat predominates, use Gardeniae Fructus *(zhī zǐ)*, Lophatheri Herba *(dàn zhú yè)*, and Akebiae Caulis *(mù tōng)*. If dampness predominates, use Dioscoreae hypoglaucae Rhizoma *(bì xiè)*, Pyrrosiae Folium *(shí wéi)*, and Benincasae Semen *(dōng guā zǐ)*.

Besides the five methods noted above that directly treat damp-heat disorders, promoting the circulation of qi is a very important indirect method. Qi stagnation is present to some degree in all damp-heat diseases, because dampness is a viscous and yin pathogenic factor that tends to stagnate the qi more readily than do other pathogenic factors. Once the qi of the Lung, Spleen, Stomach, Liver, Triple Burner, and Bladder is blocked by dampness, the transformation and transportation of water will be impaired, leading to more dampness. This is particularly true when the Spleen is involved. When there is qi stagnation, circulation of the fluids will become sluggish, generating more dampness. Moreover, qi is associated with yang, thus qi stagnation readily produces heat. All of these secondary pathological changes which result from qi stagnation will aggravate the disease. Therefore, one cannot completely eliminate damp-heat if the promotion of qi circulation is neglected in the treatment plan. Herbs used for the purpose of promoting qi circulation in these organs include Platycodi Radix *(jié gěng)*, Armeniacae Semen *(xìng rén)*, Curcumae Radix *(yù jīn)*, Aurantii Fructus immaturus *(zhǐ shí)*, Aurantii Fructus *(zhǐ ké)*, Magnoliae officinalis Cortex *(hòu pò)*, Citri reticulatae Pericarpium *(chén pí)*, Pogostemonis/Agastaches Herba *(huò xiāng)*, Eupatorii Herba *(pèi lán)*, Cyperi Rhizoma *(xiāng fù)*, Aucklandiae Radix *(mù xiāng)*, and Arecae Pericarpium *(dà fù pí)*.

When damp-heat attacks the middle burner, it can affect the digestion of food, leading to retention of food, or Spleen qi deficiency if the patient has suffered from this disorder for a long time. Herbs such as Massa medicata fermentata *(shén qū)*, Hordei Fructus germinatus *(mài yá)*, Gigeriae galli Endothelium corneum *(jī nèi jīn)*, Citri reticulatae viride Pericarpium *(qīng pí)*, and Crataegi Fructus *(shān zhā)* are often used to treat retention of food due to damp-heat in the middle burner, and Coicis Semen *(yì yǐ rén)*, Poria *(fú líng)*, Atractylodis macrocephalae Rhizoma *(bái zhú)*, and Dioscoreae Rhizoma *(shān yào)* to treat Spleen qi deficiency due to damp-heat.

11 Summerheat-Warmth

SUMMERHEAT-WARMTH (暑溫 *shǔ wēn*) is caused by an attack of the summerheat pathogen (暑溫 *shǔ rè*) and is frequently accompanied by dampness. It was first noted by Wu Tang in *Systematic Differentiation of Warm Pathogen Diseases (Wēn bìng tiáo biàn)*, published in 1798. In its early stages, summerheat-warmth (without dampness) is characterized by vigorous fever, irritability, restlessness, thirst, profuse sweating, and an excessive pulse. When it is associated with dampness, symptoms include aversion to cold, chills, fever, headache, heavy sensation in the body, body stiffness, absence of sweating, restlessness, chest distention, and a thin and greasy tongue coating. Summerheat without dampness often injures the fluids and exhausts the qi, stirs up Liver wind and invades the Pericardium. This disease only occurs in the summer.[1] Biomedical diseases such as epidemic encephalitis B, leptospirosis, and sunstroke overlap somewhat with summerheat-warmth in the Chinese diagnostic scheme.

Etiology and Pathology

Summerheat is the exogenous pathogenic factor that gives rise to summerheatwarmth. However, it does so only if the antipathogenic qi is relatively deficient, often as a result of overworking or consumption of too many cold beverages during the summer. When this is the case, the summerheat pathogen readily attacks the body. Summerheat is a type of fire, and fierce and rapid movement characterizes both heat and fire. Thus, when summerheat attacks alone (not in concert with dampness), it gives rise to qi-level Stomach heat with typical early-stage signs including vigorous fever, profuse sweat-

363

ing, thirst, and an excessive pulse. In the chapter on pediatrics from *Case Records as a Guide to Clinical Practice (Lín zhèng zhǐ nán yī àn)*,[2] Ye Gui notes that summerheat first manifests in the *yang ming*. In addition, if dampness is not involved in the attack, there are no signs or symptoms of a protective level disorder.

In the summer, dampness steams up from the earth while summerheat penetrates downward. As a result, summerheat can also attack the body in concert with dampness, resulting in the pattern of summerheat combined with dampness. In addition to the signs and symptoms mentioned above, patients will also show symptoms of dampness such as epigastric distention, generalized heaviness, muscle stiffness, and a greasy tongue coating. In general, summerheat coupled with dampness:

- Progresses at a slower rate than summerheat alone
- May begin in either the protective or qi level.

If the patient eats too many cold foods and/or sleeps outside without protection, cold will attack the exterior, and cold and summerheat will accumulate in the body, leading to a combination of protective and qi level patterns.

Factors for Identifying Summerheat-Warmth

There are three important factors for identifying summerheat-warmth:

1. Summerheat-warmth is a seasonal disease that only occurs in the summer, especially around the solstice. Thus, if a warm pathogen disease occurs in the summer, the practitioner should consider the possibility that it is summerheat-warmth.

2. At an early stage, if dampness is absent, the disease manifests as a typical pattern of Stomach heat with such signs and symptoms as vigorous fever, profuse sweating, thirst, and an excessive pulse.

3. If dampness is involved, the manifestations include fever, aversion to cold, headache, absence of sweating, generalized sensation of heaviness, muscle stiffness, epigastric distention, irritability, and a greasy tongue coating.

After diagnosing the illness as summerheat-warmth, the following points are used to differentiate the specific pattern:

- Are there signs of injury to the fluids such as thirst and a red tongue with little coating?

- Are there signs of exhaustion of qi such as fatigue, profuse sweating, shortness of breath or difficult and shallow breathing, and a scattered pulse?

- Are there signs of dampness such as epigastric distention, nausea, loose stools, heavy sensation in the extremities, muscle stiffness, and a greasy tongue coating?

Progression of Summerheat-Warmth

- *Fire and heat injure the qi as well as the fluids.* When there is no involvement of dampness, summerheat is no exception to this rule. Sharing these qualities, more than other exogenous pathogenic factors, summerheat very often leads to patterns of injury to the fluids and exhaustion of qi, or even collapse of the fluids and qi.

- *In five phase theory, summerheat is related to the Heart.* If the summerheat is not cleared from the qi level, it may quickly progress to the Pericardium, Heart, and the nutritive level, leading to invasion of the Pericardium. In some cases, when the summerheat is particularly fierce, especially when there is no dampness involved, and the antipathogenic qi is relatively weak, summerheat may attack the Pericardium directly, leading to blockage of the Heart by summerheat and sudden loss of consciousness such as sunstroke.

- *Summerheat can invade the vessels and force the blood out of the vessels.* Since summerheat blazes like fire, it will attack the body fiercely, and quickly progress deeper, easily reaching the Heart. Once it invades the vessels, summerheat causes the blood to move rapidly and out of control, resulting in bleeding disorders such as hemoptysis, hematemesis, epistaxis, or maculopapular rashes.

- *At a later stage of the disease, summerheat not only injures the fluids, but the Kidney and Liver yin as well.* This leads to symptoms of malnourishment of the sinews, such as spasm of the muscles and sinews.

- *Summerheat can lead to blockage of the Heart and stirring of Liver wind.* Summerheat gives rise to heat from excess. This heat can attack the Pericardium and Liver, leading to blockage of the Heart and stirring of Liver wind. The patient will exhibit a flat affect, dementia, and aphasia (due to blockage of the Heart spirit) coupled with trembling, stiffness (due to stirring of Liver wind from the excessive heat) or paralysis (due to malnourishment of the sinews resulting from obstruction of the channels by wind-phlegm). However, while this presentation is somewhat similar to that of wind-stroke, in many cases recovery can be relatively quick if the problem is treated in a timely manner.[3]

Treatment Principles

In differentiating summerheat-warmth and determining the principles of treatment, the practitioner must ascertain whether dampness is present. This will affect the course, prognosis, and treatment of these two quite different disorders.

Generally, the treatment principle for summerheat-warmth is to disperse and clear the summerheat. The fluids and the qi must also be protected, especially if there is no dampness. If dampness is involved, every effort should be made to separately resolve dampness and heat. Only after they are separately resolved can heat, as well as dampness, be easily eliminated.

It is critical that the practitioner treat qi level summerheat-warmth patterns immediately in order to prevent the disease from progressing directly to the Pericardium. If there is invasion of the Pericardium or stirring of Liver wind, one must clear summerheat from the Pericardium, open the orifices, cool the Liver, and extinguish the Liver wind. Promoting urination is a good way of eliminating both summerheat and dampness from the body. In the later stages, the practitioner should enrich the yin and tonify the qi, as well as clear the remnants of summer-heat. And if there is obstruction of the channels by wind-phlegm, one should transform the phlegm and remove blood stasis.

In the early seventeenth-century book *Revised and Expanded Complete Treatise on Summerheat Damage (Zēng dìng shāng shǔ quán shū)*, Zhang He-Teng proposed the following treatment methods for summerheat without dampness, which have proven to be very effective:

- For heat from excess in the Stomach, clear the heat from the qi level and vent summerheat with acrid and cool herbs.
- For injured fluids or yin, clear the heat and generate fluids and/or enrich yin with sweet and cold herbs.
- For summerheat that is nearly resolved, leaving extensive injury to the fluids and qi as a result of the initial attack, tonify the qi and generate fluids with sweet and sour herbs. Alternatively, clear heat and generate fluids with sour and bitter herbs.[4]

Differentiation and Treatment of Summerheat-Warmth without Dampness

Summerheat Attacking the Stomach

Manifestations. There are two concurrent aspects to this pattern:

1. *Heat from excess in the Stomach* with vigorous fever, restlessness, irritability, flushed face, labored breathing, significant sweating, red tongue with dry and yellow coating, and a flooding, rapid pulse.

2. *Injury to the fluids and qi* with thirst, slight aversion to cold, slight chills in the upper and/or middle back, and a big but hollow pulse.

NOTE: Two different pulses are possible with this pattern. Clinically, a flooding, big but hollow pulse is rarely seen. Instead, the pulse will reflect injury to the qi either by being hollow, or by the presence of another deficient-type quality such as thin or frail. When these occur the patient will also have slight aversion to cold or slight chills on the upper and/or middle back.

Several of the signs and symptoms listed here are similar to those of other patterns. For example, slight aversion to cold is similar to aversion to cold from an attack of exterior wind-cold. Slight chills on the upper and/or middle back is similar to the chilled back associated with yang deficiency. A flushed face is similar to malar flush, which occurs with yin deficiency. These somewhat subtle differences are important and must be recognized. In general, the accompanying signs and symptoms will make the differentiation clear.

Slight aversion to cold is not due to wind-cold when it is associated with thirst, irritability, profuse sweating, and a hollow or other deficient pulse. It is due to summerheat in the Stomach and qi level, causing profuse sweating and injuring both the qi (especially the protective qi) and fluids. The treatment for this type of aversion to cold is to clear summerheat from the Stomach. (See Table 11.1.)

For chills on the back, pay attention to the accompanying signs and symptoms. The presence of slight chills on the upper and/or middle back coupled with irritability, thirst, profuse sweating, and a hollow or other deficient pulse indicates that summerheat in the Stomach and qi level is causing profuse sweating, which injures both the qi and fluids. On the other hand, chills on the back associated with listlessness and fatigue, coupled with restless sleep, absence of thirst, and a feeble and weak pulse indicate yang qi deficiency and cold in the Kidney. The treatment principle here is to warm and tonify the Kidney yang. (See Table 11.2.)

Table 11.1	Slight Aversion to Cold vs. Aversion to Cold	
Pathology	**Signs and Symptoms**	**Treatment Principles**
▶ SLIGHT AVERSION TO COLD		
Heat from excess in Stomach and qi level causes profuse sweating that injures both the qi (especially protective qi) and fluids; interior heat pattern	Restlessness, thirst, and a flooding, big, but hollow pulse	Clear summerheat from the Stomach in the qi level
▶ AVERSION TO COLD		
Obstruction of protective qi; exterior cold pattern	Headache, little or no sweating, floating pulse	Release the exterior signs and symptoms

Table 11.2	Slight Chills on the Back vs. Chills on the Back	
Pathology	**Signs and Symptoms**	**Treatment Principles**
▶ SLIGHT CHILLS ON THE BACK		
Heat from excess in the Stomach and qi level causes profuse sweating that injures both the qi and fluids—interior heat	Restlessness, thirst, and a flooding, big but hollow pulse	Clear summerheat from the Stomach in the qi level
▶ CHILLS ON THE BACK		
Deficiency of Kidney yang and excess yin—interior cold	Listlessness with a desire for sleep, no thirst, and a feeble, weak pulse	Warm and tonify Kidney yang

The pathway of the foot *yang ming* Stomach channel begins on the face. It is therefore possible for a patient with summerheat in the Stomach to present with a flushed face coupled with thirst, irritability, and a flooding pulse. This is quite different from malar flush, which is caused by heat from Kidney yin deficiency. The latter condition presents with evening fever, a deep-red tongue with less than normal coating, and a thin, rapid pulse. (See Table 11.3.)

Pathology. Summerheat attacking the Stomach with injury to the fluids and qi.

Table 11.3	Flushed Face vs. Malar Flush	
Pathology	**Signs and Symptoms**	**Treatment Principles**
▶ FLUSHED FACE		
Upward steaming of summerheat from the Stomach in the qi level	Thirst, restlessness, flooding pulse	Clear summerheat from the Stomach in the qi level
▶ MALAR FLUSH		
Exhaustion of Kidney yin leading to floating heat from deficiency	Evening fever, deep-red tongue with less than normal coating, thin and rapid pulse	Enrich Kidney yin and clear heat from deficiency

NOTE: In this pattern, summerheat is the embodiment of pure heat. It therefore readily injures the qi and fluids. Due to the intensity of the heat, not only are the qi and fluids injured, but the spirit of the Heart is also disturbed, leading to irritability.

Treatment principles. Clear and disperse summerheat, tonify the qi, and generate fluids.

Formula No. 1:
For an attack on the Stomach by summerheat without injury to the fluids and qi, use:

> **WHITE TIGER DECOCTION** *(bái hǔ tāng)*
>
> See Chapter 7 for more information about this formula.

Because summerheat is such a fierce pathogen and attacks the Stomach, it readily injures the qi and fluids. To prevent this, as early as possible use a large dosage of Gypsum fibrosum *(shí gāo)* and Anemarrhenae Rhizoma *(zhī mǔ)* to disperse and clear the summerheat. You can use up to 60g of Gypsum fibrosum *(shí gāo)* and 15g of Anemarrhenae Rhizoma *(zhī mǔ)*. In addition, Setariae (Oryzae) Fructus germinatus *(gǔ yá)* and Lablab Semen album *(bái biǎn dòu)* can be added to protect the Stomach and Spleen.

Formula No. 2:
For an attack on the Stomach by summerheat when both the fluids and qi have been injured, use:

> **WHITE TIGER PLUS GINSENG DECOCTION** *(bái hǔ jiā rén shēn tāng)*
>
> SOURCE: *Systematic Differentiation of Warm Pathogen Diseases*
>
> Gypsum fibrosum *(shí gāo)* 30g
> Nonglutinous rice *(gěng mǐ)* 9g
> Ginseng Radix *(rén shēn)* 9g
> Anemarrhenae Rhizoma *(zhī mǔ)* 15g
> Honey-toasted Glycyrrhizae Radix preparata *(zhì gān cǎo)* 9g

ANALYSIS OF FORMULA: White Tiger Decoction *(bái hǔ tāng)* is an effective formula for dispersing and clearing heat from the Stomach. According to *Discussion of Cold Damage (Shāng hán lùn)*, Ginseng Radix *(rén shēn)* is an important herb for tonifying the qi, generating fluids, and calming the spirit. The difference between this formula and that of the same name in *Discussion of Cold Damage* is an increase in the dosage of Anemarrhenae Rhizoma *(zhī mǔ)* to 15g. This is because the condition here has relatively more heat.

MODIFICATIONS: The basic formula can be modified as follows:

- Herbs can be added that disperse and clear summerheat, such as Lonicerae Flos *(jīn yín huā)*, Forsythiae Fructus *(lián qiào)*, and Lophatheri Herba *(dàn zhú yè)*.

- For some associated dampness (epigastric distention, nausea and vomiting, and a greasy tongue coating) coupled with slight aversion to cold, add the aromatic herbs Pogostemonis/Agastaches Herba *(huò xiāng)* and Eupatorii Herba *(pèi lán)* to transform the dampness.

- For summerheat that attacks the protective level as well as the qi level (sore throat, headache, body aches, and absence of sweating), add Moslae Herba *(xiāng rú)*, Sojae Semen preparatum *(dàn dòu chǐ)*, and Forsythiae Fructus *(lián qiào)* to eliminate the summerheat from the exterior.

- For stirring of Liver wind (severe headache and slight trembling of the limbs), add Saigae tataricae Cornu *(líng yáng jiǎo)*, Uncariae Ramulus cum Uncis *(gōu téng)*, Chrysanthemi Flos *(jú huā)*, and Cicadae Periostracum *(chán tuì)* to cool the Liver and extinguish Liver wind.

- For summerheat that injures the qi and fluids and leads to rebellion of Stomach qi (nausea, burping, hiccup, or vomiting), use Lophatherum and Gypsum Decoction *(zhú yè shí gāo tāng)*.[5]

Case study: White Tiger plus Ginseng Decoction *(bái hǔ jiā rén shēn tāng)*

First visit. After returning home from a site-seeing trip, the patient, a 35-year-old male, felt extremely tired. The following morning he suffered from head and body aches, aversion to cold, fever, spontaneous sweating, and thirst. He was treated by a traditional Chinese physician who prescribed herbs to release an exterior pattern. However, after taking the herbal formula, his symptoms worsened. He experienced a severe headache marked by intense stabbing pain. He also had a fever, sweating, and irritability, and lost consciousness. His pulse was big and flooding, and he had a thin, white tongue coating. His temperature was 38.5°C. At this point the diagnosis was changed to attack by summerheat and injury to the fluids due to mistaken induction of sweating. The treatment principles were to clear summerheat, slightly tonify the qi, and support the fluids. The formula selected was a modified version of White Tiger plus Ginseng Decoction *(bái hǔ jiā rén shēn tāng)* with the following ingredients and dosage: Gypsum fibrosum *(shí gāo)* (50g), Anemarrhenae Rhizoma *(zhī mǔ)* (20g), Codonopsis Radix *(dǎng shēn)* (40g), Honey-toasted Glycyrrhizae Radix preparata *(zhì gān cǎo)* (15g), nonglutinous rice *(gěng mǐ)* (30g), and Ophiopogonis Radix *(mài mén dōng)* (20g).

Second visit. After taking two packets of herbs, the headache, aversion to cold, and fever were much reduced. The sweating, irritability, thirst, and loss of consciousness were gone. The tongue body was slightly pale with a thin and white coating. The temperature had decreased to 37.2°C. The patient had good energy and appetite. He took another three packets of the herbs, after which all of his signs and symptoms were resolved.[6]

INJURY TO THE FLUIDS AND QI BY SUMMERHEAT

Manifestations. There are two concurrent aspects to this pattern:

1. *Summerheat attacking the qi level* with fever, irritability, yellow urine, and spontaneous sweating.
2. *Summerheat injuring the fluids and qi* with thirst, fatigue, listlessness, shallow breathing, and a weak pulse.

NOTE: Compared with the previous pattern (attack on the Stomach by summer-heat), this pattern exhibits not only severe injury to the qi and fluids of the Stomach, but also injury to the qi of the Lung, as evidenced by the spontaneous sweating and shallow breathing.

Pathology. Constrained summerheat injuring the fluids and qi.

Treatment principles. Clear summerheat, tonify the qi, and generate fluids.

Formula:

WANG'S DECOCTION TO CLEAR SUMMERHEAT AND AUGMENT THE QI *(Wáng shì qīng shǔ yì qì tāng)*
SOURCE: *Warp and Woof of Warm-Heat Pathogen Diseases*[7]
Panacis quinquefolii Radix *(xī yáng shēn)* 9g
Dendrobii Herba *(shí hú)* 9g
Ophiopogonis Radix *(mài mén dōng)*...........................6g
Coptidis Rhizoma *(huáng lián)* 2.4g
Lophatheri Herba *(dàn zhú yè)* 9g
Nelumbinis Caulis *(lián gěng)* 9g
Anemarrhenae Rhizoma *(zhī mǔ)* 9g
Glycyrrhizae Radix *(gān cǎo)* 3g
Nonglutinous rice *(gěng mǐ)* 9g
Citrulli Exocarpium *(xī guā pí)* 12g

(handwritten margin note: years ago used for people who are HIV +)

ANALYSIS OF FORMULA: This formula encompasses the principles of dispersing and clearing summerheat, tonifying the qi, and producing fluids. Citrulli Exocarpium *(xī guā pí)*, Coptidis Rhizoma *(huáng lián)*, Anemarrhenae Rhizoma *(zhī mǔ)*, Nelumbinis Caulis *(lián gěng)*, and Lophatheri Herba *(dàn zhú yè)* disperse and clear summerheat. Both Lophatheri Herba *(dàn zhú yè)* and Citrulli Exocarpium *(xī guā pí)* are important components because they clear heat and promote urination, which is an effective method for draining summerheat from the body. Panacis quinquefolii Radix *(xī yáng shēn)*, Ophiopogonis Radix *(mài mén dōng)*, Dendrobii Herba *(shí hú)*, and nonglutinous rice *(gěng mǐ)* tonify the qi and generate fluids. If Panacis quinquefolii Radix *(xī yáng shēn)* is not available, substitute Glehniae/Adenophorae Radix *(shā shēn)* (60g).

The practitioner must weigh the relative importance of summerheat versus injury to the qi and fluids when modifying the formula. If summerheat is predominant, either:

- Increase the dosage of herbs that clear summerheat, such as Anemarrhenae Rhizoma *(zhī mǔ)*, Citrulli Exocarpium *(xī guā pí)*, and Lophatheri Herba *(dàn zhú yè)*; or

- Add Lonicerae Flos *(jīn yín huā)* and Gypsum fibrosum *(shí gāo)*.

If injury to the qi and fluids is predominant, either:

- Increase the dosage of those herbs that tonify the qi and generate fluids, such as Panacis quinquefolii Radix *(xī yáng shēn)*, Dendrobii Herba *(shí hú)*, Ophiopogonis Radix *(mài mén dōng)*, and nonglutinous rice *(gěng mǐ)*; or

- Add Dioscoreae Rhizoma *(shān yào)* and Glehniae/Adenophorae Radix *(shā shēn)*, and reduce the dosage of Coptidis Rhizoma *(huáng lián)*, since it is bitter and can produce dryness.

MODIFICATIONS: The basic formula can be modified as follows:

- For strong thirst, flushed face, and vigorous fever, add Gypsum fibrosum *(shí gāo)* to enhance the action of the other herbs in dispersing and clearing summerheat.

- For severe injury to the qi and fluids, add more herbs to tonify the qi, such as Ginseng Radix *(rén shēn)* or Astragali Radix *(huáng qí)*. The dosage of Coptidis Rhizoma *(huáng lián)* should be reduced significantly, as too much bitterness will further injure the qi and fluids.

Comparison. Both this formula and White Tiger Plus Ginseng Decoction *(bái hǔ jiā rén shēn tāng)* tonify the antipathogenic qi and eliminate pathogenic factors. That is, they simultaneously clear summerheat, tonify the qi, and generate fluids. However, White Tiger Plus Ginseng Decoction *(bái hǔ jiā rén shēn tāng)* more strongly tonifies qi while this one more strongly generates fluids.

Case study: Wang's Decoction to Clear Summerheat and Augment the Qi
(Wáng shì qīng shǔ yì qì tāng)

First visit. August 20. Two weeks previously, this 38-year-old female patient became exhausted while caring for a sick child. She has since felt a sense of distention in her head, dizziness, aversion to cold, fever, and sweating. In addition, her whole body has felt achey, especially the lower back (she has a history of lumbar osteophytes). Although she was hungry, she did not want to eat. She yawns frequently. After taking some Western medicine, the aversion to cold disappeared. But she still had a fever (38°C) and continued to sweat. She also developed chest distention and shortness of breath with a tendency to exhale strongly. Her soles and palms felt hot and her stomach felt empty. She had frequent belching, and scanty, yellow urine that burned. She had a red tongue with a slightly yellow coating that was thick at the root and peeled off at the front. Her pulse was thin and frail. The diagnosis was attack of summerheat that had injured the qi. The prescription was a modified version of Wang's Decoction to Clear Summerheat and Augment the Qi *(Wáng shì qīng shǔ yì qì tāng)*: Ginseng Radix *(rén shēn)* (4.5g), Ophiopogonis Radix *(mài mén dōng)* (10g), Anemarrhenae Rhizoma *(zhī mǔ)* (10g), Coptidis Rhizoma *(huáng lián)* (4.5g), Schisandrae Fructus *(wǔ wèi zǐ)* (10g), Nelumbinis Folium *(hé yè)*(10g), Dendrobii Herba *(shí hú)* (10g), Talcum *(huá shí)* (6g), Glycyrrhizae Radix *(gān cǎo)* (6g), Coicis Semen *(yì yǐ rén)* (18g), Citrulli Exocarpium *(xī guā pí)* (10g), Lonicerae Flos *(jīn yín huā)* (10g), and Lablab Semen album *(bái biǎn dòu)*(10g). Three packets of herbs were given to the patient.

Second visit: August 31. After finishing the three packets of herbs, the fever, sweating, hot sensation in the palms and soles, and scanty, yellow, burning urine were gone. Her chest symptoms and empty sensation in the stomach were much reduced, but she still had a poor appetite and occasional belching. Her tongue was slightly red, and the yellow, greasy coating on the root had disappeared. Her pulse was unchanged. She now was occasionally vomiting clear liquids, as the qi deficiency had led to Stomach qi rebellion. A modified version of Ginseng Decoction to Nourish the Stomach *(rén shēn yǎng wèi tāng)*[8] was prescribed: Codonopsis Radix *(dǎng shēn)* (18g), Atractylodis macrocephalae Rhizoma *(bái zhú)* (10g), Poria *(fú líng)* (10g), Amomi Fructus *(shā rén)* (6g), Amomi Fructus rotundus *(bái dòu kòu)* (4.5g), Massa medicata fermentata *(shén qū)* (10g), Hordei Fructus germinatus *(mài yá)* (10g), Citri reticulatae Pericarpium *(chén pí)* (10g), Glycyrrhizae Radix *(gān cǎo)* (1.5g), nonglutinous rice *(gěng mǐ)* (30g), and Terra flava usta *(zào xīn tǔ)* (60g). Three packets of herbs were given to the patient.

Third visit: September 3. After finishing the three packets of herbs, she no longer vomited. The shortness of breath with a tendency to exhale deeply, along with the empty sensation in her stomach, were also gone. She still had chest distention, poor appetite, and occasional belching. Her tongue was pale and her pulse was thin. A modified version of Six Gentlemen Decoction *(liù jūn zǐ tāng)*[9] was prescribed to tonify the Spleen qi, resolve phlegm, and direct the Stomach qi downward: Codonopsis Radix *(dǎng shēn)* (24g), Poria *(fú líng)* (18g), Pinelliae Rhizoma preparatum *(zhì bàn xià)* (10g), Atractylodis macrocephalae Rhizoma *(bái zhú)* (10g), Glycyrrhizae Radix *(gān cǎo)* (3g), Citri reticulatae Pericarpium *(chén pí)* (6g), Inulae Flos *(xuán fù huā)* (10g), Haematitum *(dài zhě shí)* (15g), Zingiberis Rhizoma recens *(shēng jiāng)* (2.4g), and Jujubae Fructus *(dà zǎo)* (2 pieces). After taking four packets of these herbs, all remaining signs and symptoms had resolved.[10]

IMMINENT COLLAPSE OF FLUIDS AND QI

Manifestations. There are three concurrent aspects to this pattern:

1. *Qi collapse* with persistent sweating following the resolution of a fever, and a pulse that feels big at the superficial level, but disappears on even slight finger pressure (this is one definition of a scattered pulse).

2. *Imminent collapse of Lung qi* with short, shallow, and difficult breathing.

3. *Injury to the fluids* with thirst, dry throat, and a red tongue and lips.

NOTE: This pattern is not as severe as that of collapse of yang qi. However, if it is not treated promptly and correctly, it can progress to collapse of yang qi.

There are two types of persistent sweating, one of which belongs to the category of cold damage and the other to the category of warm pathogen disease. Persistent sweating due to collapse of yang qi in disorders caused by cold will be accompanied by cold extremities and a feeble pulse. For these disorders, the practitioner should restore the yang. Persistent sweating in warm pathogen diseases is caused by extreme exhaustion of the qi and fluids, leading to an imminent collapse of both the qi and yin. This will be accompanied by shortness of breath or shallow breathing, thirst, dry throat, and a pale tongue with less coating. For these disorders, one should tonify the qi, enrich the yin, and preserve the yin and qi. (See Table 11.4.)

Pathology. Exhausted fluids and qi which are on the verge of collapse.

NOTE: The pathological changes seen in this pattern occur after the summerheat, which has caused significant damage to the qi and fluids, has been dispelled. This is strictly a condition of deficiency, without any signs or symptoms of summerheat. Generally speaking, the disappearance of fever is a good sign because it indicates that the warm-heat pathogen is gone. The abatement of fever in this pattern occurs quickly and dramatically, but the sweating, instead of gradually ceasing, persists. Persistent sweating not only injures the fluids, but the qi as well. The sweating, together with the weakened

Table 11.4	Persistent Sweating in Cold Damage vs. Warm Pathogen Diseases		
Pathology	**Signs and Symptoms**	**Treatment Principles**	**Formulas**
▶ COLD DAMAGE			
Exterior collapse of yang qi	Cold extremities, feeble pulse	Restore yang qi and arrest the collapse	Ginseng and Aconite Accessory Root Decoction (*shēn fù tāng*)
▶ WARM PATHOGEN DISEASES			
Extreme exhaustion of qi and fluids with imminent collapse	Short, shallow, and labored breathing, thirst, dry throat, pale tongue with less coating	Tonify the qi, enrich the yin, and preserve the yin and qi	Generate the Pulse Powder (*shēng mài sǎn*)

fluids and qi, can lead to a vicious cycle: the more one sweats, the greater the damage to the fluids and qi; and the more severe the qi deficiency, the worse the sweating will be.

Treatment principles. Tonify the qi, enrich the yin, and preserve the yin and qi to prevent collapse of qi and fluids.

Formula:

GENERATE THE PULSE POWDER *(shēng mài sǎn)*

SOURCE: *Origins of Medicine*[11]

Ginseng Radix *(rén shēn)* 9g
Ophiopogonis Radix *(mài mén dōng)* 6g
Schisandrae Fructus *(wǔ wèi zǐ)* 3g

ANALYSIS OF FORMULA: Generate the Pulse Powder *(shēng mài sǎn)* is a key formula for dealing with emergency conditions due to the collapse of qi and fluids. The practitioner can prevent the collapse of yang qi by enriching and conserving the yin and fluids, which in turn will help maintain the yang. With their sour and sweet flavors, Ophiopogonis Radix *(mài mén dōng)* and Schisandrae Fructus *(wǔ wèi zǐ)* produce and preserve the yin and fluids. Ginseng Radix *(rén shēn)* tonifies the source qi, which can stop the sweating. However, one must *not* use this formula where there is summerheat with dampness because the sour and sweet flavors from these herbs will encourage the retention of dampness in the body. If summerheat is still present, another formula to clear and disperse summerheat must be administered at the same time.

In China this formula is available both as an oral mixture and as an injection. For best results, it is important that the ratio of herbs in this formula be maintained. Even though it varies from the original text, the correct ratio of Ginseng Radix *(rén shēn)* to Ophiopogonis Radix *(mài mén dōng)* to Schisandrae Fructus *(wǔ wèi zǐ)* is now thought to be 1:1:0.5.[12]

MODIFICATIONS: The basic formula can be modified as follows:

- For persistent summerheat, use herbs like Gypsum fibrosum *(shí gāo)*, Anemarrhenae Rhizoma *(zhī mǔ)*, Lonicerae Flos *(jīn yín huā)*, and Forsythiae Fructus *(lián qiào)* to simultaneously clear and disperse summerheat.

- For treating the underlying disease that has progressed to collapse of yang qi, add Aconiti Radix lateralis preparata *(zhì fù zǐ)*, Fossilia Ossis Mastodi *(lóng gǔ)*, and Ostreae Concha *(mǔ lì)* to this formula, or use Ginseng, Aconite Accessory Root, Dragon Bone and Oyster Shell Decoction *(shēn fù lóng mù tāng)*[13] as a substitute for the formula.

ADMINISTRATION: According to Wu Tang, one should continue to administer this formula until the patient's pulse is no longer scattered.

Case study: Generate the Pulse Powder *(shēng mài sǎn)*

First visit: May 20. This 27-year-old female patient suffered from a cough with yellow, viscous sputum since February. She now feels very tired, and very hot at night. In addition, she has dribbling urination, urinates two to three times a night, has a strong thirst for cold beverages, headache over the temples, can be agitated, and dreams excessively. Her tongue had a red tip with purple edges, and reduced coating in the center. Her pulse was rapid and thin, and wiry on the left. The diagnosis was Lung and Stomach yin deficiency with Kidney qi deficiency. She was given a modified version of Generate the Pulse Powder *(shēng mài sǎn)* to tonify qi and nourish yin: Ginseng Radix *(rén shēn)* (15g), Ophiopogonis Radix *(mài mén dōng)* (12g), Schisandrae Fructus *(wǔ wèi zǐ)* (12g), and Rubi Fructus *(fù pén zǐ)* (15g). Three packets of herbs were given to the patient. She was instructed to cook the decoction so that each packet would last two days.

Second visit: May 27. Her energy was very good, there was no more urination at night, and the dribbling had diminished. She was no longer hot at night, but still had a thirst for cold beverages. There was only a slight headache over the temples. She was able to relax, and slept well. The tip of the tongue was red, and there was a slight yellow coating, reduced in the center. Her left pulse was wiry and thin, and her right pulse was wiry and slippery in the right distal and middle positions, and thin and wiry in the proximal position. The same basic treatment was continued, but Panacis quinquefolii Radix *(xī yáng shēn)* was substituted for Ginseng Radix *(rén shēn)*, as there was quite a bit of interior heat and the improvement in the qi had been more substantial than the improvement in the yin. Three packets of herbs were given to the patient.

Third visit: June 3. No change in the dribbling of urine. In addition, she ate very spicy Thai food two days before, which precipitated a mild sensation of heat at night, loose stools, and a return of the fatigue. Her tongue was tender and sore with a bright red tip and a slightly yellow coating that was reduced over the middle. Her pulse was slightly rapid, thin on the left, and wiry on the right. The previous formula was prescribed, but modified because now there was more heat due to eating the very spicy food: Asparagi Radix *(tiān mén dōng)* (12g), Gypsum fibrosum *(shí gāo)* (12g), and Rehmanniae Radix *(shēng dì huáng)* (12g) were added, and the dosage of Rubi Fructus *(fù pén zǐ)* was reduced to 9g. One packet of herbs was given to the patient.

Fourth visit: Her energy was excellent. There was no more dribbling of urine, she slept soundly, the hot sensations had disappeared, and her stools and thirst were normal. The pulse was slightly rapid, thin on the left, while submerged and wiry at the distal and middle positions, and thin at the right proximal position. The tongue was pink with a slightly yellow coating. The previous formula was again prescribed, but Gypsum fibrosum *(shí gāo)* and Rubi Fructus *(fù pén zǐ)* where removed, and Setariae (Oryzae) Fructus germinatus *(gǔ yá)* (9g) was added.[14]

INVASION OF THE PERICARDIUM BY SUMMERHEAT

Manifestations. There are three concurrent aspects to this pattern:

1. *A history of prolonged exposure to intense heat.* Examples include walking for a long distance under direct sunlight, playing for a long period under the hot rays of the sun, or working in front of a furnace in a steel factory.

2. *Invasion of the Pericardium by summerheat and blockage of the Heart* with loss of consciousness, delirium, and a stiff tongue with difficulty speaking or sudden coma and cold extremities.

3. *General signs and symptoms caused by summerheat* such as fever, irritability, labored breathing, yellow urine, and a rapid pulse.

Pathology. Summerheat invading the Pericardium, leading to blockage of the Heart.

Treatment principles. Clear summerheat from the Pericardium and open the orifices.

Emergency treatment. Under these conditions, the practitioner should:

- Carry the patient to a location where there is fresh and cool air.
- Needle LI-11 *(qū chí)*, GV-26 *(rén zhōng)*, PC-3 *(qū zé)*, and M-UE-1 *(shí xuān)*, or bleed BL-40 *(wěi zhōng)* or M-UE-1 *(shí xuān)*.

Here LI-11 *(qū chí)*, GV-26 *(rén zhōng)*, and M-UE-1 *(shí xuān)* are used to clear heat and open the orifices. PC-3 *(qū zé)* and BL-40 *(wěi zhōng)* are used to drain summerheat from the Pericardium.

Formulas:
Clear the Nutritive Level Decoction *(qīng yíng tāng)*, Calm the Palace Pill with Cattle Gallstone *(ān gōng niú huáng wán)*, Greatest Treasure Special Pill *(zhì bǎo dān)*, or Purple Snow Special Pill *(zǐ xuě dān)*. See Chapter 8 for further discussion of these formulas.

MODIFICATIONS: For phlegm with sounds of sputum in the throat, add *Bambusae Concretio silicea (tiān zhú huáng)*, Bambusae Succus *(zhú lì)*, Trichosanthis Pericarpium *(guā lóu pí)*, and Arisaema cum Bile *(dǎn nán xīng)* to transform the phlegm. Make a decoction from these herbs and take it with the above pills.

STIRRING OF LIVER WIND BY EXCESS SUMMERHEAT

Manifestations. There are three concurrent aspects to this pattern:

1. *General signs and symptoms of summerheat* such as high fever, bright-red tongue with dry, yellow coating, and a wiry, rapid pulse.

2. *Stirring of Liver wind* with convulsion, rigidity of the trunk, trismus, and opisthotonos.

3. *Blockage of the Heart by phlegm and fire* with loss of consciousness.

NOTE: This pattern is seen most often in children with weak constitutions. It is almost identical to the pattern of stirring of internal wind due to heat from excess in the Liver. Both are caused by the stirring of Liver wind as a result of extreme heat, and the treatment principles are almost the same. One difference is that the pattern here occurs in the summer, while the latter pattern occurs in the spring. Since this pattern results from internal wind that occurs in the summer, it is also called summerheat wind (暑風 *shǔ fēng*) or summerheat seizures (暑癇 *shǔ xián*). A second difference between them is that the condition of blockage of the Heart spirit in this pattern is more severe than in the pattern of stirring of internal wind due to heat from excess in the Liver. This is because summerheat is closely related to the Heart. A third difference is that the pattern here can either present gradually in the progression of summerheat-warmth, or it may have an acute onset due to sudden attack on the Pericardium by summerheat, leading to stirring of Liver wind. (This is especially common in children.) By contrast, the latter pattern can only have an acute onset.

Pathology. Summerheat leading to stirring of Liver wind.

Treatment principles. Clear summerheat and extinguish Liver wind.

Formula:

Antelope Horn and Uncaria Decoction *(líng jiǎo gōu téng tāng)*

This pattern is caused by the stirring of Liver wind as a result of extreme heat, and this formula is suitable for clearing summerheat and extinguishing Liver wind. See Chapter 8 for further discussion of this formula.

MODIFICATIONS: The basic formula can be modified as follows:

- For any heat from excess in the Stomach, add Gypsum fibrosum *(shí gāo)* and Anemarrhenae Rhizoma *(zhī mǔ)*.

- For heat that has combined with dry stool in the Large Intestine, add Rhei Radix et Rhizoma *(dà huáng)* and Natrii Sulfas *(máng xiāo)*.

- For delirium and convulsions, which reflects blockage of the Heart spirit, use Purple Snow Special Pill *(zǐ xuě dān)*.[15]

- For phlegm (manifested here as a gurgling sound in the throat), add Arisaema cum Bile *(dǎn nán xīng)*, Bambusae Concretio silicea *(tiān zhú huáng)*, and Bambusae Succus *(zhú lì)*.

- For convulsions that are hard to control with this formula, add Scorpio *(quán xiē)*, Scolopendra *(wú gōng)*, and Pheretima *(dì lóng)* to enhance its action in extinguishing Liver wind and relieving the convulsions.

Invasion of the Blood Level by Summerheat

Manifestations. There are two concurrent aspects to this pattern:

1. *Out of control bleeding due to fire and toxin* with maculopapular rashes, hematemesis, and epistaxis. The blood is purple or dark in color.

2. *Blockage of the Heart by summerheat* with fever, irritability, coma, and delirium.

NOTE: Generally in warm pathogen diseases, blood that is purple or dark in color indicates that heat has turned into fire and toxin and forced blood out of the vessels. When the condition is severe, the patient may suffer from stirring of Liver wind, which can lead to convulsion or opisthotonos. Compared with the previous pattern, this one is much more severe.

Maculas caused by intense heat in both the qi and blood levels are discussed in Chapters 5, 7, and 8. There are several important differences in the pathology and treatment of the maculas seen in this pattern and in the pattern of intense heat in both the qi and blood levels, which are outlined in Table 11.5.

Pathology. Summerheat transforming into fire and toxin which leads to uncontrolled bleeding and blockage of the Heart.

Treatment principles. Cool the blood, resolve toxicity, clear summerheat from the Heart, and open the orifices.

Table 11.5	Maculas Associated with Invasion of Blood Level by Summerheat vs. Intense Heat in Both Qi and Blood Levels		
Pathology	**Signs and Symptoms**	**Treatment**	**Formulas**
▶ INVASION OF BLOOD LEVEL BY SUMMERHEAT			
Summerheat transforms into fire and toxin, leading to bleeding	Fever, maculas that are purplish and black, restlessness, coma, delirium	Cool the blood, resolve toxicity, clear summerheat from the Pericardium, and open the orifices	Magical Rhinoceros Special Pill (*shén xī dān*) and Calm the Palace Pill with Cattle Gallstone (*ān gōng niú huáng wán*)
▶ INTENSE HEAT IN BOTH THE QI AND BLOOD LEVELS			
Intense heat in both the qi and blood levels forces blood out of the vessels	Vigorous fever, restlessness, thirst, maculas that are red	Clear heat from the qi and blood levels	Modified Jade Woman Decoction (*jiā jiǎn yù nǚ tāng*), Transform Maculas Decoction (*huà bān tāng*), or Clear Epidemics and Overcome Toxin Drink (*qīng wēn bài dú yǐn*)

Formula No. 1:

> ### MAGICAL RHINOCEROS SPECIAL PILL *(shén xī dān)*[16]
>
> SOURCE: *Warp and Woof of Warm-Heat Pathogen Diseases*

Rhinocerotis Cornu *(xī jiǎo)* 180g

Acori tatarinowii Rhizoma *(shí chāng pǔ)* 180g

Scutellariae Radix *(huáng qín)* 180g

Forsythiae Fructus *(lián qiào)* 300g

Rehmanniae Radix *(shēng dì huáng)* 500g

Isatidis/Baphicacanthis Radix *(bǎn lán gēn)* 270g

Scrophulariae Radix *(xuán shēn)* 210g

Trichosanthis Radix *(tiān huā fěn)* 120g

Arnebiae Radix/Lithospermi Radix *(zǐ cǎo)* 120g

Lonicerae Flos *(jīn yín huā)* 500g

Sojae Semen preparatum *(dàn dòu chǐ)* 240g

Succus Faecalis Aureus *(jīn zhī)* [17] 300g

ANALYSIS OF FORMULA: Rhinocerotis Cornu *(xī jiǎo)*, Lonicerae Flos *(jīn yín huā)*, Forsythiae Fructus *(lián qiào)*, Scrophulariae Radix *(xuán shēn)*, Succus Faecalis Aureus *(jīn zhī)*, Scutellariae Radix *(huáng qín)*, Isatidis/Baphicacanthis Radix *(bǎn lán gēn)*, Rehmanniae Radix *(shēng dì huáng)*, Arnebiae Radix/Lithospermi Radix *(zǐ cǎo)*, and Sojae Semen preparatum *(dàn dòu chǐ)* collectively cool the blood and treat the maculopapular rash. Trichosanthis Radix *(tiān huā fěn)* generates fluids. Acori tatarinowii Rhizoma *(shí chāng pǔ)*, an aromatic herb, opens the orifices.

This formula is effective at resolving toxicity. This is important because once the heat is cleared and the toxicity resolved, blood circulation and the spirit of the Heart will return to normal. Among the twelve herbs in this formula, eight resolve toxicity: Bubali Cornu *(shuǐ niú jiǎo)*, Scutellariae Radix *(huáng qín)*, Forsythiae Fructus *(lián qiào)*, Succus Faecalis Aureus *(jīn zhī)*, Isatidis/Baphicacanthis Radix *(bǎn lán gēn)*, Scrophulariae Radix *(xuán shēn)*, Arnebiae Radix/Lithospermi Radix *(zǐ cǎo)*, and Lonicerae Flos *(jīn yín huā)*. However, this formula does not effectively open the orifices. Calm the Palace Pill with Cattle Gallstone *(ān gōng niú huáng wán)* is therefore added for this purpose.

Formula No. 2:

> ### CALM THE PALACE PILL WITH CATTLE GALLSTONE *(ān gōng niú huáng wán)*

See Chapter 7 for further discussion of this formula.

MODIFICATIONS: The basic formula can be modified as follows:

- For convulsion and opisthotonos, add Saigae tataricae Cornu *(líng yáng jiǎo)* and Uncariae Ramulus cum Uncis *(gōu téng)*, or Stop Spasms Powder *(zhǐ jìng sǎn)*,[18] which contains Scorpio *(quán xiē)* and Scolopendra *(wú gōng)*.

- For phlegm (manifested here in a gurgling sound in the throat), add Bambusae Concretio silicea *(tiān zhú huáng)*, Bambusae Succus *(zhú lì)*, and Arisaema cum Bile *(dǎn nán xīng)*.

- For concurrent signs and symptoms of heat from excess in the qi level, add herbs that treat the qi level pattern (e.g., Gypsum *[shí gāo]*) or a formula like Clear Epidemics and Overcome Toxin Drink *(qīng wēn bài dú yǐn)*, discussed in Chapter 8. It should be noted that although some of the herbs in Magical Rhinoceros Special Pill *(shén xī dān)* address heat in the qi level, the formula is not sufficiently strong under these conditions.

Case study: Magical Rhinoceros Special Pill *(shén xī dān)*

First visit: July 29. This 19-year-old male patient had a long-standing appetite for spicy food and a history of constrained fire with episodes of hemoptysis. During a recent bout of hot weather, the patient had another attack of coughing up blood. He self-treated with powdered Notoginseng Radix *(sān qī)* dissolved in yellow wine. However, this only aggravated the problem, and he was now coughing up to a bowl of deep-red blood, and had a high fever. He looked tired and had trouble keeping his eyes open. His pulse was hollow and the body of the tongue was red. The diagnosis was summerheat provoking fire from constraint, which forced blood out of the vessels. The principles of treatment were to clear the summerheat, cool the blood, and stop the bleeding. Magical Rhinoceros Special Pill *(shén xī dān)* with other herbs were prescribed: one pill was ground into a powder and taken with a decoction made from fresh Rehmanniae Radix recens *(xiān dì huáng)* (18g), dry-fried Paeoniae Radix alba *(chǎo bái sháo)* (9g), charred Moutan Cortex *(mǔ dān pí tàn)* (3g), Agrimoniae Herba *(xiān hè cǎo)* (30g), and Imperatae Rhizoma *(bái máo gēn)* (60g). A packet of herbs was given to the patient.

Second visit: After finishing the herbs, the fever and bleeding were gone. His pulse was moderate in the distal and middle positions, and wiry and tight over LU-5 *(chǐ zé)*. His tongue was red with a thin coating. The treatment plan was altered to enriching the yin and cooling the blood: Rehmanniae Radix *(shēng dì huáng)* (30g), Rehmanniae Radix preparata *(shú dì huáng)* (30g), fresh Rehmanniae Radix *(xiān dì huáng)* (30g), Scrophulariae Radix *(xuán shēn)* (15g), Glehniae/Adenophorae Radix *(shā shēn)* (15g), Asparagi Radix *(tiān mén dōng)* (15g), Ophiopogonis Radix *(mài mén dōng)*

(15g), Imperatae Rhizoma *(bái máo gēn)* (30g), Agrimoniae Herba *(xiān hè cǎo)* (30g), and Ziziphi spinosae Semen *(suān zǎo rén)* (24g). Two packets of herbs were given to the patient.[19]

Injury to the Heart and Kidney by Summerheat

Manifestations. There are two concurrent aspects to this pattern:

1. *Hyperactivity of overabundant Heart heat* with a hot sensation in the chest, restlessness, irritability, and a bright-red tongue with a dry and yellow coating.

2. *Injury to the yin of the Liver and Kidney* with severe thirst, numbness in the extremities, and a rapid and thin pulse. The numbness in this pattern results from malnourishment of the sinews due to yin deficiency of the Liver and Kidney.

NOTE: This pattern is very common in the later stage of summerheat-warmth. Frequently, numbness is caused by obstruction of the channels and collaterals by phlegm. However, in this pattern there are no signs or symptoms of phlegm, such as a thick or greasy tongue coating. Rather, there is injury to the yin of the Liver and Kidney with such signs and symptom as severe thirst, dry tongue coating, and a thin, rapid pulse.

Pathology. Summerheat injuring the Liver and Kidney yin leading to disharmony between the Heart and Kidney. This in turn leads to failure of the Kidney yin to enrich the Heart coupled with malnourishment of the sinews.

NOTE: Normally, the fire (or yang) of the Heart should warm the water (or yin) of the Kidney. This prevents cold from accumulating in the Kidney. In turn, the water in the Kidney should balance the fire of the Heart in order to prevent hyperactivity of Heart fire. This natural and healthy state is called [proper] communication between the Heart and Kidney. However, when summerheat invades the Heart and Kidney, it can cause the Heart yang to become more active, which will injure Kidney yin. This will lead to failure of the Kidney yin to balance the Heart yang, resulting in disharmony between the Heart and Kidney.

Treatment principles. Clear heat from the Heart and enrich the Liver and Kidney yin.

Formula:

Coptis and Mume Decoction *(lián méi tang)*

SOURCE: *Systematic Differentiation of Warm Pathogen Diseases*

Coptidis Rhizoma *(huáng lián)* 6g

Mume Fructus *(wū méi)* 9g

Ophiopogonis Radix *(mài mén dōng)* 9g

Rehmanniae Radix *(shēng dì huáng)* 9g

Asini Corii Colla *(ē jiāo)* 6g

ANALYSIS OF FORMULA: In this pattern there is a one-to-one correspondence be-tween injury to the Kidney yin and hyperactivity of the Heart yang: the more the yin is injured, the more hyperactive the yang becomes, and vice versa. Coptis and Mume Decoction *(lián méi tang)* concurrently treats both the Heart and Kidney. It clears heat and drains fire from the Heart while enriching the Kidney and Liver yin.

Coptidis Rhizoma *(huáng lián)* and Mume Fructus *(wū méi)*, with their bitter and sour flavors (respectively), clear heat from the Heart. Rehmanniae Radix *(shēng dì huáng)*, Ophiopogonis Radix *(mài mén dōng)*, Asini Corii Colla *(ē jiāo)*, and Mume Fructus *(wū méi)*, with their sweet and sour flavors, enrich the yin of the Liver and Kidney. In this way, the formula adjusts and harmonizes the relationship between the Heart and the Kidney. In addition, the formula enriches the Liver yin in order to moist-en the sinews, which alleviates the thirst, restlessness, irritability, and numbness.

Comparison. This formula is actually a modified form of Coptis and Ass-Hide Gelatin Decoction *(huáng lián ē jiāo tāng)*, discussed in Chapter 8. Both formulas treat dis-harmony between the Heart and Kidney. However, Coptis and Ass-Hide Gelatin Decoction *(huáng lián ē jiāo tāng)* combines Coptidis Rhizoma *(huáng lián)* and Scutellariae Radix *(huáng qín)*, and is effective at clearing heat and draining fire from the Heart. By contrast, Coptis and Mume Decoction *(lián méi tang)* combines Coptidis Rhizoma *(huáng lián)* with Mume Fructus *(wū méi)* to clear heat with their bitter and sour flavors, and combines Mume Fructus *(wū méi)* with Ophiopogonis Radix *(mài mén dōng)* and Rehmanniae Radix *(shēng dì huáng)* to enrich the yin with their sour and sweet flavors. This method is called 'clearing heat with the sour and bitter flavors and enriching yin with the sour and sweet flavors.'

REMNANTS OF HEAT COMBINED WITH OBSTRUCTION OF THE COLLATERALS BY PHLEGM AND BLOOD STASIS

Manifestations. There are four concurrent aspects to this pattern:

1. *Remnants of heat and deficiency of qi and yin* with a low-grade, persistent fever.

2. *Obstruction to the collaterals by phlegm and blood stasis* with rigidity of the limbs.

3. *Phlegm and blood stasis blocking the Heart* with a slow reaction to stimuli, dull affect, and dementia.

4. *Stirring of Liver wind due to Liver yin deficiency* with trembling and spasms of the hands and feet.

Pathology. Remnants of heat combined with obstruction of the collaterals and blockage of the Heart by phlegm and blood stasis, and stirring of Liver wind.

Treatment principles. Eliminate the remnants of heat, transform phlegm, invigorate the collaterals, dispel blood stasis from the collaterals, and extinguish the Liver wind.

Formula:

MODIFIED THREE-SHELL POWDER *(sān jiǎ sǎn jiā jiǎn)*

SOURCE: *Systematic Differentiation of Damp- Heat*[20]

Eupolyphaga/Stelophaga *(tǔ biē chóng)* 9g
Trionycis Carapax *(biē jiǎ)* 12g
Manitis Squama *(chuān shān jiǎ)*[21] 9g
Bupleuri Radix *(chái hú)* 6g
Persicae Semen *(táo rén)* 12g
Bombyx batryticatus *(bái jiāng cán)* 6g

ANALYSIS OF FORMULA: The herbs in this formula can be divided into four groups:

1. Bupleuri Radix *(chái hú)* especially dispels the remnants of heat from the collaterals.

2. Trionycis Carapax *(biē jiǎ)* enriches the yin and extinguishes Liver wind.

3. Persicae Semen *(táo rén)*, in concert with Eupolyphaga/Stelophaga *(tǔ biē chóng)*, removes blood stasis from the collaterals.

4. Bombyx batryticatus *(bái jiāng cán)*, in concert with Manitis Squama *(chuān shān jiǎ)*, disperses the remnants of heat and eliminates phlegm from the collaterals.

MODIFICATIONS: The basic formula can be modified as follows:

• To enhance the action of eliminating the remnants of heat, add Artemisiae annuae Herba *(qīng hāo)*, Cynanchi atrati Radix *(bái wéi)*, and Lycii Cortex *(dì gǔ pí)*.

• To remove phlegm and blood stasis from the channels and collaterals, add Arisaema cum Bile *(dǎn nán xīng)*, Typhonii Rhizoma preparatum *(zhì bái fù zǐ)*, Zaocys *(wū shāo shé)*, Sinapis Semen *(bái jiè zǐ)*, and *Carthami Flos (hóng huā)*.

Differentiation and Treatment of Summerheat Combined with Dampness

SUMMERHEAT AND DAMPNESS COLLECTING INTERNALLY WHILE A COLD PATHOGEN FETTERS THE EXTERIOR

Manifestations. There are two concurrent aspects to this pattern:

1. *Interior collection of summerheat and dampness* with fever, epigastric distention, irritability, and a greasy tongue coating.
2. *Exogenous cold in the exterior* with body aches, chills, aversion to cold, and absence of sweating.

NOTE: This type of pattern is seen mostly in the early stage of summerheat-warmth when the summerheat is associated with dampness. It is initially caused by an attack of summerheat and dampness, and is closely followed by an attack of exogenous cold. The cold is prompted by overexposure to wind.[22] The exogenous cold causes the summerheat with dampness to collect internally. The resulting pattern—chills, aversion to cold, fever, and absence of sweating—is also seen in the *tai yang* pattern due to wind-cold, described in six-stage theory. One can distinguish between them by ascertaining whether there is epigastric distention, irritability, and a greasy tongue coating, all of which are indicative of dampness and summerheat.

Pathology. Summerheat and dampness collecting inside the body, combined with an attack of exogenous cold excess.

Treatment principles. Release the exterior by dispersing exogenous cold, clearing interior summerheat, and transforming dampness.

NOTE: In order to provide a precise and effective treatment, the practitioner must ascertain whether summerheat or exogenous cold predominates, or if they are equally balanced. This determination will influence which of the three formulas listed below is appropriate. Table 11.6 compares the three formulas based on the relative strength of the summerheat and cold.

Formula No. 1:

MOSLA POWDER *(xiāng rú sǎn)*[23]

SOURCE: *Formulary of the Bureau of Medicines of the Taiping Era*

Moslae Herba *(xiāng rú)* . . . . 480g[24]
Magnoliae officinalis Cortex *(hòu pò)* 240g
Lablab Semen album *(bái biǎn dòu)* 240g

Table 11.6	Summerheat Attack: Differentiation and Treatment	
Signs and Symptoms	**Treatment Principles**	**Formulas**
▶ MORE COLD AND LESS SUMMERHEAT		
More aversion to cold than fever, absence of sweating, floating pulse, epigastric distention, nausea, vomiting, white and greasy tongue coating	Release the exterior with acrid and warm herbs, and transform dampness with bitter, aromatic, and warm herbs	Mosla Powder *(xiāng rú sǎn)*
▶ COLD EQUAL TO SUMMERHEAT		
Body aches, aversion to cold and absence of sweating, fever, epigastric distention, restlessness, greasy tongue coating	Release exterior cold with acrid and warm herbs, clear interior summerheat, and transform dampness with bitter, aromatic, and warm herbs	Newly Augmented Mosla Drink *(xīn jiā yù nǔ jiān)* [modified]
▶ MORE SUMMERHEAT AND LESS COLD		
Fever, absence of sweating, slight chills and aversion to cold, restlessness, thirst, loose stools with foul smell, uncomfortable sensation in anus	Release exterior cold with acrid and warm herbs, clear summerheat with bitter and cold herbs, and transform dampness with bitter, aromatic, and warm herbs	Coptis and Mosla Drink *(huáng lián xiāng rú yǐn)*

ANALYSIS OF FORMULA: This formula is used when cold, *not* summerheat, is the predominant factor. (See further discussion of this formula immediately below.)

Formula No. 2:

> ### NEWLY AUGMENTED MOSLA DRINK *(xīn jiā xiāng rú yǐn)*
>
> SOURCE: *Systematic Differentiation of Warm Pathogen Diseases*
>
> Moslae Herba *(xiāng rú)* 6g
> Lonicerae Flos *(jīn yín huā)* 9g
> Lablab Flos *(biān dòu huā)*[25] 9g
> Magnoliae officinalis Cortex *(hòu pò)* 6g
> Forsythiae Fructus *(lián qiào)* 6g

ANALYSIS OF FORMULA: This formula is a modified version of the first formula, and is used when summerheat and cold are equally balanced. Lablab Flos *(biān dòu huā)*, Lonicerae Flos *(jīn yín huā)*, and Forsythiae Fructus *(lián qiào)* are added to that formula, and Lablab Semen album *(bái biǎn dòu)* is removed.

Moslae Herba *(xiāng rú)* is the principal herb in both formulas. With its acrid flavor and warm nature, Moslae Herba *(xiāng rú)* releases the exterior signs and symptoms by dispersing exogenous cold and exterior dampness. It also clears summerheat.[26] Moslae Herba *(xiāng rú)* is the most suitable herb for dealing with the combination of summerheat, dampness, and exogenous cold.

Magnoliae officinalis Cortex *(hòu pò)* and Lablab Flos *(biān dòu huā)* enhance the action of Moslae Herba *(xiāng rú)* in transforming interior dampness, while Lonicerae Flos *(jīn yín huā)*, Forsythiae Fructus *(lián qiào)*, and Lablab Flos *(biān dòu huā)* strengthen its action in dispersing summerheat. The latter disperses and clears summerheat, and transforms dampness. However, Lablab Flos *(biān dòu huā)* is difficult to obtain, and Lablab Semen album *(bái biǎn dòu)* can be substituted for it. The only concern with this substitution is that Lablab Semen album *(bái biǎn dòu)* may trap summerheat in the body when it is associated with dampness. This is because Lablab Semen album *(bái biǎn dòu)* acts to tonify the qi of the Spleen. To reduce the possibility of this side effect, the dosage of Magnoliae officinalis Cortex *(hòu pò)* and Forsythiae Fructus *(lián qiào)* should be greater than that of Lablab Semen album *(bái biǎn dòu)*.

According to Wu Tang, the practitioner should use this formula to induce a mild sweat in the patient. However, once the sweating has begun, use of the formula must be stopped.

> If there is sweating after taking this formula, stop taking it, even though the decoction is not yet finished. However, if the patient does not sweat after taking this formula, the patient should continue taking the formula until sweating occurs. If there is still no sweating when the patient has finished the decoction, the practitioner must refill the prescription in order to induce sweating.[27]

From this passage, it should be clear that sweating is the preferred method for dispersing the summerheat with dampness in this pattern. However, if the patient has still not experienced any sweating after having finished the decoction, instead of repeating the formula, try using an external method which I have developed to assist the formula in inducing sweating. Cook Artemisiae annuae Herba *(qīng hāo)* (30g), Menthae haplocalycis Herba *(bò hé)* (15g), Bombycis Faeces *(cán shā)* (20g), Zingiberis Rhizoma recens *(shēng jiāng)* (15 slices), Atractylodis Rhizoma *(cāng zhú)* (20g), and Allii fistulosi Bulbus *(cōng bái)* (20g). Soak a piece of gauze in the decoction and rub it all over the body (except for the head), or take a bath in the strained decoction.

MODIFICATIONS: The basic formula can be modified as follows:

- For significant signs and symptoms of dampness such as abdominal bloating, loose stools, and scanty urine, add Pogostemonis/Agastaches Herba *(huò xiāng)*, Eupatorii Herba *(pèi lán)*, Talcum *(huá shí)*, and Tetrapanacis Medulla *(tōng cǎo)*.

- If summerheat predominates with such signs and symptoms as strong thirst, insomnia, and soreness on the tongue, add Lophatheri Herba *(dàn zhú yè)*, Gypsum fibrosum *(shí gāo)*, Citrulli Exocarpium *(xī guā pí)*, and Nelumbinis Folium *(hé yè)* to clear the summerheat.

- For cough, add Trichosanthis Pericarpium *(guā lóu pí)* and Armeniacae Semen *(xìng rén)*.

Formula No. 3:

COPTIS AND MOSLA DRINK *(huáng lián xiāng rú yǐn)*[28]

SOURCE: *Book to Safeguard Life Arranged According to Pattern*[29]

Moslae Herba *(xiāng rú)*	30g[30]
Magnoliae officinalis Cortex *(hòu pò)*	15g
Lablab Semen album *(bái biǎn dòu)*	15g
Coptidis Rhizoma *(huáng lián)*	9g

ANALYSIS OF FORMULA: This formula is used when summerheat—*not* cold—is the predominant factor.

Case study: Newly Augmented Mosla Drink *(xīn jiā xiāng rú yǐn)*

The patient, a one-year-old boy, suffered from a common cold for one week during the summer. At the time of his first visit he had a fever. His father was a Western-trained physician who gave the child antibiotics, but to no effect. His father said that they had placed the child's bed next to an open window during the night because the weather was so hot. His son, therefore, had been exposed to wind, and the following morning he developed a high fever (up to 39°C) and dark-yellow urine, but was not sweating. Upon examination, the veins on both index fingers were purple. A traditional Chinese physician diagnosed this as an attack of exogenous cold and accumulated summerheat in the body. The principles of treatment were to disperse the exogenous cold and clear the interior summerheat. He used a modified version of Newly

Augmented Mosla Drink *(xīn jiā xiāng rú yǐn)*: Moslae Herba *(xiāng rú)* (3g), Lablab Semen album *(bái biǎn dòu)* (6g), Magnoliae officinalis Cortex *(hòu pò)* (3g), Coptidis Rhizoma *(huáng lián)* (1.5g), Talcum *(huá shí)* (3g), Glycyrrhizae Radix *(gān cǎo)* (1.5g), Lonicerae Flos *(jīn yín huā)* (3g), Forsythiae Fructus *(lián qiào)* (3g), and fried Gardeniae Fructus *(chǎo zhī zǐ)* (1.5g). A single packet of herbs was decocted, strained, and taken in one day, divided into three doses. After finishing this packet of herbs, the patient began to sweat, and all the signs and symptoms were soon resolved. Treatment was then concluded.[31]

SUMMERHEAT AND DAMPNESS ATTACKING THE LUNG AND PROTECTIVE LEVEL

Manifestations. There are three concurrent aspects to this pattern:

1. *General signs and symptoms of summerheat* with fever, thirst, and a rapid pulse.

2. *Summerheat attacking the Lung and protective level* with a nonproductive cough, chest distention, chills, aversion to cold, and a white tongue coating.

3. *Summerheat coupled with dampness,* which is a combination that blocks the qi mechanism, and specifically the normal ascent of qi. The resulting signs and symptoms are dizziness, heavy sensation in the head, greasy tongue coating, and a soggy pulse.

NOTE: In *Discussion of Seasonal Diseases (Shí bìng lùn)* the late-nineteenth-century author Lei Feng refers to this pattern as a common cold in the summer due to an attack of summerheat (冒暑 *mào shǔ*).[32] It is a mild and superficial pattern.

Pathology. Summerheat and dampness attacking the Lung and protective level.

Treatment principles. Clear summerheat, transform dampness, and disseminate the Lung qi.

Formula No. 1:

> **MULBERRY LEAF AND CHRYSANTHEMUM DRINK** *(sāng jú yǐn)*

To this formula, add 10g each of Artemisiae annuae Herba *(qīng hāo)* and Peucedani Radix *(qián hú)*. For further discussion of Mulberry Leaf and Chrysanthemum Drink *(sāng jú yǐn)*, see Chapter 7.

ANALYSIS OF FORMULA: This formula is used if the Lung signs and symptoms predominate. Artemisiae annuae Herba *(qīng hāo)* is added to disperse and clear summerheat, while Peucedani Radix *(qián hú)* is used to clear heat from the Lung and to stop the coughing.

Formula No. 2:

> ### AUGMENTED LEI'S DECOCTION TO CLEAR, COOL, AND SCOUR OUT SUMMERHEAT (*Léi shī qīng liáng dí shǔ tāng jiā wèi*)

SOURCE: *Discussion of Seasonal Diseases*

Talcum *(huá shí)* 9g

Glycyrrhizae Radix *(gān cǎo)* 2.4g

Tetrapanacis Medulla *(tōng cǎo)* 3g

Artemisiae annuae Herba *(qīng hāo)* 4.5g

Lablab Semen album *(bái biǎn dòu)* 3g

Forsythiae Fructus *(lián qiào)* 9g

Poria *(fú líng)* 9g

Citrulli Exocarpium *(xī guā pí)* ....1 piece

ANALYSIS OF FORMULA: This formula is used if protective level signs and symptoms predominate. Since this pattern is situated in the upper burner, one must clear summerheat and disseminate the Lung qi with light herbs. Artemisiae annuae Herba *(qīng hāo)*, Forsythiae Fructus *(lián qiào)*, and Citrulli Exocarpium *(xī guā pí)* are light herbs that clear summerheat. Lablab Semen album *(bái biǎn dòu)* tonifies the Spleen and transforms dampness. Talcum *(huá shí)*, Glycyrrhizae Radix *(gān cǎo)*, Tetrapanacis Medulla *(tōng cǎo)* and Poria *(fú líng)* clear heat and leach out dampness through the urine. Trichosanthis Semen *(guā lóu rén)* and Armeniacae Semen *(xìng rén)* are used to disseminate the Lung qi and direct it downward.[33] Clinically, Trichosanthis Pericarpium *(guā lóu pí)* is usually substituted for Trichosanthis Semen *(guā lóu rén)* as it is superior in disseminating the Lung qi. However, no substitution is made if the patient also experiences constipation due to failure of the Lung to direct its qi downward to the Large Intestine.

MODIFICATIONS: The basic formula can be modified as follows:

- For irritability and thirst, which indicate that summerheat predominates, add Lonicerae Flos *(jīn yín huā)* and Nelumbinis Folium *(hé yè)*, and increase the dosage of Forsythiae Fructus *(lián qiào)*.

- For nausea or vomiting, add Pinelliae Rhizoma preparatum *(zhì bàn xià)*, Bambusae Caulis in taeniam *(zhú rú)*, and Pogostemonis/Agastaches Herba *(huò xiāng)* to regulate the function of the Stomach.

- For diarrhea, add Puerariae Radix *(gé gēn)* to stop the diarrhea by raising the Spleen qi and clearing the summerheat.

Injury to the Collaterals of the Lung by Summerheat with Dampness

Manifestations. There are three concurrent aspects to this pattern:

1. *Injury to the collaterals of the Lung, and blood stasis in the collaterals of the Lung* with hemoptysis, labored breathing or flaring of the nostrils, and a purplish face.

2. *Summerheat disturbing the spirit of the Heart* with fever, thirst, irritability, or even muddled consciousness.

3. *Summerheat associated with dampness* with heaviness or fuzziness of the head and blurred vision.

NOTE: According to *Systematic Differentiation of Warm Pathogen Diseases*, this pattern is also called bleeding from the Lung due to attack of summerheat (暑瘵 *shǔ zhài*).[34] Both the qi and blood levels are affected; however, most aspects of this disorder relate to the Lung.

In mild cases there is cough with bloody sputum, a heavy or fuzzy sensation in the head, blurred vision, thirst, and irritability. In severe cases there is a persistent cough with blood, palpitations or shortness of breath, and even muddled consciousness. In this pattern, it is summerheat—*not* dampness—that predominates.

Pathology. Summerheat with dampness injuring the collaterals of the Lung, leading to bleeding.

Treatment principles. Clear heat, cool the blood, dispel blood stasis, and transform dampness.

NOTE: Under these circumstances, it is contraindicated to exclusively tonify, or to only use herbs that stop bleeding, because this is a pattern of excess coupled with heat: herbs that tonify qi will exacerbate the heat, and those that stop bleeding may exacerbate the blood stasis.

Normally, when bleeding is due to heat, the treatment is to directly cool the blood. This occurs with formulas such as Rhinoceros Horn and Rehmannia Decoction (*xī jiǎo dì huáng tāng*), discussed below and in Chapter 8. However, that approach is inappropriate here, since the herbs that are commonly used to cool the blood are bitter and cold. If they are used in a patient with summerheat and dampness, these pathogens will stagnate in the body and the problem will worsen. The proper treatment approach is to clear summerheat and transform dampness. One must focus on eliminating the exogenous pathogenic factor—summerheat—and to that end should clear heat from the collaterals of the Lung and transform dampness using light and cool herbs.

Formula No. 1:

CLEAR THE COLLATERALS DRINK PLUS APRICOT KERNEL, COIX,
AND TALCUM *(qīng luò yǐn jiā xìng rén yì yǐ huá shí tāng)*

SOURCE: *Systematic Differentiation of Warm Pathogen Diseases*

Lonicerae Flos *(jīn yín huā)* 6g

Nelumbinis Folium *(hé yè)* 6g

Citrulli Exocarpium *(xī guā pí)* 6g

Armeniacae Semen *(xìng rén)* 6g

Talcum *(huá shí)* 9g

Lablab Flos *(biān dòu huā)*[35] 6g

Luffae Fructus Retinervus *(sī guā luò)* 6g

Lophatheri Folium immaturus *(zhú yè juǎn xīn)*[36] 6g

Coicis Semen *(yì yǐ rén)* 9g

ANALYSIS OF FORMULA: In this formula the combination of Lonicerae Flos *(jīn yín huā)*, Citrulli Exocarpium *(xī guā pí)*, and Lophatheri Folium immaturus *(zhú yè juǎn xīn)* clears summerheat through urination. Nelumbinis Folium *(hé yè)*, Coicis Semen *(yì yǐ rén)*, and Lablab Flos *(biān dòu huā)* transform dampness. Coicis Semen *(yì yǐ rén)* and Talcum *(huá shí)* resolve dampness by draining through urination. Armeniacae Semen *(xìng rén)* is used to direct the Lung qi downward and to help resolve the dampness. Luffae Fructus Retinervus *(sī guā luò)* guides the other herbs to the collaterals of the Lung.

According to the source text, the use of fresh ingredients maximizes the formula's results. However, it is usually difficult to find them. Therefore, for best results, double the dosages. In addition, because this formula is not sufficiently strong by itself to deal with this pattern, one should enhance its effects by adding Ophiopogonis Radix *(mài mén dōng)* (10g) and Anemarrhenae Rhizoma *(zhī mǔ)* (12g).

Hemoptysis can be caused by an attack on the Lung by summerheat transforming into toxin. In this type of case there is no dampness. Therefore, in addition to clearing summerheat, one must also cool the blood and resolve toxicity. The ideal formula for this purpose is the combination of Rhinoceros Horn and Rehmannia Decoction *(xī jiǎo dì huáng tāng)* and Honeysuckle and Forsythia Powder *(yín qiào sǎn)*, discussed in Chapters 8 and 7 respectively. However, Schizonepetae Herba *(jīng jiè)*, Sojae Semen preparatum *(dàn dòu chǐ)*, and Menthae haplocalycis Herba *(bò hé)* should be omitted from Honeysuckle and Forsythia Powder *(yín qiào sǎn)* because there are no exterior signs or symptoms. In addition, Gardeniae Fructus *(zhī zǐ)*, Scutellariae Radix *(huáng qín)*, Platycladi Cacumen *(cè bǎi yè)*, and Nelumbinis Nodus rhizomatis *(ǒu jié)* should be added to enhance the other herbs' action in clearing summerheat and cooling the blood.

MODIFICATIONS: The basic formula can be modified as follows:

- For massive bleeding, add Notoginseng Radix *(sān qī)* and Ginseng Radix *(rén shēn)* to stop the bleeding and tonify the qi. In traditional Chinese medical theory, qi commands the blood. One must immediately stop the bleeding and tonify the qi to prevent the collapse of qi, should massive bleeding continue. How does one know that this is necessary, since the general rule is that herbs that tonify or bind should *not* be used in the presence of an active pathogenic factor? When heavy bleeding severely injures the qi and leads to shortness of breath, facial pallor, extreme fatigue, pale tongue body, and a thin and frail pulse, one should simultaneously tonify qi and stop the bleeding. This is because, by this point, there is a vicious cycle whereby the bleeding continuously injures the qi (and can even lead to qi collapse) while the resulting qi deficiency aggravates the bleeding. Even when the bleeding is initially due to summerheat with dampness, since the situation here is critical, one must focus on the bleeding in order to save the patient's life.
- For bleeding that is difficult to stop, combine Clear Epidemics and Overcome Toxin Drink *(qīng wēn bài dú yǐn)*,[37] which clears heat, resolves toxicity, and removes blood stasis, with Generate the Pulse Powder *(shēng mài sǎn)*,[38] which stops the bleeding by tonifying the qi.
- If the patient experiences collapse of the qi due to massive bleeding, immediately administer 60g of Ginseng Radix *(rén shēn)*.[39] If there are also signs of cold from yang collapse, provide Ginseng and Aconite Accessory Root Decoction *(shēn fù tāng)*.[40]

ACCUMULATION OF SUMMERHEAT AND DAMPNESS IN THE MIDDLE BURNER

Manifestations. There are two concurrent aspects to this pattern:

1. *Heat from excess in the Stomach* with vigorous fever, irritability, restlessness, thirst, profuse sweating, and a flooding pulse.
2. *Dampness in the Spleen* with epigastric distention and heaviness of the body.

NOTE: It is very important to ascertain whether heat or dampness predominates in patterns of combined heat and dampness. In this pattern, there is more heat than dampness.

Pathology. Accumulation of summerheat and dampness in the middle burner, heat predominating.

Treatment principles. Clear summerheat from the Stomach with acrid, bitter, and cold herbs and transform dampness in the Spleen with bitter and slightly warm herbs.

Formula:

> ### WHITE TIGER PLUS ATRACTYLODES DECOCTION (*bái hǔ jiā cāng zhú tāng*)
>
> SOURCE: *Book to Safeguard Life Arranged According to Pattern*
>
> Gypsum fibrosum (*shí gāo*) . . . . .500g[41]
> Anemarrhenae Rhizoma (*zhī mǔ*) 180g
> Atractylodis Rhizoma (*cāng zhú*). 90g
> Nonglutinous rice (*gěng mǐ*) 90g
> Honey-toasted Glycyrrhizae Radix preparata (*zhì gān cǎo*) 60g

ANALYSIS OF FORMULA: White Tiger Decoction (*bái hǔ tāng*), discussed in Chapter 7, disperses and clears summerheat from the Stomach. Because summerheat is very likely to be accompanied by some degree of dampness, Atractylodis Rhizoma (*cāng zhú*) is added. With its bitter flavor and slightly warm nature, it serves to dry and transform dampness affecting the Spleen.

MODIFICATIONS: The basic formula can be modified as follows:

- For significant dampness in the middle burner, add the following aromatic and bland herbs: Pogostemonis/Agastaches Herba (*huò xiāng*), Eupatorii Herba (*pèi lán*), Talcum (*huá shí*), Sojae Semen germinatum (*dà dòu juǎn*), and Tetrapanacis Medulla (*tōng cǎo*).
- For injury to the qi and fluids by summerheat with such symptoms as lassitude, fatigue, feverish body, shallow breathing, irritability, yellow urine, thirst, and spontaneous sweating, Li Gao's Decoction to Clear Summerheat and Augment the Qi (*Lǐ shī qīng shǔ yì qì tāng*)[42] would be a good choice.[43]

Case study: White Tiger plus Atractylodes Decoction (*bái hǔ jiā cāng zhú tāng*)

First visit: August 15. This 23-year-old male patient had a fever of one day's duration and was treated with Honeysuckle and Forsythia Powder (*yín qiào sǎn*). After taking the formula and sweating, the fever declined from 39.5°C to 38.3°C. However, by the following afternoon the fever had gone up again to 39.8°C. The patient presented with a flushed face, strong thirst for cold beverages, a heavy sensation in his head and body, slight nausea, epigastric distention, and a reduced appetite. He had a normal bowel movement on the day of his first visit, but his urine was scanty, dark, and yellow. He felt restless yet tired. His tongue was red with a slightly yellow and greasy coating, and his pulse was rapid and slippery. The diagnosis was attack of summerheat with dampness, leading to the rebellion of Stomach qi. A modified version of White Tiger plus Atractylodes Decoction (*bái hǔ jiā cāng zhú tāng*) was prescribed: Gypsum fibrosum *(shí gāo)* (30g), Anemarrhenae Rhizoma *(zhī mǔ)* (15g), nonglutinous rice *(gěng mǐ)* (10g), Honey-toasted Glycyrrhizae Radix preparata *(zhì gān cǎo)* (3g), Atractylodis Rhizoma *(cāng zhú)* (12g), and Tetrapanacis Medulla *(tōng cǎo)* (6g). Two packets of the herbs were given to the patient. He was instructed to take one packet of herbs each day, by dividing the strained decoction into six doses and drinking one dose every four hours.

Second visit: August 17. After finishing the first packet, the patient sweated slightly and his fever went down to 37.3°C. The heavy sensation in his head and body was significantly reduced by that evening. Except for slight fatigue, all signs and symptoms were alleviated by the time he had finished the second packet of herbs. At this point, Panacis quinquefolii Radix *(xī yáng shēn)* (10g) was given to the patient to tonify the qi and enrich the yin.[44]

SUMMERHEAT AND DAMPNESS SPREAD THROUGH THE THREE BURNERS

Manifestations. There are four concurrent aspects to this pattern:

1. *Summerheat and dampness in the upper burner* with coughing of blood-tinged sputum, chest distention, and diminished hearing or deafness.
2. *Summerheat and dampness in the middle burner* with abdominal distention, watery diarrhea, slight thirst, and a yellow tongue coating with profuse saliva.
3. *Summerheat and dampness in the lower burner* with low back pain, scanty and dark yellow or cloudy urine, or yellow, foul-smelling vaginal discharge.
4. *General signs and symptoms of summerheat* with fever, flushed face, and a red tongue.

NOTE: In this pattern, summerheat is the predominant factor, primarily affecting the qi level of the involved burners. Generally speaking, diminished hearing or deafness is associated with Gallbladder heat or Kidney deficiency, but in this pattern there are no signs of dysfunction in these organs. Hearing loss from heat in the Gallbladder is accompanied by alternating chills and fever, bitter taste, dry throat, and/or a wiry pulse. Hearing loss associated with Kidney deficiency is accompanied by weakness and soreness of the low back, or a warmer sensation in the soles and palms than on the back of the hands and top of the feet, and slight but persistent fever. By contrast, the deafness here is caused by the steaming of summerheat and dampness upward into the clear orifices.

Pathology. Summerheat and dampness attacking the qi level in all three burners; heat predominates.

Treatment principles. Clear summerheat and eliminate dampness by disseminating and unblocking the movement of qi and fluids in the three burners.

Formula:

THREE MINERALS DECOCTION *(sān shí tāng)*

SOURCE: *Systematic Differentiation of Warm Pathogen Diseases*

Talcum *(huá shí)* 9g
Gypsum fibrosum *(shí gāo)* 15g
Glauberitum *(hán shuǐ shí)* 9g
Armeniacae Semen *(xìng rén)* 9g
Bambusae Caulis in taeniam *(zhú rú)* 6g
Lonicerae Flos *(jīn yín huā)* 9g
Tetrapanacis Medulla *(tōng cǎo)* 6g
Succus Faecalis Aureus *(jīn zhī)* [45] . . . . 1 cup

ANALYSIS OF FORMULA: Armeniacae Semen *(xìng rén)* helps eliminate dampness by promoting the downward-directed action of the Lung. Gypsum fibrosum *(shí gāo)* and Bambusae Caulis in taeniam *(zhú rú)* clear summerheat from the middle burner. Talcum *(huá shí)*, Tetrapanacis Medulla *(tōng cǎo)*, and Glauberitum *(hán shuǐ shí)* clear heat and discharge dampness from the lower burner by promoting urination. Lonicerae Flos *(jīn yín huā)* and Succus Faecalis Aureus *(jīn zhī)* clear summerheat and resolve toxicity.

MODIFICATIONS: Other herbs should be added depending on the location of most of the signs and symptoms, whether that be in the upper, middle, or lower burner:

- For significant signs and symptoms of summerheat in the upper burner (cough with sticky, thick, and yellow sputum), add Trichosanthis Pericarpium *(guā lóu pí)*, Sojae Semen germinatum *(dà dòu juǎn)*, and Phragmitis Rhizoma *(lú gēn)*.

- For severe bleeding accompanied by sputum, add Imperatae Rhizoma *(bái máo gēn)* and Nelumbinis Nodus rhizomatis *(ǒu jié)*.

- For significant signs and symptoms of dampness in the middle burner (nausea, vomiting, diarrhea, epigastric distention), add aromatic and bitter herbs, such as Atractylodis Rhizoma *(cāng zhú)*, Pogostemonis/Agastaches Herba *(huò xiāng)*, Magnoliae officinalis Cortex *(hòu pò)*, and Eupatorii Herba *(pèi lán)*, to transform dampness.

- For significant signs and symptoms of heat in the middle burner (strong thirst for cold beverages, and a yellow, thick, but dry tongue coating), add Coptidis Rhizoma *(huáng lián)* and Magnoliae officinalis Cortex *(hòu pò)*.

- For distention of the lower abdomen combined with scanty and dark yellow urine, add Plantaginis Herba *(chē qián cǎo)*, Tetrapanacis Medulla *(tōng cǎo)*, and Liquidambaris Fructus *(lù lù tōng)* to strengthen Bladder's function of discharging urine.

Summary

Summerheat-warmth results from an attack on the body by summerheat. It is often coupled with dampness, and occurs during the summer season. As an exogenous pathogenic factor, summerheat is characterized by fire and heat, and is therefore apt to injure the fluids and exhaust the qi. Summerheat-warmth alone, without dampness, is the most quickly progressing of all the warm pathogen diseases, even more so than wind-warmth. In biomedical terms, this pattern is often equivalent to sunstroke. By contrast, summerheat-warmth in concert with dampness progresses relatively slowly. However, once the dampness and summerheat transform into pure heat, the progression of the illness and the treatment principles are identical to those of summerheat-warmth without dampness. (See Tables 11.7 and 11.8.)

Table 11.7	Differentiation and Treatment of Summerheat Without Dampness	
Patterns	**Treatment Principles**	**Formulas**
Summerheat attacking the Stomach	Clear and disperse summerheat, tonify the qi, and generate fluids	White Tiger Decoction (*bái hǔ tāng*) or White Tiger plus Ginseng Decoction (*bái hǔ jiā rén shēn tāng*)
Injury to fluids and qi by summerheat	Clear summerheat, tonify the qi, and generate fluids	Wang's Decoction to Clear Summerheat and Augment the Qi (*Wáng shì qīng shǔ yì qì tāng*)
Imminent collapse of fluids and qi	Tonify the qi, enrich the yin, and preserve the yin and qi to prevent collapse of qi and fluids	Generate the Pulse Powder (*shēng mài sǎn*)
Invasion of Pericardium by summerheat	Clear summerheat from the Pericardium and open the orifices	Clear the Nutritive Level Decoction (*qīng yíng tāng*), Calm the Palace Pill with Cattle Gallstone (*ān gōng niú huáng wán*), Purple Snow Special Pill (*zǐ xuě dān*), or Greatest Treasure Special Pill (*zhì bǎo dān*)
Stirring of Liver wind by excess summerheat	Clear summerheat and extinguish Liver wind	Antelope Horn and Uncaria Decoction (*líng jiǎo gōu téng yǐn*)
Invasion of blood level by summerheat	Cool the blood, resolve toxicity, clear summerheat from the Heart, and open the orifices	Magical Rhinoceros Special Pill (*shén xī dān*)

Table 11.7, cont.		
Injury to Heart and Kidney by summerheat	Clear heat from the Heart and enrich the Liver and Kidney yin	Coptis and Mume Decoction (*lián méi tāng*)
Remnants of heat combined with obstruction of collaterals by phlegm and blood stasis	Eliminate the remnants of heat, transform phlegm, invigorate the collaterals, dispel blood stasis from the collaterals, and extinguish Liver wind	Modified Three-Shell Powder

Table 11.8	Differentiation and Treatment of Summerheat with Dampness	
Patterns	**Treatment Principles**	**Formulas**
Interior stagnant summer- heat and dampness associated with attack of exogenous cold	Release the exterior by dispersing exogenous cold, clearing interior summerheat, and transforming dampness	Newly Augmented Mosla Drink (*xīn jiā xiāng rú yǐn*), Mosla Powder (*xiāng rú sǎn*), or Coptis and Mosla Drink (*huáng lián xiāng rú yǐn*)
Summerheat and dampness attacking the Lung and protective level	Clear summerheat, transform dampness, and disseminate the Lung qi	Mulberry Leaf and Chrysanthemum Drink (*sāng jú yǐn*) or Augmented Lei's Decoction to Clear, Cool, and Scour Out Summerheat (*lèi shī qīng liáng dí shǔ tāng jiā wèi*)
Injury to collaterals of Lung by summerheat with dampness	Clear heat, cool the blood, dispel blood stasis, and transform dampness	Clear the Collaterals Drink Plus Apricot Kernel, Coix, and Talcum (*qīng luò yǐn jiā xìng rén yì yǐ huá shí tāng*), or Rhinoceros Horn and Rehmannia Decoction (*xī jiǎo dì huáng tāng*) plus Honeysuckle and Forsythia Powder (*yín qiào sǎn*)
Accumulation of summer- heat and dampness in the middle burner (heat predominates)	Clear summerheat and transform dampness with acrid, bitter, cold, and slightly warm herbs	White Tiger Plus Atractylodes Decoction (*bái hǔ jiā cāng zhú tāng*)
Summerheat and dampness spread throughout three burners (heat predominates)	Clear summerheat and eliminate dampness by disseminating and unblocking the movement of qi and fluids in the three burners	Three Stone Decoction (*sān shí tāng*)

Endnotes

1. According to Chapter 31 of *Basic Questions*, a disease caused by the warm-heat pathogen which occurs between the beginning of summer and the summer solstice is called a warm pathogen disease, and that which occurs between the summer solstice and the end of the summer is called summerheat-warmth. Anonymous, *Yellow Emperor's Inner Classic: Basic Questions (Huáng Dì nèi jīng sù wèn)*. Beijing: People's Health Publishing House, 1963: 186.

2. Ye Gui, *Case Records as a Guide to Clinical Practice (Lín zhèng zhǐ nán yī àn)*. Shanghai: Shanghai Science and Technology Publishing House, 1959: 734. Note that Wang Shi-Xiong (approximately 1808-1867) selected this chapter, and, using another of Ye Gui's appellations, called it *Ye Xiang-Yan's Differentiating Lurking Pathogens and Externally-Contracted [Diseases] During Three Seasons (Yè Xiāng-Yán sān shí fú xié wài gǎn piàn)*, which he included in his book *Warp and Woof of Warm-Heat Pathogen Diseases (Wēn rè jīng wěi)*. It can be found in Lu Zhen, *Collection of Modern Rare Books of Chinese Medicine: Warm Pathogen Disease Volume (Jīn dài zhōng yī zhēn běn jí: wēn bìng fèn cè)*. Hangzhou: Zhejiang Science and Technology Publishing House, 1987: 80.

3. There is some overlap between the biomedically-diagnosed disease epidemic encephalitis B and the pattern of obstruction of wind and phlegm in summerheat-warmth.

4. Zhang He-Teng (Zhang Feng-Kui, active 1623), *Revised and Expanded Complete Treatise on Summerheat Damage (Zēng dìng shāng shǔ quán shū)*, annotated by Ye Lin (Ye Zi-Yu, date unknown), Chapter 2: 7, 9. This can be found in Cao Bing-Zhang (ed.), *Compendium of Medicine in China (Zhōng guó yī xué dà chéng)*. Shanghai: Shanghai Science and Technology Publishing House, 1990. See also Ye Gui, *Case Records as a Guide to Clinical Practice (Lín zhèng zhǐ nán yī àn)*. Shanghai: Shanghai Science and Technology Publishing House, 1959: 736.

5. This formula was first introduced by Zhang Ji in *Discussion of Cold Damage*. It includes Lophatheri Herba *(dàn zhú yè)* (9 g), Gypsum fibrosum *(shí gāo)* (30g), Ginseng Radix *(rén shēn)* (9g), Ophiopogonis Radix *(mài mén dōng)* (15g), Pinelliae Rhizoma preparatum *(zhì bàn xià)* (9g), nonglutinous rice *(gēng mǐ)* (12g), and Honey-toasted Glycyrrhizae Radix preparata *(zhì gān cǎo)*(3g).

6. Dong Jian-Hua et al., *Selected Case Studies from Famous Modern Chinese Doctors (Zhōng guó xiàn dài míng zhōng yī yī àn jīng huá)*. Beijing: Beijing Publishing House, 1990: 2097. This case study was reported by Sun Yun-Zhong.

7. The dosages come from Meng Shu-Jiang et al., *Warm Pathogen Diseases (Wēn bìng xué)*. Shanghai: Shanghai Science and Technology Publishing House, 1985: 66. Wang Meng-Yin neither named this formula nor specified the dosages.

8. It was first recorded in *Formulary of the Bureau of Medicines of the Taiping Era (Tàipíng huì mín hé jì jú fāng)* written by Chen Shi-Wen et al. Beijing: People's Health Publishing House, 1959: 37. It contains Pinelliae Rhizoma preparatum *(zhì bàn xià)* (30g), Magnoliae officinalis Cortex *(hòu pò)* (30g), Atractylodis Rhizoma *(cāng zhú)* (30g), Pogostemonis/ Agastaches Folium *(huò xiāng yè)* (15g), Tsaoko Fructus *(cǎo guǒ)* (15g), Poria *(fú líng)* (15g), Ginseng Radix *(rén shēn)* (15g), Honey-toasted Glycyrrhizae Radix preparata *(zhì gān cǎo)* (7.5g), Citri reticulatae Pericarpium *(chén pí)* (22.5g), Zingiberis Rhizoma recens *(shēng jiāng)* (7 slices), and Mume Fructus *(wū méi)* (1 piece).

9. This formula was first recorded in the thirteenth century in Chen Zi-Ming, *Great Collection of Fine Formulas for Women (Fù rén liáng fāng dà quán)*. Shanghai: Shanghai Great Achievement Press, 1926: 45.

10. Chengdu College of Traditional Chinese Medicine, *Selected Case Studies from Veteran Traditional Chinese Doctors (Lǎo zhōng yī yī àn xuǎn, dì èr jí)*, vol. 2. Chengdu: Chengdu College of Traditional Chinese Medicine, 1980: 40. This case study was reported by Song Lu-Bing.

11. Zhang Yuan-Su (Zhang Ji-Gu), *Origins of Medicine (Yī xué qǐ yuán)*, annotated by Ren Ying-Qiu. Beijing: People's Health Publishing House, 1978: 198.

12. Generate the Pulse Powder *(shēng mài sǎn)* is commonly used today. According to recent research reports, two basic biomedical functions of this formula have been borne out in laboratory and clinical research. One function is to elevate blood pressure. The second is to prevent shock. See Ma You-Du, *New Explanation of Medical Formulas (Yī fāng xīn jiě)*. Shanghai: Shanghai Science and Technology Publishing House, 1980: 32-132.

13. This is Ginseng and Aconite Accessory Root Decoction *(shēn fù tāng)*, which was discussed in Chapter 7, with the addition of Fossilia Ossis Mastodi *(lóng gǔ)* (10-20g) and Ostreae Concha *(mǔ lì)* (10-20g).

14. Author's own case study.

15. See Chapter 7.

16. According to the source text, all ingredients in this formula, except Rhinocerotis Cornu *(xī jiǎo)*, Succus Faecalis Aureus *(jīn zhī)*, and Rehmanniae Radix *(shēng dì huáng)*, should be ground into powder, then mixed with Rhinocerotis Cornu *(xī jiǎo)* powder, Succus Faecalis Aureus *(jīn zhī)*, and juice from Rehmanniae Radix *(shēng dì huáng)*, and made into a pill. This pill is generally available in Chinese pharmacies. If given as a decoction, the dosages are adjusted as follows: Bubali Cornu *(shuǐ niú jiǎo)* (3060g), Acori tatarinowii Rhizoma *(shí chāng pǔ)* (9-15g), Scutellariae Radix *(huáng qín)* (9-15g), Forsythiae Fructus *(lián qiào)* (18-24g), Rehmanniae Radix *(shēng dì huáng)* (18-24g), Isatidis/Baphicacanthis Radix *(bǎn lán gēn)* (24-30g), Arnebiae Radix/Lithospermi Radix *(zǐ cǎo)* (15-24g), Lonicerae Flos *(jīn yín huā)* (24-30g), Sojae Semen preparatum *(dàn dòu chǐ)* (9-12g), Isatidis Folium *(dà qīng yè)*(30g) (substituting for Succus Faecalis Aureus *[jin zhi]*), Trichosanthis Radix *(tiān huā fěn)* (12-15g).

17. Nowadays, this is a rarely used substance derived from human feces, which strongly clears heat and resolves toxicity. See Appendix C for further details. At present, Isatidis Folium *(dà qīng yè)* or Coptidis Rhizoma *(huáng lián)* are usually substituted for it.

18. Guangzhou College of Traditional Chinese Medicine, *Formulas (Fāng jì xué)*. Shanghai: Shanghai Science and Technology Publishing House, 1979: 196. It contains equal amounts of Scolopendra *(wú gōng)* and Scorpio *(quán xiē)*.

19. Dong Jian-Hua et al., *Selected Case Studies from Famous Modern Chinese Doctors*, 337. This case study was reported by Wei Chang-Chun.

20. The source text did not provide dosages. Those listed here are the author's recommendations.

21. Because Manitis Squama *(chuān shān jiǎ)* is no longer available due to the endangered species status of pangolins, we can increase the dosage of Eupolyphaga/Stelophaga *(tǔ biē chóng)* up to 12g or 15g and use it as a substitute.

22. Wind refers not only to natural wind, such as that coming through an open window or what one is exposed to by sleeping outside, but also to drafts of any kind, including those from the vents of air conditioners.

23. Also known as Mosla Powder *(xiāng rú sǎn)*.

24. According to the source text, all three herbs should be ground into coarse powder and cooked: 9g of the formula with 0.3g wine. Take as a decoction. Clinically, it is not necessary to give such a large dosage of herbs, because it is an acute disease, and just a few days would be enough to cure the disease if the treatment is correct. The following dosages are recommended by the author: Moslae Herba *(xiāng rú)* (9-15g), Lablab Semen album *(bái biǎn dòu)* (6-12g), and Magnoliae officinalis Cortex *(hòu pò)* (6-12g).

25. This is the flower of the plant from which Lablab Semen album *(bái biǎn dòu)* is derived. It is sweet, aromatic, and neutral and enters the Spleen and Stomach channels. It clears summerheat, transforms dampness, and harmonizes the Stomach. It is commonly used for problems due to summerheat and dampness such as fever, diarrhea or dysenteric disorders, as well as vaginal discharge. The normal dosage is 3-9g.

26. In fact, Moslae Herba *(xiāng rú)*, which is warm and acrid, only treats the dampness that often accompanies summerheat. It is therefore most appropriate for treating yin-type summerheat in which dampness is predominant. But we can also use it for yang-type summerheat as its dispersing action, when combined with other herbs, helps push out summerheat that has been trapped by dampness and cold in the exterior.

27. Wu Tang, *Systematic Differentiation of Warm Pathogen Diseases (Wēn bìng tiáo biàn)*. Beijing: People's Health Publishing House, 1963: 32

28. This formula is known by various names. It was called Molsa Powder *(xiāng rú sǎn)* in the source text, and Four-Substance Decoction with Mosla *(sì wèi xiāng rú yǐn)* in *Medical Formulas Collected and Analyzed (Yī fāng jí jiě)*.

29. This book was written by Zhu Gong and published in 1108.

30. The dosages here are from Wang Ang, *Medical Formulas Collected and Analyzed (Yī fāng jí jiě)*. Shanghai: Shanghai Science and Technology Publishing House, 1959: 171.

31. Dong Jian-Hua et al., *Selected Case Studies from Famous Modern Chinese Doctors*, 1157. This case study was reported by Xiong Liao-Sheng.

32. Lei Feng, *Discussion of Seasonal Diseases (Shí bìng lùn)*. Beijing: People's Health Publishing House, 1956: 63.

33. The base formula was used in the source text to treat diarrhea from summerheat with dampness attacking the Spleen. This modification for treating the common cold in the summer due to an attack of summerheat was made in the source text by adding Trichosanthis Semen *(guā lóu rén)* and Armeniacae Semen *(xìng rén)*.

34. The earliest usage of the word *zhài* to mean disease was in the *Classic of Poetry (Shī jīng)*. It also has this meaning in the early Tang dynasty work *Important Formulas Worth a Thousand Gold Pieces for any Emergency (Bèi jí qiān jīn yào fāng)*. Later, in such works as *Teachings of (Zhu) Dan-Xi (Dān-Xī xīn fǎ)*, it was used as a synonym for Lung consumption (肺癆 *fèi láo*), a disease marked with wasting and coughing of blood. This is the sense of the word intended here by Wu Tang.

35. See n. 25 above.

36. This is the immature leaf of Lophatheri Herba *(dàn zhú yè)* and is difficult to find outside of East Asia. We recommend substituting Lophatheri Herba *(dàn zhú yè)*.

37. See Chapter 8.

38. See Chapter 7.

39. This is known as Unaccompanied Ginseng Decoction *(dú shēn tāng)* and was first mentioned in *Collected Treatises of [Zhang] Jing-Yue (Jǐng-Yuè quán shū)* written by Zhang Jie-Bing (Zhang Jing-Yue) and published in 1624.

40. See Chapter 7.

41. The source text suggests grinding the herbs into powder and cooking 15g of the powder each time for a day. The dosages for the ingredients in this formula are too high to apply clinically, and the following are recommended instead: Gypsum fibrosum *(shí gāo)* (24-30g), Anemarrhenae Rhizoma *(zhī mǔ)* (12-15g), Atractylodis Rhizoma *(cāng zhú)* (9-15g), nonglutinous rice *(gěng mǐ)* (9-12g), and Honey-toasted Glycyrrhizae Radix preparata *(zhì gān cǎo)* (3-6g).

42. Li Gao (Li Dong-Yuan), *Discussion of Spleen and Stomach (Pí wèi lùn)*. Beijing: People's Health Publishing House, 1976: 217. The formula consists of Astragali Radix *(huáng qí)* (9g), Atractylodis Rhizoma *(cāng zhú)* (9g), Cimicifugae Rhizoma *(shēng má)* (9g), Ginseng Radix *(rén shēn)* (4.5g), Alismatis Rhizoma *(zé xiè)* (4.5g), Massa medicata fermentata *(shén qū)* (4.5g), Citri reticulatae Pericarpium *(chén pí)* (4.5g), Atractylodis macrocephalae Rhizoma *(bái zhú)* (4.5g), Angelicae sinensis Radix *(dāng guī)* (2.7g), Honey-toasted Glycyrrhizae Radix preparata *(zhì gān cǎo)* (2.7g), Citri reticulatae viride Pericarpium *(qīng pí)* (2.7g), Phellodendri Cortex *(huáng bǎi)* (2.7g), Puerariae Radix *(gé gēn)* (2.7g), and Schisandrae Fructus *(wǔ wèi zǐ)* (9 pieces).

43. Wang Shi-Xiong, *Warp and Woof of Warm-Heat Pathogen Diseases (Wēn rè jīng wěi)*. This title is reproduced in Lu Zhen, *Collection of Modern Rare Books of Chinese Medicine: Warm Pathogen Disease Volume*, 120-21.

44. Author's own case study.

45. This medicine was discussed in the context of the formula Magical Rhinoceros Special Pill *(shé xī dān)* above. Isatidis Folium *(dà qīng yè)* is usually substituted.

12 Damp-Warmth

D AMP-WARMTH (濕溫 *shī wēn*) is caused by an attack of a damp-heat pathogen (濕熱 *shī rè*). The term damp-warmth was first mentioned in *Classic of Difficulties (Nán jīng)* but was not described at length until the eighteenth century.[1] It is characterized by contained fever, heavy sensation in the body, generalized lassitude, chest and epigastric distention, poor appetite, yellow, greasy tongue coating, and a moderate pulse. While theoretically it should only appear in the late summer or early autumn, it may in fact occur at any time.

Given its association with dampness, damp-warmth progresses slowly. Like other warm pathogen diseases, it can progress from the protective level to the qi, nutritive, or blood levels. However, it tends to remain in the qi level, and its pathological center is the Spleen and Stomach.

Before continuing with our discussion of damp-warmth, we should consider the differences between it and the pattern of internally-generated damp-heat in internal medicine. Although they share several signs and symptoms, they are in fact quite different. Damp-warmth is mainly caused by a combination of two external pathogenic factors, dampness and heat, and primarily occurs in the late summer and early autumn. (See Chapter 3 for further details.) By contrast, the pattern of internal damp-heat is caused by a combination of internal pathogenic factors, that is, internal dampness and heat, resulting from a disharmony in the yin and yang organs. The pattern of internal damp-heat can cause many problems such as jaundice, colitis, diarrhea, bloody stools, urinary dysfunction, vaginal discharge, eczema, and abdominal pain.

Despite these differences, the patterns of internal damp-heat and damp-warmth nevertheless share the same pathology (failure of the Spleen to transform and transport) and display certain similar signs and symptoms (poor appetite, epigastric distention, abdominal bloating). They also manifest similar bowel difficulties: bowel movements may be loose, but only every two or three days; or, if they occur one or more times a day, evacuation feels incomplete, even if the stool is soft.

Table 12.1	Internal Damp-Heat vs. Damp-Warmth	
Etiology	**Pathology**	**Signs and Symptoms**
▶ INTERNAL DAMP-HEAT		
Dysfunction of the Spleen and Stomach in transporting and transforming of fluids	Begins in Spleen and Stomach and can affect many organs	Either no fever or a low- grade fever, jaundice, stool containing mucus and blood, slow and split urine stream with thick and white urethral discharge at the end of urination, foul and smelly vaginal discharge, and/or red, itchy, and weeping skin eruptions
▶ DAMP-WARMTH		
Attack of external dampness and heat	Mostly in the qi level (Spleen and Stomach), but can progress to any level and even affect Heart or Pericardium	Early stage: fever and aversion to cold; middle stage: vesicles and muddled consciousness; late stage: maculas, convulsion, and delirium

Biomedical diseases such as typhoid, paratyphoid, leptospirosis, and influenza overlap somewhat with the Chinese medical diagnosis of damp-warmth, and can be treated with the same methods outlined in this chapter.

Etiology and Pathology

There are two distinct etiologies for damp-warmth:

1. Externally-contracted damp-heat

2. Internally-generated damp-heat

The former is attributable to damp-heat attacking the body through the skin and muscles during the late summer or early autumn, or to a sudden attack after eating improper foods, which thereby enter through the mouth. By 'improper foods' is meant the overconsumption of foods that are much too cold, spicy, or greasy, or the regular consumption of such foods over time. The latter is caused by dysfunction of the Spleen in transforming and transporting, resulting in the accumulation of food and fluids in the middle burner. According to Xue Xue (Xue Sheng-Bai, 1681–1770) in *Systematic Differentiation of Damp-Heat (Shī rè tiáo biàn)*, "The patient first develops internal dampness from injury to the Spleen. Then external dampness [and heat] attacks the body due to its attraction to internal dampness, and the patient suffers from damp-warmth."[2] How does this occur? Since both external and internal dampness pertain to earth, they resonate with each other. Clinically, not everyone who suffers from damp-warmth has a clear history of pre-existing injury to the Spleen with internal dampness. In such individuals, the external dampness aspect of damp-heat impairs the transportive and transformative functions of the Spleen, and quickly generates manifestations of internal dampness.

Compared with other warm pathogen diseases, damp-warmth has several distinguishing features:

- *Damp-warmth is relatively complex.* Damp-warmth patterns are caused by a combination of two pathogens, one yang (heat) and one yin (dampness). Sometimes these two pathogens affect the body equally, while at other times one will predominate. Clinically, it is extremely important to understand this and to ascertain the relative strength of the pathogens in the patient you are treating, as this will have a major impact on treatment. It is true that dampness may also accompany summerheat; however, summerheat is usually the predominant pathogen. Moreover, summerheat is limited to the summer season (see Table 12.4).

- *Damp-warmth begins relatively deeply.* According to five-phase theory, dampness prevails in late summer, the season related to earth. The Stomach and Spleen also pertain to earth. Thus, an invasion of damp-heat readily affects the Spleen and Stomach (middle burner). Most of the other types of warm pathogen disease attack the Lung and/or protective level first, which is more superficial relative to the middle burner.

- *Damp-warmth usually affects two organs simultaneously.* Because damp-heat usually relates to both external and internal dampness during its early stage, from its onset it affects both the protective and qi levels (including the Spleen and Stomach). Manifestations include aversion to cold, chills, fever, epigastric distention, lassitude, loose stools, abdominal bloating, a sensation of heaviness or numbness in the body, muscle soreness, dry mouth with no desire to drink, and a white tongue coating, which may be greasy.

As just noted, damp-warmth may occur either with equal measures of dampness and heat, or with a predominance of one or the other pathogen. This leads to two subcategories: damp-predominant and heat-predominant. The predominance of one or the other pathogen is related to the strength of the Spleen and Stomach qi. When the qi is strong, the damp-heat pathogen will constrain it and transform it into heat. In this case, either heat will predominate or dampness and heat will be equal. When heat predominates, the Stomach is the focus of pathology, with a feverish body, irritability, thirst, epigastric distention, red tongue with a yellow, greasy coating, and a rapid pulse that is either soggy or slippery.

On the other hand, if the qi of the Stomach and Spleen is weak, then the inability of the Spleen to transform and transport fluids will produce even more dampness, leading to a pattern in which dampness predominates. In this case, the Spleen is the focus of pathology, with headache with a heavy sensation in the head, aversion to cold, chills, generalized aches, contained fever[3] (especially in the afternoon), poor appetite, abdominal bloating, irregular bowel movements or ones that, while loose, feel incomplete, a white, greasy tongue coating, and a soggy, moderate pulse. Xue Xue described this division of damp-warmth patterns in *Systematic Differentiation of Damp-Heat:* "Most damp-heat diseases are located in the *yang ming* [Stomach] and *tai yin* [Spleen]. If the middle qi is replete [excesive], the disease will be located in the *yang ming;* if the middle qi is deficient, the disease will enter the *tai yin.*"[4]

- *Damp-warmth progresses relatively slowly.* Dampness is a viscous and sluggish pathogen. Diseases with a significant component of dampness, such as damp-warmth, progress slowly, and by the same token, are relatively slow to depart.

- *Damp-warmth requires relatively complicated treatment.* This follows from the characteristics of damp-warmth described above. When treating damp-warmth we must ascertain the relative strength of the two pathogens in order to effectively treat the disorder. First, because one pathogen is yin and the other is yang, treatment which helps with one aspect of the disease may make the other aspect worse. Second, dampness is a viscous pathogenic factor with form, which is more tenacious and difficult to treat than a formless pathogen such as heat. Third, external dampness can injure the Spleen and set up a vicious cycle whereby the more dampness there is, the more the Spleen is impaired, resulting in even more dampness. This makes treatment more difficult. Finally, the resulting Spleen deficiency reduces the production of qi and blood and thereby weakens the antipathogenic qi. Taken together, these factors make the treatment of damp-warmth relatively difficult and prolonged.

Factors for Identifying Damp-Warmth

There are four important factors for identifying damp-warmth:

1. Damp-warmth usually appears in late summer or early autumn.

2. In the early stages of damp-warmth, there are signs and symptoms of blockage of the antipathogenic qi, especially the protective qi, as well as disturbance of the Spleen and Stomach. These include contained fever, aversion to cold, chills, a heavy sensation in the head and body, chest and epigastric distention, greasy tongue coating, and a soggy and moderate pulse.

3. Because dampness is tenacious, the disease will progress slowly and will affect the individual for a relatively long period of time. This type of disease can remain in the qi level for a long time.

4. Miliaria alba[5] commonly appear during the development of damp-warmth.

These variables—blockage of antipathogenic qi, disturbance of the Spleen and Stomach, and the emergence of miliaria alba—are important indicators for the diagnosis of damp-warmth. Clinically, if any one of them occurs acutely in the late summer or early autumn, a diagnosis of damp-warmth may be established.

However, it is not enough to simply diagnose damp-warmth. The practitioner must then make a more precise differentiation, based on the following factors:

- *Nature of the predominant factor: dampness or heat.* The successful treatment of damp-warmth is completely dependent on precisely determining the relative balance of dampness and heat. This is true whether it is a pattern of internal damp-heat or externally-generated damp-warmth. (See Table 12.2.)

- *Location of the dampness.* If the dampness is situated in the upper burner, the patient will present with fever (especially a persistent and contained fever), aversion to cold, heaviness and pain in the head, dizziness, a plugged sensation in the ears, chest distention, and lethargy. If it is situated in the middle burner, there will be abdominal and epigastric distention or abdominal pain, poor appetite, nausea, belching, vomiting, flatulence, loose stools, generalized lassitude, and a thick, greasy tongue coating. And if it resides in the lower burner, there will be scanty or turbid urine or difficult urination, and sweating in the groin area or excessive vaginal discharge. (See Table 12.3.)

- *Nature of the pattern: damp-warmth versus summerheat combined with dampness.* Both damp-warmth and the pattern of summerheat combined with dampness may appear during the summer. They are both caused by the same two external pathogens, dampness and heat. Although they progress quite differently, their early manifestations are very similar. Accurate differentiation is therefore important. (See Table 12.4.)

Table 12.2	Determining Whether Dampness or Heat Predominates in Damp-Warmth	
	Dampness Predominates	**Heat Predominates**
FEVER:	Contained fever that occurs in the afternoon	High fever that does not diminish after sweating
BEHAVIOR:	Lethargic and indifferent	Restless
HEAD & BODY:	Head and body are heavy, painful, and stiff	Distending pain or soreness throughout the body
CHEST, EPIGASTRIUM, & ABDOMEN:	Distention in chest, epigastrium, and abdomen	Distending epigastric pain
STOOLS AND URINE:	Loose or watery stools, turbid urine	Loose and foul-smelling stools, uncomfortable sensation around anus, scanty and dark-yellow urine
MOUTH AND TONGUE:	No thirst but profuse saliva; white, greasy, and slippery, tongue coating	Bitter taste, bad breath, significant thirst, red tongue body with coating that is yellow, thick, greasy, or turbid
PULSE:	Soggy and slippery	Slippery and rapid

Table 12.3	Location of Dampness in the Three Burners
Location	**Signs and Symptoms**
Upper burner	Contained fever that is especially persistent, aversion to cold, heaviness and pain in the head, dizziness, chest distention, lethargy
Middle burner	Abdominal and epigastric distention, poor appetite, nausea, vomiting, loose stools, generalized lassitude, thick and/or greasy tongue coating
Lower burner	Scanty or turbid urine or urinary dysfunction

Table 12.4	Damp-Warmth vs. Summerheat Combined with Dampness	
Type	**Common Aspects**	**Different Aspects**
Damp-warmth	Heat and dampness with fever, aversion to cold, headache, chest and epigastric distention	Dampness predominates (at first) with contained fever, heavy sensation in body, generalized lassitude, white and greasy tongue coating, soggy and moderate pulse
Summerheat combined with dampness	Same as above.	High fever, cough or hemoptysis, thirst, restlessness or even muddled consciousness, flooding and rapid pulse

Progression of Damp-Warmth

Generally speaking, the progression of damp-warmth is slower than other warm pathogen diseases, and its course is more drawn out. Damp-warmth presents with two basic lines of progression:

1. Damp-heat to dry-heat and injury of the yin

2. Damp-heat to cold-dampness and injury of the yang qi.

Clinically, damp-heat may not follow either of these progressions. It may remain as damp-heat, which often leads to jaundice, or may transform into phlegm-heat and veil the orifices of the Heart.

In its early stage, a protective level pattern may appear because the external damp-heat pathogen attacks the exterior. However, the duration of such a pattern is transient, without special characteristics, and is often associated with accumulation of dampness in the Spleen, leading to a pattern with both protective and qi level involvement. This short-lived and unremarkable exterior pattern leads some practitioners to mistakenly conclude that there is no protective level pattern in damp-warmth, and that the disease has started in the qi level.

When heat without dampness attacks the Lung and protective level there will be a high fever, aversion to cold, chills, headache, and cough. These symptoms readily attract the attention of the patient and practitioner. By contrast, the early stage of damp-warmth presents with relatively mild contained fever, lassitude, chest and epigastric distention, and a poor appetite. A patient may be slow to report these symptoms, as one may experience them as less acute and severe and therefore unworthy of mention.

Also, unlike those warm pathogen diseases that result from heat alone, damp-warmth seldom quickly invades the Pericardium or the nutritive level. Yet, although it may appear to be mild and have a slow progression, damp-warmth can in fact be severe, even fatal, and is not easy to treat, even at an early stage. Its progression was summarized by Zhang Nan, who wrote in *A Stick to Awaken Physicians (Yī mén bàng hè)* that, because both the Stomach and Spleen pertain to earth in five-phase theory, they are of the same category and call upon each other. For this reason, while a damp-heat pathogen may be received from the outside at the beginning, in the end it will migrate to the Spleen and Stomach.[6]

As the protective level signs disappear, damp-warmth will have completely progressed to the qi level. Once there, damp-warmth patterns become very complicated and usually end up lingering in the body for a long period of time. As previously noted, damp-warmth can be divided into three subtypes based on the relative strength of the middle qi: more dampness than heat, more heat than dampness, and equal parts dampness and heat. However, regardless of the type, it is the center of the body (Spleen and Stomach) that is the pathological focus of the disease, and from this center it will disrupt other parts of the body:

- If damp-heat invades the Liver and Gallbladder, blocking the secretion of bile, there will be jaundice.
- If damp-heat steams upward and veils the Pericardium or blocks the Heart spirit, there will be muddled consciousness and delirium.
- If damp-heat flows downward to the Bladder and affects its qi activity, there will be urinary dysfunction.
- If damp-heat steams out to the exterior, miliaria alba will emerge.

When it exists for a relatively long time, damp-heat can transform into heat and fire and progress to the nutritive and blood levels. Its pathology and manifestations in the nutritive and blood levels are similar to those warm pathogen diseases caused by heat alone:

- Maculas
- Bleeding symptoms caused by heat pushing the blood outside the vessels
- Loss of consciousness due to the blockage of the spirit of the Heart
- Convulsions due to the stirring of Liver wind
- Bloody stools.

The last symptom is a special feature of damp-heat that has transformed into pure heat and fire. They invade the channel of the Large Intestine and cause bloody stools.

There are three more possible patterns that appear in a later stage of damp-warmth, where dampness predominates. In the first pattern, there is a reduction in damp-heat coupled with deficiency of antipathogenic qi. This type presents as the

remnants of damp-heat with Spleen qi deficiency. In the second pattern, the dampness injures the Kidney yang, leading to retention of pathological fluids. In the third
pattern, the damp-heat is responsible for heavy bleeding in the Large Intestine, leading to the collapse of qi.

Treatment Principles

Dampness is characterized by stickiness, stagnation, and tenacity. Of all the external
pathogenic factors, dampness is the most difficult to treat, and when it combines
with heat, it is even more difficult to resolve. It is said that combining dampness
with heat is like mixing oil with wheat flour. As described by Xue Xue in *Systematic
Differentiation of Damp-Heat*:

> Heat with dampness blazes more intensely; dampness with heat becomes more
> turbulent. When dampness and heat are separate, the disease is mild and [rela-
> tively] moderate. When dampness and heat come together, the disease is intense
> and [relatively] severe.[7]

Therefore, the treatment principle for damp-warmth is to separately resolve the heat
and the dampness as thoroughly as possible. But how can they be 'separately' resolved? If one attempts only to clear the heat with bitter and cold herbs, the dampness will become worse, as these herbs injure the yang qi. And if one attempts only to
eliminate dampness through draining, drying, and transforming dampness, the herbs
used for this purpose injure the yin. In the words of Wu Tang, "If [the practitioner]
only clears heat, dampness will not retreat; if [the practitioner] only dispels dampness, the heat will blaze brighter."[8] To get around this dilemma, the practitioner must
simultaneously clear heat and eliminate dampness. This is the only way to isolate
dampness from heat, also known as separately resolving dampness and heat. For best
results, follow these guidelines:

- *Treat according to the location of the dampness and heat in the three burners.*
  It is very important to select a treatment method that is based on the location
  of the heat and dampness. The practitioner should pay more attention to
  dampness when treating damp-warmth because it is dampness that serves as the
  foundation to which heat attaches. Unless the dampness is eliminated, the heat
  cannot be cleared. Table 12.5 shows how to select a treatment approach based
  on the location of the dampness.

- *Treat according to the location of the dampness and heat in the different levels.* In
  general, the practitioner must focus on the qi level when treating damp-warmth.
  In the early stage of damp-warmth, dampness predominates, so treatment
  should focus on transforming dampness in conjunction with clearing heat in

Table 12.5	Treatment of Dampness in Damp-Warmth Based on Location
Location	**Treatment Principles**
Upper burner	Transform dampness by disseminating and directing Lung qi downward
Middle burner	Dispel dampness by warming the Spleen and Stomach and promoting their transportive and transformative functions
Lower burner	Leach out dampness with bland herbs

order to isolate the heat. If the patient suffers from a combination of protective and qi level patterns, use acrid and aromatic herbs, and slightly cold herbs, to transform and disperse damp-heat in the protective and qi levels. Promoting qi circulation and clearing heat will play an important role when damp-warmth reaches the qi level.

• *Treat the predominant pathogenic factor: dampness and/or heat.* If dampness predominates, eliminate the dampness with bitter, acrid, and warm herbs. If heat is more severe than dampness, clear the heat with bitter, acrid, and cold herbs. Yet, irrespective of whether heat or dampness predominates, leach out the dampness through urination with bland herbs (in combination with the other methods) because *both* heat and dampness can be discharged via the urine. Of course, if heat predominates, the focus of treatment should still be on clearing the heat. (See Table 12.6.)

If the damp-heat transforms into pure heat and fire, the treatment options are the same as for those warm pathogen diseases which are caused by heat alone:

• Clear heat and generate fluids when there is heat from excess and injury to the fluids in the Stomach.

Table 12.6	Treatment of Heat in Damp-Warmth Based on Location
Location	**Specific Treatment Principles**
Upper burner	Dispel and disperse heat
Lower burner	Discharge heat

- Purge heat and dry stools for severe constipation with dry stools and heat in the Large Intestine.

- Cool the blood and stop the bleeding for bloody stools caused by an invasion of the blood level and injury to the collaterals in the Large Intestine.

- Warm the Kidney yang and promote urination for water retention due to injury to the Kidney yang by dampness.

- Strongly tonify and restore the qi for qi collapse.

According to Wu Tang, an important method for eliminating dampness is to promote qi circulation, especially for the Lung.[9] In damp-warmth the circulation of qi is blocked by the dampness, which can produce further dampness in the middle burner, or even Liver qi stagnation and blood stasis. Based on my own understanding and experience, qi is not only the commander of blood, but also of the fluids. Once qi circulation is normalized in the organs, especially the Spleen and Stomach, there will be no further production of dampness, and the existing dampness will be transformed. Therefore, no matter where the dampness is situated, the movement of qi should be promoted.

How do these herbs transform dampness? There are a few ways in which dampness can be transformed and eliminated from the body:

- Dampness can be transported to the Triple Burner and Bladder by strengthening qi circulation, after which it is discharged in the form of urine. The patient may notice an increase in the volume of urine after taking a formula for a week or two. Alternatively, the urine may be more turbid.

- Dampness can be warmed and evaporated by the circulating qi, which is yang in nature, and discharged through the act of passing gas. Thus, the patient may notice an increase in flatulence after having taken a formula for a week or two.

- Dampness can be warmed, evaporated, and discharged through the pores in the skin by normal circulation of the protective qi. Thus, when dampness is situated in the exterior, the patient may sweat slightly for a couple hours after taking a formula.

The patient should notice that accompanying signs and symptoms have improved in conjunction with the increase in urination, flatulence, or slight sweating. In general, the practitioner should promote the natural directional flow of the Lung qi to treat dampness in the upper burner, the Spleen and Stomach to treat dampness in the middle burner, and the Bladder to treat dampness in the lower burner. Use acrid and bitter herbs such as Armeniacae Semen *(xìng rén)* and Platycodi Radix *(jié gěng)* to disseminate the Lung qi and direct it downward. Use bitter herbs such as Aurantii Fructus immaturus *(zhǐ shí)*, Magnoliae officinalis Cortex *(hòu pò)*, and Citri reticulatae Pericarpium *(chén pí)* to direct the Stomach qi downward, and acrid herbs like Amomi Fructus rotundus *(bái dòu kòu)*, Eupatorii Herba *(pèi lán)*, and Pogostemonis/Agastaches Herba *(huò xiāng)* to lift the Spleen qi. Use bland and/or bitter herbs such as Polyporus *(zhū líng)*, Alismatis Rhizoma *(zé xiè)*, Talcum *(huá shí)*, and Coicis Semen *(yì yǐ rén)* to drain the Bladder.

Contraindications for Treating the Early Stage of Damp-Warmth

In his book *Systematic Differentiation of Warm Pathogen Diseases (Wēn bìng tiáo biàn)*, written in 1798, Wu Tang warned of three things when treating the early stage of damp-warmth.[10] If these warnings are ignored, treatment will be unsuccessful.

1. *It is contraindicated to use sweating to rid the body of dampness.*[11] Signs and symptoms associated with the early stage of damp-warmth often include headache, generalized aches, chills, aversion to cold, and fever. This is somewhat similar to the presentation of the exterior *tai yang* wind-cold pattern described in *Discussion of Cold Damage (Shāng hán lùn)*,[12] which is commonly treated by inducing sweating with acrid and warm herbs. How does the practitioner distinguish between them?

   • The best way is to ascertain whether the tongue coating is greasy, and if there is a sensation of heaviness in the head and body. If these symptoms are present, they are caused by an attack of dampness associated with heat, rather than by wind-cold.

   • Chills associated with wind-cold will be more severe than those due to stagnation of the protective qi caused by dampness. In addition, chills due to dampness may worsen in the afternoon, while those associated with wind-cold rarely do.

   • Finally, a headache caused by wind-cold is always associated with a stiff neck, while a headache caused by stagnation of the protective qi due to dampness is very often accompanied by a heavy sensation in the head.

According to Wu Tang, if one induces sweating to treat the pattern of dampness combined with heat, this could result in acute deafness and loss of consciousness caused by the dampness steaming upward and attacking the Triple Burner and Gallbladder channels, or veiling the Pericardium or blocking the Heart.[13]

2. *It is contraindicated to expel the dampness through purging.* In the early stage of damp-warmth, chest and epigastric distention may appear. Some physicians associate this with retention of food in the Large Intestine. However, this type of

chest and epigastric distention is actually caused by stagnation of qi due to accumulation of dampness in the middle burner. This distinction is easy to make when there are no symptoms pointing to retention of food, such as belching with a fetid odor.

According to Wu Tang, if one uses purging to treat dampness combined with heat, this will lead to severe watery diarrhea.[14]

3. *It is contraindicated to enrich yin.* In some cases, an afternoon or evening fever may appear. This can be easily confused with a yin deficiency-induced fever, which also commonly occurs at that time of day. However, a careful differentiation must be made. Pay particular attention to the tongue coating. If it is greasy (and perhaps thick), the fever is caused by dampness.[15] If there is little tongue coating, coupled with a hot sensation in the palms and soles, malar flush, and a thin and rapid pulse, the fever is caused by yin deficiency.

According to Wu Tang, if herbs that enrich the yin (and thus produce moisture) are used to treat dampness, they will only exacerbate and prolong the damp condition.[16]

Differentiation and Treatment of Damp-Warmth with Dampness Predominant

ATTACK ON THE PROTECTIVE LEVEL BY DAMPNESS

Manifestations. There are two concurrent aspects to this pattern:[17]

1. *Blockage of the protective qi by dampness* with aversion to cold, chills, absence of sweating, a white, thin, greasy tongue coating, and a soggy pulse.
2. *Obstruction of the channels by dampness* with a heavy or painful sensation in the body or joints.

NOTE: If the dampness has not transformed into heat, there will be an absence of sweating, and fever will rarely appear. However, if the dampness has transformed into heat, there will be fever, which is not diminished even after sweating.

Pathology. Dampness attacking the protective level, leading to blockage of the protective qi and obstruction of the channels.

Treatment principles. The goals vary depending on the pathology. For dampness only, disperse the dampness with acrid and aromatic herbs. For dampness coupled with heat, transform the dampness with aromatic herbs, and leach out dampness and drain heat with bland and cold herbs.

Formula No. 1: [18]

> ### XUE'S ACRID AND AROMATIC FORMULA TO RELEASE THE EXTERIOR
> *(Xuē shì xīn xiāng jiě biǎo fāng)*

SOURCE: *Systematic Differentiation of Damp-Heat*

Pogostemonis/Agastaches Herba *(huò xiāng)*..................9g

Moslae Herba *(xiāng rú)* 6g

Menthae haplocalycis Herba *(bò hé)* 6g

Notopterygii Rhizoma seu Radix *(qiāng huó)* 3g

Atractylodis Radicis Cortex *(cāng zhú pí)*[19].................6g

Arctii Fructus *(niú bàng zǐ)* 6g

ANALYSIS OF FORMULA: This formula is indicated for dampness that has not yet transformed into heat. Pogostemonis/Agastaches Herba *(huò xiāng)* and Cortex Atractylodis Rhizomatis *(cang zhu pi)* are aromatic herbs that transform dampness and promote qi circulation. It is hard to obtain Atractylodis Radicis Cortex *(cāng zhú pí)*, and it can be replaced with Atractylodis Rhizoma *(cāng zhú)* (12g). Moslae Herba *(xiāng rú)* and Notopterygii Rhizoma seu Radix *(qiāng huó)*, which are acrid and warm, disperse dampness from the exterior, activate the channels, and relieve pain. Menthae haplocalycis Herba *(bò hé)* and Arctii Fructus *(niú bàng zǐ)*, which are acrid and cool, work with Notopterygii Rhizoma seu Radix *(qiāng huó)* and Moslae Herba *(xiāng rú)* to disperse dampness and slightly promote sweating to let dampness out of the body. Notopterygii Rhizoma seu Radix *(qiāng huó)* strongly promotes sweating, so its dosage should be small; if there is no headache, it can be omitted entirely.

Formula No. 2:

> ### XUE'S FORMULA TO RELEASE THE EXTERIOR, LEACH OUT DAMPNESS, AND DRAIN HEAT *(Xuē shì jiě biǎo shēn shī xiè rè fāng)*

SOURCE: *Systematic Differentiation of Damp-Heat*

Pogostemonis/Agastaches Folium *(huò xiāng yè)*[20] 6g

Talcum *(huá shí)* 6g

Atractylodis Radicis Cortex *(cāng zhú pí)* 6g

Tetrapanacis Medulla *(tōng cǎo)* 6g

Nelumbinis Folium *(hé yè)*.....................6g

Sojae Semen germinatum *(dà dòu juǎn)* 9g

Poriae Cutis *(fú líng pí)* 6g

Platycodi Radix *(jié gěng)*.....................6g

ANALYSIS OF FORMULA: This formula is indicated for dampness that has gradually transformed into heat. Atractylodis Radicis Cortex *(cāng zhú pí)*, Pogostemonis/ Agastaches Folium *(huò xiāng yè)*, and Nelumbinis Folium *(hé yè)* are aromatic herbs that disperse and transform dampness. Talcum *(huá shí)*, Sojae Semen germinatum *(dà dòu juǎn)*, Poriae Cutis *(fú líng pí)*, and Tetrapanacis Medulla *(tōng cǎo)* leach out dampness and drain heat. Platycodi Radix *(jié gěng)* disseminates the Lung qi to help disperse dampness in the exterior and drain damp-heat through urination; the Lung governs the protective qi and exterior as well as the water pathways. In this condition, the dampness has gradually transformed into heat, thus the acrid and warm herbs present in Xue's Acrid and Aromatic Formula to Release the Exterior *(Xuē shì jiě biǎo shēn shī xiè rè fāng)* have been omitted. Atractylodis Rhizoma *(cāng zhú)* can be substituted for Atractylodis Radicis Cortex *(cāng zhú pí)*, as Atractylodis Radicis Cortex *(cāng zhú pí)* is difficult to obtain.

DAMPNESS HINDERING THE QI MECHANISM OF THE PROTECTIVE AND QI LEVELS

Manifestations. There are two concurrent aspects to this pattern:

1. *Dampness hindering the protective qi in the exterior* with a contained fever that is especially intense in the afternoon, chills, aversion to cold, heavy sensation and pain in the head and body, and slight sweating.

2. *Dampness hindering the qi in the qi level* with chest and epigastric distention, a white, greasy tongue coating, and a soggy, moderate pulse.

The predominance of dampness here is evident in the contained fever, chest and epigastric distention, white and greasy tongue coating, heavy sensation in the head as if it is wrapped in a wet towel, and soggy and moderate pulse.[21]

NOTE: Three aspects of this condition are easily confused with other disorders. First, the fever, chills, aversion to cold, headache, and slight sweating can be mistaken for a *tai yang* wind-cold exterior pattern. However, the pulse is neither floating nor tight, and the neck is not stiff. Rather, dampness here leads to chest and epigastric distention.

Second, chest and epigastric distention can be mistaken for the retention of food. However, with retention of food, there are generally no exterior signs and symptoms, and the patient will belch with a fetid odor, and have a poor appetite or acid reflux; in addition, the tongue coating will be thick and greasy. By contrast, with stagnation of qi in the protective and qi levels due to dampness, the patient will have exterior signs and symptoms, a sensation of heaviness, and a white and greasy tongue coating.

Third, an afternoon fever can occur in three different patterns:

1. *Yang ming organ pattern (severe constipation with dry stools and heat in the Large Intestine).* The fever here is caused by the flourishing of qi in the Large Intestine, because qi in the *yang ming* flourishes (according to the Chinese clock) between the hours of *shēn* to *yǒu*, or 3 P.M. to 7 P.M. However, this is usually accompanied by distending pain in the abdomen, dry and hard stools, a yellow and dry tongue coating, and a submerged and forceful pulse.

2. *Yin deficiency.* This type of fever occurs in the afternoon, which is the 'yin within yang' time of day. Additionally, this form of heat, situated in yin areas of the body such as the soles and palms, will become intense during the relatively yin time of day, hence afternoon fevers. Other signs and symptoms of yin deficiency are night sweats, a red tongue with less than normal coating or no coating at all, or a cracked tongue body.

3. *Damp-warmth.* Fever due to damp-warmth is quite similar to that of yin deficiency. However, the presentation will be different because of the different pathogenic factor. For damp-warmth, the tongue coating must be greasy, and the pulse soggy or slippery. There will also be many symptoms that are characteristic of dampness, such as chest and epigastric distention and a heavy sensation in the body.

Pathology. Stagnation of protective qi and dysfunction of the Spleen's transforming and transporting functions. Dampness is the predominant factor.

Treatment principles. Disperse, transform, and leach out dampness in both the exterior and interior with acrid, aromatic, and bland herbs.

Formula No. 1:

PATCHOULI/AGASTACHE, MAGNOLIA BARK, PINELLIA, AND PORIA DECOCTION (huò pò xià líng tāng)

SOURCE: *Bases of Medicine*[22]

Pogostemonis/Agastaches Herba *(huò xiāng)* .6g
Pinelliae Rhizoma preparatum *(zhì bàn xià)* 4.5g
Poria rubra *(chì fú líng)* 9g
Armeniacae Semen *(xìng rén)* 9g
Coicis Semen *(yì yǐ rén)* 12g
Amomi Fructus rotundus *(bái dòu kòu)* 1.8g
Polyporus *(zhū líng)* 4.5g
Sojae Semen preparatum *(dàn dòu chǐ)* 9g
Magnoliae officinalis Cortex *(hòu pò)* 3g
Alismatis Rhizoma *(zé xiè)* 4.5g

ANALYSIS OF FORMULA: This formula is designed for treating protective and qi level disorders caused by an attack of dampness. Sojae Semen preparatum *(dàn dòu chǐ)*, Armeniacae Semen *(xìng rén)*, and Amomi Fructus rotundus *(bái dòu kòu)* treat dampness in the protective level by disseminating the Lung qi and causing it to descend. Thus, the dampness will be eliminated through the normal qi activity of the Lung. Pogostemonis/Agastaches Herba *(huò xiāng)*, Pinelliae Rhizoma preparatum *(zhì bàn xià)*, and Magnoliae officinalis Cortex *(hòu pò)* transform and dry dampness with their bitter and acrid flavors and warm nature. Thus, the circulation of qi in the middle burner will normalize following the elimination of dampness. With their bland flavor, Polyporus *(zhū líng)*, Alismatis Rhizoma *(zé xiè)*, Coicis Semen *(yì yǐ rén)*, and Poria rubra *(chì fú líng)* drain urine and thereby provide an avenue for dampness to exit the body. This formula combines herbs that transform dampness with an aromatic flavor, herbs that dry dampness with a bitter flavor and warm nature, and herbs that leach out dampness with a bland flavor to eliminate both exterior and interior dampness.

Formula No. 2:

THREE-NUT DECOCTION *(sān rén tāng)*

SOURCE: *Systematic Differentiation of Warm Pathogen Diseases*

Armeniacae Semen *(xìng rén)*	15g
Amomi Fructus rotundus *(bái dòu kòu)*	6g
Magnoliae officinalis Cortex *(hòu pò)*	6g
Pinelliae Rhizoma preparatum *(zhì bàn xià)*	15g
Coicis Semen *(yì yǐ rén)*	18g
Tetrapanacis Medulla *(tōng cǎo)*	6g
Lophatheri Herba *(dàn zhú yè)*	6g
Talcum *(huá shí)*	18g

ANALYSIS OF FORMULA: The best way to evaluate this formula is by comparing the formulas described above. Both formulas:

- Dispel dampness by disseminating the Lung qi and causing it to descend.
- Transform dampness by improving the transportive and transformative functions of the Spleen.
- Dry and transform dampness with bitter, aromatic, and warm herbs.
- Leach out dampness via the urine with bland herbs.

In other words, both formulas can be used to treat stagnation of qi in the protective and qi levels due to dampness. On what basis, then, does the practitioner choose between them to treat the pattern correctly? Their differences can be summarized in two words: heat and level. If the dampness has gradually transformed into heat, and if the qi level is principally involved, use Three-Nut Decoction *(sān rén tāng)*. This is because it includes Lophatheri Herba *(dàn zhú yè)* and Talcum *(huá shí)* to clear heat in both the upper and lower burners in addition to draining dampness, and a large dosage of Armeniacae Semen *(xìng rén)* to direct the Lung qi downward and help leach out dampness. Large dosages of these three herbs are used because dampness has transformed into heat primarily involving the qi level of the middle burner. In addition, because the presence of heat can injure the yin, fewer and weaker herbs to leach out dampness are used in this formula. Specifically, it contains Tetrapanacis Medulla *(tōng cǎo)* instead of the Polyporus *(zhū líng)*, Alismatis Rhizoma *(zé xiè)*, and Poria rubra *(chì fú líng)* that are present in Patchouli/Agastache, Magnolia Bark, Pinellia, and Poria Decoction *(huò pò xià líng tāng)*.

However, if there are significant protective-level signs and symptoms (heavy sensation in the head and body, generalized aches, chills) and there are no indications that the dampness has gradually transformed into heat, use Patchouli/Agastache, Magnolia Bark, Pinellia, and Poria Decoction *(huò pò xià líng tāng)*. This is because it incorporates Pogostemonis/Agastaches Herba *(huò xiāng)* combined with Sojae Semen preparatum *(dàn dòu chǐ)* to eliminate exterior signs and symptoms in the protective level.

MODIFICATION: For significant signs and symptoms of heat, add Lonicerae Flos *(jīn yín huā)*, Forsythiae Fructus *(lián qiào)*, and Artemisiae annuae Herba *(qīng hāo)* to clear the heat.

Case study: Patchouli/Agastache, Magnolia Bark, Pinellia, and Poria Decoction
(huò pò xià líng tāng)

First visit: July 31. This 29-year-old male patient suffered from fever, aversion to cold, epigastric distention, and poor appetite for three days. On the fourth day his condition worsened. His temperature went up to 40.2°C and he experienced muddled consciousness and delirium. He was diagnosed at a hospital with typhus. The patient did not want to be hospitalized and came for Chinese herbal treatment.

His head felt distended, heavy, and painful, and he had chest distention, concentrated urine, cold extremities, and constipation. The patient still had a slight aversion to cold, sweating, and muddled consciousness with delirium at night. His temperature was 39.5°C. His mind was clear, he had a dry mouth with no desire to drink water, and a red tongue with a white, greasy, and slightly thick coating. His face was yellow without luster and his pulse was thin and rapid. The diagnosis was stagnation of dampness in the exterior and interior of the body, leading to damp-heat veiling the spirit. The treatment principles were to transform and leach out dampness, clear heat, and open the orifice. A modified version of Patchouli/Agastache,

Magnolia Bark, Pinellia, and Poria Decoction *(huò pò xià líng tāng)* was chosen: fresh Pogostemonis/Agastaches Herba *(huò xiāng)* (30g), fresh Eupatorii Herba *(pèi lán)* (30g), Pinelliae Rhizoma preparatum *(zhì bàn xià)* (10g), Lablab Semen album *(bái biǎn dòu)*(10g), Magnoliae officinalis Cortex *(hòu pò)* (10g), Armeniacae Semen *(xìng rén)*(10g), Coicis Semen *(yì yǐ rén)* (20g), Amomi Fructus rotundus *(bái dòu kòu)* (10g), Tetrapanacis Medulla *(tōng cǎo)* (10g), Nelumbinis Folium *(hé yè)*(10g), and Atractylodis Rhizoma *(cāng zhú)* (10g), along with Greatest Treasure Special Pill *(zhì bǎo dān)*[23] (one pill divided into several portions and swallowed with the decoction).

Second visit: August 3. Over the course of taking three packets of the formula, the patient's temperature went down to 38.2°C, he had no delirium, and urination increased. The distending headache and heavy sensation, slight aversion to cold, and cold extremities were unchanged. The day before his second visit his temperature had been down to 37.8°C; he still had a heavy sensation in his head, sticky sweat, slight aversion to cold, a dry mouth with no desire to drink, and chest distention. He had bouts of delirium that night. On the day of his visit his temperature was up to 39.4°C and his limbs felt heavy and achy. His tongue was red with a white, slightly thick coating that was greasy at the root. His pulse was still thin and rapid. At this point heat predominated. Atractylodis Rhizoma *(cāng zhú)* was removed from the formula and Scutellariae Radix *(huáng qín)* (10g) was added. Two packets of these herbs were given to the patient.

Third visit: August 5. The patient's temperature was normal in the morning and was 38.2°C in the afternoon. There had been no delirium. His headache and chest distention were significantly reduced. His aversion to cold was gone, but his urine was still yellow and his head still felt distended. Several crystal-like miliaria alba had appeared on his neck. While the yellow and greasy coating had disappeared, his tongue was still red and now had a white, slightly dry coating. His pulse was soggy and moderate. The appearance of miliaria alba was a good sign, as it showed that damp-heat was being expelled to the surface. The treatment principles now were to disperse damp-heat and promote qi circulation: fresh Pogostemonis/Agastaches Herba *(huò xiāng)* (30g), fresh Eupatorii Herba *(pèi lán)* (30g), Tetrapanacis Medulla *(tōng cǎo)* (10g), Amomi Fructus rotundus *(bái dòu kòu)* (10g), Coicis Semen *(yì yǐ rén)* (20g), Armeniacae Semen *(xìng rén)*(10g), Arecae Pericarpium *(dà fù pí)* (10g), Scutellariae Radix *(huáng qín)* (10g), Sojae Semen germinatum *(dà dòu juǎn)* (10g), Lablab Semen album *(bái biǎn dòu)*(10g), and Lophatheri Herba *(dàn zhú yè)* (10g).

After taking more than ten packets of these herbs over the course of a month, all signs and symptoms were gone. His energy gradually improved, and he walked into the room like a normal person. But he still had epigastric distention, poor appetite, and complained that food had no taste. Nourish the Stomach Decoction with Aucklandia and Amomum *(xiāng shā yǎng wèi tāng)*[24] was used to tonify the Spleen and Stomach. The patient totally recovered and went back to work in January.[25]

Case study: Three-Nut Decoction *(sān rén tāng)*

First visit: September 20. This 29-year-old male patient suffered from fever for over four months. His temperature ranged from 37–38°C. He had been hospitalized and a number of tests had been performed, all of which were negative. The treatment he received in the hospital had no effect, and he had been discharged.

His head and body felt heavy and his fever was worse in the afternoon. He had lassitude and chest distention. His appetite was poor, and although he was thirsty, he had no desire to drink. His bowel movements and urination were normal. He had a slightly yellow face, a pale tongue with a white, greasy coating, and a soggy, slightly rapid pulse. The diagnosis was accumulation of damp-heat in the qi level. The principles of treatment were to clear heat, drain and transform dampness, and promote the circulation of qi. A modified version of Three-Nut Decoction *(sān rén tāng)* was prescribed: Coicis Semen *(yì yǐ rén)* (25g), Armeniacae Semen *(xìng rén)*(15g), Amomi Fructus rotundus *(bái dòu kòu)* (15g), Tetrapanacis Medulla *(tōng cǎo)* (7.5g), Lophatheri Herba *(dàn zhú yè)* (7.5g), Magnoliae officinalis Cortex *(hòu pò)* (10g), Pinelliae Rhizoma preparatum *(zhì bàn xià)* (15g), Talcum *(huá shí)* (20g), and Luffae Fructus Retinervus *(sī guā luò)* (20g). Two packets of these herbs were given to the patient.

Second visit. After taking the herbs for two days, the patient's fever was gone and the other signs and symptoms were much ameliorated. The white, greasy tongue coating was significantly reduced. Because the formula appeared to be working, two more packets of the same herbs were given to the patient.

Third visit. All signs and symptoms were gone except that the patient still felt tired. This was attributed to the Spleen deficiency. He was given ten Strengthen the Spleen Pills *(jiàn pí wán)*[26] and instructed to take one pill with a decoction made from Zingiberis Rhizoma recens *(shēng jiāng)* and Jujubae Fructus *(dà zǎo)* three times a day. The patient was cured after finishing the pills.[27]

ACCUMULATION OF TURBID DAMPNESS IN THE MEMBRANE SOURCE

Manifestations. There are two concurrent aspects to this pattern:

1. *A struggle between antipathogenic qi and turbid dampness in the membrane source* with alternating chills and fever, where the chills predominate and are associated with trembling of the body, and a white, thick, greasy, and slightly dry tongue coating that looks just like a fine white powder on the tongue.

2. *Predominance of dampness* with nausea, vomiting, epigastric distention, and a heavy sensation in the hands and feet.

NOTE: Progression of damp-heat to the qi level is a primary characteristic of damp-warmth, as stagnation and turbidity are characteristic of dampness. The type of pattern that occurs depends upon the patient's physical constitution. If the middle burner qi is strong enough, the Stomach will be involved and heat will predominate. If the middle burner qi is weak, the Spleen will be involved and dampness will predominate. Obviously, dampness is predominant in the pattern mentioned above. While it may seem that there is no heat present, there actually is. The dampness is so severe that it compresses the heat inside the body, thereby masking the signs and symptoms of heat. Yet this heat will incubate inside the body and eventually emerge. According to He Lian-Chen in *Revised and Expanded Discussion of Warm-Heat Pathogen Diseases (Chóng dìng guǎng wēn rè lùn*, subjective and objective heat in the chest and abdomen and scanty, turbid, yellow urine accompany this pattern.[28]

Pathology. A struggle between antipathogenic qi and turbid dampness in the membrane source, leading to the ascension of Stomach qi.

Treatment principles. Dispel and disperse the turbid dampness from the membrane source.

Formula No 1:

LEI'S FORMULA TO DISSEMINATE AND VENT [DAMPNESS AND HEAT] FROM THE MEMBRANE SOURCE *(Léi shì xuān tòu mó yuán fāng)*

SOURCE: *Discussion of Seasonal Diseases*[29]

Magnoliae officinalis Cortex *(hòu pò)* 3g
Arecae Semen *(bīng láng)* 4.5g
Tsaoko Fructus *(cǎo guǒ)* 2.4g
Scutellariae Radix *(huáng qín)* 3g
Glycyrrhizae Radix *(gān cǎo)* 1.5g
Pogostemonis/Agastaches Folium *(huò xiāng yè)*[30] 3g
Pinelliae Rhizoma preparatum *(zhì bàn xià)* 4.5g
Zingiberis Rhizoma recens *(shēng jiāng)* . . . . 3 pieces

ANALYSIS OF FORMULA: This formula addresses problems in the membrane source. Magnoliae officinalis Cortex *(hòu pò)*, Arecae Semen *(bīng láng)*, and Tsaoko Fructus *(cǎo guǒ)* are special herbs that can reach the membrane source directly, promoting the circulation of qi and drying dampness. Pogostemonis/Agastaches Herba *(huò xiāng)*, Pinelliae Rhizoma preparatum *(zhì bàn xià)*, and Zingiberis Rhizoma recens *(shēng jiāng)* transform dampness in the middle burner and assist the actions of the previous three herbs. Scutellariae Radix *(huáng qín)* clears heat. Glycyrrhizae Radix *(gān cǎo)* acts to harmonize the other herbs and harmonizes the function of the Stomach. Caution should be exercised when using this formula because it is warm and dry: once the dampness is eliminated, heat may present. At that point, the focus of the treatment should be changed to clearing heat.

MODIFICATION: For a patient with constitutional yang deficiency, add Zingiberis Rhizoma *(gān jiāng)* and Amomi Fructus rotundus *(bái dòu kòu)*.

Formula No. 2:

REACH THE SOURCE DRINK *(dá yuán yǐn)*

SOURCE: *Discussion of Warm Epidemics*[31]

Magnoliae officinalis Cortex *(hòu pò)* 3g

Arecae Semen *(bīng láng)* 6g

Tsaoko Fructus *(cǎo guǒ)* 1.5g

Scutellariae Radix *(huáng qín)* 3g

Glycyrrhizae Radix *(gān cǎo)* 1.5g

Anemarrhenae Rhizoma *(zhī mǔ)* 3g

Paeoniae Radix alba *(bái sháo)* 3g

ANALYSIS OF FORMULA: This formula is used when most of the dampness has transformed into heat and the heat has injured the fluids, resulting in a high fever and a deep-red tongue with a dry, thick coating that looks just like coarse powder on the tongue. This formula can be seen as a simple modification of the previous formula. Pogostemonis/Agastaches Herba *(huò xiāng)*, Pinelliae Rhizoma preparatum *(zhì bàn xià)*, and Zingiberis Rhizoma recens *(shēng jiāng)* have been removed because those dampness-treating herbs are too warm and aromatic and can injure the fluids. Anemarrhenae Rhizoma *(zhī mǔ)* and Paeoniae Radix alba *(bái sháo)* have been added to clear heat and enrich the yin.

MODIFICATIONS: The basic formula can be modified as follows:

- To enhance the formula's effect, add Acori tatarinowii Rhizoma *(shí chāng pú)* and Coptidis Rhizoma *(huáng lián)*.
- For hypochondriac pain, bitter taste, vomiting, and alternating chills and fever due to heat affecting the *shao yang* channel, add Bupleuri Radix *(chái hú)* (3g) (source text).
- For back pain and neck pain due to heat affecting the *tai yang* channel, add Notopterygii Rhizoma seu Radix *(qiāng huó)* (3g) (source text).
- For pain in the eye and above the eyebrow due to heat affecting the *yang ming* channel, add Puerariae Radix *(gé gēn)* (3g) (source text).

Case study: Reach the Source Drink *(dá yuán yǐn)*

First visit: March 12. This 10-year-old male child suffered from chills and high fever that were mild in the morning and worse in the evening. He also had a headache, chest distention, nausea and vomiting, thirst with no desire to drink, irritability, restlessness, and scanty, dark-yellow urine. While the frequency of his bowel movements had declined, they were loose. Even though the patient had sweated after taking acetaminophen, he still had a fever. He had been purged successfully with Chinese herbs, but this did not affect the fever. In addition, injections of penicillin had no effect.

By the time the patient came to our clinic he had been sick for nine days. Besides the signs and symptoms mentioned above, he had a white, greasy tongue coating and a soggy, rapid pulse. The diagnosis was accumulation of damp-heat in the membrane source. The principle of treatment was to eliminate damp-heat from the membrane source with aromatic herbs. A modified version of Reach the Source Drink *(dá yuán yǐn)* was prescribed: Magnoliae officinalis Cortex *(hòu pò)* (7.5g), Scutellariae Radix *(huáng qín)* (5g), Paeoniae Radix alba *(bái sháo)* (10g), Anemarrhenae Rhizoma *(zhī mǔ)* (5g), Tsaoko Fructus *(cǎo guǒ)* (5g), Talcum *(huá shí)* (10g), Eupatorii Herba *(pèi lán)* (4g), Puerariae Radix *(gé gēn)* (10g), Glycyrrhizae Radix *(gān cǎo)* (5g), and Bupleuri Radix *(chái hú)* (5g). Three packets of the herbs were given to the patient for cooking as a decoction.

Second visit: March 17. After taking the first packet of herbs the quantity of urine increased and the nausea and vomiting disappeared. After the second packet, he could eat food. After the third packet, the fever was gone and the headache and chest distention were significantly improved. However, his bowel movements were still sluggish. Eupatorii Herba *(pèi lán)* and Puerariae Radix *(gé gēn)* were removed, and Arecae Semen *(bīng láng)* (2.5g) added. Three packets of the herbs were given to the patient.

Third visit: March 20. After finishing the herbs, all signs and symptoms were resolved.[32]

ACCUMULATION OF DAMPNESS IN THE SPLEEN, STOMACH, AND TRIPLE BURNER

Manifestations. There are two concurrent aspects to this pattern:

1. *Accumulation of dampness in the Triple Burner* with alternating chills and fever, dizziness, chest distention, and scanty or dark urine.

NOTE: The Triple Burner is *shao yang* and located at the half interior, half exterior level. When dampness attacks the Triple Burner, it can constrain the qi and also negatively affect the ability of the protective qi to reach the exterior. This leads to chills. The struggle between yang qi and dampness, along with the qi constraint, can produce fever.

> 2. *Accumulation of damp-heat in the Spleen and Stomach* with epigastric and abdominal distention, nausea or vomiting at times, a yellow, greasy tongue coating, and a soggy and slippery pulse.

NOTE: Alternating chills and fever can occur both in the *shao yang* pattern of the six stages (described in *Discussion of Cold Damage*) and the pattern mentioned above. While the mechanism in the two patterns is similar, there are some differences. From an organ perspective, the *shao yang* pattern is located in the Gallbladder and is caused by an attack of wind-cold (without dampness), which leads to contention between wind-cold and the antipathogenic qi that produces heat in the Gallbladder. In addition to alternating chills and fever, the presentation includes a bitter taste, dry throat, distention or pain in the hypochondriac or costal regions, and a thin tongue coating. The pattern here is primarily located in the Triple Burner and is due to an attack of damp-heat, in which dampness is predominant. Because of the Triple Burner's relation to the qi mechanism and fluid metabolism, along with the presence of dampness, this pattern includes abdominal distention, scanty or dark urine, and a yellow and greasy tongue coating. The tongue coating is an especially useful marker for distinguishing between these two patterns. In the *shao yang* pattern, the tongue coating will be thin because it is caused by wind-cold initially, and has not yet fully affected water metabolism. The pattern here has aspects of both dampness and heat, thus the tongue coating will be yellow and greasy.

Pathology. Dampness accumulating in the Spleen, Stomach, and Triple Burner, leading to dysfunction of the organs' qi mechanisms.

Treatment principles. Clear heat and eliminate dampness by improving the qi mechanisms of the Triple Burner and Spleen, and direct the Stomach qi downward.

Formula:

WARM THE GALLBLADDER DECOCTION *(wēn dǎn tāng)*
SOURCE: *Discussion of Illnesses, Patterns, and Formulas Related to the Unification of the Three Etiologies*[33]
Bambusae Caulis in taeniam *(zhú rú)* 6g
Pinelliae Rhizoma preparatum *(zhì bàn xià)* 6g

Aurantii Fructus immaturus *(zhǐ shí)* 6g

Jujubae Fructus *(dà zǎo)* . . . . 1 piece

Citri reticulatae Pericarpium *(chén pí)* 9g

Poria *(fú líng)* 4.5g

Honey-toasted Glycyrrhizae Radix preparata *(zhì gān cǎo)* 3g

Zingiberis Rhizoma recens *(shēng jiāng)* . . . . 5 pieces

ANALYSIS OF FORMULA: In this formula, Pinelliae Rhizoma preparatum *(zhì bàn xià)* and Poria *(fú líng)* dry and leach out dampness, and Citri reticulatae Pericarpium *(chén pí)* and Aurantii Fructus immaturus *(zhǐ shí)* promote qi circulation and help resolve dampness.

Bambusae Caulis in taeniam *(zhú rú)* and Aurantii Fructus immaturus *(zhǐ shí)*, which are cold in nature, clear heat, direct the Stomach qi downward, and transform dampness by regulating the circulation of qi. Pinelliae Rhizoma preparatum *(zhì bàn xià)* and Zingiberis Rhizoma recens *(shēng jiāng)* direct the Stomach qi downward to treat nausea or vomiting. Glycyrrhizae Radix *(gān cǎo)*, Zingiberis Rhizoma recens *(shēng jiāng)*, and Jujubae Fructus *(dà zǎo)* are used to harmonize the function of the Stomach and Spleen. The idea of using this formula in the treatment of this condition originates with Ye Gui, who also mentioned an alternative method: simply use Armeniacae Semen *(xìng rén)*, Magnoliae officinalis Cortex *(hòu pò)*, and Poria *(fú líng)*.[34] According to Zhao Shao-Qin, who teaches at Beijing University of Traditional Chinese Medicine, Warm the Gallbladder Decoction *(wēn dǎn tāng)* can promote qi circulation, transform dampness, and leach out dampness; it is suitable for the type of damp-heat in the Triple Burner in which dampness predominates. If dampness and heat are present in equal measure, herbs to clear heat should be added; Scutellaria and Coptis Two-Cured Decoction *(qín lián èr chén tāng)*[35] is a more appropriate choice in that context.

MODIFICATIONS:

- For constipation, add Arecae Pericarpium *(dà fù pí)* and Magnoliae officinalis Cortex *(hòu pò)*.
- For nausea, belching, or vomiting, add Perillae Folium *(zǐ sū yè)*.

DISTURBANCE OF THE FUNCTION OF THE SPLEEN AND STOMACH IN THE MIDDLE BURNER BY DAMP-HEAT

Manifestations. There are two concurrent aspects to this pattern:

1. *Disturbance of the Spleen and Stomach* with distention in the chest, epigastrium, and abdomen, nausea, a need to vomit, and loose stools.

2. *Predominance of dampness* with contained fever, absence of thirst, dry mouth with a desire to drink only a little or a preference for warm beverages, turbid urine, and a white and greasy tongue coating.

NOTE: Dampness predominates here, so much so that it seems as if there are no heat symptoms. The dominant dampness overcomes the heat, the only trace of which can be found in the contained fever.

Pathology. Damp-heat accumulating in the middle burner, leading to failure of the Spleen to transport and transform; and rebellious Stomach qi.

Treatment principles. Dry and transform dampness with aromatic, bitter, and warm herbs, and direct the Stomach qi downward with bitter herbs.

Formula No. 1:

LEI'S FRAGRANT AND AROMATIC FORMULA TO TRANSFORM TURBIDITY
(Léi shì fāng xiāng huà zhuó fāng)

SOURCE: *Discussion of Seasonal Diseases*

Pogostemonis/Agastaches Herba *(huò xiāng)*[36] 3g
Pinelliae Rhizoma preparatum *(zhì bàn xià)* 4.5g
Arecae Pericarpium *(dà fù pí)*. 3g
Citri reticulatae Pericarpium *(chén pí)* 4.5g
Eupatorii Folium *(pèi lán yè)*[37] 3g
Nelumbinis Folium *(hé yè)*. 9g
Magnoliae officinalis Cortex *(hòu pò)* 2.4g

ANALYSIS OF FORMULA: In this pattern there is damp-heat in the middle burner, with dampness predominant. The practitioner should be cautious in using cold or cool herbs since they can block qi circulation and congeal the dampness. According to Zhang Nan in his book *A Stick to Awaken Physicians (Yī mén bàng hè)*:

> The ascending and descending qi in the Triple Burner depends on the function of the Spleen. If the qi circulation in the middle burner is normal, the qi circulation in the upper and lower burners will be normal. On the one hand, weakness of the Spleen qi can produce interior dampness; on the other hand, excessive dampness can impair the function of the Spleen, lead to the accumulation of turbid dampness, and block the qi, resulting in distention [in the chest, epigastrium, and abdomen]. Although there is heat, the dampness predominates and no dry tongue coating is presented. At this time we should first dispel and leach out the dampness, then clear heat. If done otherwise, cold and cool herbs to clear heat will congeal and trap the dampness.[38]

This formula reflects three basic methods for eliminating interior dampness:

1. Dry dampness with bitter and warm herbs such as Magnoliae officinalis Cortex *(hòu pò)*.

2. Transform dampness with aromatic herbs like Pogostemonis/Agastaches Folium *(huò xiāng yè)*, Eupatorii Folium *(pèi lán yè)*, and Nelumbinis Folium *(hé yè)*.

3. Promote the circulation of qi to assist in eliminating dampness with herbs that rectify the qi, such as Citri reticulatae Pericarpium *(chén pí)* and Arecae Pericarpium *(dà fù pí)*.

In addition, Pinelliae Rhizoma preparatum *(zhì bàn xià)* dries dampness and directs the Stomach qi downward. The prescribed dosage for the ingredients in this formula is small and can be increased by one-third.

Formula No. 2:

> ### THIRD MODIFICATION OF RECTIFY THE QI POWDER
> *(sān jiā jiǎn zhèng qì sǎn)*

SOURCE: *Systematic Differentiation of Warm Pathogen Diseases*

Pogostemonis/Agastaches Herba *(huò xiāng)* 9g
Magnoliae officinalis Cortex *(hòu pò)* 6g
Armeniacae Semen *(xìng rén)* 9g
Poriae Cutis *(fú líng pí)* 9g
Citri reticulatae Pericarpium *(chén pí)* 4.5g
Talcum *(huá shí)* 15g

ANALYSIS OF FORMULA: The indication for Third Modification of Rectify the Qi Powder *(sān jiā jiǎn zhèng qì sǎn)* is dampness that has gradually transformed into heat. The signs and symptoms are epigastric distention, increased thirst, yellow tongue coating, and a red tongue body. Pogostemonis/Agastaches Herba *(huò xiāng)*, Magnoliae officinalis Cortex *(hòu pò)*, Citri reticulatae Pericarpium *(chén pí)*, and Poriae Cutis *(fú líng pí)* are used to transform, dry, and leach out dampness and promote qi circulation, Talcum *(huá shí)* is chosen to drain heat as well as dampness, and Armeniacae Semen *(xìng rén)* to direct the Lung qi downward to help discharge dampness through urination. According to Wu Tang, Poriae Cutis *(fú líng pí)* is cold and is highly effective in draining dampness as well as heat.[39]

MODIFICATIONS: In *Systematic Differentiation of Warm Pathogen Diseases*, Wu Tang discussed two modifications of this formula:

- For significant epigastric and abdominal distention and loose stools with no sense of completion after bowel movement, remove Talcum *(huá shí)* and add Massa medicata fermentata *(shén qū)*, Hordei Fructus germinatus *(mài yá)*, Artemisiae scopariae Herba *(yīn chén)*, and Arecae Pericarpium *(dà fù pí)* (source text).

- For body aches, loose stools, epigastric distention, and a white tongue coating, remove Armeniacae Semen *(xìng rén)* and Talcum *(huá shí)*, and add Sojae Semen germinatum *(dà dòu juǎn)*, Tetrapanacis Medulla *(tōng cǎo)*, Coicis Semen *(yì yǐ rén)*, and Aristolochiae fangchi Radix *(guǎng fáng jǐ)* (source text).[40]

Actually, in the source text these two modifications are called First Modification of Rectify the Qi Powder *(yī jiā jiǎn zhèng qì sǎn)* and Second Modification of Rectify the Qi Powder *(èr jiā jiǎn zhèng qì sǎn)*. Because all three formulas are very commonly used for damp-heat in the middle burner, we need to distinguish among them. A summary comparison of the three formulas is provided in Table 12.7.

Table 12.7	Comparison of Three Modifications of Rectify the Qi Powder		
Pathology	**Signs and Symptoms**	**Treatment Principles**	**Main Modifications***
▶ FIRST MODIFICATION OF RECTIFY THE QI POWDER			
Failure of Spleen and Stomach due to accumulation of dampness in the middle burner	Epigastric and abdominal distention, loose stools without a sense of completion after bowel movement	Promote Spleen's transportive and transformative functions, promote digestion	Arecae Pericarpium *(dà fù pí)*, Massa medicata fermentata *(shén qū)*, Hordei Fructus germinatus *(mài yá)*
▶ SECOND MODIFICATION OF RECTIFY THE QI POWDER			
Combination of exterior dampness in the channels and collaterals and interior dampness in the middle burner; dampness is more severe	Body aches, loose stool, epigastric distention and a white tongue coating	Promote the Spleen's transportive and transformative functions, eliminate dampness from the channels and collaterals, discharge dampness by diuresis	Stephaniae tetrandrae Radix *(hàn fáng jǐ)*, Coicis Semen *(yì yǐ rén)*, Tetrapanacis Medulla *(tōng cǎo)*
▶ THIRD MODIFICATION OF RECTIFY THE QI POWDER			
Dampness has gradually transformed into heat due to stagnation of dampness and qi	Yellow, greasy tongue coating, dark urine	Clear heat, enhance the action of the formula in eliminating dampness	Talcum *(huá shí)*, Armeniacae Semen *(xìng rén)*

*The common herbs are Pogostemonis/Agastaches Herba *(huò xiāng)*, Magnoliae officinalis Cortex *(hòu pò)*, Citri reticulatae Pericarpium *(chén pí)*, and Poria *(fú líng)*

Comparison. Compared with Lei's Fragrant and Aromatic Formula to Transform Turbidity, the Third Modification of Rectify the Qi Powder *(sān jiā jiǎn zhèng qì sǎn)* has a stronger action in draining dampness but is weaker in dispersing heat from constraint, because it contains Poriae Cutis *(fú líng pí)*, Talcum *(huá shí)*, and Armeniacae Semen *(xìng rén)*, and does not have Eupatorii Folium *(pèi lán yè)* and Nelumbinis Folium *(hé yè)*.

ACCUMULATION OF DAMPNESS IN THE BLADDER

Manifestations. There are four concurrent aspects to this pattern:

1. *Dysfunction of the Bladder* with retention of urine or difficult urination.
2. *Dampness steaming to the middle burner* with nausea and vomiting.
3. *Dampness steaming to the upper burner* with distention in the head and muddled consciousness.
4. *Interior dampness* with thirst but little desire to drink, a white and greasy tongue coating, and a soggy pulse.

NOTE: This is an acute and severe pattern of damp-warmth marked by retention of urine and loss of consciousness. Although there is difficult urination (or no urine) in both this pattern and that of heat from excess in the Small Intestine, leading to a failure to distribute fluids, the two patterns are quite different. Here, dampness predominates and there is no burning and painful urination; there is nausea, vomiting, and muddled consciousness. By contrast, in the other pattern, heat predominates and urination is burning and painful; there is also irritability, restlessness, dry lips, and a bright-red tongue with less than normal coating.

Pathology. Accumulation of damp-heat in the Bladder affecting the upper burner (Heart) and middle burner (Stomach).

NOTE: Retention of urine, nausea or vomiting, and muddled consciousness reflect the involvement of all three burners. The damp-heat, however, is located in the lower burner. In *Systematic Differentiation of Damp-Heat*, Xue Xue observes that, because there is much dampness but little heat, it veils above (affecting the Heart) and flows below (affecting the Bladder).[41]

Treatment principles. Leach out dampness and open the orifices.

Formula No. 1:

> **PORIA PEEL DECOCTION** *(fú líng pí tāng)*
>
> SOURCE: *Systematic Differentiation of Warm Pathogen Diseases*

Poriae Cutis *(fú líng pí)* 15g
Coicis Semen *(yì yǐ rén)* 15g
Polyporus *(zhū líng)* 9g
Arecae Pericarpium *(dà fù pí)* 9g
Tetrapanacis Medulla *(tōng cǎo)* 9g
Lophatheri Herba *(dàn zhú yè)* 6g

ANALYSIS OF FORMULA: Dampness predominates in this pattern, and the Bladder's function of discharging urine is severely impaired. The only way to eliminate the dampness and heat is through urination. Poriae Cutis *(fú líng pí)* and Polyporus *(zhū líng)* strongly eliminate dampness through urination. Lophatheri Herba *(dàn zhú yè)*, Tetrapanacis Medulla *(tōng cǎo)*, and Coicis Semen *(yì yǐ rén)* discharge both dampness and heat through urination. Arecae Pericarpium *(dà fù pí)* eliminates dampness by promoting the circulation of qi, which is important because normal qi circulation is critical for the elimination of dampness.

Poria Peel Decoction *(fú líng pí tāng)* focuses only on draining damp-heat. Blockage of the Heart by damp-heat steaming upward is not addressed by this formula. Instead, the formula must be combined with Liquid Styrax Pill *(sū hé xiāng wán)* to open the orifices.

Formula No. 2:

LIQUID STYRAX PILL *(sū hé xiāng wán)*

SOURCE: *Formulary of the Bureau of Medicines of the Taiping Era*

Styrax *(sū hé xiāng)* 30g
Borneolum *(bīng piàn)* 30g
Aristolochiae Radix *(qīng mù xiāng)* 60g
Aquilariae Lignum resinatum *(chén xiāng)* 60g
Caryophylli Flos *(dīng xiāng)* 60g
Piperis longi Fructus *(bì bá)* 60g
Cinnabaris *(zhū shā)* 60g
Chebulae Fructus *(hē zǐ)* 60g
Moschus *(shè xiāng)* 60g
Benzoinum *(ān xī xiāng)* 60g
Santali albi Lignum *(tán xiāng)* 60g
Olibanum *(rǔ xiāng)* 30g
Cyperi Rhizoma *(xiāng fù)* 60g
Rhinocerotis Cornu *(xī jiǎo)* 60g
Atractylodis macrocephalae Rhizoma *(bái zhú)* 60g

ANALYSIS OF FORMULA: Since this formula contains so many precious and expensive herbs, it is seldom prescribed, although it can often be purchased from a fully stocked Chinese herbal pharmacy. The formula consists primarily of aromatic and warm herbs. Collectively, they open the orifices, promote qi circulation, and transform turbid dampness. In this pattern, the turbid dampness has attacked the orifices and blocked the passage of clear yang. These herbs penetrate the turbidity and open the channels and collaterals.

NOTE: The majority of ingredients in Liquid Styrax Pill *(sū hé xiāng wán)* are warm and acrid. The indication for this formula is blockage of the Heart by damp-heat or phlegm-heat in which dampness, or phlegm, predominates. Clinically, if heat predominates, the practitioner should instead prescribe Greatest Treasure Special Pill *(zhì bǎo dān)*.[42]

DAMPNESS OBSTRUCTING THE INTESTINAL PATHWAY WITH A BREAKDOWN IN TRANSPORTATION

Manifestations. There is only one aspect to this pattern:

- *Accumulation of dampness in the Large Intestine* with a hard and distended area in the lower abdomen, muddled thinking, constipation, and a thick, greasy tongue coating. Clinically, epigastric distention and nausea or vomiting may present.

NOTE: The constipation in this pattern is caused by stagnation of qi in the Large Intestine due to obstruction by dampness, rather than the combination of dry stool and heat. The presentation includes only distention and hardness in the lower abdomen with a thick and greasy tongue coating; there is no abdominal pain, tidal fever, or dry, yellow tongue coating. The stools can be either soft and formed or dry and hard; the latter occurs if they have not been passed for several days due to obstruction of qi in the Large Intestine by dampness. However, the presence of dry and hard stools does not mean that there is heat in the Large Intestine. Also, muddled thinking or epigastric distention and nausea or vomiting is a result of qi stagnation in the Large Intestine leading to qi stagnation in the middle or upper burner, or even the rebellion of Stomach qi.

Pathology. Dampness accumulating in the Large Intestine, leading to qi stagnation with a breakdown in the transportive function of the Large Intestine. There is also a slight veiling of the Pericardium by dampness.

Treatment principles. Promote the circulation of qi in the Large Intestine and transform and leach out dampness through urination.

Formula:

> ### DISSEMINATE THE CLEAR AND GUIDE OUT THE TURBID DECOCTION
> *(xuān qīng dǎo zhuó tāng)*

SOURCE: *Systematic Differentiation of Warm Pathogen Diseases*

Polyporus *(zhū líng)* 15g

Bombycis Faeces *(cán shā)* 12g

Glauberitum *(hán shuǐ shí)* 18g

Poria *(fú líng)* 15g

Gleditsiae Spina *(zào jiǎo cì)* 9g

ANALYSIS OF FORMULA: Bombycis Faeces *(cán shā)* and Gleditsiae Spina *(zào jiǎo cì)* are the main herbs. The first transforms the thickening dampness (also called damp turbidity) in the Large Intestine. This is also known as guiding out the turbid. The second herb promotes the circulation of qi in the Large Intestine. This is called disseminating the clear qi. Polyporus *(zhū líng)*, Poria *(fú líng)*, and Glauberitum *(hán shuǐ shí)* clear heat and leach out dampness from the lower burner. According to Wu Tang, this formula should be taken until the patient has regular bowel movements.[43]

Since the pattern is not the result of dry stool and heat in the Large Intestine, bitter and cold herbs that purge are not used. If they were, not only would the dampness fail to be discharged completely, but the Spleen qi or yang would be injured as well.

Differentiation and Treatment of Equal Parts Dampness and Heat

ACCUMULATION OF DAMP-HEAT IN THE MIDDLE BURNER

Manifestations. There are two concurrent aspects to this pattern:

1. *Accumulation of dampness in the middle burner* with chest and epigastric distention, nausea, and vomiting.

2. *Equal parts dampness and heat in the body* with fever, thirst, irritability, a fever that does not diminish after sweating, scanty urination, a yellow and greasy tongue coating, and a soggy and rapid pulse.

NOTE: Fever, irritability, and chest and epigastric distention are common symptoms of a damp-warmth pattern in which there are equal parts dampness and heat. Clinically, if dampness predominates the patient will present with a contained fever, muddled thinking, and chest and epigastric distention; irritability is absent. If heat predominates, there will be no chest distention or muddled thinking, but there will be fever and irritability. There may also be diarrhea due to an attack on the Spleen by damp-heat, leading to failure of the Spleen qi to ascend.

Pathology. Steaming of damp-heat obstructing qi circulation in the middle burner.

Treatment principles. Lift Spleen qi and transform dampness with acrid herbs, and clear heat and direct the Stomach qi downward with bitter herbs.

NOTE: Bitter and acrid herbs are used here in concert because the main problem is failure of the Spleen and Stomach qi to lift and descend, respectively. The bitter herbs direct the qi downward by restoring the downward-directing function of the Stomach, while the acrid herbs raise the qi and restore the lifting function of the Spleen.

Formula No. 1:

COPTIS AND MAGNOLIA BARK DRINK *(lián pò yǐn)*

SOURCE: *Discussion of Sudden Turmoil Disorders*[44]

Coptidis Rhizoma *(huáng lián)* 3g
Magnoliae officinalis Cortex *(hòu pò)* 6g
Acori tatarinowii Rhizoma *(shí chāng pǔ)* 3g
Phragmitis Rhizoma *(lú gēn)* 60g
Pinelliae Rhizoma preparatum *(zhì bàn xià)* 3g
Sojae Semen preparatum *(dàn dòu chǐ)* 9g
Gardeniae Fructus *(zhī zǐ)* 9g

---

ANALYSIS OF FORMULA: This formula incorporates the basic treatment method of separately resolving dampness and heat. Sojae Semen preparatum *(dàn dòu chǐ)* disperses the Lung qi to promote the circulation of qi and eliminate dampness. The acrid, bitter, and warm herbs Magnoliae officinalis Cortex *(hòu pò)*, Acori tatarinowii Rhizoma *(shí chāng pǔ)*, and Pinelliae Rhizoma preparatum *(zhì bàn xià)* treat the dampness by strengthening the Spleen, lifting the Spleen qi, and drying dampness. Coptidis Rhizoma *(huáng lián)* and Gardeniae Fructus *(zhī zǐ)*, which are bitter and cold, drain heat. The combination of Magnoliae officinalis Cortex *(hòu pò)* and Pinelliae Rhizoma preparatum *(zhì bàn xià)* direct the Stomach qi downward. Finally, a large amount of Phragmitis Rhizoma *(lú gēn)* can clear heat, generate fluids, and leach out dampness and drain heat through the urine.

MODIFICATIONS: The basic formula can be modified as follows:

- To enhance the heat-clearing and dampness-transforming effects of this formula, add Scutellariae Radix *(huáng qín)* and Talcum *(huá shí)*.
- For the eruption of miliaria alba, add Coicis Semen *(yì yǐ rén)* and Lophatheri Herba *(dàn zhú yè)*.

Formula No. 2:

UNRIPE BITTER ORANGE PILL TO GUIDE OUT STAGNATION
(zhǐ shí dǎo zhì wán)

SOURCE: *Clarifying Doubts about Damage from Internal and External Causes*[45]

Aurantii Fructus immaturus *(zhǐ shí)* 15g
Rhei Radix et Rhizoma *(dà huáng)* 30g
Massa medicata fermentata *(shén qū)* 15g
Poria *(fú líng)* 9g
Scutellariae Radix *(huáng qín)* 9g
Coptidis Rhizoma *(huáng lián)* 9g
Atractylodis macrocephalae Rhizoma *(bái zhú)* 9g
Alismatis Rhizoma *(zé xiè)* 6g

ANALYSIS OF FORMULA: Aurantii Fructus immaturus *(zhǐ shí)*, in concert with Rhei Radix et Rhizoma *(dà huáng)*, eliminates retained food as well as heat in the Large Intestine by purging. Scutellariae Radix *(huáng qín)*, Coptidis Rhizoma *(huáng lián)*, Poria *(fú líng)*, and Alismatis Rhizoma *(zé xiè)* clear heat and eliminate dampness. Massa medicata fermentata *(shén qū)* and Atractylodis macrocephalae Rhizoma *(bái zhú)* eliminate retained food and transform dampness by strengthening the function of the Spleen.

NOTE: We have mentioned that one should not purge in the early stage of damp-warmth. However, it is appropriate to moderately purge when damp-heat combines with retained food in the Large Intestine. Otherwise, there is no way to eliminate these pathogenic factors from the body. Do remember, however, that only *moderate* purging is recommended, not strong purging as one might expect from using a formula like Major Order the Qi Decoction *(dà chéng qì tāng)*. That formula has a strong purgative action due to the very large dosage of Rhei Radix et Rhizoma *(dà huáng)* (30g). Li Gao, the author of the source text, noted that the dosages in the formula recommended above should be tailored to the constitution of the patient.[46] Nowadays, when Rhei Radix et Rhizoma *(dà huáng)* is used to treat food stagnation (as in this case) the dosage ranges from 6–12g. The appearance of a normal bowel movement with formed stool is a sign that the dampness and food stagnation have been substantially reduced. At that point, use of this formula should be discontinued.

Comparison. Both Coptis and Magnolia Bark Drink *(lián pò yǐn)* and Unripe Bitter Orange Pill to Guide Out Stagnation *(zhǐ shí dǎo zhì wán)* can be used to treat accumulation of damp-heat in the middle burner. The focus of the former is only on the middle burner while the latter also treats food retention in the Large Intestine, which manifests with incomplete and irregular bowel movements.

ERUPTION OF MILIARIA ALBA DUE TO STEAMING OF DAMP-HEAT

Manifestations. There are three concurrent aspects to this pattern:

1. *Steaming of dampness* with the eruption of miliaria alba and fever even after sweating.
2. *Obstruction of qi by damp-heat* with a heavy feeling and achy body, muddled thinking, and chest and epigastric distention.
3. *Dysfunction of the Spleen and Stomach by damp-heat* with nausea, vomiting, loose stools, a yellow, greasy tongue coating, and a soggy, rapid pulse.

NOTE: The eruption of miliaria alba is regarded as a positive sign since it demonstrates that the antipathogenic qi is discharging damp-heat through the muscle layer and skin. Normally, these eruptions occur following sweating and are generally located on the neck, chest, and abdomen. Because dampness is tenacious, such eruptions must occur several times before the damp-heat is fully discharged. If the antipathogenic qi is strong, the miliaria alba will appear pale, lustrous, and full of fluid. On the other hand, if the qi and fluids are exhausted, the miliaria alba will be pale but will lack luster, and will contain only a small amount of fluid.

Pathology. Steaming of damp-heat, leading to obstruction of qi and dysfunction of the Spleen and the Stomach.

Treatment principles. Clear heat, leach out dampness, and disperse damp-heat.

Formula:

COIX AND LOPHATHERUS POWDER *(yì yǐ zhú yè sǎn)*

SOURCE: *Systematic Differentiation of Warm Pathogen Diseases*

Coicis Semen *(yì yǐ rén)*	15g
Talcum *(huá shí)*	15g
Forsythiae Fructus *(lián qiào)*	9g
Tetrapanacis Medulla *(tōng cǎo)*	4.5g
Lophatheri Herba *(dàn zhú yè)*	9g
Amomi Fructus rotundus *(bái dòu kòu)*	4.5g
Poria *(fú líng)*	15g

ANALYSIS OF FORMULA: According to Wu Tang, this formula:

> eliminates exterior heat [and dampness] with acrid and cool herbs, and leaches out dampness [and heat] with acrid and bland herbs. In this way, the pathogens in the exterior will be dispersed with normal qi circulation, while the interior pathogens will be discharged through urination.[47]

In this formula, the bland herbs Coicis Semen *(yì yǐ rén)*, Talcum *(huá shí)*, Poria *(fú líng)*, and Tetrapanacis Medulla *(tōng cǎo)* leach out dampness and clear heat, letting damp-heat exit via the urine. Amomi Fructus rotundus *(bái dòu kòu)* transforms dampness and harmonizes the function of the Spleen and Stomach. Forsythiae Fructus *(lián qiào)* and Lophatheri Herba *(dàn zhú yè)*, acrid and cool herbs, vent heat through the exterior.

MODIFICATION: To enhance the action of this formula, add Arctii Fructus *(niú bàng zǐ)*, Akebiae Caulis *(mù tōng)*, and Menthae haplocalycis Herba *(bò hé)*.

Comparison. This formula can be viewed as a modification of Three-Nut Decoction *(sān rén tāng)*. Armeniacae Semen *(xìng rén)*, Pinelliae Rhizoma preparatum *(zhì bàn xià)*, and Magnoliae officinalis Cortex *(hòu pò)* are removed from that formula, and Poria *(fú líng)* and Forsythiae Fructus *(lián qiào)* are added. Since this is a pattern of damp-heat in the middle burner steaming out to the exterior, removing Pinelliae Rhizoma preparatum *(zhì bàn xià)*, Armeniacae Semen *(xìng rén)*, and Magnoliae officinalis Cortex *(hòu pò)* prevents the formula from producing heat, while adding Forsythiae Fructus *(lián qiào)* and Poria *(fú líng)* enhances the formula's ability to clear heat and leach out dampness. Therefore, compared with Three-Nut Decoction *(sān rén tāng)*, this formula can more effectively disperse heat from the exterior. Coix and Lophatherus Powder *(yì yǐ zhú yè sǎn)* is an important formula for treating miliaria alba.

OBSTRUCTION OF THE CHANNELS BY DAMP-HEAT

Manifestations. There are two concurrent aspects to this pattern:

1. *Steaming of damp-heat* with fever and sweating or a fever with shivering, a yellow, gray tongue coating, and a soggy, rapid pulse.

2. *Obstruction of the channels by damp-heat* with a heavy feeling and painful limbs, and swollen and painful joints.

Pathology. Damp-heat obstructing the channels.

NOTE: This condition is actually painful obstruction caused by damp-heat affecting the relatively superficial aspects of the body including the skin, muscles, and joints. It often occurs in those who work in very hot and humid environments where external dampness and heat can attack the body. Compared with other damp-warmth patterns, this one is more limited to the exterior and presents with signs and symptoms associated with obstruction of the channels by damp-heat.

Treatment principles. Clear heat and transform dampness, and promote qi and blood circulation to relieve pain.

Formula:

DISBAND PAINFUL OBSTRUCTION DECOCTION *(xuān bì tāng)*

SOURCE: *Systematic Differentiation of Warm Pathogen Diseases*

Stephaniae tetrandrae Radix *(hàn fáng jǐ)* 15g
Talcum *(huá shí)* 15g
Gardeniae Fructus *(zhī zǐ)* 9g
Pinelliae Rhizoma preparatum *(zhì bàn xià)* 9g
Phaseoli Semen *(chì xiǎo dòu)* 9g
Armeniacae Semen *(xìng rén)* 15g
Forsythiae Fructus *(lián qiào)* 9g
Coicis Semen *(yì yǐ rén)* 15g
Bombycis Faeces *(cán shā)* 9g

ANALYSIS OF FORMULA: Damp-heat obstructs qi circulation, leading to obstruction of the blood. This formula uses a large dosage of Armeniacae Semen *(xìng rén)* to direct the Lung qi downward, help the Lung govern the water pathways, and leach out damp-heat. Armeniacae Semen *(xìng rén)* and Talcum *(huá shí)* together drain damp-heat. Stephaniae tetrandrae Radix *(hàn fáng jǐ)* eliminates dampness in the channels and collaterals.[48] Forsythiae Fructus *(lián qiào)*, Coicis Semen *(yì yǐ rén)*, and Phaseoli Semen *(chì xiǎo dòu)* clear damp-heat from the channels. Pinelliae Rhizoma preparatum *(zhì bàn xià)* and Bombycis Faeces *(cán shā)* transform dampness, and Gardeniae Fructus *(zhī zǐ)* enhances the function of Forsythiae Fructus *(lián qiào)* and Talcum *(huá shí)* in clearing heat.

MODIFICATIONS: The basic formula can be modified as follows:

- For severe joint pain, add Cinnamomi Ramulus *(guì zhī)*, Curcumae longae Rhizoma *(jiāng huáng)*, Erythrinae Cortex *(hǎi tóng pí)*, and Paeoniae Radix rubra *(chì sháo)*.
- For severe swelling of the joints, add Atractylodis Rhizoma *(cāng zhú)* and Dioscoreae hypoglaucae Rhizoma *(bì xiè)*.

STEAMING OF DAMP-HEAT IN THE TRIPLE BURNER

Manifestations. There are four concurrent aspects to this pattern:

1. *Obstruction of damp-heat in the upper burner* with chest distention.
2. *Obstruction of damp-heat in the middle burner* with epigastric distention, nausea, and vomiting.
3. *Obstruction of damp-heat in the lower burner* with loose stools and scanty, dark urine.
4. *Heat from excess with slight injury to the fluids* with afternoon fever, sweating, irritability and thirst, a gray, greasy tongue coating, and a soggy, rapid pulse.

Pathology. Steaming of damp-heat in the Triple Burner.

Treatment principles. Clear heat and transform dampness in the Triple Burner.

Formula:

APRICOT KERNEL AND TALCUM DECOCTION *(xìng rén huá shí tāng)*
SOURCE: *Systematic Differentiation of Warm Pathogen Diseases*

Armeniacae Semen *(xìng rén)* 9g
Citri reticulatae Exocarpium rubrum *(jú hóng)* 4.5g
Curcumae Radix *(yù jīn)* 6g
Magnoliae officinalis Cortex *(hòu pò)* .6g
Scutellariae Radix *(huáng qín)* 6g
Talcum *(huá shí)* 9g
Coptidis Rhizoma *(huáng lián)* 3g
Tetrapanacis Medulla *(tōng cǎo)* 3g
Pinelliae Rhizoma preparatum *(zhì bàn xià)* 9g

ANALYSIS OF FORMULA: In this formula, Armeniacae Semen *(xìng rén)* and Curcumae Radix *(yù jīn)* promote qi circulation in the upper burner to resolve dampness. Magnoliae officinalis Cortex *(hòu pò)*, Citri reticulatae Exocarpium rubrum *(jú hóng)*, and Pinelliae Rhizoma preparatum *(zhì bàn xià)* promote qi circulation in the middle burner to resolve dampness. Scutellariae Radix *(huáng qín)* and Coptidis Rhizoma *(huáng lián)* dry dampness and clear heat in the middle burner. Talcum *(huá shí)* and Tetrapanacis Medulla *(tōng cǎo)* leach out dampness and drain heat. Citri reticulatae Exocarpium rubrum *(jú hóng)* is stronger at drying dampness than Citri reticulatae Pericarpium *(chén pí)*, while the latter herb is relatively stronger at promoting the proper movement of qi. Because in this pattern the fluids have been injured, I would recommend Citri reticulatae Pericarpium *(chén pí)* here.

Comparison. This formula and Coptis and Magnolia Bark Drink *(lián pò yǐn)* treat dampness and heat when they exist in equal parts. However, Apricot Kernel and Talcum Decoction *(xìng rén huá shí tāng)* affects all three burners and uses four common methods for treating the dampness: promoting qi circulation, transforming dampness, drying dampness, and draining dampness. By contrast, Coptis and Magnolia Bark Drink *(lián pò yǐn)* works mainly on the middle burner by focusing on directing the Stomach qi downward and lifting the Spleen qi to dry and transform dampness.

Veiling of the Pericardium by Phlegm Due to Damp-Heat

Manifestations. There are two concurrent aspects to this pattern:

1. *Veiling of the Pericardium by phlegm* with muddled consciousness, delirium, or, when the condition is severe, loss of consciousness.
2. *Damp-heat in the qi level* with fever, a yellow and greasy tongue coating, and a soggy and rapid pulse.

NOTE: It is important to distinguish this pattern from that of invasion of the Pericardium by heat because these two patterns share the same location as well as some signs, such as loss of consciousness (see Table 12.8). The principal differences concern the tongue, as well as the severity and extent of the changes in consciousness.

Table 12.8	Veiling of Pericardium by Phlegm vs. Invasion of Pericardium by Heat
Pathology	**Signs and Symptoms***
▶ VEILING OF PERICARDIUM BY PHLEGM	
Damp-heat situated in qi level and Pericardium is veiled by phlegm due to damp-heat	Mild abnormal consciousness, occasional loss of consciousness or delirium, yellow and greasy tongue coating
▶ INVASION OF PERICARDIUM BY HEAT	
Heat is situated in the nutritive level and Pericardium is invaded by heat	Severe abnormal consciousness, continuous coma or delirium, cold extremities, deep-red tongue

*In common: both patterns are situated in the Pericardium and share the symptom of abnormal consciousness.

443

Pathology. Phlegm from the steaming of damp-heat veiling the Pericardium.

Treatment principles. Clear heat, transform dampness, and eliminate phlegm to open the orifices.

Formula:

ACORUS AND CURCUMA DECOCTION *(chāng pǔ yù jīn tāng)*

SOURCE: *Complete Book of Warm Pathogen Diseases*[49]

Acori tatarinowii Rhizoma *(shí chāng pǔ)* 9g
Curcumae Radix *(yù jīn)* 6g
Forsythiae Fructus *(lián qiào)* 6g
Gardeniae Fructus *(zhī zǐ)* 9g
Akebiae Caulis *(mù tōng)* 4.5g
Lophatheri Herba *(dàn zhú yè)* 9g
Moutan Cortex *(mǔ dān pí)* 9g
Bambusae Succus *(zhú lì)* 15g
Junci Medulla *(dēng xīn cǎo)* 6g
Jade Pivot Pill *(yù shū dān)*[50] 1.5g

ANALYSIS OF FORMULA: Gardeniae Fructus *(zhī zǐ)*, Forsythiae Fructus *(lián qiào)*, Moutan Cortex *(mǔ dān pí)*, and Lophatheri Herba *(dàn zhú yè)* clear heat. Acori tatarinowii Rhizoma *(shí chāng pǔ)*, Curcumae Radix *(yù jīn)*, Bambusae Succus *(zhú lì)*, and Jade Pivot Pill *(yù shū dān)* transform dampness and phlegm to open the orifices. Akebiae Caulis *(mù tōng)* and Junci Medulla *(dēng xīn cǎo)* conduct heat downward and discharge it through the urine.

ADMINISTRATION: By itself, Acorus and Curcuma Decoction *(chāng pǔ yù jīn tāng)* is not strong enough to open the orifices. Therefore, one Liquid Styrax Pill *(sū hé xiāng wán)* should be taken twice a day with this decoction.

MODIFICATIONS: The basic formula can be modified as follows:

- If heat predominates, substitute Greatest Treasure Special Pill *(zhì bǎo dān)*[51] for Liquid Styrax Pill *(sū hé xiāng wán)*.

- For stirring of Liver wind due to stagnation of damp-heat and production of fire by damp-heat with convulsions, add herbs that extinguish internal wind such as Pheretima *(dì lóng)*, Uncariae Ramulus cum Uncis *(gōu téng)*, and Mori Ramulus *(sāng zhī)*.

Differentiation and Treatment of Damp-Warmth with Heat Predominant

STAGNATION OF QI ACTIVITY BY DAMP-HEAT

Manifestations. There are three concurrent aspects to this pattern:

1. *Steaming of damp-heat* with fever, heavy and foggy head, generalized soreness and lassitude, and a yellow and greasy tongue coating.
2. *Stagnation of qi activity in the Triple Burner* with signs and symptoms in all three burners:
   • Upper burner: chest distention
   • Middle burner: abdominal distention, nausea, vomiting, thirst; jaundice may also be observed
   • Lower burner: scanty and dark urine.
3. *Damp-heat transforming into toxin* with high fever and a swollen and sore throat.

NOTE: A soggy and rapid pulse often accompanies this pattern. If damp-heat forces out the bile in the Gallbladder, yang-type jaundice will present.

Pathology. Dampness and heat steaming together, obstructing the qi mechanism and brewing into heat-toxin.

Treatment principles. Clear heat, resolve toxicity, and transform dampness with aromatic, bitter, and cold herbs.

Formula:

SWEET DEW SPECIAL PILL TO ELIMINATE TOXIN *(gān lù xiāo dú dān)*

SOURCE: *Warp and Woof of Warm-Heat Pathogen Diseases*[52]

Forsythiae Fructus *(lián qiào)*	120g
Scutellariae Radix *(huáng qín)*	300g
Menthae haplocalycis Herba *(bò hé)*	120g
Belamcandae Rhizoma *(shè gān)*	120g
Fritillariae cirrhosae Bulbus *(chuān bèi mǔ)*	150g
Talcum *(huá shí)*	450g
Akebiae Caulis *(mù tōng)*	150g
Artemisiae scopariae Herba *(yīn chén)*	330g
Pogostemonis/Agastaches Herba *(huò xiāng)*	120g
Acori tatarinowii Rhizoma *(shí chāng pǔ)*	180g
Amomi Fructus rotundus *(bái dòu kòu)*	120g

ANALYSIS OF FORMULA: Pogostemonis/Agastaches Herba *(huò xiāng)*, Acori tatarinowii Rhizoma *(shí chāng pǔ)*, and Amomi Fructus rotundus *(bái dòu kòu)* are aromatic herbs that transform dampness. Forsythiae Fructus *(lián qiào)*, Scutellariae Radix *(huáng qín)*, and Belamcandae Rhizoma *(shè gān)* clear heat and resolve toxicity. Menthae haplocalycis Herba *(bò hé)* and Fritillariae cirrhosae Bulbus *(chuān bèi mǔ)* eliminate dampness by dispersing the Lung qi and promoting its circulation. Talcum *(huá shí)*, Akebiae Caulis *(mù tōng)*, and Artemisiae scopariae Herba *(yīn chén)* leach out dampness via the urine.

MODIFICATIONS: The basic formula can be modified as follows:

- For nausea and vomiting, add Zingiberis Rhizomatis Succus *(jiāng zhī)* [ginger juice], Bambusae Caulis in taeniam *(zhú rú)*, and Pinelliae Rhizoma preparatum *(zhì bàn xià)*.

- For severe irritability, restlessness, and thirst, add Gardeniae Fructus *(zhī zǐ)*, Phragmitis Rhizoma *(lú gēn)*, and Lophatheri Herba *(dàn zhú yè)*.

- For body aches, add Erythrinae Cortex *(hǎi tóng pí)* and Coicis Semen *(yì yǐ rén)*.

- For the eruption of miliaria alba, add Coicis Semen *(yì yǐ rén)* and Lophatheri Herba *(dàn zhú yè)*.

Case study: Sweet Dew Special Pill to Eliminate Toxin *(gān lù xiāo dú dān)*

This 2-year-old male first came to our clinic in the summer of 1939. He had contracted summerheat associated with dampness. However, the previous practitioner had treated with the heat-clearing method, which had congealed the dampness and made things worse. The patient had fever, muddled consciousness, vomiting, and a poor appetite along with chest and abdominal distention. Urination and bowel movements had ceased. The previous practitioner believed that there was no hope to save the boy and his father had gone to prepare a coffin for him. At the same time, his mother brought him to our clinic to see what we could do. In addition to the signs and symptoms noted above, the patient had a red tongue with a greasy, slippery coating and a soggy, rapid pulse. The diagnosis was summerheat and dampness constraining and stagnating in the middle burner and affecting the upper and lower burners, leading to a breakdown in the transformation of qi by the Triple Burner such that the pathogens had no avenue through which to exit the body.

The principles of treatment were to disperse heat, transform dampness, transform phlegm, and open the orifices. A modified version of Sweet Dew Special Pill to Eliminate Toxin *(gān lù xiāo dú dān)* was prescribed: Pogostemonis/Agastaches Herba *(huò xiāng)* (6g), Acori tatarinowii Rhizoma *(shí chāng pǔ)* (5g), Curcumae Radix *(yù jīn)* (5g), Armeniacae Semen *(xìng rén)*(5g), Amomi Fructus rotundus *(bái dòu kòu)* (5g), Eupatorii Herba *(pèi lán)* (6g), Scutellariae Radix *(huáng qín)* (6g), Forsythiae

Fructus *(lián qiào)* (9g), Gardeniae Fructus *(zhī zǐ)* (5g), Artemisiae scopariae Herba *(yīn chén)* (6g), Talcum *(huá shí)* (9g), and Bambusae Caulis in taeniam *(zhú rú)* (6g). The patient's mother was told to cook the herbs immediately and administer three spoonfuls at a time, frequently. After taking the decoction twice, the young boy urinated and had a bowel movement. His mental status also cleared up. His mother was very happy and took her son and the herbs back home. Three days later, the patient returned for a visit. All signs and symptoms were gone and the boy was able to play around as he pleased. He was then given herbs to harmonize the Spleen and Stomach and clear any remnants of the pathogen, after which he was cured.[53]

HEAT FROM EXCESS IN THE STOMACH ACCOMPANIED BY DAMPNESS IN THE SPLEEN

Manifestations. There are two concurrent aspects to this pattern:

1. *Heat in the Stomach* with a vigorous fever, profuse sweating, and thirst.

2. *Dampness in the Spleen* with chest and epigastric distention, heavy sensation in the body, a slightly yellow, greasy tongue coating, and a slippery, rapid pulse.

Pathology. Heat from excess in the Stomach accompanied by dampness in the Spleen.

Treatment principles. Clear heat in the Stomach with acrid and cold herbs, and transform dampness in the Spleen with bitter and slightly warm herbs.

Formula:

WHITE TIGER PLUS ATRACTYLODES DECOCTION *(bái hǔ jiā cāng zhú tāng)*

See Chapter 11 for further discussion of this formula.

MODIFICATIONS: The basic formula can be modified as follows:

- For strong thirst, add Trichosanthis Radix *(tiān huā fěn)* and Phragmitis Rhizoma *(lú gēn)*.
- For body aches, add Coicis Semen *(yì yǐ rén)*, Sojae Semen germinatum *(dà dòu juǎn)*, and Erythrinae Cortex *(hǎi tóng pí)*.
- For abdominal bloating, add Magnoliae officinalis Cortex *(hòu pò)* and Perillae Caulis *(zǐ sū gěng)*.
- For a bitter taste, nausea, and vomiting, add Pinelliae Rhizoma preparatum *(zhì bàn xià)*, Bambusae Caulis in taeniam *(zhú rú)*, and Scutellariae Radix *(huáng qín)*.

SEVERE CONSTIPATION WITH DRY STOOL AND HEAT COUPLED WITH DAMPNESS IN THE LARGE INTESTINE

Manifestations. There are two concurrent aspects to this pattern:

1. *Severe constipation with dry stool and heat in the Large Intestine* with fever, red face, dry mouth and throat, thirst for cold beverages, constipation (dry and hard stools), a yellow, dry tongue coating, and a submerged, excessive pulse.

2. *Residual dampness* with epigastric distention.

NOTE: This pattern often follows one of equal parts dampness and heat, and represents the gradual transformation of dampness into heat. Clinically, the presence of epigastric distention alone would not be enough to identify dampness, because severe constipation with qi stagnation in the Large Intestine might lead to the failure of the Stomach qi to descend, resulting in epigastric distention. Therefore, we must consider the history as well as the other symptoms in order to identify this pattern.

Pathology. Damp-heat gradually transforming into dryness and heat in the Large Intestine.

Treatment principles. Purge heat and transform dampness.

Formula:

MINOR ORDER THE QI DECOCTION *(xiǎo chéng qì tāng)*
SOURCE: *Discussion of Cold Damage*
Rhei Radix et Rhizoma *(dà huáng)* 12g
Aurantii Fructus immaturus *(zhǐ shí)* 6g
Magnoliae officinalis Cortex *(hòu pò)* 6g

ANALYSIS OF FORMULA: Minor Order the Qi Decoction *(xiǎo chéng qì tāng)* treats severe constipation with dry stools and heat coupled with qi obstruction in the Large Intestine. In this condition, there is both clumping of heat and dry stools in the Large Intestine as well as dampness, with heat predominating. The dryness and heat in the Large Intestine has developed from damp-heat. As a result, strong purging is not suitable because the turbid, tenacious dampness must be purged several times before it can be discharged. Yet the Spleen qi will be injured if the patient is subjected to repeated strong purging. Under these circumstances, I would modify the formula by using 6-9g of Rhei Radix et Rhizoma *(dà huáng)*. In this way, the for-mula's purging action is reduced, and its functions of promoting qi circulation and transforming dampness are enhanced.

MODIFICATIONS: The basic formula can be modified as follows:

- For epigastric and abdominal pain with a deep-yellow or gray and yellow tongue coating, add Arecae Semen *(bīng láng)*, Citri reticulatae viride Pericarpium *(qīng pí)*, Polygoni multiflori Radix *(hé shǒu wū)*, and Natrii Sulfas *(máng xiāo)*.[54]

- For severe thirst caused by heat from excess, add Trichosanthis Radix *(tiān huā fěn)*, Scrophulariae Radix *(xuán shēn)*, and Phragmitis Rhizoma *(lú gēn)*.

Differentiation and Treatment of the Remnants of Dampness and Heat

REMNANTS OF DAMPNESS AND HEAT

Manifestations. Slight epigastric distention, hunger with no desire to eat, and a thin and slightly greasy tongue coating.

NOTE: This pattern appears most often when damp-heat has lingered for a long time in the qi level; the heat is almost gone, but some dampness remains.

Pathology. Remnants of dampness and heat along with partial recovery of the Stomach and Spleen.

Treatment principles. Eliminate the remnants of dampness and heat with aromatic, light, and cool herbs.

Formula:

FIVE LEAVES AND REED DECOCTION *(wǔ yè lú gēn tāng)*

SOURCE: *Systematic Differentiation of Damp-Heat*[55]

Pogostemonis/Agastaches Folium *(huò xiāng yè)*[56] 9g

Menthae haplocalycis Folium *(bò hé yè)*[57] 3g

Nelumbinis Folium *(hé yè)*.......................................9g

Eriobotryae Folium *(pí pá yè)* 6g

Eupatorii Folium *(pèi lán yè)*[58] 9g

Phragmitis Rhizoma *(lú gēn)*.....................................6g

Benincasae Semen *(dōng guā zǐ)* 6g

ANALYSIS OF FORMULA: In this formula, the aromatic herbs Pogostemonis/Agastaches Folium *(huò xiāng yè)*, Nelumbinis Folium *(hé yè)*, and Eupatorii Folium *(pèi lán yè)* transform the remnants of dampness and restore function to the Stomach and Spleen. The light and cool herbs Menthae haplocalycis Folium *(bò hé yè)*, Eriobotryae Folium *(pí pá yè)*, and Phragmitis Rhizoma *(lú gēn)* disperse the remnants of heat. Benincasae Semen *(dōng guā zǐ)* has a mild action in leaching out dampness via the urine.

In this pattern most of the damp-heat is gone but the qi of the Stomach and Spleen has not yet recovered. As a result, avoid the use of any bitter or cold herb, or a large dosage of any herb, to prevent further injury to the Spleen and Stomach qi. Xue Xue noted that this condition is

> due to remnants of damp-heat veiling and blocking the clear yang such that the Stomach qi fails to transport. We must use very light herbs to disseminate qi in the upper burner, while bitter and heavy herbs are not suitable for this condition at all.[59]

All five of the leaves in this formula are very light and aromatic herbs that disseminate qi, and promote the function of the Spleen and Stomach. Thus, it is better to use the leaves instead of the whole plant. Of course, if the leaves of these herbs are not available, Pogostemonis/Agastaches Herba *(huò xiāng)*, Eupatorii Herba *(pèi lán)*, and Menthae haplocalycis Herba *(bò hé)* can be substituted.

Differentiation and Treatment of Deteriorated Patterns of Damp-Heat

BLOODY STOOLS DUE TO FIRE AND TOXIN INJURING THE COLLATERALS OF THE LARGE INTESTINE

Manifestations. High fever, restlessness, bright-red bloody stools, and a deep-red tongue.

Pathology. Fire and toxin injuring the collaterals of the Large Intestine. This occurs when damp-heat transforms into dry-heat, which in turn becomes fire and toxin which invade the blood level and force blood out of the vessels. When the yang qi in the middle burner is fairly strong but damp-heat still manages to attack the *yang ming* (Large Intestine and Stomach), it will gradually transform into heat or dryness. From here it can become fire or toxin, just like warm pathogen diseases without dampness.

Treatment principles. Cool the blood, resolve the toxicity, and stop the bleeding.

Formula:

RHINOCEROS HORN AND REHMANNIA DECOCTION *(xī jiǎo dì huáng tāng)*

See Chapter 8 for further discussion.

MODIFICATIONS: The basic formula can be modified as follows:

- To enhance the effectiveness of this formula to stop bleeding, add *Sanguisorbae Radix (dì yú)*, Platycladi Cacumen *(cè bǎi yè)*, and Rubiae Radix *(qiàn cǎo gēn)*.

- For scanty, yellow urine, add Gardeniae Fructus *(zhī zǐ)*, Coptidis Rhizoma *(huáng lián)*, and Lophatheri Herba *(dàn zhú yè)*.

- According to Xue Xue, Ginseng Radix *(rén shēn)* and Astragali Radix *(huáng qí)* can be used after the fire and toxin have been eliminated and the bleeding stopped.

OVERABUNDANT DAMPNESS WITH FEEBLE YANG

Manifestations. There are three concurrent aspects to this pattern:

1. *Failure of the yang to warm the exterior* with an intolerance of cold and chills.

2. *Malnourishment of the spirit due to deficiency of the Heart yang* with palpitations and listlessness.

3. *Deficiency of the Spleen and Kidney yang, leading to overflow of water and dampness* with a puffy face, edema of the limbs, scanty urination, and a deep and thin pulse.

NOTE: This pattern is often seen in the later stage of damp-warmth in which damp-heat has transformed into cold-dampness and has injured the yang of the Heart, Spleen, and Kidney. This occurs when excessive dampness has injured the yang, which usually occurs in patients with underlying yang deficiency, or when bitter, cold herbs have been overused or used inappropriately.

Pathology. Heart, Spleen, and Kidney yang deficiency leading to overflowing of water and dampness.

Treatment principles. Warm the Heart, Spleen, and Kidney yang, and discharge the retained water and dampness.

Formula:

TRUE WARRIOR DECOCTION *(zhēn wǔ tāng)*

SOURCE: *Discussion of Cold Damage*

Aconiti Radix lateralis preparata *(zhì fù zǐ)* 9g
Poria *(fú líng)* 9g
Zingiberis Rhizoma recens *(shēng jiāng)* 9g
Atractylodis macrocephalae Rhizoma *(bái zhú)* 6g
Paeoniae Radix alba *(bái sháo)* 9g

ANALYSIS OF FORMULA: Aconiti Radix lateralis preparata *(zhì fù zǐ)* warms the Spleen, Heart, and Kidney yang. Atractylodis macrocephalae Rhizoma *(bái zhú)* and Poria *(fú líng)* tonify the Spleen and leach out dampness. Zingiberis Rhizoma recens *(shēng jiāng)* disperses water and dampness. Paeoniae Radix alba *(bái sháo)* separates dampness and water and controls the hot nature of Aconiti Radix lateralis preparata *(zhì fù zǐ)*.

MODIFICATION: For significant qi deficiency, add Ginseng Radix *(rén shēn)*.

COLLAPSE OF YANG QI FOLLOWING MASSIVE BLEEDING

Manifestations. Persistent heavy bleeding, pale face without luster, profuse sweating, cold extremities, pale tongue, and a faint, thin pulse.

Pathology. Collapse of yang qi following massive bleeding. Above, we discussed a pattern in which damp-heat transforms into fire and toxin and causes bleeding. If the bleeding is severe, the yang qi will follow the blood out, leading to the collapse of yang. If heavy bleeding is allowed to go unchecked, this pattern can occur quickly, regardless of the etiology of the bleeding.

Treatment principles. Tonify qi and arrest the collapse.

Formula:

UNACCOMPANIED GINSENG DECOCTION *(dú shēn tāng)*

SOURCE: *Collected Treatises of [Zhang] Jing-Yue*

ANALYSIS OF FORMULA: According to the early eighteenth-century author Cheng Guo-Peng (Cheng Zhong-Ling), "Blood, which has form, cannot be produced quickly enough. However, qi, which does not have form, should be restored as soon as possible."[60] Otherwise the patient will die regardless of the strength of the blood-enriching herbs, because if qi is not immediately restored, not only will the blood continue to be lost, but the qi will collapse as well. Recovering from this collapse will be difficult. Also, during this emergency, it is suitable to select as few herbs as possible. Only in this way can the yang qi be restored and the bleeding stopped quickly. Otherwise, the other herbs will impair the effect of ginseng to tonify the qi and arrest the collapse. In addition, regardless of which herbal strategy is selected, in our present situation such patients should be sent immediately to the emergency room.

Summary

Damp-warmth is a warm pathogen disease caused by damp-heat that occurs mostly during the late summer or early autumn. Damp-warmth has a slower onset and progression than other warm pathogen diseases. Likewise, it often takes longer to cure and is more difficult to treat than other warm pathogen diseases.

Depending on the condition of the body's yang qi, the damp-warmth will be centered more in the Stomach or in the Spleen. That is, if the yang qi in the middle burner is strong, the disease will more likely be situated in the Stomach. In that case, heat will predominate. If the yang qi in the middle burner is weak, the disease will more likely be situated in the Spleen, and dampness will predominate.

To treat damp-warmth, the first task is to determine whether dampness or heat predominates, and then to separately resolve the dampness and the heat. Dampness can be transformed with aromatic herbs, dried with bitter and warm herbs, or bitter and cold herbs, and leached out with bland herbs. In addition, the practitioner should consider moving the qi in the middle burner. Qi in the Spleen should ascend, and qi in the Stomach should descend; acrid herbs that lift the qi and bitter herbs that direct the qi downward should be used in concert to restore proper qi movement in the middle burner. On the other hand, if the dampness attacks the membrane source, it is important that it be dispersed; acrid herbs that disperse and move qi should be used for this purpose. On balance, a key treatment principle for all damp-warmth patterns is to promote the circulation of qi. This is because when the qi does not circulate, the fluids cannot move; dampness thereupon accumulates and cannot reach the Bladder to exit the body. A summary of damp-warmth is provided in Table 12.9.

Table 12.9	Differentiation and Treatment of Damp-Warmth	
Patterns	**Treatment Principles**	**Formulas**
▶ DAMP-WARMTH WITH DAMPNESS AS PREDOMINANT FACTOR		
Attack on protective level by dampness	Disperse dampness with acrid and aromatic herbs, transform dampness with aromatic herbs, leach out dampness and drain heat with bland and cold herbs	• Xue's Acrid and Aromatic Formula to Release the Exterior (*Xuē shì xīn xiāng jiě biǎo fāng*) • Xue's Formula to Release the Exterior, Leach Out Dampness, Drain Heat (*Xuē shì jiě biǎo shèn shī xiè rè fāng*)
Dampness hindering the qi mechanism of the protective and qi levels	Disperse, transform, and leach out dampness in the exterior and interior with acrid, aromatic, and bland herbs	• Patchouli/Agastache, Magnolia Bark, Pinellia, and Poria Decoction (*huò pò xià líng tāng*) • Three-Nut Decoction (*sān rén tāng*)
Accumulation of turbid dampness in the membrane source	Dispel and disperse turbid dampness from the membrane source	• Lei's Formula to Disseminate and Vent [Dampness and Heat] from the Membrane Source (*Léi shì xuān tòu mó yuán fāng*) • Reach the Source Drink (*dá yuán yǐn*)
Accumulation of dampness in the Spleen, Stomach, and Triple Burner	Clear heat and eliminate dampness by improving the qi mechanism of the Spleen and Triple Burner, direct the Stomach qi downward	Warm the Gallbladder Decoction (*wēn dǎn tāng*)
Disturbance of Spleen and Stomach functions in the middle burner by dampness	Dry and transform dampness with aromatic, bitter, and warm herbs, and direct Stomach qi downward with bitter herbs	• Lei's Fragrant and Aromatic Formula to Transform Turbidity (*Léi shì fāng xiāng huàa zhuó fāng*) • Third Modification of Rectify the Qi Powder (*sān jiā jiǎn zhèng qì sǎn*)
Accumulation of dampness in the Bladder affecting the orifices	Leach out dampness and open the orifices	• Poria Peel Decoction (*fú líng pí tāng*) • Liquid Styrax Pill (*sū hé xiāng wán*)

Table 12.9, cont.		
Dampness obstructing the Intestinal pathway with a breakdown in transportation	Promote the circulation of qi in the Large Intestine and transform dampness, and leach out dampness by urination	Disseminate the Clear and Guide out the Turbid Decoction (*xuān qīng dǎo zhuó tāng*)

▶ DAMP-WARMTH WITH EQUAL PARTS OF DAMPNESS AND HEAT

Accumulation of damp-heat in the middle burner	Lift Spleen qi and transformdampness with acrid herbs, and clear heat and direct Stomach qi downward with bitter herbs; dry the dampnessin the middle burner and moderately purge damp-heat with food retentionin the Large Intestine	• Coptis and Magnolia Bark Drink (*lián pò yǐn*) • Unripe Bitter Orange Pill to Guide Out Stagnation (*zhǐ shí dǎo zhì wán*)
Eruption of vesicles due to steaming of damp-heat	Clear heat and leach out dampness, and disperse damp-heat	Coix and Lophatherus Powder (*yì yǐ zhú yè sǎn*)
Obstruction of channels by damp-heat	Clear heat and transform dampness, and promote qi and blood circulation to relieve pain	Disband Painful Obstruction Decoction (*xuān bì tāng*)
Steaming of damp-heat in Triple Burner	Clear heat and transform dampnessin the Triple Burner	Apricot Kernel and Talcum Decoction (*xìng rén huá shí tāng*)
Veiling of Pericardium by phlegm due to damp-heat	Clear heat and transform dampness, and eliminate phlegm to open the orifices	Acorus and Curcuma Decoction (*chāng pǔ yù jīn tāng*)

▶ DAMP-WARMTH WITH HEAT AS PREDOMINANT FACTOR

Stagnation of qi activity from damp-heat that has transformed into toxin	Clear heat, resolve toxicity, and transform dampness with aromatic, bitter, and cold herbs	Sweet Dew Special Pill to Eliminate Toxin (*gān lù xiāo dú dān*)
Heat from excess in Stomach accompanied by dampness in Spleen	Clear heat in Stomach with acrid and cold herbs, and transform dampness in Spleen with bitter and slightly warm herbs	White Tiger plus Atractylodes Decoction (*bái hǔ jiā cāng zhú tāng*)

Table 12.9, cont.		
Severe constipation with dry stools and heat coupled with dampness in the Large Intestine (damp-heat gradually transforms into dryness in Large Intestine)	Purge heat and transform dampness	Minor Order the Qi Decoction (*xiǎo chéng qì tāng*)
▶ REMNANTS OF DAMPNESS AND HEAT		
Remnants of dampness and heat (with only partial recovery of Stomach and Spleen function)	Eliminate remaining dampness and heat with aromatic, light, and cool herbs	Five Leaves and Reed Decoction (*wǔ yè lú gēn tāng*)
▶ DETERIORATED PATTERNS OF DAMP-HEAT		
Bloody stools due to fire and toxin injuring collaterals of Large Intestine	Cool the blood, resolve toxicity, and stop the bleeding	Rhinoceros Horn and Rehmannia Decoction (*xī jiǎo dì huáng tāng*)
Overabundant dampness with feeble yang (yang deficiency of Heart, Spleen, and Kidney leading to overflowing of water and dampness)	Warm the Heart, Spleen, and Kidney yang, discharge retainedwater and dampness	True Warrior Decoction (*zhēn wǔ tāng*)
Collapse of yang qi following massive bleeding	Tonify qi and arrest the collapse	Unaccompanied Ginseng Decoction (*dú shēn tāng*)

Endnotes

1. *Systematic Differentiation of Damp-Heat Disorders (Shī rè tiáo biàn)*, written by Xue Xue around 1770, is regarded as the first book to systematically discuss damp-warmth.

2. Song Zhao-Qi (Song You-Fu), *Distinguishing [Aspects] of Southern Diseases (Nán bìng bié jiàn)*. Shanghai: Shanghai Health Publishing House, 1958(2): 3. This book is one source for the text of *Systematic Differentiation of Damp-Heat Disorders*.

3. This is a type of fever, usually persistent, wherein the patient feels hot, but the skin may not feel warm until it is pressed for a few seconds. The temperature might not be measurably elevated. For more information on this type of fever, see Chapter 5.

4. Song Zhao-Qi, *Distinguishing [Aspects] of Southern Diseases,* Chapter 2: 2.

5. Miliaria alba manifest as small vesicles that look like crystals. See Chapter 5 for further details.

6. Wang Shi-Xiong, *Warp and Woof of Warm-Heat Pathogen Diseases (Wēn rè jīng wěi),* reproduced in Lu Zhen, *Collected Rare Recent Books on Chinese Medicine: Warm Pathogen Disease Section (Jīn dài zhōng yī zhēn běn jí: wēn bìng fèn cè).* Hangzhou: Zhejiang Science and Technology Publishing House, 1987: 100.

7. Song Zhao-Qi, *Distinguishing [Aspects] of Southern Diseases,* Chapter 2: 10.

8. Wu Tang, *Systematic Differentiation of Warm Pathogen Diseases (Wēn bìng tiáo biàn).* Beijing: People's Health Publishing House, 1963: 96.

9. Ibid., 40.

10. Ibid.

11. In fact, inducing a slight sweat with a combination of cool and warm and acrid herbs is a good method for getting rid of dampness. What Wu is arguing against here is to induce sweating by using *only* acrid and warm herbs that strongly induce sweating. This was common practice during his time. See Chapter 1 for more information about the history of treating externally-contracted diseases in China.

12. Zhang Ji, *Discussion of Cold Damage (Shāng hán lùn).* Shanghai: Shanghai Science and Technology Publishing House, 1983: 12.

13. Wu Tang, *Systematic Differentiation of Warm Pathogen Diseases,* 40.

14. Ibid. It is true that in general, as noted here, one should not use the purging method for damp-heat, especially that affecting the Spleen and Stomach. However, in the author's experience, when the situation requires a route out of the body for resolution of the disease—as with food retention, clumping of damp-heat, dryness, and dry stool, or blood stasis in the Large Intestine—a mild purging method is appropriate.

15. There are some exceptions to this rule. For example, Ran Pin-Zhen, a well-respected professor who taught internal medicine at Chengdu College of Traditional Chinese Medicine for many years, would frequently change his diagnosis from damp-heat to yin deficiency if the treatment was not having the desired effect. Often when he did this, after the patient took the yin-enriching herbs, their thick tongue coating would recede and reveal a stripped red tongue. This would be accompanied by a marked improvement in the patient's condition.

16. Wu Tang, *Systematic Differentiation of Warm Pathogen Diseases,* 40.

17. As is clear from the discussion below, this pattern is due to dampness without any heat, at least in the beginning. It is included here because the dampness in this pattern (and the one that follows) can easily block the protective qi and very quickly transform into damp-heat. The treatment is then the same as that for damp-warmth.

18. In the original source, formulas no. 1 and 2 were not named and no dosages were listed for the ingredients. The names and dosages are found in Song Nai-Guang et al., *Warm Pathogen Diseases (Wēn bìng xué).* Beijing: Learning Garden Publishing House, 1995: 101.

19. Nothing is known about this herb except for this particular use by Xue Xue. While there is a theoretical rationale for using the cortex of the herb, as the peel, bark, or skin of a plant or fruit is often used to treat skin and exterior conditions, at present Atractylodis Rhizoma *(cāng zhú)* is used to dry dampness and eliminate wind.

20. Pogostemonis/Agastaches Folium *(huò xiāng yè)* is sweet, acrid, and slightly warm, and enters the Lung and Spleen channels. Its functions are similar to those of Pogostemonis/Agastaches Herba *(huò xiāng)*, but as the leaves are light and have a relatively mild aroma, their usage focuses more on releasing, disseminating, and dispersing.

21. If there is a predominance of heat, as opposed to dampness, the above signs and symptoms will not appear.

22. Shi-Shou Tang, *Bases of Medicine (Yī yuán)*. Nanjing: Jiangsu Science and Technology Publishing House: 94. The source text provides neither a name nor dosages for this formula. That information comes from Meng Shu-Jiang et al., *Warm Pathogen Diseases (Wēn bìng xué)*. Shanghai: Shanghai Science and Technology Publishing House, 1985: 79.

23. See Chapter 7 for further information.

24. There are two formulas with the name Nourish the Stomach Decoction with Aucklandia and Amomum *(xiāng shā yǎng wèi tāng)*. The first one was recorded in 1587 by Gong Ting-Xian (Gong Zi-Cai) in his *Restoration of Health from the Myriad Diseases (Wàn bìng huí chūn)*. Beijing: People's Health Publishing House, 1984: 106. It contains Cyperi Rhizoma *(xiāng fù)* (2.4g), Amomi Fructus *(shā rén)* (2.4g), Atractylodis Rhizoma *(cāng zhú)* (2.4g), Magnoliae officinalis Cortex *(hòu pò)* (2.4g), Citri reticulatae Pericarpium *(chén pí)* (2.4g), Ginseng Radix *(rén shēn)* (1.5g), Atractylodis macrocephalae Rhizoma *(bái zhú)* (3g), Poria *(fú líng)* (2.4g), Aucklandiae Radix *(mù xiāng)* (1.5g), Amomi Fructus rotundus *(bái dòu kòu)* (2.1g), and a little bit of Glycyrrhizae Radix *(gān cǎo)*. The other was recorded in 1772 in Shen Jin-Ao (Shen Qian-Lu), *Wondrous Lantern for Peering into the Origin and Development of Miscellaneous Diseases (Zá bìng yuán liú xī zhú)*. Beijing: China Traditional Chinese Medicine and Pharmacology Publishing House, 1994: 440. It contains Atractylodis macrocephalae Rhizoma *(bái zhú)* (3g), Citri reticulatae Pericarpium *(chén pí)* (3g), Poria *(fú líng)* (3g), Pinelliae Rhizoma preparatum *(zhì bàn xià)* (3g), Cyperi Rhizoma *(xiāng fù)* (2.1g), Amomi Fructus *(shā rén)* (2.1g), Aucklandiae Radix *(mù xiāng)* (2.1g), Aurantii Fructus immaturus *(zhǐ shí)* (2.1g), Amomi Fructus rotundus *(bái dòu kòu)* (2.1g), Pogostemonis/Agastaches Herba *(huò xiāng)* (2.1g), Magnoliae officinalis Cortex *(hòu pò)* (2.1g), Glycyrrhizae Radix *(gān cǎo)* (0.9g), Zingiberis Rhizoma recens *(shēng jiāng)* (3 slices), and Jujubae Fructus *(dà zǎo)* (2 pieces). It is unknown which version was used here.

25. Beijing Traditional Chinese Hospital, *Compilation of Experiences from Famous Veteran Traditional Chinese Doctors*, vol. 2 *(Míng lǎo zhōng yī jīng yàn quán biān, xià cè)*. Beijing: Beijing Publishing House, 1994: 253-54. This is a case by Wu Yin-Nan.

26. This was first recorded by Wang Ken-Tang (Wang Yu-Tai) in his book *Indispensable Tools for Pattern Treatment (Zhèng zhì zhǔn shéng)*, and contains Atractylodis macrocephalae Rhizoma *(bái zhú)* (75g), Poria *(fú líng)* (60g), Ginseng Radix *(rén shēn)* (45g), Dioscoreae Rhizoma *(shān yào)* (30g), Myristicae Semen *(ròu dòu kòu)* (30g), Crataegi Fructus *(shān zhā)* (30g), Massa medicata fermentata *(shén qū)* (30g), Hordei Fructus germinatus *(mài yá)* (30g), Aucklandiae Radix *(mù xiāng)* (22.5g), Citri reticulatae Pericarpium *(chén*

pí) (30g), Amomi Fructus *(shā rén)* (30g), Coptidis Rhizoma *(huáng lián)* (22.5g), and Glycyrrhizae Radix *(gān cǎo)* (22.5g).

27. Dong Jian-Hua et al., *Selected Case Studies from Famous Modern Chinese Doctors (Zhōng guó xiàn dài míng zhōng yī yī àn jīng huá)*. Beijing: Beijing Publishing House, 1990: 2000. This case was reported by Ke Li-Min.

28. He Lian-Chen, *Revised and Expanded Discussion of Warm-Heat Pathogen Diseases (Chóng dìng guǎng wēn rè lùn.* Beijing: People's Health Publishing House, 1960: 7.

29. Lei Feng, *Discussion of Seasonal Diseases (Shí bìng lùn)*. Beijing: People's Health Publishing House, 1956: 94.

30. See n. 20 above.

31. Wu You-Xing, *Discussion of Warm Epidemics (Wēn yì lùn)*. Shenyang: Liaoning Science and Technology Publishing House, 1997: 2.

32. Dong Jian-Hua et al., *Selected Case Studies from Famous Modern Chinese Doctors*, 2099. This case was reported by Sun Yun-Zhong.

33. This was written by Chen Yan in 1174. The formula is actually a modification of one with the same name orginally recorded by Sun Si-Miao in *Important Formulas Worth a Thousand Gold Pieces for any Emergency (Bèi jí qiān jīn yào fāng)*, published in 652. The original formula contained Pinelliae Rhizoma preparatum *(zhì bàn xià)* (6g), Bambusae Caulis in taeniam *(zhú rú)* (6g), Aurantii Fructus immaturus *(zhǐ shí)* (6g), Citri reticulatae Pericarpium *(chén pí)* (9g), Zingiberis Rhizoma recens *(shēng jiāng)* (12g), and Glycyrrhizae Radix *(gān cǎo)* (3g).

34. Tang Da-Lie, *Collection of Papers of Physicians from Wu (Wú yī huì jiǎng)*. Shanghai: Shanghai Science and Technology Publishing House, 1983: 4.

35. Yu Gen-Chu (Yu Zhao-Yuan), *Revised Popular Guide to the Discussion of Cold Damage (Chóng ding tōng sú shāng hán lùn)*. Hangzhou: New Medicine Press, 1956: 1. This formula contains Scutellariae Radix *(huáng qín)* (6g), Pinelliae Rhizoma preparatum *(zhì bàn xià)* (4.5g), Bambusae Caulis in taeniam *(zhú rú)* (6g), Poria rubra *(chì fú líng)* (3g), Coptidis Rhizoma *(huáng lián)* (2.4g), Citri reticulatae Pericarpium *(chén pí)* (4.5g), Aurantii Fructus immaturus *(zhǐ shí)* (4.5g), Jade Powder *(bì yù sǎn)* (6g) [which contains Indigo naturalis *(qīng dài)*, Talcum *(huá shí),* and Glycyrrhizae Radix *(gān cǎo)*], Zingiberis Rhizomatis Succus *(jiāng zhī)* (2 drops), and Bambusae Succus *(zhú lì)* (2 spoonfuls).

36. See n. 20 above.

37. It is acrid and neutral and enters the Spleen and Stomach channels. The leaves have a clear, light aroma with milder properties than Eupatorii Herba *(pèi lán)*. It is used to resolve summerheat, transform dampness, and eradicate filth. Indicated for fever, chills, aversion to cold, headache, poor appetite, epigastric distention, nausea, vomiting, and a sweet, sticky taste in the mouth.

38. This book was preserved in Wang Shi-Xiong's *Warp and Woof of Warm-Heat Pathogen Diseases (Wēn rè jīng wěi)*. It is reproduced in Lu Zhen, *Collected Rare Recent Books on Chinese Medicine: Warm Pathogen Disease Section (Jīn dài zhōng yī zhēn běn jí: wēn bìng fèn cè)*. Hangzhou: Zhejiang Science and Technology Publishing House, 1987: 71.

39. Wu Tang, *Systematic Differentiation of Warm Pathogen Diseases*, 94.

40. See n. 48 below.

41. Song Zhao-Qi, *Distinguishing [Aspects] of Southern Diseases*, Chapter 2: 10.

42. See Chapter 7 for further details.

43. Wu Tang, *Systematic Differentiation of Warm Pathogen Diseases*, 102.

44. This was published by Wang Shi-Xiong in 1838.

45. This was published by Li Gao in 1231.

46. Li Gao (Li Dong-Yuan), *Clarifying Doubts about Damage from Internal and External Causes (Nèi wài shāng biàn huò lùn)*. Nanjing: Jiangsu Science and Technology Publishing House, 1982: 61.

47. Wu Tang, *Systematic Differentiation of Warm Pathogen Diseases*, 98.

48. The source text did not specify which herb known as *fang ji* should be used: Aristolochiae fangchi Radix *(guǎng fáng jǐ)* or Stephaniae tetrandrae Radix *(hàn fáng jǐ)*. Both herbs eliminate wind-dampness, promote urination, and relieve pain. Traditionally, Aristolochiae fangchi Radix *(guǎng fáng jǐ)* is regarded as stronger in eliminating wind-dampness and relieving pain, which is more suitable for this case. However, over the past ten years there has been some question as to whether the small amount of the known nephrotoxin aristolochic acid in this herb has been responsible for renal damage in some patients. As of May, 2000 the U.S. Federal Drug Administration has issued a warning in this regard not only for Aristolochiae fangchi Radix *(guǎng fáng jǐ)*, but for any herb that could be confused with one containing aristolochic acid, such as Stephaniae tetrandrae Radix *(hàn fáng jǐ)*. Although there has been discussion about the clinical implications of this matter and whether the harm from this herb is theoretical or real, at the present time I would suggest that to ensure patient safety, neither of these herbs be should used until the matter is resolved. Clinically, Dioscoreae hypoglaucae Rhizoma *(bì xiè)* can be used as a substitute here.

49. This book was written by Shi Yi-Ren and published in 1933.

50. Jade Pivot Pill *(yù shū wán)* is a patent formula that includes Cremastrae/Pleiones Pseudobulbus *(shān cí gū)* (90g), Galla chinensis *(wǔ bèi zǐ)* (90g), Arnebiae Radix/ Lithospermi Radix Realgar *(xióng huáng)* (30g), *Knoxiae Radix/Euphorbiae pekinensis Radix (dà jǐ)* (45g), Moschus *(shè xiāng)* (9g), Cinnabaris *(zhū shā)* (30g), and Euphorbiae lathyridis Semen *(qiān jīn zǐ)* (30g). The last substance is also known as *xù suì zǐ*. It is acrid, warm, and toxic and enters the Lung, Stomach, and Bladder channels. It is a purgative that expels water while also breaking up masses due to blood stasis. In addition, it kills parasites and is used for snakebite. Like several of the other substances in this pill, it should not be used during pregnancy or in the debilitated. Note that while this medicine contains several toxic substances, their dosages are well below the maximum safe daily dose, and they are used for a very brief time period.

51. See Chapter 7 for further details.

52. The source text recommends that all ingredients be dried in the sun and ground into powder. Swallow 12g of the powder by boiled water, twice a day. These dosages are too high to be practical clinically, and we suggest the following instead: Talcum *(huá shí)* (12-15g), Artemisiae scopariae Herba *(yīn chén)* (15-24g), Scutellariae Radix *(huáng qín)* (12-15g), Acori tatarinowii Rhizoma *(shí chāng pǔ)* (12-15g), Fritillariae cirrhosae Bulbus *(chuān*

bèi mǔ) (9-12g), Akebiae Caulis *(mù tōng)* (9-12g), Pogostemonis/Agastaches Herba *(huò xiāng)* (12-15g), Belamcandae Rhizoma *(shè gān)* (12-15g), Forsythiae Fructus *(lián qiào)* (15-18g), Menthae haplocalycis Herba *(bò hé)* (6-9g), and Amomi Fructus rotundus *(bái dòu kòu)* (6-9g).

53. Chongqing Traditional Chinese Medicine Research Institute, *Traditional Chinese Medicine and Acute Conditions Report (Zhōng yī jí zhèng tōng xùn)*. Chongqing: Chonging Traditional Chinese Medicine Research Institute, 1985(8): 6. This case was reported by Liu Du-Xing.

54. This modification was discussed by Ye Gui in *Discussion of Warm-Heat Disorders (Wēn rè lùn)*.

55. The name and dosages for the formula and its ingredients come from the Teaching and Research Section of Warm Pathogen Diseases, Chengdu College of Traditional Chinese Medicine, *Self-Study Textbook for Chinese Medicine: Warm Pathogen Diseases (Zhōng yī zì xué jiào cái: Wēn bìng xué)*. Chengdu, Chengdu College of Traditional Chinese Medicine, 1985: 97.

56. See n. 20 above.

57. This is acrid and cool, and enters the Lung and Liver channels. It has the same actions as Menthae haplocalycis Herba *(bò hé)*, but is stronger at inducing sweating.

58. See n. 37 above.

59. Song Zhao-Qi, *Distinguishing [Aspects] of Southern Diseases*, Chapter 2: 9.

60. Cheng Guo-Peng, *Medical Revelations (Yī xué xīn wù)*. Tianjin: Tianjin Science and Technology Publishing House, 1999: 33-34.

13 Lurking Summerheat

W
ANG KEN-TANG (WANG Yu-Tan, 1549–1613) first introduced the term lurking summerheat (伏暑 *fú shǔ*) in *Indispensable Tools for Pattern Treatment (Zhèng zhì zhǔn shéng)*.[1] Lurking summerheat occurs when a summerheat pathogen attacks during the summer, incubates inside the body, and is then induced to emerge by an attack from a secondary external pathogen in either the autumn or winter. Since the disease appears after the initial attack, it is also known as lurking summerheat that manifests in autumn (伏暑 秋發 *fú shǔ qiū fā)*, winter-extruding lurking summerheat (冬越伏暑 *dōng yuè fú shǔ)*, or delayed discharge (晚發 *wǎn fā)*. When the disease finally manifests, it has a sudden onset. It is generally serious, and the course of the disease is protracted.

In its early stage, lurking summerheat may be similar to a common cold with chills, aversion to cold, fever, and body aches. However, it will be accompanied by other signs and symptoms:

- *Those from lurking summerheat with dampness*, such as fever, irritability, restlessness, thirst, epigastric distention, scanty, dark-yellow urine, and a greasy tongue coating.

- *Those from dry-heat transformed from lurking summerheat with dampness*, such as fever, dry mouth, irritability, restlessness, and a deep-red tongue with less than normal coating.

Later, the pattern changes and the signs and symptoms are similar to those of malarial disorders, but with irregular fever and chills. As it progresses, the chills and aversion to cold abate, and the fever becomes worse in the evening and subsides in the early morning hours after some sweating. There is a burning sensation in the chest and abdomen, bowel movements that are loose yet feel incomplete, and which leave an uncomfortable sensation around the anus after evacuation.

In Chapter 8 we discussed another kind of lurking warm pathogen disease, spring-warmth. Both spring-warmth and lurking summerheat are caused by lurking external pathogens. However, the season of onset and the quality of the external pathogens associated with these two diseases are quite different. Spring-warmth results from an initial attack of cold in the winter, and its onset is in the spring. By contrast, lurking summerheat results from an initial attack of summerheat that combines with dampness, and its onset is in the autumn or winter. The presentation of spring-warmth includes dry mouth, thirst, irritability, restlessness, fever, and scanty and dark-yellow urine. By contrast, the presentation of lurking summerheat includes one of two presentations:

- Lurking summerheat with dampness, which is accompanied by fever, irritability, thirst, epigastric distention, scanty, dark-yellow urine, and a greasy tongue coating,

- Lurking summerheat with dampness that has transformed into dry-heat that invades the nutritive level, with fever, dry mouth, restlessness, and a deep-red tongue with little coating.

Table 13.1	Lurking Summerheat vs. Spring-Warmth
Pathology	**Signs and Symptoms**
LURKING SUMMERHEAT	
Attack by summerheat with dampness during the summer, or dry-heat that has trans- formed from summerheat with dampness; onset in autumn or winter	Fever, restlessness, thirst, epigastric distention, scanty and dark-yellow urine, greasy tongue coating or fever, dry mouth, restlessness, deep-red tongue with little coating
SPRING-WARMTH	
Attack by cold in the winter; onset in spring	Dry mouth, thirst, restlessness, fever, scanty and dark-yellow urine

The biomedical diagnoses of such diseases as influenza, encephalitis B, epidemic hemorrhagic fever, and leptospirosis overlap somewhat with lurking summerheat in Chinese medicine, and can be treated with the same methods outlined in this chapter.

Etiology and Pathology

Summerheat combines with dampness and attacks the body during the course of the summer. Factors that facilitate the pathogen's incubation in the body include its association with dampness, which is turbid and hard to eliminate, and weak antipathogenic qi. Subsequent to its incubation, an attack by a secondary external pathogen, such as wind-cold or wind-heat, during the autumn or winter induces the lurking summerheat pathogen to emerge.

An individual need not exhibit signs and symptoms of weak antipathogenic qi in the early stage of the illness. Rather, the obvious factors are an accumulation of internal damp-heat and the history of an attack during the summer by externally-contracted dampness. It is this external dampness that combines with the summer-heat pathogen to attack the body of one with compromised antipathogenic qi. Theoretically, therefore, those without pre-existing internal damp-heat cannot contract lurking summerheat. In the clinic, however, we find that while individuals with constitutional damp-heat are more likely to contract this disorder, lurking summer-heat can occur in others as well, probably due to underlying qi deficiency that has not yet manifested.

Where in the body does the pathogen incubate, and why? Most practitioners believe that lurking summerheat incubates in the Spleen because, according to five-phase theory, both dampness and the Spleen pertain to the earth phase. When external dampness attacks the body, the internal dampness that is already present will attract it to the Spleen; as a result, the signs and symptoms will be those of qi level Spleen patterns. Wu Tang had a slightly different take on this. He noted that, due to qi deficiency, the disease settles internally in the bones and marrow, while externally it settles between the interstices and muscles.[2] This conception emphasizes the deep, lurking nature of the disorder, and suggests that its treatment is usually prolonged.

In addition, since dampness causes the circulation of qi to stagnate, the disease usually appears as a qi level pattern in its early stages. On the other hand, if the patient has underlying yin deficiency, the summerheat with dampness will likely transform into heat and dryness, and the disease will present as a nutritive level pattern. Yet regardless of which level it affects, because it must be induced to manifest by a secondary external pathogen, at the very beginning there will be some protective level manifestations. According to Wu Tang, the sooner the secondary attack occurs, the milder the pattern, and the more time that elapses before the secondary attack, the more severe the pattern.[3]

Finally, should internal damp-heat accumulate while lurking summerheat resides within the body, an attack by external pathogens during the autumn or winter will result in a combination of an externally-contracted pattern and an internal-ly-generated damp-heat pattern. The external attack can exacerbate the internal damp-heat, and because dampness is characterized by stickiness and stagnation, this can have the effect of trapping lurking summerheat inside the body. This may start a vicious cycle that can continue for an extended period of time.

Factors for Identifying Lurking Summerheat

There are two important factors for identifying lurking summerheat:

1. *Lurking summerheat manifests only in the autumn or winter,* although summerheat with dampness only attacks during the summer.
2. *Lurking summerheat has a sudden onset and is characterized by an accumulation of lurking summerheat combined with dampness, or its transformation into dryheat.*[4] If the onset of the disease is in the qi level, fever, irritability, thirst, chest distention, and a greasy tongue coating will appear. If the onset is in the nutritive level, there will be fever, dry mouth, restlessness, and a deep-red tongue with little coating. However, regardless of the level in which the onset of the disease occurs, there will be signs and symptoms of the initial stage of an exterior pattern, such as aversion to cold.

Alternating chills and fever is a symptom that can occur with malarial disorders, *shao yang* stage disorders, as well as lurking summerheat in the Triple Burner. However, in malarial disorders it occurs with some regularity, while in lurking summerheat it comes irregularly. Also, *shao yang* patterns generally do not present with signs of dampness, such as chest and abdominal distention or a greasy tongue coating, because the Gallbladder rather than the Triple Burner is most involved. Moreover, the *shao yang* pattern can occur in any season, unlike lurking summer-heat, which manifests only in the autumn or winter.

Progression of Lurking Summerheat

Regardless of whether the onset of the disease involves the qi or nutritive level, the early stage of lurking summerheat will also display exterior (protective level) signs and symptoms because of the external pathogen which has induced its appearance. Once the exterior pattern has abated, lurking summerheat coupled with dampness will attack the qi level, leading to steaming of damp-heat in the qi level. There are two patterns of lurking summerheat in the qi level:

1. *Lurking summerheat coupled with dampness remains in the Triple Burner and presents with alternating chills and fever.* Upper burner symptoms include chest distention; middle burner symptoms include epigastric distention, abdominal bloating and nausea; and lower burner symptoms include scanty, turbid urine.

2. *Lurking summerheat coupled with dampness specifically invades the middle burner.* The pathology and manifestations will be almost the same as that of summerheat-warmth or damp-warmth, that is, there will be more dampness than heat. Symptoms include epigastric and chest distention, gas, bloating, loose stools, and a loss of appetite.

The treatment of these two patterns is similar to the corresponding patterns in the summerheat-warmth and damp-warmth categories, respectively.

If lurking summerheat initially attacks the protective and nutritive levels *and* the protective level pattern abates, the disease may remain in the nutritive level. Alternatively, the disease may progress to the blood level, presenting with signs and symptoms of bleeding or disturbance of the spirit.

Treatment Principles

Because the underlying conditions will vary, so too will the treatment principles. When lurking summerheat is found in the qi level, focus on clearing lurking summerheat and transforming dampness. If a second external pathogen is also present, leading to a combination of exterior and interior patterns, focus on releasing the exterior pattern, clearing lurking summerheat, and transforming the dampness. If lurking summerheat emerges in the *shao yang* aspect of the qi level, clear heat from the *shao yang* and drain dampness, because the *shao yang* here means the Triple Burner, which circulates water and qi. When lurking summerheat attacks the Intestines, the best way to eliminate it is to purge damp-heat, clear heat, and transform dampness.

When lurking summerheat appears in the nutritive level, focus on enriching the yin and clearing heat from the nutritive level. If there is invasion of the Pericardium or stirring of Liver wind, see the corresponding treatments in Chapters 7, 8, and 11 for further details.

Treatment should focus on the interior pattern even in the early stage, when there may be a coexisting exterior pattern. According to He Lian-Chen (He Bing-Yuan, 1860-1929) in his commentary[5] to *Revised Popular Guide to the Discussion of Cold Damage (Chóng dìng tōng sú shāng hán lùn)*, written by Yu Gen-Chu (Yu Zhao-Yuan, 1734-1799), the important thing to remember when treating lurking summerheat is to focus on dampness, heat, deficiency, and excess. He Lian-Chen observed that "The key point in treating lurking summerheat is to first determine the level of dampness and heat, then the level of deficiency and excess."[6]

How does one identify dampness, heat, deficiency and excess? Yu Gen-Chu provided general guidelines in *Revised Popular Guide to the Discussion of Cold Damage*: "If lurking summerheat occurs in the qi level, it is caused by dampness and is a condition of excess. If it occurs in the nutritive level, it is caused by dryness [heat] and is a condition of deficiency."[7] In other words, lurking summerheat has more of a damp aspect when it appears in the qi level, and, at this level, the antipathogenic qi is still strong and the condition is one of excess. On the other hand, lurking summerheat has more of a dry (heat) aspect when it appears in the nutritive level because it is more likely to transform into fire and injure the yin at this level.

Differentiation and Treatment of the Initial Onset of Lurking Summerheat

COEXISTENCE OF PROTECTIVE AND QI LEVEL PATTERNS OF LURKING SUMMERHEAT

Manifestations. There are three concurrent aspects to this pattern:

1. *Wind-cold attacks the exterior* with fever, chills, aversion to cold, headache, general body aches, and the absence of sweating.

2. *Internal constraint of lurking summerheat* with irritability, thirst, and scanty and dark-yellow urine, a rapid pulse.

3. *Obstruction of qi by dampness* with chest distention, greasy tongue coating, and a soggy pulse.

NOTE: If the secondary attack is one of wind-cold, the result is likely to be the coexistence of protective and qi level patterns, described here. If the secondary attack is one of wind-heat, the result is likely to be the coexistence of protective and nutritive level patterns, described below. This is because wind-heat has a tendency to move rapidly around the body, causing the lurking summerheat with dampness to quickly transform into dry-heat and then progress to a deeper level with greater speed than does wind-cold. The herbal formulas for treating these two conditions also differ, and are based on the specific pathogens involved in the secondary attack and their progression.

The coexistence of protective and qi level patterns of lurking summerheat often occurs in the autumn or winter and is easy to confuse with the exterior pattern caused by wind-cold. This is because both present with exterior signs and symptoms such as fever, chills, aversion to cold, headache, general body aches, and the absence of sweating. You can distinguish between them by focusing on the signs and symptoms of lurking summerheat with dampness, such as thirst, scanty and dark urine, and a greasy tongue coating.

Pathology. Wind-cold attack that activates a preexisting lurking summerheat pathogen coupled with dampness.

Treatment principles. Release the exterior with acrid, warm herbs; clear lurking summerheat with bitter, cold herbs; and transform dampness with bitter, warm herbs.

Formula:

> **Coptis and Mosla Drink** *(huáng lián xiāng rú yǐn)*[8]
>
> source: *Book to Safeguard Life Arranged According to Pattern*
>
> Moslae Herba *(xiāng rú)* . . . . .30g[9]
> Magnoliae officinalis Cortex *(hòu pò)* 15g
> Lablab Semen album *(bái biǎn dòu)* 15g
> Coptidis Rhizoma *(huáng lián)* 9g

analysis of formula: Moslae Herba *(xiāng rú)*, with its acrid flavor and warm nature, disperses external wind-cold and eliminates the exterior signs and symptoms. Coptidis Rhizoma *(huáng lián)*, with its bitter flavor and cold nature, clears lurking summerheat and reduces irritability. Lablab Semen album *(bái biǎn dòu)* and Magnoliae officinalis Cortex *(hòu pò)* transform dampness. (This formula is also discussed in Chapter 11.)

modifications: The basic formula can be modified as follows:

- For a tongue coating that is not greasy, remove Magnoliae officinalis Cortex *(hòu pò)* and add Forsythiae Fructus *(lián qiào)*.

- For severe epigastric and chest distention, add Pogostemonis/Agastaches Herba *(huò xiāng)* and Eupatorii Herba *(pèi lán)*.

- According to Wu Tang, if wind-heat activates a preexisting lurking summerheat pathogen coupled with dampness, leading to chills, fever, cough, absence of sweating, thirst, and a white tongue coating, use Honeysuckle and Forsythia Powder *(yín qiào sǎn)* modified by adding Talcum *(huá shí)* and Armeniacae Semen *(xìng rén)* and removing Arctii Fructus *(niú bàng zǐ)*.[10]

Coexistence of Protective and Nutritive Level Patterns of Lurking Summerheat

Manifestations. There are two concurrent aspects to this pattern:

1. *Wind-heat attacking the surface* with fever, chills, slight aversion to cold, headache, and a little sweating.
2. *Injury to the nutritive level yin by dry-heat, which has transformed from lurking summerheat with dampness,* with restlessness, dry mouth with no desire to drink, red tongue with little coating, and a floating, thin, and rapid pulse.

Pathology. Wind-heat attack that activates preexisting lurking summerheat with dampness and transforms it into dry-heat, which injures nutritive level yin.

Treatment principles. Release the exterior with acrid, cool herbs, clear heat from the nutritive level, and enrich the yin.

Formula:

AUGMENTED HONEYSUCKLE AND FORSYTHIA POWDER *(jiā wèi yín qiào sǎn)*

SOURCE: *Systematic Differentiation of Warm Pathogen Diseases*

This is Honeysuckle and Forsythia Powder*(yín qiào sǎn)*[11] with the addition of Rehmanniae Radix *(shēng dì huáng)*, Moutan Cortex *(mǔ dān pí)*, Paeoniae Radix rubra *(chì sháo)*, and Ophiopogonis Radix *(mài mén dōng)*.

ANALYSIS OF FORMULA: Lonicerae Flos *(jīn yín huā)*, Lophatheri Herba *(dàn zhú yè)*, and Forsythiae Fructus *(lián qiào)* disperse and vent the heat from the nutritive level. Schizonepetae Herba *(jīng jiè)*, Sojae Semen preparatum *(dàn dòu chǐ)*, and Menthae haplocalycis Herba *(bò hé)* disperse wind-heat. Rehmanniae Radix *(shēng dì huáng)* and Ophiopogonis Radix *(mài mén dōng)* enrich the yin. Moutan Cortex *(mǔ dān pí)* and Paeoniae Radix rubra *(chì sháo)* clear heat in the nutritive level.

Table 13.2	Coptis and Mosla Drink vs. Augmented Honeysuckle and Forsythia Powder	
Pathology	**Signs and Symptoms**	**Treatment Principles**
▶ COPTIS AND MOSLA DECOCTION *(huáng lián xiāng rú yǐn)*		
Secondary attack by wind-cold; the lurking summerheat is associated with dampness; protective and qi level patterns	Fever, chills, aversion to cold, headache, absence of sweating, chest distention, scanty and dark-yellow urine, and a greasy tongue coating	Disperse exterior cold, clear interior lurking summerheat; transform dampness
▶ AUGMENTED HONEYSUCKLE AND FORSYTHIA POWDER *(jiā wéi yín qiào sǎn)*		
Secondary attack by wind-heat; the exterior heat is more intense while the lurking summerheat is not associated with dampness; protective or nutritive level patterns	Restlessness, dry mouth with no desire to drink, fever, chills, headache, slight sweating, and a red tongue with little coating	Release the exterior with acrid herbs; clear lurking summerheat from the nutritive level; enrich the yin

Table 13.3	Protective/Qi Level Patterns Compared with Protective/Nutritive Level Patterns*	
Pattern	**Pathology**	**Signs and Symptoms**
Protective/qi level patterns	Steaming up and constraint by lurking summerheat and dampness	Thirst, chest distention, dizziness, greasy tongue coating
Protective/nutritive level patterns	Injury to the yin by heat	Dry mouth with no desire to drink, red tongue wit little coating

*Common points: simultaneous exterior and interior patterns

MODIFICATIONS: The basic formula can be modified as follows:

- To enhance the yin-enriching aspect of this formula, add Polygonati odorati Rhizoma *(yù zhú)* and Scrophulariae Radix *(xuán shēn)*.
- For delirium, skin eruptions, and a deep-red tongue, use Clear the Nutritive Level Decoction *(qīng yíng tāng)*[12] modified by adding Sojae Semen preparatum *(dàn dòu chǐ)* and Menthae haplocalycis Herba *(bò hé)* to disperse heat from constraint in the nutritive level.

Differentiation and Treatment of Lurking Summerheat in the Qi Level

CONSTRAINT OF LURKING SUMMERHEAT AND DAMPNESS IN THE TRIPLE BURNER

Manifestations. There are four concurrent aspects to this pattern:

1. *The struggle between antipathogenic qi and lurking summerheat and dampness* with irregular, alternating fever and chills, where the fever is more intense than the chills.
2. *Obstruction of the qi mechanism of the Triple Burner by lurking summerheat and dampness* with chest distention, epigastric distention, thirst, irritability, restlessness, scanty urine, and a greasy, yellow tongue coating.
3. *Dampness-related problems increasing during the yin time of day* with fever that increases in the afternoon and is even higher in the evening.

4. *Severe dampness restraining heat from dispersing* with fever that diminishes a little after slight sweating from the chest and abdomen; the fever does, however, continue. Severe dampness contains the lurking summerheat deep within the body and inhibits the dispersion of heat.

NOTE: Constraint of lurking summerheat and dampness in the Triple Burner presents with half-exterior and half-interior signs and symptoms. It is therefore similar to the *shao yang* stage of the six stages described in *Discussion of Cold Damage*, as well as malarial disorders, and damp-heat in the membrane source. (See Table 13.4 for a comparison of these conditions.)

Table 13.4	Comparison of Constraint of Lurking Summerheat and Dampness in Triple Burner with Other Common Causes of Alternating Fever and Chills
Pattern	**Signs and Symptoms***
Constraint of lurking summerheat and dampness in the Triple Burner	Fever is more intense than chills, chest distention, restlessness, thirst, greasy and yellow tongue coating; after sweating there is decrease in temperature, but chest and abdomen remain hot
Shao yang stage of the six stages	Bitter taste, sore throat, dizziness, hypochondriac or costal pain, nausea or vomiting, poor appetite, white tongue coating, wiry pulse
Malarial disorders	Shivering; temperature as well as other signs and symptoms disappear after sweating but reappear after fixed time; feels fatigued after attack
Damp-heat in the membrane source	More chills than fever, heavy sensation in body with body aches, and white, thick, greasy, and slippery tongue coating that looks like white powder over the tongue

*Common symptoms: alternating fever and chills

Pathology. Lurking summerheat and dampness constrain the Triple Burner, leading to obstruction of the qi mechanism.

Treatment principles. Clear lurking summerheat from the Triple Burner and transform dampness.

Formula:

> **SWEET WORMWOOD AND SCUTELLARIA DECOCTION TO CLEAR THE GALLBLADDER** *(hāo qín qīng dǎn tāng)*

SOURCE: *Revised Popular Guide to Discussion of Cold Damage*

Artemisiae annuae Herba *(qīng hāo)* 4.5–6g
Scutellariae Radix *(huáng qín)* 4.5–9g
Bambusae Caulis in taeniam *(zhú rú)* 9g
Pinelliae Rhizoma preparatum *(zhì bàn xià)* 4.5g
Aurantii Fructus *(zhǐ ké)* 4.5g
Citri reticulatae Pericarpium *(chén pí)* 4.5g
Poria rubra *(chì fú líng)* 9g
Jasper Powder *(bì yù sǎn)*[13] 9g

ANALYSIS OF FORMULA: Artemisiae annuae Herba *(qīng hāo)* and Scutellariae Radix *(huáng qín)* clear lurking summerheat from the Triple Burner. Bambusae Caulis in taeniam *(zhú rú)*, Pinelliae Rhizoma preparatum *(zhì bàn xià)*, Aurantii Fructus *(zhǐ ké)*, and Citri reticulatae Pericarpium *(chén pí)* transform dampness by promoting the circulation of qi. Poria rubra *(chì fú líng)* and Jasper Powder *(bì yù sǎn)*, which includes Glycyrrhizae Radix *(gān cǎo)*, Talcum *(huá shí)*, and Indigo naturalis *(qīng dài)*, serve to conduct the lurking summerheat from the Triple Burner downward, and to clear heat and discharge dampness via the urine.

MODIFICATIONS: The basic formula can be modified as follows:

- For significant heat with insomnia and severe restlessness, add Gardeniae Fructus *(zhī zǐ)* and Coptidis Rhizoma *(huáng lián)*.
- For significant dampness with severe abdominal bloating, add Amomi Fructus rotundus *(bái dòu kòu)*, Tetrapanacis Medulla *(tōng cǎo)*, and Sojae Semen germinatum *(dà dòu juǎn)*.
- For jaundice, add Artemisiae scopariae Herba *(yīn chén)*, Curcumae Radix *(yù jīn)*, and Gardeniae Fructus *(zhī zǐ)*.
- For nausea and vomiting, add Eriobotryae Folium *(pí pá yè)*, and increase the dosage of Bambusae Caulis in taeniam *(zhú rú)* and Pinelliae Rhizoma preparatum *(zhì bàn xià)*.

DAMP-HEAT COMBINED WITH RETENTION OF FOOD IN THE STOMACH AND LARGE INTESTINE

Manifestations. There are two concurrent aspects to this pattern:

1. *Steaming-up of lurking summerheat and dampness and retention of food in the Stomach* with fever, burning sensation in the chest and abdomen, nausea, vomiting, and a yellow, greasy tongue coating.
2. *Constraint of lurking summerheat and dampness with retention of food in the Large Intestine impairing its transportive function* with stools that are not well-formed and abdominal bloating. The color and consistency of the stools is like a yellow and red jam, and there is an uncomfortable sensation around the anus following evacuation.

NOTE: The stools in this pattern could be sticky or hard to pass. Alternatively, the patient may not experience a sense of completion after the bowels are evacuated. These symptoms are due to the sticky and turbid nature of dampness.

Pathology. Constraint from damp-heat with retention of food in the Stomach and Large Intestine, leading to a breakdown of the transportive function of the Large Intestine and rebellious Stomach qi.

Treatment principles. Guide out the damp-heat and retained food with mild purging, clear the heat, and transform the dampness.

Formula:

UNRIPE BITTER ORANGE DECOCTION TO GUIDE OUT STAGNATION *(zhǐ shí dǎo zhì tāng)*

SOURCE: *Revised Popular Guide to Discussion of Cold Damage*

Aurantii Fructus immaturus *(zhǐ shí)* 6g

Rhei Radix et Rhizoma *(dà huáng)* 4.5g

Crataegi Fructus *(shān zhā)* 9g

Arecae Semen *(bīng láng)* 4.5g

Magnoliae officinalis Cortex *(hòu pò)* 4.5g

Coptidis Rhizoma *(huáng lián)* .1.8g

Massa medicata fermentata *(shén qū)* 9g

Forsythiae Fructus *(lián qiào)* 4.5g

Arnebiae Radix/Lithospermi Radix *(zǐ cǎo)* 9g

Akebiae Caulis *(mù tōng)* 2.4g

Glycyrrhizae Radix *(gān cǎo)* 1.5g

ANALYSIS OF FORMULA: In this pattern there is constraint of damp-heat as well as food retention in the Stomach and Large Intestine. The function of the yang organs will be normal if the movement and circulation of their qi is normal, in particular, the downward-directing of qi by the Stomach and Large Intestine. In this instance, use mild purging to remove the damp-heat and retained food in the Large Intestine.

Unripe Bitter Orange Decoction to Guide Out Stagnation *(zhǐ shí dǎo zhì tāng)* contains bitter herbs that direct the qi of the Stomach and Large Intestine downward, and acrid herbs that promote the circulation of qi.

Rhei Radix et Rhizoma *(dà huáng)*, Aurantii Fructus immaturus *(zhǐ shí)*, Magnoliae officinalis Cortex *(hòu pò)*, and Arecae Semen *(bīng láng)*, with their bitter taste, mildly purge the damp-heat and retained food from the Large Intestine, and promote the circulation of qi. Crataegi Fructus *(shān zhā)* and Massa medicata fermentata *(shén qū)* promote digestion and remove food stagnation from the Stomach. Coptidis Rhizoma *(huáng lián)*, Forsythiae Fructus *(lián qiào)*, Arnebiae Radix/Lithospermi Radix *(zǐ cǎo)*, and Glycyrrhizae Radix *(gān cǎo)* clear heat. Akebiae Caulis *(mù tōng)* discharges heat and dampness via the urine and enhances the actions of the other herbs in this formula.

Major Order the Qi Decoction *(dà chéng qì tāng)* should never be used for treating this pattern because there is no clumping of dry stool and heat in the Large Intestine. Its use will injure the Spleen yang.

Table 13.5	Constraint of Lurking Summerheat and Dampness in Stomach and Large Intestine vs. Severe Constipation with Dry Stools and Heat in Large Intestine	
Pattern	**Pathology**	**Signs and Symptoms***
Constraint of lurking summerheat and dampness in the Stomach and Large Intestine	Dampness becomes stronger during the yin times of day	Chest distention, fever worsens in the afternoon and evening, and greasy, yellow tongue coating
Severe constipation with dry stools and heat in the Large Intestine	Interior excess pattern of severe constipation with dry stools and heat in the Large Intestine	Fever that worsens between 3 and 7 P.M., dry and yellow tongue coating

*Common symptoms: temperature increases in the afternoon

ADMINISTRATION: The damp-heat and retained food in the Large Intestine is not easily removed through mild purging because dampness is characterized by stickiness and stagnation. Therefore, it is recommended that one prescribe frequent mild purging for this pattern until the damp-heat and retained food are eliminated. Consider the following three markers to help decide when to stop the mild purging; when two of the markers appear, it is time to stop the purging:

1. When the fever or hot sensation is gone.

2. When the stools become well-formed.
3. When the tongue coating becomes normal.

MODIFICATIONS: The basic formula can be modified as follows:

- If there is vomiting and nausea, add Pinelliae Rhizoma preparatum *(zhì bàn xià)* and Bambusae Caulis in taeniam *(zhú rú)*.
- If there is severe abdominal bloating, add Arecae Pericarpium *(dà fù pí)*.

Differentiation and Treatment of Lurking Summerheat in the Nutritive and Blood Levels

TRANSFER OF LURKING SUMMERHEAT FROM THE HEART AND NUTRITIVE LEVEL TO THE SMALL INTESTINE

Manifestations. There are three concurrent aspects to this pattern:

1. *Injury to the nutritive level yin by lurking summerheat* with fever that is mild in the daytime and severe at night, a dry mouth, but no desire to drink.

2. *Disturbance of the Heart spirit by lurking summerheat* with restlessness and insomnia.

3. *Transfer of lurking summerheat from the Heart to the Small Intestine* with scanty, dark-yellow urine that is hot and painful to excrete.

NOTE: Painful urination not only indicates that heat has transferred from the Heart to the Small Intestine, but also that the body is trying to discharge the heat via the urine. One should support this trend when choosing the treatment strategy, that is, by promoting the draining of heat through urination.

Pathology. Lurking summerheat is being transmitted from the Heart and nutritive level to the Small Intestine.

Treatment principles. Clear lurking summerheat from the Heart and cool the nutritive level, and drain heat from the Small Intestine through the urine.

Formula:

> GUIDE OUT THE RED AND CLEAR THE HEART DECOCTION
> *(dǎo chì qīng xīn tāng)*

> SOURCE: *Revised Popular Guide to Discussion of Cold Damage*

Rehmanniae Radix *(shēng dì huáng)* 18g
Poriae Sclerotium pararadicis *(fú shén)* 6g
Akebiae Caulis *(mù tōng)* 1.5g
Ophiopogonis Radix *(mài mén dōng)* 3g
Moutan Cortex *(mǔ dān pí)* 6g
Lophatheri Herba *(dàn zhú yè)* 4.5g
Nelumbinis Plumula *(lián zǐ xīn)* .... 30 pieces
Junci Medulla *(dēng xīn cǎo)* .... 28 pieces
Augment the Primal Powder *(yì yuán sǎn)*[14] 9g
Infantis Urina *(tóng biàn)*[15] .... 1 cup

ANALYSIS OF FORMULA: This formula is based on Guide Out the Red Powder *(dǎo chì sǎn)*[16] but also includes Ophiopogonis Radix *(mài mén dōng)*, Nelumbinis Plumula *(lián zǐ xīn)*, Moutan Cortex *(mǔ dān pí)*, Junci Medulla *(dēng xīn cǎo)*, Poriae Sclerotium pararadicis *(fú shén)*, and Infantis Urina *(tóng biàn)*. In this formula, Rehmanniae Radix *(shēng dì huáng)*, Ophiopogonis Radix *(mài mén dōng)*, and Moutan Cortex *(mǔ dān pí)* clear lurking summerheat from the Heart and cool the nutritive level. Poriae Sclerotium pararadicis *(fú shén)* and Nelumbinis Plumula *(lián zǐ xīn)* clear lurking summerheat from the Heart and calm the spirit. Akebiae Caulis *(mù tōng)*, Lophatheri Herba *(dàn zhú yè)*, Junci Medulla *(dēng xīn cǎo)*, Infantis Urina *(tóng biàn)*, and Augment the Primal Powder *(yì yuán sǎn)* conduct lurking summerheat in the Heart downward and discharge it via the urine.

MODIFICATION: For canker sores in the mouth or sores on the tongue, add Coptidis Rhizoma *(huáng lián)*.

VEILING OF THE PERICARDIUM BY PHLEGM-HEAT COMBINED WITH OBSTRUCTION OF THE COLLATERALS

Manifestations. There are three concurrent aspects to this pattern:

1. *Injury to yin by lurking summerheat* with fever that worsens at night.
2. *Lurking summerheat attacking the blood level leading to blood stasis and obstruction of the collaterals* with dry mouth but no desire to drink, and a deep-red tongue without coating, which looks dry but is moist to the touch, or a purple tongue with saliva.
3. *Production of phlegm from heat congealing fluids in the collaterals, leading to veiling of the Pericardium by phlegm-heat* with muddled consciousness or coma, and delirium.

NOTE: The attack on the blood level here only means obstruction of the channels, which leads to blood stasis. It does not refer to a blood level pattern.

Pathology. Phlegm-heat veiling the Pericardium with stasis of the blood in collaterals due to lurking summerheat.

Treatment principles. Clear heat and resolve phlegm in the nutritive and blood levels, open the orifices, and remove obstruction from the collaterals.

Formula:

> ### Rhinoceros and Rehmannia Drink to Clear the Collaterals
> *(xī dì qīng luò yǐn)*
>
> source: *Revised Popular Guide to Discussion of Cold Damage*
>
> Bubali Cornu *(shuǐ niú jiǎo)*[17] 30-120g
> Moutan Cortex *(mǔ dān pí)* 6g
> Forsythiae Fructus *(lián qiào)* 4.5g
> Bambusae Succus *(zhú lì)* . . . . .2 spoonfuls
> Rehmanniae Radix *(shēng dì huáng)* 24g
> Persicae Semen *(táo rén)* . . . . 9 pieces
> Paeoniae Radix rubra *(chì sháo)* 4.5g
> Imperatae Rhizoma *(bái máo gēn)* 30g
> Junci Medulla *(dēng xīn cǎo)* 1.5g
> Acori tatarinowii Rhizoma *(shí chāng pǔ)* . . . . .9g[18]
> Zingiberis Rhizomatis Succus *(jiāng zhī)* . . . . .2 drops

analysis of formula: This formula is based on Rhinoceros Horn and Rehmannia Decoction *(xī jiǎo dì huáng tāng)*,[19] which both cools and promotes movement of the blood. Among the herbs that are added, Persicae Semen *(táo rén)* and Imperatae Rhizoma *(bái máo gēn)* invigorate the blood and remove obstruction from the collaterals; Forsythiae Fructus *(lián qiào)* and Junci Medulla *(dēng xīn cǎo)* clear heat from the Pericardium; and Acori tatarinowii Rhizoma *(shí chāng pǔ)*, Bambusae Succus *(zhú lì)*, and Zingiberis Rhizomatis Succus *(jiāng zhī)* resolve phlegm and open the orifices.

modifications: For severe coma or delirium, add one-half pill of Calm the Palace Pill with Cattle Gallstone *(ān gōng niú huáng wán)*.[20]

Summary

Lurking summerheat pathogen causes an acute febrile disease. Summerheat with dampness attacks and then incubates in the body during the summer; a subsequent attack by a secondary external pathogen induces it to emerge during the autumn or winter. It then presents with signs and symptoms of interior summerheat and internal dampness, as well as exterior signs and symptoms.

The onset of this disease varies according to the constitution of the patient and the nature of the secondary pathogenic factor. If dampness is present or there is an attack of wind-cold, the onset of the disease will occur in the qi level. If lurking summerheat with dampness has transformed into dry-heat, or there is an attack of wind-heat, the onset of the disease will usually occur in the nutritive level. The treatment principles for this disorder are to eliminate exterior signs and symptoms, clear lurking summerheat, and transform the dampness inside the body, as summarized in Table 13.6.

Table 13.6	Differentiation and Treatment of Lurking Summerheat	
Patterns	**Treatment Principles**	**Formulas**
▶ INITIAL ONSET PATTERNS		
Protective/qi level patterns from attack of wind-cold that activates pre-existing lurking summerheat with dampness	Release the exterior with acrid, warm herbs, clear lurking summerheat with bitter, cold herbs, and transform dampness with bitter, warm herbs	Coptis and Mosla Drink (*huáng lián xiāng rú yǐn*)
Protective/nutritive level patterns from attack of wind-heat that activates pre-existing lurking summerheat with dampness and transforms into dry-heat, which injures nutritive level yin	Release the exterior with acrid, cool herbs, clear heat from the nutritive level, and enrich the yin	Augmented Honeysuckle and Forsythia Powder (*jiā wéi yín qiào sǎn*)
▶ QI LEVEL PATTERNS		
Lurking summerheat with dampness constrains Triple Burner, leading to obstruction of the qi mechanism	Clear lurking summerheat from the Triple Burner and transform dampness	Sweet Wormwood and Scutellaria Decoction to Clear the Gallbladder (*hāo qín qīng dǎn tāng*)
Damp-heat with retention of food constrains the Stomach and Large Intestine, leading to a breakdown of the transportive function of the Large Intestine and rebellious Stomach qi	Guide out damp-heat and retained food with mild purging, clear heat, and transform dampness	Unripe Bitter Orange Decoction to Guide Out Stagnation (*zhǐ shí dǎo zhì wán*)

Table 13.6, cont.		
▶ NUTRITIVE AND BLOOD LEVEL PATTERNS		
Lurking summerheat transmitted from Heart and nutritive level to Small Intestine	Clear lurking summerheat from the Heart, cool the nutritive level, drain heat from the Small Intestine via the urine	Guide out the Red and Clear the Heart Decoction (*dǎo chì qīng xīn tāng*)
Veiling of Pericardium by phlegm-heat associated with obstruction of the collaterals	Clear heat and resolve phlegm in the nutritive and blood levels, open the orifices, and remove obstruction in the collaterals	Rhinoceros and Rehmannia Drink to Clear the Collaterals (*xī dì qīng luò yǐn*)

Endnotes

1. Wang Ken-Tang, *Indispensable Tools for Pattern Treatment: Miscellaneous Disease Section (Zhèng zhì zhǔn shéng: zá bìng)*. Shanghai: Shanghai Science and Technology Publishing House, 1959: 20.

2. Wu Tang, *Systematic Differentiation of Warm Pathogen Diseases (Wēn bìng tiáo biàn)*. Beijing: People's Health Publishing House, 1963: 38.

3. Ibid.

4. The conventional idea that the dry-heat is the result of a transformation from summerheat with dampness is often hard to confirm in the clinic. In my own experience, the only real clue is the history. That is, these patients have a history of contracting summerheat with dampness the previous summer.

5. Yu Gen-Chu, *Revised Popular Guide to the Discussion of Cold Damage (Chóng dìng tōng sú shāng hán lùn)*. Hangzhou: New Medicine Press, 1956: 256. He Lian-Chen's commentary is included in all modern editions of this book.

6. Ibid.

7. Teaching and Research Section of Warm Pathogen Diseases, Chengdu College of Traditional Chinese Medicine, *Self-Study Textbook for Chinese Medicine: Warm Pathogen Diseases (Zhōng yī zì xué jiào cái: Wēn bìng xué)*. Chengdu: Chengdu College of Traditional Chinese Medicine, 1985: 2.

8. This formula has a variety of names. It was called Mosla Powder (*xiāng rú sǎn*) in the source text, Coptis and Mosla Drink (*huáng lián xiāng rú yǐn*) in the *Teachings of [Zhu] Dan-Xi (Dān-Xī xīn fǎ)*, and Four-Substance Decoction with Mosla (*sì wèi xiāng rú yǐn*) in *Medical Formulas Collected and Analyzed (Yī fāng jí jiě)*.

9. The dosages come from Wang Ji, *Medical Formulas Collected and Analyzed (Yī fāng jí jiě)*, Shanghai: Shanghai Science and Technology Publishing House, 1959: 171.

10. Wu Tang, *Systematic Differentiation of Warm Pathogen Diseases*, 39.

11. See Chapter 7.

12. Ibid.

13. It was first recorded in Liu Wan-Su, *Formulas from the Discussion Illuminating the Yellow Emperor's Basic Questions (Huáng Dì sù wèn xuán míng lùn fāng)*. This book is reproduced in Shanghai Publishing House of Ancient Literature, ed., *Collected Medical Books from the Four Bibliographic Divisions (Sì kù yī xué cóng shū)*. Shanghai: Shanghai Ancient Literature Publishing House, 1991: 814. It contains Talcum *(huá shí)* (18g), Glycyrrhizae Radix *(gān cǎo)* (3g), and Indigo naturalis *(qīng dài)*.

14. Ibid. It contains Talcum *(huá shí)* (18g) and Glycyrrhizae Radix *(gān cǎo)* (3g).

15. This is the urine of children. It is salty and cool and enters the Lung, Liver, and Kidney channels. It enriches yin, drains fire, stops bleeding, and dispels blood stasis. It is used for such problems as fever from yin deficiency, cough or vomiting with blood, and dizziness from blood stasis in the Womb after childbirth.

16. This was first recorded in Qian Yi, *Craft of Medicines and Patterns for Children (Xiǎo ér yào zhèng zhēn jué)*. Shenyang: Liaoning Science and Technology Publishing House, 1997: 14. It contains Rehmanniae Radix *(shēng dì huáng)*, Akebiae Caulis *(mù tōng)*, Lophatheri Herba *(dàn zhú yè)*, and Glycyrrhizae Radix *(gān cǎo)*.

17. According to *Revised Popular Guide to Discussion of Cold Damage*, four spoonfuls of ground Rhinocerotis Cornu *(xī jiǎo)* should be used in this formula. Since Rhinocerotis Cornu *(xī jiǎo)* is from an endangered species, Bubali Cornu *(shuǐ niú jiǎo)* is a good substitute, with a dosage of 30–120g.

18. According to the source text, fresh Acori tatarinowii Rhizomatis Succus *(shí chāng pú zhī)* should be used. Because this is very hard to obtain in most places, 9g of Acori tatarinowii Rhizoma *(shí chāng pǔ)* is a good substitute.

19. See Chapter 8.

20. See Chapter 7.

Bibliography

Anonymous. *Yellow Emperor's Inner Classic: Basic Questions (Huáng Dì nèi jīng: Sù wèn)* 黃帝內經素問. Beijing: People's Health Publishing House, 1963. (Primarily compiled from Eastern Han sources.)

Anonymous. *Yellow Emperor's Inner Classic: Divine Pivot (Huáng Dì nèi jīng: Líng shū)* 黃帝內經靈樞. Beijing: People's Health Publishing House, 1963. (Primarily compiled from Eastern Han sources.)

Beijing College of Traditional Chinese Medicine. *Beijing College of Traditional Medicine Collection of First Class Graduate Papers (Běijīng zhōng yī xué yuàn shōu jiè yán jiū shēng lùn wén huì biān)* 北京中醫學院首屆研究生論文彙編. Beijing: Beijing College of Traditional Chinese Medicine, 1981.

Beijing College of Traditional Chinese Medicine. *Chinese Medical History* (4th ed.) *(Zhōng guó yī xué shǐ)* 中國醫學史. Shanghai: Shanghai Science and Technology Publishing House, 1978.

Beijing Traditional Chinese Hospital. *Compilation of Experiences from Famous Veteran Traditional Chinese Doctors,* vol. 2 *(Míng lǎo zhōng yī jīng yàn quán biān)* 名老中醫經驗全編下冊. Beijing: Beijing Publishing House, 1994.

Bensky D, Barolet R. *Chinese Herbal Medicine: Formulas and Strategies.* Seattle: Eastland Press, 1990.

Cao Bing-Zhang, ed. *Compendium of Medicine in China (Zhōng guó yī xué dà chéng)* 中國醫學大成. Shanghai: Shanghai Science and Technology Publishing House, 1990.

Cao Bing-Zhang. *Guide to Distinguishing Tongues (Biàn shé zhǐ nán)* 辨舌指南. Nanjing: Jiangsu People's Publishing House, 1962.

Cao Jia-Da. *Records of Experiences with Classic Formulas (Jīng fāng shí yàn lù)* 經方實驗錄. Shanghai: Shanghai Science and Technology Publishing House, 1979.

Chao Yuan-Fang. *Discussion of the Origins of Symptoms of Disease (Zhū bìng yuán hòu lùn)* 諸病原侯論. Beijing: People's Health Publishing House, 1992. (Originally published in 610.)

Chen Guang-Song. *Annotation and Correction of the Discussion of Warm-Heat Pathogen Disorders (Wēn rè lùn jiān zhèng)* 溫熱論筬正. Reproduced in Qiu Qing-Yuan, ed. *Collection of Rare Medical Books, vol. 2 (Zhēn běn yī shū jí chéng)* 珍本醫書集成. Bejing: Chinese Medicine and Pharmacology Publishing House, 1996.

Chen Ming, Zhang Yin-Sheng, ed. *Selected Case Studies from Famous Doctors who Specialize in Cold Damage (Shāng hán míng yī yàn àn jīng xuǎn)* 傷寒名醫驗案精選. Beijing: Learning Garden Publishing House, 1998.

Chen Nian-Zu. *Simple Annotation of the Discussion of Cold Damage (Shāng hán lùn qiǎn zhǔ)* 傷寒論淺注. Fuzhou: Fujian Science and Technology Publishing House, 1987. (Originally published in 1803.)

Chen Ping-Bo. *Collected Guides for Warm-Heat Pathogen Diseases (Wēn rè bìng zhǐ nán jí)* 溫熱病指南集. Reproduced in Cao Bing-Zhang, ed. *Compendium of Medicine in China (Zhōng guó yī xué dà chéng)* 中國醫學大成. Shanghai: Shanghai Science and Technology Publishing House, 1990. (Originally published in 1809.)

Chen Shi-Gong. *Orthodox Lineage of External Medicine (Wài kē zhèng zōng)* 外科正宗. Tianjin: Tianjin Science and Technology Publishing House, 1999. (Originally published in 1617.)

Chen Shi-Wen, Chen Cheng, Pei Zong-Yuan, eds. *Imperial Grace Formulary of the Tai Ping Era (Tài ping huì mín hé jì jú fāng)* 太平惠民和劑局方. Beijing: People's Health Publishing House, 1959. (Originally published in 1078.)

Chen Yan. *Discussion of Illnesses, Patterns, and Formulas Related to the Unification of the Three Etiologies (Sān yīn jí yī bìng zhèng fāng lùn)* 三因極一病證方論. Beijing: People's Health Publishing House, 1957. (Originally published in 1174.)

Chen Ze-Lin, Chen Mei-Fang. *Research on Tongue Diagnosis (Shé zhěn yán jiù)* 舌診研究. Shanghai: Shanghai Science and Technology Publishing House, 1982.

Chen Zi-Ming. *Great Collection of Fine Formulas for Women (Fù rén liáng fāng dà quán)* 婦人良方大全. Shanghai: Great Achievement Press, 1934. (Originally published in 1237.)

Cheng Guo-Peng. *Medical Revelations (Yī xué xīn wù)* 醫學心悟. Tianjin: Tianjin Science and Technology Publishing House, 1999. (Originally published in 1732.)

Cheng Wu-Ji. *Annotation and Explanation of the Discussion of Cold Damage (Zhù jiě shāng hán lùn)* 注解傷寒論. Beijing: People's Health Publishing House, 1963. (Originally published in 1144.)

Chengdu College of Traditional Chinese Medicine. *Selected Case Studies from Veteran Doctors,* vol. 1 *(Lǎo zhōng yī yī àn xuǎn)* 老中醫醫案選. Chengdu: Chengdu College of Traditional Chinese Medicine, 1978.

Chengdu College of Traditional Chinese Medicine. *Selected Case Studies from Veteran Traditional Chinese Doctors,* vol. 2 *(Lǎo zhōng yī yī àn xuǎn)* 老中醫醫案選. Chengdu: Chengdu College of Traditional Chinese Medicine, 1980.

Chinese Academy of Traditional Chinese Medicine. *Collected Medical Experience of Pu Fu-Zhou (Pú Fǔ-Zhōu yī liǎo jīng yàn jí)* 蒲輔周醫療經驗集. Beijing: People's Health Publishing House, 1976.

Chinese National Administrative Bureau for Traditional Chinese Medicine Editorial Panel for Chinese Materia Medica. *Chinese Materia Medica (Zhōng huá běn cǎo)* 中華本草. Shanghai: Shanghai Science and Technology Publishing House, 1996.

Chongqing Traditional Chinese Medicine Research Institute. *Traditional Chinese Medicine and Acute Conditions Report,* vol. 6 *(Zhōng yī jí zhèng tōng xùn)* 中醫急症通訊. Chongqing: Chongqing Traditional Chinese Medicine Research Institute, 1985.

Dai Tian-Zhang. *Discussion of Widespread Warm Epidemics (Guǎng wēn yì lùn)* 廣溫議論. Reproduced in Cao Bing-Zhang, ed. *Compendium of Medicine in China (Zhōng guó yī xué dà chéng)* 中國醫學大成. Shanghai: Shanghai Science and Technology Publishing House, 1990. (Originally published in 1774.)

Ding Gan-Ren. *Outline of the Presentation and Treatment of Throat Granular Disorder (Hóu shā zhèng zhì gài yào)* 喉痧政治概要. Reproduced in Lu Zhen et al., eds. *Collected Rare Recent Books on Chinese Medicine: Warm Pathogen Disease Section (Jīn dài zhōng yī zhēn běn jí: wēn bìng fèn cè)* 今代中醫珍本集溫病分冊. Hangzhou: Zhejiang Science and Technology Publishing House, 1987.

Dong Jian-Hua et al., eds. *Selected Case Studies from Famous Modern Chinese Doctors (Zhōng guó xiàn dài míng zhōng yī yī àn jīng huá).* 中國現代名醫中醫醫案精華. Beijing: Beijing Publishing House, 1990.

Dong Jian-Hua. "Features, Range, and Clinical Differentiation for Warm Pathogen Disease" *(Wēn bìng tè diǎn fàn wéi jí qí lín chuáng biàn zhèng)* 溫病特點範圍及麒臨床辨證. In Fang Yao-Zhong, Xu Jia-Song, eds. *Collection of Lectures on Warm Pathogen Diseases (Wēn bìng huì jiǎng)* 溫病匯講. Beijing: People's Health Publishing House, 1986.

Du Qing-Bi. *Ao's Golden Mirror Collection (Aó shì jīn jìng lù)* 敖氏金鏡錄. (Originally published in 1341.) Reproduced in Great Achievement Press, ed. *Xue's Case Studies (Xuē shì yī ān)* 薛氏醫案. Shanghai: Great Achievement Press, 1926.

Fang Yao-Zhong, Xu Jia-Song, eds. *Collection of Lectures on Warm Pathogen Disease (Wēn bìng huì jiǎng)* 溫病匯講. Beijing: People's Health Publishing House, 1986.

Gansu People's Publishing House. *A Selection of Chinese Case Studies and Medical Discussions (Zhōng yī yī àn yī huà jí jǐn)* 中醫醫案醫話集錦. Lanzhou: Gansu People's Publishing House, 1980.

Gong Ting-Xian. *Restoration of Health from the Myriad Diseases (Wàn bìng huí chūn)* 萬病回春. Beijing: People's Health Publishing House, 1984. (Originally published in 1587.)

Guangzhou College of Traditional Chinese Medicine. *Formulas (Fāng jì xué)* 方劑學. Shanghai: Shanghai Science and Technology Publishing House, 1979.

Guo Wei-Feng, Zhou Zhong-Ying. Identification and significance of qi level heat being transmitted to the nutritive level in exogenous febrile diseases with severe symptoms *(Wài gǎn rè bìng zhòng zhèng qì rè chuán yíng de biàn shì jí qí yì)* 外感熱並重正氣熱傳營的辨試及其意義. *Journal of Traditional Chinese Medicine* 1999(8):457

Guo Yong. *Supplement to What has been Lost from [Discussion of] Cold Damage (Shāng hán bǔ wáng lùn)* 傷寒補亡論. (Originally published in 1181.) Reproduced in Institute of Chinese Medical Literature of Shanghai College of Traditional Chinese Medicine, ed., *Historical Collection of Rare Chinese Medical Books (Lì dài zhōng yī zhēn běn jí chéng)* 歷代中醫珍本集成. Shanghai: Joint Publishing Company, 1990.

Guo Zi-Guang. Informal discussion on the concept of toxin *(Màn tán dú de gài niàn)* 漫談毒的概念. *Zhejiang Journal of Traditional Chinese Medicine* 1985(5):227

Hanson M. "Inventing a Tradition in Chinese Medicine." Ph.D. dissertation, University of Pennyslvania, 1997.

He Lian-Chen. *Revised and Expanded Discussion of Warm-Heat Pathogen Diseases (Chóng dìng guǎng wēn rè lùn)* 重訂廣溫熱論. Beijing: People's Health Publishing House, 1960. (Originally published in 1907.)

He Lian-Chen. *Revised Classified Case Studies from Nationally Famous Doctors (Chóng dìng quán guó míng yī yàn àn lèi biān)* 重訂全國名醫驗案類編. Shanghai: Shanghai Science and Technology Press, 1959.

Hu Ding-Bang. "Initial Discussion about the Onset and Progression Principles of Warm Pathogen Diseases" *(Shì lùn wēn rè bìng fā bìng jí chuán biàn guī lù)* 試論溫熱並發病及傳變規律. In Beijing College of Traditional Chinese Medicine. *Selected Papers for Thirty Year Anniversary of Foundation of Beijing College of Traditional Chinese Medicine*

(Běijīng zhōng yī xué yuàn sān shí nián lùn wén xuǎn) 北京中醫學院三十年論文選. Beijing: Chinese Ancient Medical Literature Publishing House, 1986.

Huang Gong-Xiu. *Seeking Accuracy in the Materia Medica (Běn cǎo qiú zhēn)* 本草求真. Shanghai: Shanghai Science and Technology Publishing House, 1959. (Originally published in 1769.)

Huang Xing-Yuan, Tian Ling-Qun. "General Description of Research and Study on Protective, Qi, Ying, and Blood Theory in Warm Pathogen Diseases" *(Wēn bìng wèi qì yíng xuè yán jiù gài kuàng)* 溫病衛氣營學研究概況. In Fang Yao-Zhong, Xu Jia-Song, eds. *Collection of Lectures on Warm Pathogen Diseases (Wēn bìng huì jiǎng)* 溫病匯講. Beijing: People's Health Publishing House, 1986.

Hubei College of Traditional Chinese Medicine. *Explanation of the Essentials from the Golden Cabinet (Jīn guì yào lüè shì yì)* 金櫃要略釋義. Wuhan: Hunan People's Publishing House, 1963.

Hubei College of Traditional Chinese Medicine. *Selected Readings from the Discussion of Cold Damage* (4th ed.) *(Shāng hán lùn xuǎn dú)* 傷寒論選讀. Shanghai: Shanghai Science and Technology Publishing House, 1980.

Institute of Chinese Medical Literature of the Shanghai College of Traditional Chinese Medicine. *Historical Collection of Rare Chinese Medical Books (Lì dài zhōng yī zhēn běn jí chéng)* 歷代中醫珍本集成. Shanghai: Shanghai Joint Publishing Company, 1990.

Jiang Bao-Su, *Thirteen Chapter Precis of Medicine (Yī lüè shí sān piān)* 醫略十三篇. In Qiu Qing-Yuan, ed. *Collection of Rare Chinese Medical Books,* vol. 2 *(Zhēn běn yī shū jí chéng)* 珍本醫書集成. Bejing: Chinese Medicine and Pharmacology Publishing House, 1996.

Jiang Chun-Hua. Ye tian-shi's theory and treatment for warm pathogen disease and internal disease *(Yè Tiān-Shì de wēn bìng hé zá bìng de lǐ lùn yǔ zhì liáo)* 葉天士的溫病和雜病的理論與治療. *New Medicine Journal* 1978(8):8

Ke Qin. *Collected Writings on Renewal of the Discussion of Cold Damage (Shāng hán lái sū jí)* 傷寒來蘇集. Shanghai: Shanghai Science and Technology Publishing House, 1959. (Originally published in the early 18th century.)

Lei Feng. *Discussion of Seasonal Diseases (Shí bìng lùn)* 時病論. Beijing: People's Health Publishing House, 1956. (Originally published in 1882.)

Li An-Qing. *Outline of Warm-Heat Pathogen Diseases (Wēn rè bìng gāng yào)* 溫熱病綱要. Zhengzhou: Henan People's Publishing House, 1956.

Li Chan. *Introduction to Medicine (Yī xué rù mén)* 醫學入門. Beijing: Chinese Traditional Medicine Publishing House, 1994. (Originally published in 1575.)

Li Gao. *Clarifying Doubts about Damage from Internal and External Causes (Nèi wài shāng biàn huò lùn)* 內外傷辨惑論. Nanjing: Jiangsu Science and Technology Publishing House, 1982. (Originally published in 1247.)

Li Gao. *Discussion of the Spleen and Stomach (Pí wèi lùn)* 脾胃論. Beijing: People's Health Publishing House, 1976. (Originally published in the 13th century.)

Li Shi-Zhen. *Grand Materia Medica (Běn cǎo gang mù)* 本草綱目. Beijing: People's Health Publishing House, 1982. (Originally published in 1590.)

Lin Zhi-Nan. "Looking at the Application of the Method of Dispersing and Draining Heat from Constraint in Treating Warm Pathogen Diseases from [Analyzing] Ascending and Descending Powder" *(Cóng shēng jiàng sǎn kàn xuān xiè yù rè fǎ zài wēn bìng zhōng de yùn yòng)* 從升降散看宣泄鬱熱法在溫病中的運用. In *Collection of First-Level Graduate Papers at Beijing College of Traditional Chinese Medicine (Běijīng zhōng yī xué yuàn shǒu jiè yán jiū shēng lùn wén huì biān)* 北京中醫學院首屆研究生論文彙編. Beijing: Beijing College of Traditional Chinese Medicine, 1981.

Ling Yi-Kui et al. *Chinese Materia Medica (Zhōng yào xué)* 中藥學. Shanghai: Shanghai Science and Technology Publishing House, 1984.

Liu Bao-Yi. *Encountering the Sources of Warm-Heat Pathogen Diseases (Wēn rè féng yuán)* 溫熱逢原. Beijing: People's Health Publishing House, 1959. (Originally published during the late Qing dynasty.)

Liu Ji-Ren. *New Treatise on Lurking Pathogens (Fú xié xīn shū)* 伏邪新書. (Originally published during the Qing dynasty.) In Cao Bing-Zhang, ed. *Compendium of Medicine in China (Zhōng guó yī xué dà chéng)* 中國醫學大成. Shanghai: Shanghai Science and Technology Publishing House, 1990.

Liu Wan-Su. *Collection of Writings on the Mechanism of Disease, Suitability of Qi, and the Safeguarding of Life as Discussed in Basic Questions (Sù wèn bìng jī qì yí bǎo míng jí)* 素問病機宜保名集. Shanghai: Shanghai Ancient Literature Publishing House, 1991. (Originally published in 1186.)

Liu Wan-Su. *Direct Investigation of Cold Damage (Shāng hán zhí gé)* 傷寒直格. Shanghai: Shanghai Ancient Literature Publishing House, 1991. (Originally published in the 12th century.)

Liu Wan-Su. *Formulas from the Discussion Illuminating the Yellow Emperor's Basic Questions (Huáng Dì sù wèn xuán míng lùn fāng)* 黃帝素問宣明論方. Shanghai: Shanghai Ancient Literature Publishing House, 1991. (Originally published in 1172.)

Liu Wan-Su. *Mysterious Mechanism at the Origin of Pathology in Basic Questions (Sù wèn xuān jí yuán bìng shì)* 素問玄機原病式. Beijing: People's Health Publishing House, 1983. (Originally published in 1152.)

Lou Jie. *Guide to Warm Pathogen Diseases (Wēn bìng zhǐ nán)* 溫病指南. This book was edited by Li An-Qing who changed its name to *Outline of Warm-Heat Pathogen Diseases (Wēn
rè bìng gāng yào)* 溫熱病綱要. Zhengzhou: Henan People's Publishing House, 1956.

Lu Mao-Xiu. *Medical Texts from the Shibu Studio (Shì bǔ zhāi yī shū)* 世補齋醫書. (Originally
published in 1884.) Reproduced in Hu Guo-Chen, ed. *Compendium of Complete Books
from Famous Ming-Qing Physicians (Míng-Qīng míng yī quán shū dà chéng)* 明清名醫全
書大成. Beijing: Traditional Chinese Medicine Publishing House, 1999.

Lu Ting-Zhen. *Systematic Differentiation of the Six Etiologies (Liù yīn tiáo biàn)* 六因條
辨. (Originally published in 1868.) Reproduced in Qiu Qing-Yuan, ed. *Collection of
Rare Chinese Medical Books (Zhēn běn yī shū jí chéng)* 珍本醫書集成. Bejing: Chinese
Medicine and Pharmacology Publishing House, 1996.

Lu Zhen et al., eds. *Collected Rare Recent Books on Chinese Medicine: Warm Pathogen Disease
Section (Jīn dài zhōng yī zhēn běn jí: wēn bìng fèn cè)* 今代中醫珍本集溫病分冊.
Hangzhou: Zhejiang Science and Technology Publishing House, 1987.

Ma You-Du. *New Explanation of Medical Formulas (Yī fāng xīn jiě)* 醫方新解. Shanghai:
Shanghai Science and Technology Publishing House, 1980.

Meng Shu-Jiang et al. *Teaching Reference Books for Traditional Chinese Medical Colleges: Warm
Pathogen Diseases (Gāo děng zhōng yī yuàn xiào jiào xué cān kǎo shū: wēn bìng xué)* 高等
中醫院校教學參考書溫病學. Beijing: People's Health Publishing House, 1989.

Meng Shu-Jiang et al. *Warm Pathogen Diseases (Wēn bìng xué)* 溫病學. Shanghai: Shanghai
Science and Technology Publishing House, 1985.

Meng Shu-Jiang. "Discussion of Several Issues Relating to Warm Pathogen Diseases" *(Duì wēn
bìng xué zhōng yǒu guān wèn tí de tǎo lùn)* 對溫病學中有關問題的討論. In Fang
Yao-Zhong, Xu Jia-Song, ed. *Collection of Lectures on Warm Pathogen Diseases (Wēn bìng
huì jiǎng)* 溫病匯講. Beijing: People's Health Publishing House, 1986.

Meng Yong-Li, Shen Guo-Nan, Li Xiao-Lu. *Modern Research and Clinical Application of the
Discussion of Cold Damage (Shāng hán lùn xiàn dài yán jiù yǔ lín chuáng yìng yòng)* 傷寒
論現代研究與臨床應用. Beijing: Learning Garden Publishing House, 1998.

Outline of Chinese Medical Literature Editorial Panel. *Outline of Chinese Medical Literature
(Zhōng guó yī jí tí yào)* 中國醫籍提要. Changchun: Jilin Science and Technology
Publishing House, 1984.

Pang An-Shi. *General Discussion of Discussion of Cold Damage (Shāng hán zǒng bìng lùn)* 傷
寒總病論. (Originally published in 1100.) Reproduced in Institute of Chinese Medical
Literature of the Shanghai College of Traditional Chinese Medicine, ed. *Historical Collection
of Rare Chinese Medical Books (Lì dài zhōng yī zhēn běn jí chéng)* 歷代中醫珍本集成.
Shanghai: Joint Publishing Company, 1990.

Peng Jian-Zhong, Yang Lian-Zhu. *Selected Case Studies from Zhao Shao-Qin (Zhào Shào-Qín lín zhèng yàn àn jīng xuǎn)* 趙紹琴臨證驗案精選. Beijing: Learning Garden Publishing House, 1996.

Qian Yi. *Craft of Medicinal Treatment for Childhood Disease Patterns (Xiǎo ér yào zhèng zhēn jú)* 小兒藥證真訣. (Originally published in 1119.) Shenyang: Liaoning Science and Technology Publishing House, 1997.

Qin Bo-Wei. *Medical Lecture Notes of [Qin] Qian-Zhai (Qiān-Zhāi yī xué jiǎng gǎo)* 謙齋醫學講稿. Shanghai: Shanghai Science and Technology Publishing House, 1964.

Qin Yue-Ren [traditional attribution]. *Classic of Difficulties (Nán jīng)* 難經. (Probably complied during the Eastern Han.) Beijing: People's Health Publishing House, 1979.

Ren Ying-Qiu. *Doctrines of the Various Schools of Chinese Medicine* (4th ed.) *(Zhōng yī gè jiā xué shuō)* 中醫各家學說. Shanghai: Shanghai Science and Technology Publishing House, 1980.

Research and Study Section on Basic Theory of the Beijing College of Traditional Chinese Medicine. *Tongue Diagnosis in Chinese Medicine (Zhōng yī shé zhěn)* 中醫舌診. Beijing: People's Health Publishing House, 1980.

Shanghai College of Traditional Chinese Medicine. *Selected Essays from Traditional Chinese Medicine Teacher's Training Seminar (Zhōng yī shī xùn bān lùn wén xuǎn)* 中醫師訓班論文選. Shanghai: Shanghai College of Traditional Chinese Medicine, 1980.

Shen Jin-Ao. *Wondrous Lantern for Peering into the Origin and Development of Miscellaneous Diseases (Zá bìng yuán liú xī zhú)* 雜病源流犀燭. Beijing: Traditional Chinese Medicine and Pharmacology Publishing House, 1994. (Originally published in 1773.)

Shen Qing-Fa. "On the Venting Method in Warm Pathogen Diseases" *(Lùn wēn bìng de tòu fǎ)* 論溫病的透法. In *Selected Essays from Traditional Chinese Medicine Teacher's Training Seminar (Zhōng yī shī xùn bān lùn wén xuǎn)* 中醫師訓班論文選. Shanghai: Shanghai College of Traditional Chinese Medicine, 1980.

Shen Zhong-Li et al., eds. *Collected Clinical Writings of Ding Gan-Ren (Dīng Gān-Rén lín zhèng yī jí)* 丁甘仁臨證一集. Shanghai University of Traditional Chinese Medicine Publishing House, 2000.

Shi Shou-Tang. *Bases of Medicine (Yī yuán)* 醫原. Nanjing: Jiangsu Science and Technology Publishing House, 1983. (Originally published in 1862.)

Shi Yi-Ren. *Cold Damage and Warm Pathogen Diseases in Chinese Medicine (Zhōng yī shāng hán yǔ wēn bìng)* 中醫傷寒與溫病. Shanghai: Shanghai Qian Qin Tang Press, 1956.

Shi Yi-Ren. *Complete Book of Warm Pathogen Diseases (Wēn bìng quán shū)* 溫病全書. Shanghai: The Masses Press, 1936.

Sichuan Cooperative Panel on Research and Study of Protective, Qi, Ying, and Blood in Warm Pathogen Diseases, ed. *Collection of Literature About Research and Study of Protective, Qi, Ying, and Blood Theory in Warm Pathogen Diseases (Zhōng yī wēn bìng wèi qì yíng xuè lǐ lùn yán jiù zī liào huì biān)* 中醫溫病衛氣營血理論研究資料彙編. Chengdu: Sichuan Cooperative Panel on Research and Study of Protective, Qi, Ying, and Blood in Warm Pathogen Diseases, 1980.

Song Lu-Bing. "Brief Discussion of Two Types of Warm Pathogen Diseases and Their Pathologies and Treatment Principles" *(Wēn bìng de liǎng dà lèi bié jí qí bìng jī zhì zé jiǎn lùn)* 溫病的兩大類別及期病機治則簡論. In *Collection of Literature About Research and Study of Protective, Qi, Ying, and Blood Theory in Warm Pathogen Diseases (Zhōng yī wēn bìng wèi qì yíng xuè lǐ lùn yán jiù zī liào huì biān)* 中醫溫病衛氣營血理論研究資料彙編. Sichuan: Sichuan Cooperative Panel on Research and Study of Protective, Qi, Ying, and Blood [Levels] in Warm Pathogen Diseases, 1980.

Song Nai-Guang et al. *Warm Pathogen Diseases (Wēn bìng xue)* 溫病學. Beijing: Learning Garden Publishing House, 1995.

Song Zhao-Qi. *Distinguishing [Aspects] of Southern Diseases (Nán bìng bié jiàn).* 南病別鑒. Shanghai: Shanghai Health Publishing House, 1958. (Originally published in 1878.)

Sun Si-Miao. *Important Formulas Worth a Thousand Gold Pieces for Any Emergency (Bèi jí qiān jīn yào fāng)* 備急千金要方. Beijing: People's Health Publishing House, 1982. (Originally published in the 7th century.)

Tang Da-Lie. *Collection of Papers of Physicians from Wu (Wú yi huì jiǎng)* 吳醫匯講. Shanghai: Shanghai Science and Technology Publishing House, 1983. (Originally published from 1792-1801.)

Tao Hong-Jing. *Collection of Commentaries on the Classic of Materia Medica (Běn cǎo jīng jí zhù)* 本草經集注. Beijing: People's Health Publishing House, 1994. (Originally published in 494.)

Tao Hua. *Six Texts on Cold Damage (Shāng hán liù shū)* 傷寒論六書. Beijing: People's Health Publishing House, 1957. (Originally published in 1445.)

Teaching and Research Section on *Discussion of Cold Damage* of the Nanjing College of Traditional Chinese Medicine. *Translation and Explanation of Discussion of Cold Damage (Shāng hán lùn yì shì)* 傷寒論譯釋. Shanghai: Shanghai Science and Technology Publishing House, 1980.

Teaching and Research Section on Formulas of the Shanghai College of Traditional Chinese Medicine. *Clinical Handbook of Chinese Medicine (Zhōng yào lín chuáng shǒu cè)* 中藥臨床手冊. Shanghai: Shanghai People's Publishing House, 1977.

Teaching and Research Section on Warm Pathogen Diseases of the Chengdu College of Traditional Chinese Medicine. *Self-Study Book for Chinese Medicine: Warm Pathogen Diseases (Zhōng yī zì xué jiào cài: wēn bìng xué)* 中醫自學教材溫病學. Chengdu: Chengdu College of Traditional Chinese Medicine, 1985.

491

Teaching Hospital of the Chengdu College of Tradtional Chinese Medicine. *Selected Data 2 (Zī liǎo xuǎn biān 2)* 資料選編 2. Chengdu: Teaching Hospital of the Chengdu College of Traditional Chinese Medicine, 1979.

Wan You-Sheng. Establish differentiation system for febrile disease by uniting the theory of warm pathogen diseases and the theory of cold damage under eight parameters *(Bā gāng tǒng yī hán wēn zhèng zhì, jiàn lì rè bìng xué kē tǐ xì)* 八綱統一寒溫證治建立熱病學科體系. *Journal of Beijing College of Traditional Chinese Medicine,* 1983(3): 2–5

Wang Ang. *Medical Formulas Collected and Analyzed (Yī fāng jí jiě)* 醫方集解. Shanghai: Shanghai Science and Technology Publishing House, 1959. (Originally published in 1682.)

Wang Ken-Tang. *Indispensable Tools for Pattern Treatments (Zhèng zhì zhǔn shéng)* 證治准繩. Shanghai: Shanghai Science and Technology Publishing House, 1959. (Originally published in 1602.)

Wang Lu. *Discourse on Tracing Back to the Medical Classics (Yī jīng sù huí jí)* 醫經溯迴集. Nanjing: Jiangsu Science and Technology Press, 1984. (Originally published in 1368.)

Wang Qi et al. *Modern Translation and Explanation of Basic Questions (Sū wèn jīn shì)* 素問今釋. Guiyang: Guizhou People's Publishing House, 1981.

Wang Shi-Xiong. *Case Studies from Wang Meng-Ying (Wáng Mèng-Yīng yī àn)* 王孟英醫案. Beijing: Traditional Chinese Medicine and Pharmacology Publishing House, 1999.

Wang Shi-Xiong. *Warp and Woof of Warm-Heat Pathogen Diseases (Wēn rè jīng wěi)* 溫熱經緯. (Originally published in 1852.) Reproduced in Lu Zhen et al., eds. *Collected Rare Recent Books on Chinese Medicine: Warm Pathogen Disease Section (Jīn dài zhōng yī zhēn běn jí: wēn bìng fèn cè)* 今代中醫珍本集溫病分冊. Hangzhou: Zhejiang Science and Technology Publishing House, 1987.

Wang Tao. *Arcane Essentials from the Imperial Library (Wài tái mì yào)* 外台秘要. Shanghai: Shanghai Ancient Literature Publishing House, 1991. (Originally published in 752.)

Wu Qian. *Golden Mirror of the Medical Tradition (Yī zōng jīn jiàn)* 醫宗金鑑. Beijing: People's Health Publishing House, 1973. (Originally published in 1742.)

Wu Tang. *Systematic Differentiation of Warm Pathogen Diseases (Wēn bìng tiáo biàn)* 溫病條辨. Beijing: People's Health Publishing House, 1963. (Originally published in 1798.)

Wu You-Xing. *Discussion of Warm Epidemics (Wēn yì lùn)* 溫疫論. Changchun: Liaoning Science and Technology Publishing House, 1997. (Originally published in 1642.)

Wu Zhen. *Thorough Understanding of Cold Damage (Shāng hán zhǐ zhǎng)* 傷寒指掌. Shanghai: Shanghai Science and Technology Publishing House, 1959. (Originally published in 1796.)

Xia Yun. *Initial Discussion on Putrefying Throat Granular Disorder (Yì hóu shā qiǎn lùn)* 疫喉痧淺論. Reproduced in Cao Bing-Zhang, ed. *Compendium of Medicine in China (Zhōng guó yī xué dà chéng)* 中國醫學大成. Shanghai: Shanghai Science and Technology Publishing House, 1990.

Xiao De-Xin. "My Views on Uniting the Differentiation Systems of Cold [Damage] and Warm [Diseases]" *(Tǒng yī hán wēn biàn zhèng tǐ xì zhī wǒ jiàn)* 統一寒溫辨證體系之我見. In Fang Yao-Zhong, Xu Jia-Song, eds. *Collection of Lectures on Warm Pathogen Diseases (Wēn bìng huì jiǎng)* 溫病匯講. Beijing: People's Health Publishing House, 1986.

Xiao Geng-Liu. *Ordered [Approach] to Women's Diseases (Fù kē jīng lùn)* 婦科經論. Shanghai: Shanghai Health Publishing House, 1957.

Xie Zhong-Mo. *Key Points for Warm Pathogen Diseases (Wēn bìng yào yì)* 溫病要義. Beijing: People's Health Publishing House, 1956.

Xue Xue. *Systematic Differentiation of Damp-Heat Disorders (Shī rè tiáo biàn)* 濕熱條辨. (Originally published in the 18th century.) Reproduced in Song Zhao-Qi. *Distinguishing [Aspects] of Southern Diseases (Nán bìng bié jiàn)* 南病別鑒. Shanghai: Shanghai Health Publishing House, 1958.

Yang Shi-Yin. *Discussion of Formulas from Straight Directions from [Yang] Ren-Zhai (Rén-Zhāi zhí zhǐ fāng lùn)* 仁齋直指方論. Shanghai: Shanghai Publishing House of Ancient Literature, 1991. (Originally published in 1264.)

Yang Xuan. *Systematic Differentiation of Cold Damage and Warm Epidemics (Shāng hán wēn yì tiáo biàn)* 傷寒瘟疫條辨. (Originally published in 1784.) Reproduced in Yu Bo-Hai et al., eds. *Collection of Famous Books on Discussion of Cold Damage, Essentials from the Golden Cabinet, and Warm Pathogen Disease (Shāng hán jīn guì wēn bìng míng zhù jí chéng)* 傷寒金櫃溫病名著集成. Beijing: China Publishing House, 1997.

Ye Chuan et al., eds. *Collection of Famous Works by Four Outstanding Physicians of the Jin and Yuan Dynasties (Jīn yuán sì dà yī xué jiā míng zhù jí chéng)* 金元四大醫學家名著集成. Beijing: Traditional Chinese Medicine Publishing House, 1995.

Ye Gui. *Case Records as a Guide to Clinical Practice (Lín zhèng zhǐ nán yī àn)* 臨證指南醫案. Shanghai: Shanghai Science and Technology Publishing House, 1959. (Originally published in 1746.)

Ye Gui. *Differentiating Lurking Pathogens and Externally-Contracted Diseases during Three Seasons (Sān shí fú xié wài gǎn piàn)* 三時伏邪外感偏. Reproduced in Ye Gui. *Case Records as a Guide to Clinical Practice (Lín zhèng zhǐ nán yī àn)* 臨證指南醫案. Shanghai: Shanghai Science and Technology Publishing House, 1959.

Ye Gui. *Discussion of Warm-Heat Pathogen Disorders (Wēn rè lun)* 溫熱論. (Originally published in the 18th century.) Reproduced in Tang Da-Lie. *Collection of Papers of Physicians from Wu (Wú yī huì jiǎng)* 吳醫匯講. Shanghai: Shanghai Science and Technology Publishing House, 1983.

Ye Lin. *Explanation of Lurking Qi (Fú qì jiě)* 伏氣解. In Cao Bing-Zhang, ed. *Compendium of Medicine in China (Zhōng guó yī xué dà chéng)* 中國醫學大成. Shanghai: Shanghai Science and Technology Publishing House, 1990.

You Yi. *String of Pearls from the [Discussion] of Cold Damage (Shāng hán guàn zhū jí)* 傷寒貫珠集. Shanghai: Shanghai Science and Technology Publishing House, 1959. (Originally published in 1810.)

Yu Chang. *Precepts for Physicians (Yī mén fǎ lǜ)* 醫門法律. Shanghai: Shanghai Science and Technology Publishing House, 1983. (Originally published in 1658.)

Yu Chang. *Writings on the Esteemed Discussion (Shàng lùn piān)* 尚論篇. (Originally published in 1648.) Reproduced in Yu Bo-Hai et al., eds. *Collection of Famous Books on Discussion of Cold Damage, Essentials from the Golden Cabinet, and Warm Pathogen Disease (Shāng hán jīn guì wēn bìng míng zhù jí chéng)* 傷寒金櫃溫病名著集成. Beijing: China Publishing House, 1997.

Yu Gen-Chu. *Revised Popular Guide to Discussion of Cold Damage (Chóng ding tōng sú shāng hán lùn)* 重定通俗傷寒論. Hangzhou: New Medicine Press, 1956.

Yu Lin. *Achievements Regarding Epidemic Rashes (Yì zhěn yī dé)* 疫疹一得. (Originally published in 1794.) Survives in Wang Shi-Xiong. *Warp and Woof of Warm Heat Pathogen Diseases (Wēn rè jīng wěi)* 溫熱經緯. Reproduced in Lu Zhen et al., eds. *Collected Rare Recent Books on Chinese Medicine: Warm Pathogen Disease Section (Jīn dài zhōng yī zhēn běn jí: wēn bìng fèn cè)* 今代中醫珍本集溫病分冊. Hangzhou: Zhejiang Science and Technology Publishing House, 1987.

Yu Ying-Ao, Gao Yi-Min. *Selected and Classified Case Studies from Famous Modern Doctors of Traditional Chinese Medicine (Xiàn dài míng zhōng yī lèi àn xuǎn)* 現代名中醫類案選. Beijing: People's Health Publishing House, 1983.

Zhang Bo-Yu et al. *Traditional Chinese Internal Medicine* (5th ed.) *(Zhōng yī nèi kē xué)* 中醫內科學. Shanghai: Shanghai Science and Technology Publishing House, 1985.

Zhang Fa-Rong et al. *Traditional Chinese Internal Medicine (Zhōng yī nèi kē xué)* 中醫內科學. Beijing: Traditional Chinese Medicine Publishing House, 1995.

Zhang He-Teng. *Revised and Expanded Complete Treatise on Summerheat Damage (Zēng dìng shāng shǔ quán shū)* 增訂傷暑全書. In Cao Bing-Zhang, ed. *Compendium of Medicine in China (Zhōng guó yī xué dà chéng)* 中國醫學大成. Shanghai: Shanghai Science and Technology Publishing House, 1990.

Zhang Ji. *Discussion of Cold Damage (Shāng hán lùn)* 傷寒論. Beijing: People's Health Publishing House, 1983. (Originally published in the third century.)

Zhang Ji. *Essentials from the Golden Cabinet (Jīn guì yào lüè)* 金櫃要略. Beijing: People's Health Publishing House, 1963. (Originally published in the third century.)

Zhang Jie-Bin. *Appendices to the Classified Classic (Lèi jīng fù yì)* 類經附翼. Beijing: People's Health Publishing House, 1965. (Originally published in 1624.)

Zhang Jie-Bin. *Collected Treatises of [Zhang] Jing-Yue (Jǐng-Yuè quán shū)* 景岳全書. Beijing: People's Health Publishing House, 1991. (Originally published in 1624.)

Zhang Lu. *Comprehensive Medicine According to Master Zhang (Zhāng shì yī tōng)* 張氏醫通. Beijing: Chinese Medicine Publishing House, 1995. (Originally published in 1695.)

Zhang Xi-Chun. *Essays on Medicine Esteeming the Chinese and Respecting the Western (Yī xúe zhōng zhōng cān xī lù)* 醫學衷中參西錄. Shijiazhuang: Hebei People's Publishing House, 1957. (Originally published from 1918-1934.)

Zhang Yuan-Su. *Origins of Medicine,* annotated by Ren Ying-Qiu *(Yī xué qǐ yuán)* 醫學啟源. Beijing: People's Health Publishing House, 1978. (Originally published during the Yuan dynasty.)

Zhang Zhi-Wen, Liu Bi-Qing, eds. *Atlas of Tongue Diagnosis in Warm Pathogen Diseases (Wēn bìng shé zhěn tú pǔ)* 溫病舌診圖譜. Beijing: People's Health Publishing House, 1998.

Zhao Ji. *Comprehensive Recording of Sage-like Benefit from the Zhenghe Era (Zhènghé shèng jì zǒng lù)* 政和聖濟總錄. Beijing: People's Health Publishing House, 1962. (Originally published in 1117.)

Zhao Shao-Qin, Hu Ding-Bang, Liu Jing-Yuan. *Length and Breadth of Warm Pathogen Disease [Differentiation] (Wēn bìng zòng héng)* 溫病縱橫. Beijing: Beijing College of Traditional Chinese Medicine, 1979.

Zhao Xu-Chu et al. *Compendium of Modern Chinese Medicine Applications and Research: Warm Pathogen Diseases (Xiàn dài zhōng yī yào yìng yòng yǔ yán jiù dà xì: wēn bìng)* 現代中醫藥應用語研究大系溫病. Shanghai: Shanghai University of Chinese Medicine Publishing House, 1995.

Zhou Yang-Jun. *Summerheat Disease and Epidemic Disease (Wēn rè shǔ yì quán shū)* 溫熱暑疫全書. (Originally published in 1679.) In Cao Bing-Zhang, ed. *Compendium of Medicine in China (Zhōng guó yī xué dà chéng)* 中國醫學大成. Shanghai: Shanghai Science and Technology Publishing House, 1990.

Zhu Gong. *Book to Safeguard Life Arranged According to Pattern (Lèi zhèng huó rén shū)* 類證活人書. Shanghai: Commercial Press, 1957. (Originally published in 1108.)

Zhu Zhen-Heng. *Teachings of [Zhu] Dan-Xi (Dān-Xī xīn fǎ)* 丹溪心法. (Originally published in 1481.) In *Collection of Works from [Zhu] Dan-Xi (Dān-Xī yī jí)* 丹溪醫集. Beijing: People's Health Publishing House, 1993.

Table of Chinese Dynasties

Zhou	1066–221 BCE
Warring States	475–221 BCE
Qin	221-206 BCE
Western Han	206 BCE–23 CE
Eastern Han	25–220
Three Kingdoms	220–280
Jin	265–420
North and South Kingdoms	420–589
Sui	589–618
Tang	618–907
Five Dynasties	907–960
Song	960–1279
Southern Song	1127–1279
Jin	1115–1234
Yuan	1279–1368
Ming	1368–1644
Qing dynasty	1644–1911

Table of Authors

T HE CONCEPTS AND practices relating to warm pathogen diseases evolved over a period of two thousand years. A multitude of practitioners and authors contributed to these ideas in ancient China, and many of them are noted in the main text. In this appendix are the basic data about the cited authors: given (birth) name, honorific name, and dates. Both the birth and honorific names are commonly used in the Chinese literature, and most Chinese readers are familiar with the various names of the major contributors to the Chinese medical tradition. To simplify things, in this book we have just used the given names.

Given name	Honorific Name	Dates (all CE)
Cao Bing-Zhang	Cao Chi-Dian	1877–1955
Cao Jia-Da	Cao Ying-Fu	1866–1937
Chao Yuan-Fang	none noted	active 610
Chen Guang-Song	Chen Gen-Ru	active early 20th century
Chen Nian-Zu	Chen Xiu-Yuan	1753–1823
Chen Si-Gong	Chen Yu-Ren	c. 1555–1636
Chen Yan	Chen Wu-Ze	c. 1131–1189
Chen Zi-Ming	Chen Liang-Fu	1190–1270
Chen Zu-Gong	Chen Ping-Bo	active 1809
Cheng Guo-Peng	Cheng Zhong-Ling	active 1732

Given name	Honorific Name	Dates (all CE)
Cheng Wu-Ji	none noted	c. 1115–1235
Dai Tian-Zhang	Dai Lin-Jiao	1644–1722
Ding Gan-Ren	Ding Ze-Zhou	1866–1926
Du Ben	Du Bi-Qing	active 1341
Fei Bo-Xiong	Fei Jin-Qing	active 1863
Ge Hong	Ge Ya-Chuan	281–341
Gong Ting-Xian	Gong Zi-Cai	active 1587
Guo Yong	Guo Zi-He	active 1165
He Lian-Chen	He Bing-Yuan	1860–1929
Huang Gong-Xiu	Huang Jin-Fang	active 1773
Jiang Bao-Su	Jiang Wen-Zhai	active 1840
Jing De-Jian	Jing Bao-San	active 1868
Ke Qin	Ke Yun-Bo	active 1674
Lei Feng	Lei Shao-Yi	active 1882
Li Chan	Li Jian-Zhai	active 1575
Li Gao	Li Ming-Zhi	1180–1251
Liu Bao-Yi	Liu Gu-Sun	1842–1900
Liu Ji-Ren	Liu Hen-Rui	active 1898
Liu Kui	Liu Wen-Fu	active 1789
Liu Wan-Su	Liu Shou-Zhen	c. 1120–1200
Lou Jie	Lou Shou-Zhi	active 1903
Lu Mao-Xiu	Lu Jiu-Zhi	active 1866
Lu Ting-Zhen	Lu Zi-Xian	active 1868
Lu Yuan-Lei	Lu Peng-Nian	1894–1955
Pang An-Shi	Pang An-Shang	1042–1099
Pu Fu-Zhou	none noted	1888–1975
Qian Yi	Qian Zhong-Yang	1055–1117
Qin Bo-Wei	Qin Zhi-Ji	1901–1970
Ren Ying-Qiu	Ren Hong-Bing	1914–1986
Shao Deng-Yin	Shao Bu-Qing	active 1749
Shen Jin-Ao	Shen Qian-Lu	1717–1776

Given name	Honorific Name	Dates (all CE)
Shen Ming-Zong	Shen Mu-Nan	active 1693
Shen Xiao-Gu	none noted	active 1933
Shi Shou-Tang	Shi Fu-Nan	active 1861
Shi Yi-Ren	Shi Yi-Xing	1896–1966
Sun Si-Mo	none noted	c. 581–682
Tang Da-Lie	Tang Li-San	active 1801
Tang Rong-Chuan	Tang Zong-Hai	1851–1908
Tao Hong-Jing	Tao Tong-Ming	active 494
Tao Hua	Tao Jie-An	active 1445
Wang Ang	Wang Ren-An	active 1615
Wang Ji	Wang Sheng-Zhi	1463–1539
Wang Bing	none noted	active 762
Wang Ken-Tang	Wang Yu-Tai	active 1549–1613
Wang Lu	Wang An-Dao	active 1332–1391
Wang Qing-Ren	Wang Xun-Chen	1768–1831
Wang Shi-Xiong	Wang Meng-Ying	active 1808–1867
Wang Tao	none noted	active 752
Wang Xi	Wang Shu-He	active 200
Wu Qian	Wu Liu-Jie	c. 1736–1795
Wu Tang	Wu Ju-Tong	1758–1836
Wu Xi-Huang	Wu Rui-Fu	active 1920
Wu You-Xing	Wu You-Ke	c. 1582–1652
Wu Zhen	Wu Kun-An	active 1796
Xia Chun-Nong	none noted	active late 19th century
Xiao Geng-Liu	Xiao Shen-Zhai	active 1684
Xie Zhong-Mo	none noted	active 1957
Xue Xue	Xue Sheng-Bai	1681–1770
Yang Shi-Ying	Yang Deng-Fu	active 1264
Yang Xuan	Yang Yu-Heng	c. 1705–1784
Yang Zhao-Li	Yang Su-Yuan	dates unknown
Ye Gui	Ye Tian-Shi	active 1666–1745

Given name	Honorific Name	Dates (all CE)
Ye Lin	Ye Zi-Yu	active 1897
You Yi	You Zai-Jing	active 1729
Yu Chang	Yu Jia-Yan	c. 1585–1664
Yu Gen-Chu	Yu Zhao-Yuan	1734–1799
Yu Lin	Yu Shi-Yu	1736–1795
Yun Tie-Qiao	Yun Shu-Jue	1878–1935
Zhang Deng	Zhang Dan-Xian	active 1668
Zhang He-Teng	Zhang Feng-Kui	active 1623
Zhang Ji	Zhang Zhong-Jin	active late Han dynasty
Zhang Jie-Bin	Zhang Jing-Yue	active 1636
Zhang Lu	Zhang Lu-Yu	active 1689
Zhang Nan	Zhang Xu-Gu	active 1825
Zhang Xi-Chun	Zhang Shou-Fu	1860–1933
Zhang Xi-Ju	Zhang Ling-Shao	active 1712
Zhang Yuan-Su	Zhang Jie-Gu	active 1186
Zhou Yang-Jun	Zhou Yu-Zai	active 1679
Zhu Gong	Zhu Yi-Zhong	active 1108
Zhu Zhen-Heng	Zhu Yan-Xiu	1281–1358

APPENDIX C

Supplemental Case Studies

Clinical Extensions of Warm Pathogen Disease Concepts and Treatment

C LINICAL REALITY IS FLUID and requires that practitioners be flexible. Often situations in the clinic are more variable than they are presented to be in textbooks, even this one. As early as the seventh century, the famous physician Sun Si-Miao remarked, "[In general,] after studying for three years, practitioners feel that there is no disease that they cannot cure. However, after practicing for three years, they become confused and believe that there is no formula that is clinically useful."[1]

This state of affairs comes about at least in part because the presentations seen in the clinic frequently do not exactly match the herbal formulas that have been studied. Real patients, of course, have their own individual constitutions, emotions, dietary habits, and lifestyles. All of these factors contribute to making each illness specific and in some ways unique. If we focus on understanding the underlying pathologies, and on utilizing herbal formulas that are appropriate to those pathologies, this problem can in large part be resolved. Yet there will always be some distance between what is found in textbooks and what is found in the clinic. It is important for both students and practitioners to narrow this distance. One way to do so is to follow a master in the clinic and thereby obtain direct teachings about how the knowledge in textbooks and the classics can be applied in the clinic. Another method is to read case studies, which give one insight into how experienced physicians practice. This is one reason why the case study has long been one of the cornerstones of Chinese medical training.

Over the course of time, the concepts and theories of warm pathogen disease as described in this book have seeped into the fabric of Chinese medicine. Their usage has not been limited to externally-contracted diseases, but to general internal medicine as well. This, in turn, has expanded the concepts of warm pathogen disease themselves. This appendix provides several case studies that demonstrate how the ideas and concepts of warm pathogen disease theory have been extended, and a few examples of how they can be used in clinical practice.

Mulberry Leaf and Chrysanthemum Drink *(sāng jú yǐn)*

K.K., female, age 34

First visit: June 15, 1999. The chief complaint was allergies. The patient had nasal congestion, sneezing, a plugged sensation in her right ear, and itchy and watery eyes for a week since coming to Portland from Michigan to visit her parents. No dizziness and headache were reported. She had a history of irregular bowel movements with small amounts of stool. She also had anxiety attacks and was taking 25mg of Sertraline a day. The tip of her tongue was red, the tongue coating was yellow and greasy, and her pulse was thin on the left, weak in the right distal position, and slippery in the other positions on the right. The patient was nursing her six-month-old son who also had a runny nose and was sneezing.

The diagnosis was wind-heat with dampness attacking the Lung and the Liver. The treatment principle chosen was to disperse wind and heat, clear heat and eliminate dampness, and disseminate the Lung qi and direct it downward. A modified version of Mulberry Leaf and Chrysanthemum Drink *(sāng jú yǐn)*[2] was prescribed:

Mori Folium *(sāng yè)*	9g
Chrysanthemi Flos *(jú huā)*	9g
Forsythiae Fructus *(lián qiào)*	6g
Menthae haplocalycis Herba *(bò hé)*	6g
Platycodi Radix *(jié gěng)*	6g
Armeniacae Semen *(xìng rén)*	6g
Phragmitis Rhizoma *(lú gēn)*	6g
Talcum *(huá shí)*	6g
Magnoliae Flos *(xīn yí)*	9g
Angelicae dahuricae Radix *(bái zhǐ)*	6g
Glycyrrhizae Radix *(gān cǎo)*	3g

The herbs were in granular form[3] and the patient took 3g, three times a day. Acupuncture was also given at points LI-4 *(hé gǔ)*, LR-3 *(tài chòng)*, TB-5 *(wài guān)*, LU-7 *(liè quē)*, and BL-2 *(zǎn zhú)*.

Second visit: June 22, 1999. After taking the formula, the patient sweated profusely and experienced palpitations for a short time. However, the nasal congestion improved markedly, her ears felt less plugged up, and she was sneezing less. She became slightly constipated and her energy was much better. The tongue body color and coating were unchanged. She had a wiry pulse on the left side; her right distal pulse was wiry, while the middle and proximal pulses were slippery. She reported that her son had had two bouts of diarrhea, but his allergies were also much improved. The treatment principle remained the same, but the formula was modified as follows:

Mori Folium *(sāng yè)* 6g

Chrysanthemi Flos *(jú huā)* 6g

Talcum *(huá shí)* 3g

Phragmitis Rhizoma *(lú gēn)*..............................3g

Magnoliae Flos *(xīn yí)* 3g

Glycyrrhizae Radix *(gān cǎo)* 3g

The same acupuncture points were used.

Third visit: June 29, 1999. The patient had had no problems with her sinuses after the last treatment until she went out for a hike on this day. During the hike she had slight nasal congestion, but none of her other allergy symptoms. Her stools were more regular and soft and her energy was good. The yellow and greasy tongue coating was almost gone, but she had slightly less coating than normal on the front of her tongue. Her pulse was wiry and thin on the left, and slippery and wiry on the right. Her son's allergies were gone. The herbal treatment was discontinued and she was needled at the following acupuncture points: BL-2 *(zǎn zhú)*, TB-5 *(wài guān)*, LU-7 *(liè quē)*, LI-4 *(hé gǔ)*, SP-4 *(gōng sūn)*, and PC-6 *(nèi guān)*. It was recommended that she build up her Lung yin by eating pears and/or water chestnuts. A week later, the patient's sister came to see me and said that the patient's allergy problems were totally gone.[4]

Commentary: According to Wu Tang, the pathology for which Mulberry Leaf and Chrysanthemum Drink *(sāng jú yǐn)* is prescribed is wind-heat attacking the Lung, leading to failure of the Lung to disseminate and direct its qi downward. Looking at the formula superficially, it may seem that it is inappropriate for this case because cough, which is usually regarded as the cardinal symptom for its use, is absent. However, when we analyze the formula carefully, we realize that it can disseminate the Lung qi and distribute it to the throat and nasal passages, because it contains Platycodi Radix *(jié gěng)* and Menthae haplocalycis Herba *(bò hé)*. As I understand it, the qi is dispersed through the Lung by Mori Folium *(sāng yè)* and Chrysanthemi Flos *(jú huā)*, then to the throat by Platycodi Radix *(jié gěng)*, and finally to the nose by Menthae haplocalycis Herba *(bò hé)*. Therefore, this formula can impact the qi circulation in the nose and is useful for nasal problems, especially acute sinusitis and allergic rhinitis. Based on this understanding, I often use this formula combined with the acupuncture points noted above for treating acute nasal problems due to wind-heat.

Because it was humid during the time of the treatments, the wind-heat was associated with dampness; Talcum *(huá shí)* was therefore added. Magnoliae Flos *(xīn yí)* and Angelicae dahuricae Radix *(bái zhǐ)* were also added to counteract the possible congealing effect of the cold substances. At the first treatment, I did not pay close enough attention to the patient's underlying situation, which probably included qi or blood deficiency following childbirth. For this reason, the dosages of Magnoliae Flos *(xīn yí)*, Angelicae dahuricae Radix *(bái zhǐ)*, and Menthae haplocalycis Herba *(bò hé)* were too large and the resulting dispersing effect caused transient profuse sweating and palpitations. At the second visit, I removed two of these three herbs and reduced the dosage of the other one.

Disseminate the White and Order the Qi Decoction *(xuān bái chéng qì tāng)*

Mr. Wang, male, 87 years old

First visit: The patient had had a fever for seven days and had been coughing and having difficulty breathing for the last five days. His temperature had ranged from 38-39.5°C. He was hospitalized, diagnosed with pneumonia, and given an injection of gentamycin. The patient had also taken tetracycline. There was little effect from these treatments, and a traditional Chinese doctor was therefore called in to treat him.

The patient had a high fever, sweating, and cough with profuse, thick, and yellow sputum. Due to labored breathing, he was unable to sleep lying down. His mouth was dry and he had not had a bowel movement for five days. He had scanty, yellow urine, and slight abdominal distention without pain. His tongue was red with a yellow, greasy coating and his pulse was slippery and rapid. The diagnosis was warm-heat pathogen attacking the Lung and congealing the fluids into phlegm. This led to phlegm obstructing the qi in the Lung, with resulting failure of the Lung to disseminate its qi and direct it downward. Because the Lung and the Large Intestine are paired organs, failure of the Lung to descend can lead to qi stagnation in the Large Intestine, manifesting as constipation. The treatment principles called for disseminating the Lung qi, transforming phlegm, and purging heat from the Large Intestine. Fortunately, even though the patient was 87 years old, he was robust enough to be purged for a short time. The formula used was modified Disseminate the White and Order the Qi Decoction *(xuān bái chéng qì tāng):*[5]

Armeniacae Semen *(xìng rén)*	6g,
Trichosanthis Fructus *(guā lóu)*	20g
prepared Eriobotryae Folium *(zhì pí pá yè)*	15g
Gypsum fibrosum *(shí gāo)*	15g
Rhei Radix et Rhizoma *(dà huáng)* (added near end)	6g
Indigo and Clam Shell Powder *(dài gé sǎn)*[6] (put into tea bag)	10g

A packet of the herbs was given to the patient.

Second visit: The patient had three bowel movements after taking the herbs, each time with intensely foul-smelling stool. His cough and labored breathing had improved, and he no longer experienced abdominal distention. He was given two more packets of the same formula, minus Rhei Radix et Rhizoma *(dà huáng)*.

Third visit: All signs and symptoms were much improved after taking the herbs. His temperature was 37.8°C. Only a very slight cough remained, and he could sleep lying down. His tongue was red with a yellow and white coating, and his pulse was wiry, thin, and slightly slippery. The treatment principle at this time was to clear heat from the Lung and adjust the Stomach:

> Armeniacae Semen *(xìng rén)* 6g
> Platycodi Radix *(jié gěng)* 6g
> Trichosanthis Pericarpium *(guā lóu pí)* 10g
> Pinelliae Rhizoma preparatum *(zhì bàn xià)* 10g
> dry-fried Fructus Oryzae Sativae Germinantus *(chǎo gǔ yá)* 10g
> Glycyrrhizae Radix *(gān cǎo)* 6g
> Mori Cortex *(sāng bái pí)* 6g
> Phragmitis Rhizoma *(lú gēn)* 20g

Two packets of these herbs were given to the patient. After finishing the herbs, all signs and symptoms were gone and his temperature was normal. His chest x-ray was negative and he was discharged from the hospital.[7]

Commentary: This condition is commonly seen in the clinic with patients who have acute bronchitis or pneumonia. This patient had fever and a cough for five days, as the disease had progressed from the protective to the qi level, affecting the Lung and Large Intestine. If viewed from the perspective of the eight parameters, the disease had been getting worse. However, if analyzed based on the concept of the normal progression of warm pathogen diseases (see Chapter 4), the progression of heat from the Lung to the Large Intestine is not always a bad sign, as this gives the practitioner a clear avenue for eliminating the heat from the body. Therefore, treatment should *promote* this process instead of interfering with it. This is why purging heat and resolving phlegm were used in combination.

If one were to give this case just a cursory look, it does not appear to match the pattern of blockage of the Lung by phlegm and heat with clumping of stool and heat in the Large Intestine. Here the urine was scanty and yellow and there was just slight abdominal bloating. However, because that pattern does describe the pathology in this case, the corresponding treatment method should be followed.

This case was treated by Zhao Shao-Qin, a famous contemporary authority on warm pathogen diseases. From this case we can learn not only about choosing the right formula for an old man like this, but also about how to administer the formula and to modify it in response to the patient's reaction. Thus, in treating the elderly, one must be cautious in using the purging method. In this case, the elderly patient, after having a high fever for some time, probably had some underlying injury to his qi and yin. With this in mind, Dr. Zhao first prescribed just one packet of herbs, and then removed Rhei Radix et Rhizoma *(dà huáng)* immediately after the patient had a few bowel movements. This allowed for purging without any further injury to the qi and yin. As the situation improved he added Phragmitis Rhizoma *(lú gēn)* and dry-fried Fructus Oryzae Sativae Germinantus *(chǎo gǔ yá)*, demonstrating a method of how the Stomach could be protected and the yin nourished without trapping residual phlegm and heat.

Regulate the Stomach and Order the Qi Decoction *(tiáo wèi chéng qì tāng)*

First visit: August 21, 1957. Three days prior to visiting the clinic, the child, a 6-year-old male, developed a sudden fever, spiking to a temperature of 40°C. He complained of headache and poor appetite, and appeared restless. The day before, he vomited frequently, appeared sleepy and delirious, and had occasional convulsions. He received a spinal tap and the analysis of his cerebrospinal fluid showed evidence of encephalitis B. At the time of his first visit to the traditional Chinese medicine clinic, the patient also had a dry mouth and lips, and clenched his teeth so that the practitioner was unable to observe his tongue. His pulse was wiry and slippery, and his temperature was 39.7°C. The diagnosis was summerheat-warmth in which heat was predominant. The treatment principle was to clear heat from the Stomach and open the orifices with cool herbs. A modified version of White Tiger Decoction *(bái hǔ tāng)* was used:[8]

Gypsum fibrosum *(shí gāo)*	120g
Anemarrhenae Rhizoma *(zhī mǔ)*	9g
Glycyrrhizae Radix *(gān cǎo)*	9g
Lonicerae Flos *(jīn yín huā)*	15g
Forsythiae Fructus *(lián qiào)*	15g

The physician also melted one Calm the Palace Pill with Cattle Gallstone *(ān gōng niú huáng wán)*[9] into the decoction. The patient received the decoction through a naso-gastric tube.

Second visit: After taking two packets of the herbs, the patient's temperature decreased to 38°C. His convulsions and vomiting stopped. The patient was able to eat, but was still occasionally delirious and even briefly lost consciousness a few times. In addition, he had not had a bowel movement for five days. This, coupled with a submerged, rapid, and forceful pulse, and a dry and yellow tongue coating, indicated the presence of heat from excess in the Large Intestine. The physician determined that it would be appropriate to purge heat through the Large Intestine, so he combined the preceding formula with Regulate the Stomach and Order the Qi Decoction (*tiáo wèi chéng qì tāng*):[10]

Gypsum fibrosum (*shí gāo*)	60g
Scrophulariae Radix (*xuán shēn*)	9g
Glycyrrhizae Radix (*gān cǎo*)	4.5g
wine-washed Rhei Radix et Rhizoma (*jiǔ dà huáng*)	9g
Natrii Sulfas (*máng xiāo*)	4.5g
Forsythiae Fructus (*lián qiào*)	12g
Lonicerae Caulis (*rěn dōng téng*)	15g
Nelumbinis Plumula (*lián zǐ xīn*)	9g

Additionally, he added 1.2g of Purple Snow Special Pill (*zǐ xuě dān*).[11]

Third visit: After taking one packet of herbs, the patient had bowel movements and his temperature decreased to 37.5°C. Moreover, his consciousness returned to normal and the delirium was gone. He continued receiving the formula, but the physician reduced the dosage of several ingredients and added herbs to enrich the yin. Ten days later, the patient had fully recovered.[12]

Commentary: This case was treated by Liu Zhi-Ming, vice president of the All-China Traditional Chinese Medicine Association, and a senior attending physician at the China Academy of Traditional Chinese Medicine. The case demonstrates how fast summerheat-warmth with less dampness can progress due to its characteristically rapid movement. Here the disease progressed from the protective level to the qi and nutritive levels, leading to blockage of the Heart and stirring up of Liver wind, in just three days. Usually, summerheat without dampness is more likely to attack the Stomach, leading to the *yang ming* (Stomach) pattern in the qi level. But it can sometimes attack the Pericardium directly and suddenly, blocking the spirit of the Heart, or even leading to stirring up of Liver wind (see Chapters 3 and 11). Clinically, summerheat can first attack the *yang ming*, and shortly thereafter progress from the *yang ming* to the Heart or even the Liver. This case demonstrates this kind of progression. The poor appetite and severe vomiting is evidence that the Stomach was attacked before the Heart and the Liver. The summerheat was so severe in this case that not only was the spirit of the Heart blocked, but also extreme heat damaged the fluids and stirred up Liver wind. Without a large dosage of Gypsum fibrosum (*shí gāo*), it is impossible to disperse and clear extreme heat that has attacked the Heart and the Liver from the Stomach. Only someone with the level of experience of this physician could confidently prescribe 120g of Gypsum fibrosum (*shí gāo*) for a 6-year-old child.

After taking the modified White Tiger Decoction (*bái hǔ tāng*), some of the heat in the Stomach was cleared, which was evidenced in the lower temperature, and the disappearance of the convulsions and vomiting. But the patient still had delirium at times and presented with new signs and symptoms, such as constipation, dry and yellow tongue coating, and a submerged, rapid, and forceful pulse, which would be confusing to some practitioners. Among the possible questions would be, Where was the disease progressing to? Was it getting worse? And what should the next treatment be? As discussed in Chapter 4, it is always a good sign when a disease goes from the yin to the yang organs, especially to the Large Intestine where pathogens can be readily discharged from the body. Here some of the heat had been transmitted from the Stomach to the Large Intestine, which gave the practitioner a good opportunity to purge it. Therefore, Dr. Liu added Regulate the Stomach and Order the Qi Decoction (*tiáo wèi chéng qì tāng*) to follow the body's lead in purging the heat. In my own opinion, it would be better in these circumstances to use Greatest Treasure Special Pill (*zhì bǎo dān*)[13] rather than Purple Snow Special Pill (*zǐ xuě dān*), as the former medicine is stronger for opening the orifices.

Clear the Nutritive Level Decoction (*qīng yíng tāng*)

Ms. Fan, 29 years old

The patient was diagnosed with meningitis and hospitalized. She presented with a high fever, restlessness, epistaxis, and episodes of delirium during the night. In addition, during the day her consciousness alternated between being clear and muddled, and she suffered a few convulsions. Her tongue was deep red and her pulse was thin and rapid. The diagnosis was attack on the nutritive level by warm-heat pathogen, leading to stirring up of the Liver wind by extreme heat and toxin. A modified version of Clear the Nutritive Level Decoction (*qīng yíng tāng*)[14] was prescribed:

Rhinocerotis Cornu (*xī jiǎo*)	1.5g
Scrophulariae Radix (*xuán shēn*)	9g
Ophiopogonis Radix (*mài mén dōng*)	12g
fresh Rehmanniae Radix recens (*xiān dì huáng*)	25g
Salviae miltiorrhizae Radix (*dān shēn*)	9g
Coptidis Rhizoma (*huáng lián*)	3g
Folium Lophatheri Immaturus (*zhu ye juan xin*)[15]	4.5g
Lonicerae Flos (*jīn yín huā*)	9g
Forsythiae Fructus (*lián qiào*)	12g

She was also given 2.5g of Purple Snow Special Pill (*zǐ xuě dān*) to be taken with the strained decoction. After taking two packets of the formula, the patient's convulsions stopped and her consciousness returned to normal.[16]

Commentary: In the clinic it is more common to see patients with overlapping patterns rather than with just a single pattern. In this case there were signs of problems in both the nutritive level (deep-red tongue, restlessness, delirium and muddled consciousness at times) as well as the blood level (epistaxis). However, here the nutritive level condition is more severe. Invasion of the Pericardium and Heart often leads to bleeding and stirring up of the Liver. This is because the Heart is responsible for moving the blood, and the Pericardium is, along with the Liver, a *jue yin* organ. Clear the Nutritive Level Decoction *(qīng yíng tāng)* is a primary formula for treating heat in the nutritive level accompanied by some bleeding. Purple Snow Special Pill *(zǐ xuě dān)* is very effective when stirring up of Liver wind occurs after heat has invaded the Pericardium. Therefore, quick and good results came from combining both formulas, without any modifications.

This case was treated by He Ren, currently a professor at the Zhejiang College of Traditional Chinese Medicine. He is regarded as a specialist in six-stage differentiation. This case is an example of how competent practitioners use whatever approach is appropriate when treating a patient, regardless of their own predilections.

Increase the Fluids and Order the Qi Decoction *(zēng yè chéng qì tāng)*

Female, 65 years old

First visit: The patient had been sick for over twenty days since the beginning of spring with a fever. Her temperature was around 38.5°C. She had very thin musculature and a dark face that lacked luster. Her tongue was deep red, cracked, and had less saliva than normal; the tongue coating was dry, thick, and yellow. Her lips were also dry. She had a poor appetite, was thirsty for cold beverages, and was constipated. She had epigastric and abdominal distention that worsened with pressure. Her throat was red, dry, and sore. Her pulse was submerged, thin, small, and slippery, but forceful.

The history revealed that she had suffered from pulmonary tuberculosis for more than ten years with frequent night sweats and occasional low-grade fevers. Recently, she had been mistakenly treated with acrid and warm herbs several times to induce sweating for a common cold that in fact was due to wind-heat. This badly damaged her yin and fluids, and had led to an accumulation of heat in the Large Intestine with constipation. This in turn led to a vicious cycle of increasing yin deficiency leading to increasing heat; the heat led to more dryness, which in turn damaged the yin even more. The appropriate treatment principles were to purge heat from the Large Intestine while enriching the yin and fluids to moisten what has become dry. The formula prescribed was a modified version of Increase the Fluids and Order the Qi Decoction *(zēng yè chéng qì tāng):*[17]

Scrophulariae Radix *(xuán shēn)*	45g
Rehmanniae Radix *(shēng dì huáng)*	30g
Ophiopogonis Radix *(mài mén dōng)*	25g
Paeoniae Radix alba *(bái sháo)*	30g
Dendrobii Herba *(shí hú)*	25g

Natrii Sulfas *(máng xiāo)* 1.5g
   (taken with the strained decoction)

powdered Rhei Radix et Rhizoma *(dà huáng)* 1.2g
   (taken with the strained decoction)

A packet of the herbs was given to the patient.

Second visit: The morning after finishing the herbs, the patient had a bowel movement. The stool was very hard, like that of a goat, at the beginning of the bowel movement, but softened by the end. The hard, dry stool caused cracks around the anus with slight bleeding. Her temperature was 37.5°C. She still had a deep-red tongue with cracks and less than normal saliva. Her appetite had increased while the epigastric and abdominal distention had decreased. Her throat was still red, but it was less dry and sore. Her pulse was deep, thin, small, slippery, and less forceful than before. This patient had an underlying deficiency of yin that had been further damaged by both externally-contracted wind-heat and incorrect treatment. The resulting problem with bowel movements could be compared to a boat that gets stuck because the water level is too low. The first treatment enriched the yin, moistened the Large Intestine, and purged heat. Now that her stool was moving and the heat had been somewhat drained off, it was not appropriate to continue using purging substances such as Natrii Sulfas *(máng xiāo)* and Rhei Radix et Rhizoma *(dà huáng)*. Instead, the proper method was to enrich the yin and moisten the dryness with sweet and cold herbs:

Glehniae/Adenophorae Radix *(shā shēn)* 30g

Rehmanniae Radix *(shēng dì huáng)* 25g

Paeoniae Radix alba *(bái sháo)* 25g

Asini Corii Colla *(ē jiāo)* 15g
   (divided into two portion and melted in the strained decoction)

Auricularia *(hei mu er)*[18] 12g

prepared Trionycis Carapax *(zhì biē jiǎ)* .... 15g (cook first)

Ophiopogonis Radix *(mài mén dōng)* 15g

Two packets of the herbs were given to the patient.

Third visit: The patient no longer felt feverish and her temperature was 37°C. Her tongue coating was back to normal, but the tongue body was still deep red with cracks and less than normal saliva. Her appetite was normal. She had a bowel movement on each of the preceding two days, with stools of normal consistency. There was no distention in her abdomen or epigastrium. The red, dry, and painful throat symptoms were gone. Her pulse was thin, wiry, and small. The same treatment principle was followed in designing the formula:

Rehmanniae Radix *(shēng dì huáng)* 25g

Glehniae/Adenophorae Radix *(shā shēn)* 25g

Paeoniae Radix alba *(bái sháo)* 25g

Coicis Semen *(yì yǐ rén)* 15g

Lablab Semen album *(bái biǎn dòu)* 25g

Asini Corii Colla *(ē jiāo)* 12g

    (divided into two portions and melted in the strained decoction)

Ophiopogonis Radix *(mài mén dōng)* 10g

Asparagi Radix *(tiān mén dōng)* 10g

Gigeriae galli Endothelium corneum *(jī nèi jīn)* 10g

Five packets of the herbs were given to the patient. After finishing the herbs, all signs and symptoms were gone and her appetite and sleep were normal. The patient was asked to avoid spicy and greasy foods, and to eat bland food sparingly.[19]

Commentary: When heat progresses to the Large Intestine, two pathological changes occur. Heat not only injures the fluids but also interferes with the function of the Large Intestine, leading to qi stagnation and constipation. Injury of the fluids intensifies the constipation, which aggravates the qi stagnation. This in turn produces more heat, which further injures the fluids, and so on, in a vicious cycle. The key is to get the stool to move out of the Intestines, which not only opens up an avenue for heat to exit the body, but also breaks the cycle of qi stagnation and production of heat. What has puzzled practitioners is how to purge the stool from the body without further injuring the fluids. This can be done in one of two ways. Purgative substances can be combined with those that enrich the yin for a relatively direct approach. A more indirect approach would be to simply use herbs that enrich yin and moisten the Intestines such that the Large Intestine becomes moist enough for the stools to slip out.

    This case, which was treated by the physician Zhao Shao-Qin, reflects both of these strategies and how to protect the yin when treating a combination of heat and yin deficiency. Patients with underlying yin deficiency, such as this woman, are more likely to catch warm pathogen diseases. Unfortunately, she was treated improperly with acrid and warm herbs to induce sweating, which further injured the fluids. The disease then progressed to the Large Intestine, leading to clumping of heat and dry stool in the Large Intestine. At this time, besides severe yin deficiency, the heat was still quite strong, as evidenced by the fever and the red, dry, and sore throat. This situation required both purging the heat along with enriching the yin. Note that while Increase the Fluids and Order the Qi Decoction *(zēng yè chéng qì tāng)* was prescribed here, the patient was given only one packet, and the dosage of Rhei Radix et Rhizoma *(dà huáng)* and Natrii Sulfas *(máng xiāo)* was relatively small. As soon as the patient had a bowel movement, the purgatives were removed and a modified version of Increase the Fluids Decoction *(zēng yè tāng)* was prescribed to promote bowel movements by moistening the Large Intestine. The dietary recommendations given at the end of the case were for the purpose of preventing food from further injuring the yin.

Transform Maculas Decoction *(huà bān tāng)*

Adult female

First visit: The patient developed an aversion to cold, chills, fever, and headache a day after giving birth. A doctor had used acrid, warm, exterior-releasing herbs, but without effect. Then another doctor diagnosed the condition as an attack of wind-cold with underlying blood deficiency, and prescribed herbs to nourish the blood and release the exterior, also without effect.

The patient had a vigorous fever, restlessness, thirst, and a painful and swollen throat. She also had bright maculas all over her body. Her pulse was flooding and rapid, and her tongue was deep red with a yellow coating. Her white blood cell count was 18,000/mm.[3] The diagnosis was putrefying throat granular disorder due to intense heat in both the qi and blood levels. A modified version of Transform Maculas Decoction *(huà bān tāng)*[20] was prescribed:

Gypsum fibrosum *(shí gāo)*	30g
Anemarrhenae Rhizoma *(zhī mǔ)*	15g
Glycyrrhizae Radix *(gān cǎo)*	6g
Scrophulariae Radix *(xuán shēn)*	24g
Rhinocerotis Cornu *(xī jiǎo)* (cook earlier than other herbs)	10g
Lonicerae Flos *(jīn yín huā)*	15g
Forsythiae Fructus *(lián qiào)*	30g
Scutellariae Radix *(huáng qín)*	25g
Moutan Cortex *(mǔ dān pí)*	12g
Paeoniae Radix rubra *(chì sháo)*	15g

The patient was given two packets of the herbs to be taken over a period of one day (the strained decoction was to be administered every four hours, six times a day).

Second visit: After finishing two packets of the herbs, the heat condition was remarkably reduced. A slightly modified formula was continued for two more days. At that time all signs and symptoms were gone.[21]

Commentary: This case was treated by Xu You-Ling, a senior attending physician at the Chongqing Institute of Traditional Chinese Medicine. The case showed a clear progression from the protective to the qi to the nutritive level, and finally to the blood level. The patient had aversion to cold, fever, and headache due to warm-heat in the protective level, as evidenced by the fact that the acrid, warm herbs had no effect. While it is not explicitly stated in the case, it is understood that these herbs exacerbated the condition. To compound the error, herbs to nourish the blood were added. These somewhat cloying substances can readily trap warm-heat pathogens. This can cause the disease to progress to the qi and then the nutritive and blood levels, as evidenced by the vigorous fever, restlessness, thirst, maculas, and deep-red tongue. The combination of deep-red tongue and restlessness were indications of nutritive level involvement; the presence of maculas signified a blood-level condition. The combination of sore throat and maculas can be diagnosed as a case of putrefying throat granular disorder. Because the nutritive and blood levels were involved, if left untreated, or treated with insufficient strength, the heat could invade the Pericardium, leading to the blockage of the Heart spirit. Accordingly, the patient was given the decoction six times a day in order to clear the heat as quickly and efficaciously as possible, and to prevent further progression of the disease.

Antelope Horn and Uncaria Decoction *(líng jiǎo gōu téng tāng)*

Female, 30 years old

First visit: November 20, 1979. The patient had a high fever (40°C), clenched teeth, coma, and incontinence of urine and stool. Her right hand and foot were stiff and her right hand was in spasm. Her eyeballs moved involuntarily, there was a gurgling sound in the throat, and ulcers in the mouth. Although she often yawned, she was unresponsive. Her tongue coating was white, thick, and moldy-looking *(腐 fǔ)*, and her pulse was wiry and slippery. The diagnosis was damp-heat transforming into heat, stirring up internal wind and leading to blockage of the Heart spirit by extreme heat. Treatment was directed at clearing heat, eliminating dampness, opening the orifices, and extinguishing Liver wind. Modified Antelope Horn and Uncaria Decoction *(líng jiǎo gōu téng tāng)*[22] was prescribed:

Powdered Saigae tataricae Cornu *(líng yáng jiǎo)* (taken with the strained decoction)	10g
Uncariae Ramulus cum Uncis *(gōu téng)*	10g
Chrysanthemi Flos *(jú huā)*	10g
Mori Folium *(sāng yè)*	10g
Fritillariae cirrhosae Bulbus *(chuān bèi mǔ)*	10g
Acori tatarinowii Rhizoma *(shí chāng pú)*	10g
Eupatorii Herba *(pèi lán)*	10g
Isatidis/Baphicacanthis Radix *(bǎn lán gēn)*	20g
Rehmanniae Radix *(shēng dì huáng)*	10g
Paeoniae Radix alba *(bái sháo)*	10g
Glycyrrhizae Radix *(gān cǎo)*	10g

She was also given one Calm the Palace Pill with Cattle Gallstone (*ān gōng niú huáng wán*)[23] that was dissolved and taken with the strained decoction, given by nasogastric tube.

Second visit: November 22, 1979. After taking the herbs, her right foot and hand relaxed, but she was still comatose and her tongue and pulse were unchanged. A modified version of Support Longevity and Release Speech Decoction (*zī shòu jiě yǔ tāng*)[24] was then prescribed:

> Notopterygii Rhizoma seu Radix *(qiāng huó)* 5g
> Uncariae Ramulus cum Uncis *(gōu téng)* 10g
> Powdered Saigae tataricae Cornu *(líng yáng jiǎo)* 10g
>   (taken with the strained decoction)
> Ziziphi spinosae Semen *(suān zǎo rén)* 10g
> Gastrodiae Rhizoma *(tiān má)* 10g
> Acori tatarinowii Rhizoma *(shí chāng pǔ)* 10g
> Eupatorii Herba *(pèi lán)* 10g
> Bambusae Caulis in taeniam *(zhú rú)*...................... 30g

Third visit: November 24, 1979. The patient's consciousness was occasionally clear, and when that occurred she could appropriately respond to questions. She was no longer incontinent and her tongue coating was white and rough; the tip of her tongue was red. She had a slippery pulse. These symptoms showed that while the internal wind was gone, the orifices had not yet opened. Treatment was therefore directed at transforming phlegm and dampness and opening the orifices:

> Moschus *(shè xiāng)*....................................... 3g
>   (taken with the strained decoction)
> Acori tatarinowii Rhizoma *(shí chāng pǔ)* 5g
> Eupatorii Herba *(pèi lán)* 10g
> Amomi Fructus rotundus *(bái dòu kòu)* 10g
> Curcumae Radix *(yù jīn)* 10g
> Forsythiae Fructus *(lián qiào)*........................ 15g
> Bambusae Caulis in taeniam *(zhú rú)*...................... 15g

Fourth visit: November 26, 1979. The patient had a clear mind and was in a good mood. Her appetite was very good, but she was thirsty and had not had a bowel movement for several days. The tongue coating was white and the tip of her tongue was red. The pulse was moderate. The presentation was that of yin damaged by heat. Therefore the treatment method was to enrich yin, moisten the Large Intestine, clear heat from the Heart, and transform dampness. A modified version of Increased the Fluids Decoction (*zēng yè tāng*) was prescribed:

Rehmanniae Radix *(shēng dì huáng)* 10g

Scrophulariae Radix *(xuán shēn)* 10g

Ophiopogonis Radix *(mài mén dōng)* 10g

Cistanches Herba *(ròu cōng róng)* 10g

Eupatorii Herba *(pèi lán)* 10g

Curcumae Radix *(yù jīn)* 5g

Semen Forsythiae Suspensae *(lian qiao xin)* 15g

Pruni Semen *(yù lǐ rén)* 10g

Nelumbinis Plumula *(lián zǐ xīn)* 10g

The patient took this basic formula through December 14, 1979. At that time all of her problems were resolved, and she went back to work.[25]

Commentary: This case was treated by Ni Xuan-Hua, a famous doctor from the city of Zigong in Sichuan province. The case shows how to deal in an orderly fashion with different pathological conditions related to warm pathogen diseases that have led to a critical condition. The first step is always to aggressively treat the excess condition so that the patient's life can be preserved, and thereafter to enrich the yin. The patient's high fever and mouth ulcers, together with diminished consciousness, reflected the presence of extreme heat. While the tongue coating evidenced some dampness, intense heat will always injure the yin to some degree. However, there was no significant evidence of yin deficiency, and this aspect was therefore of no particular importance at this time. Rather, the blockage of the Heart spirit and stirring up of Liver wind, evidenced by clenched teeth, coma, stiffness of the right arm and leg with right hand spasms, were of more immediate concern, and were actually signs of a life-threatening condition. What is more, the patient showed slight collapse of yang qi, evidenced in the incontinence of urine and stool, as well as yawning. Thus, the urgent and important thing to do was to save the patient first by extinguishing the Liver wind and opening the orifices by combining Antelope Horn and Uncaria Decoction *(líng jiǎo gōu téng tāng)* with Calm the Palace Pill with Cattle Gallstone *(ān gōng niú huáng wán)*.

After the first treatment, the patient's wind signs and symptoms were gone, but the Heart spirit condition was unchanged. This was because the treatment was focused on extinguishing Liver wind rather than opening the orifices. From my perspective, at this time the physician did not clearly differentiate between internal and external wind. He used a modified version of Support Longevity and Release Speech Decoction *(zī shòu jiě yǔ tāng)*, which contains the acrid, warm Notopterygii Rhizoma seu Radix *(qiāng huó)*, an herb that is inappropriate in this case. Fortunately, the patient's condition did not worsen, and the physician seemed to realize his mistake and accordingly changed the treatment to clear heat, resolve phlegm, transform dampness, and open the orifices. At the final stage of treatment he chose a modified version of Increase the

Fluids Decoction *(zēng yè tāng)* to nourish the yin while clearing heat and transforming dampness until the patient had totally recovered.

Ass-Hide Gelatin and Scutellaria Decoction *(ē jiāo huáng qín tāng)*

Male, 6 years old

During the eighth month of the lunar calendar [late August or early September], the patient presented with a dry cough and diarrhea. He first developed fever and aversion to cold and had been treated by a few practitioners, but without success. At the time of this visit his body felt hot and he had an unproductive cough and thirst. He also had watery stool that contained undigested food particles. His tongue was red, the coating white, and the pulse floating and big. The diagnosis was heat being transmitted from the Lung to the Large Intestine. The treatment method was to clear heat from the Lung and moisten the Large Intestine. A modified version of Ass-Hide Gelatin and Scutellaria Decoction *(ē jiāo huáng qín tāng)*[26] was prescribed:

Asini Corii Colla *(ē jiāo)*	3g
Scutellariae Radix *(huáng qín)*	9g
Armeniacae Semen *(xìng rén)*	4.5g
Lycii Cortex *(dì gǔ pí)*	9g
Glycyrrhizae Radix *(gān cǎo)*	1.2g

After finishing the first packet of herbs, the patient's diarrhea was reduced. After finishing the second packet, his feverish body and thirst were gone. After taking another two packets, his cough was gone.[27]

Commentary: If one ignores the time of year and just focuses on the signs and symptoms, sometimes one misses important opportunities for making correct differentiation and treatment. This case is a good example. The patient first had fever and aversion to cold in September, which is the early part of autumn. While this is the time of year during which patients are prone to autumn-dryness, this fact was overlooked by the first few practitioners who saw the boy, and their treatment had no effect. Furthermore, when we think of the reasons someone develops watery diarrhea containing undigested food particles, we usually think of problems of the Spleen or even the Kidney. At first glance, cough would seem to have no relationship with this kind of diarrhea. However, if we analyze the chronological order of the appearance of the various symptoms and consider the concept of a normal pro-gression,[28] we would realize that the development of diarrhea can be a positive sign, as it shows that the body is discharging the dry-heat. In this case, the watery diarrhea containing undigested food particles is the result of the intense dry-heat that has been transmitted from the Lung to the Large Intestine, and which is forcing water and food out of the body before they have been completely absorbed or transformed. Xiao Zhuo-Ru, a famous physician active in the early part of the twentieth century in Hunan province, noted that this was a normal transmission when the Lung and Large Intestine were attacked by dry-heat. He therefore decided to encourage the body's own response and prescribed Ass-Hide Gelatin and Scutellaria Decoction *(ē jiāo huáng qín tāng)* to moisten the Lung and clear and discharge the dry-heat. For this purpose, Asini Corii Colla *(ē jiāo)* enriches the Lung yin and moistens the Large Intestine, and Scutellariae Radix *(huáng qín)*, Lycii Cortex *(dì gǔ pí)*, and Glycyrrhizae Radix *(gān cǎo)* clear Lung heat. A very interesting idea here was the use of Armeniacae Semen *(xìng rén)*, as this herb promotes bowel movements while also moistening the Lungs and directing its qi downward. By means of this extremely apt approach, this seemingly difficult case was resolved within a few days.

Three-Nut Decoction *(sān rén tāng)*

C.H., female, age 74

The chief complaint was chest pain. The patient had surgery for cancer of the left breast followed by nine months of chemotherapy. Over the course of her treatment she experienced discomfort, tightness, and a burning pain in her left breast which required very strong pain medication. The pain was like a sunburn and so severe that even the weight of clothes would make it worse. While medication controlled the pain, she was not very functional. She was dizzy, nauseous, and could not do normal housework or drive. She decided to stop the medication and to use Chinese medicine instead to control the pain.

First visit: March 12, 1998. The patient had hot flashes, attacks of sweating (either in the morning or evening), a bitter taste, slight problem with breathing on inhalation, as well as slight heartburn and stomach upset that worsened after eating. While she had daily bowel movements, they did not feel complete. She felt stressed, which made it difficult for her to get to sleep. Her energy was fine (9-10 on a scale of 1 to 10). Her tongue had a purple edge and a yellow, greasy coating. She had a slightly rapid pulse that was slippery in both middle positions, and wiry and thin in the other positions. The diagnosis was damp-heat in all three burners (affecting the Lung, Heart, Spleen, Stomach, Liver, and Large Intestine) leading to qi and blood stagnation in the Liver and Stomach channels. The chosen treatment method was to clear heat while also transforming and draining dampness. A modified version of Three-Nut Decoction *(sān rén tāng)*[29] was prescribed:

Armeniacae Semen *(xìng rén)*	9g
Amomi Fructus rotundus *(bái dòu kòu)*	12g
Coicis Semen *(yì yǐ rén)*	24g
Magnoliae officinalis Cortex *(hòu pò)*	9g

Pinelliae Rhizoma preparatum *(zhì bàn xià)* 12g

Trichosanthis Pericarpium *(guā lóu pí)* 15g

Akebiae Caulis *(mù tōng)* 12g

Talcum *(huá shí)* 9g

Scutellariae Radix *(huáng qín)* 9g

Moutan Cortex *(mǔ dān pí)* 12g

She received three packets and was told to take one packet over the course of two days. She was also given acupuncture at the following points: ST-36 *(zū sān lǐ)*, SP-6 *(sān yīn jiāo)*, LR-3 *(tài chòng)*, and LI-4 *(hé gǔ)*.

Second visit: March 19, 1998. The patient's left chest was still sensitive, but there was no burning pain. The hot flashes were gone, and she was having three bowel movements a day that felt complete. While she still had some slight heartburn, the bitter taste was gone. Urine volume had increased. Her energy remained good and she was sleeping well, except for the previous night, when she had had some difficulty getting to sleep. The tongue had a slight purple edge, and the yellow, greasy tongue coating had diminished. The pulse was unchanged.

The same formula was used again, with slight modification: Amomi Fructus rotundus *(bái dòu kòu)* was reduced to 9g, and 3g of Honey-toasted Glycyrrhizae Radix preparata *(zhì gān cǎo)* was added. Three packets of the herbs were given to the patient, with one packet to be taken every two days. The acupuncture treatment was unchanged.

Third visit: March 26, 1998. The abnormal sensitivity of the left chest was the same as the last visit (0–2 on a scale of 0–4) with slight tightness. She had mild hot flashes and one instance of acid regurgitation. She also had loose stools for three days (2–3 times/day). The quality of her sleep varied with her stress level. The edge of the tongue was purple, and the yellow, greasy tongue coating had increased. The pulse was wiry, with slippery middle positions. At this time it was decided to focus more on moving the blood:

Armeniacae Semen *(xìng rén)* 9g

Amomi Fructus rotundus *(bái dòu kòu)* 9g

Coicis Semen *(yì yǐ rén)* 24

Magnoliae officinalis Cortex *(hòu pò)* 9g

Pinelliae Rhizoma preparatum *(zhì bàn xià)* 12g

Akebiae Caulis *(mù tōng)* 15g

Trichosanthis Pericarpium *(guā lóu pí)* 15g

Artemisiae scopariae Herba *(yīn chén)* 15g

Lycopi Herba *(zé lán)* 15g

Leonuri Herba *(yì mǔ cǎo)* 15g

Chuanxiong Rhizoma *(chuān xiōng)* 12g

Moutan Cortex *(mǔ dān pí)* 12g

Three packets of the herbs were given to the patient, each to be taken over the course of two days. Acupuncture points: ST-36 *(zú sān lǐ)*, SP-6 *(sān yīn jiāo)*, SP-9 *(yīn líng quán)*, and LR-8 *(qū quán)*.

Fourth visit: April 2, 1998. The sensitivity in her left chest continued to improve (0–1 on a scale of 0-4). She had slight hot flashes, one instance of acid regurgitation, and loose stools twice a day. She had slept well except for one night, and her energy was good. She had red dots on the tip of the tongue and slightly yellow coating on the root. Her distal and middle positions were wiry and slippery, while the proximal positions were submerged. The same acupuncture treatment was continued, and the dosage of Coicis Semen *(yì yǐ rén)* was increased to 30g. She was given three packets of herbs, each packet to last two days.

Fifth visit: April 9, 1998. The abnormal sensitivity of her left chest was now between 0 and 1 (on a scale of 0–4). She had no hot flashes, the acid regurgitation had decreased, and she was sleeping well. The tongue had a purple edge and a yellow, greasy, and dry coating in the center and root. Her pulse was slightly rapid and wiry; in addition, the middle position was slippery. LI-11 *(qū chí)* was added to the list of acupuncture points, and 12g of Talcum *(huá shí)* was added to the previous formula. She was given three packets of the herbs, each packet to last two days.

Sixth visit: April 16, 1998. The patient only felt the abnormal sensitivity of her left chest in the evening, and its intensity was between 0 and 1. She reported that she now had a sharp pain under the left arm that radiated down to the hypochondriac region. Other signs and symptoms were unchanged, except that the greasy tongue coating had disappeared. LI-11 *(qū chí)* was removed from the list of acupuncture points, and LR-3 *(tài chōng)* added. Likewise, 15g of Curcumae Radix *(yù jīn)* was added to the formula. She was given three packets of the herbs, each packet to last two days.

Seventh visit: April 20, 1998. There had been no abnormal sensitivity in her left chest for three days. The acid regurgitation and pain under the left arm were gone. Otherwise she was unchanged. The last treatment was repeated.

Eighth visit: April 30, 1998. There had been no abnormal sensitivity in her left chest for ten days. No other changes were noted. She was given the same acupuncture treatment as before. The herbal treatment was discontinued.

This patient has been followed up to the present, and there has been no abnormal sensitivity or pain on her left chest.[30]

Commentary: According to Wu Tang, some aspects of the presentation of a patient with damp-heat will be similar to those of yin deficiency, such as afternoon fever. Clinically, damp-heat syndrome may often present with other signs and symptoms that are similar to those of yin deficiency. It would be easy to think that hot flashes, sweating, burning sensation in the chest, and dizziness in a 74-year-old woman who had undergone nine months of chemotherapy would be caused by the deficiency of the Kidney and Liver yin. However, the tongue coating, one of the key factors in identifying yin deficiency, fails to support this conclusion. Rather, the patient had a greasy tongue coating and slippery pulse that suggests damp-heat. A careful analysis and grouping of the presentation made it clear that all three burners were involved: discomfort, tightness, and burning pain in the left breast, insomnia, and slight difficulty with breathing (upper burner); bitter taste, slight heartburn, and stomach upset that was worse after eating (middle burner); and an incomplete feeling following bowel movements (lower burner). Therefore, the diagnosis was damp-heat in the three burners, for which Three-Nut Decoction *(sān rén tāng)* was prescribed. The first stage of treatment focused on the damp-heat. Once this had diminished, the focus gradually changed to invigorating the blood.

Endnotes

1. Sun Si-Mo, *Important Formulas Worth a Thousand Gold Pieces for Any Emergency (Bèi jí qiān jīn yào fāng)*. Beijing: People's Health Publishing House, 1982: 1.

2. Mulberry Leaf and Chrysanthemum Drink *(sāng jú yǐn)* was discussed in Chapter 7.

3. The granules were ordered from the Spring Wind Company in the United States, and the concentration was 5:1.

4. This case is one of the author's.

5. Disseminate the White and Order the Qi Decoction *(xuān bái chéng qì tāng)* was discussed in Chapter 7.

6. This contains Indigo naturalis *(qīng dài)* and powdered Meretricis/Cyclinae Concha *(gé qiào)*. It was recorded in Zhang Bo-Yu et al., *Traditional Chinese Internal Medicine (Zhōng yī nèi kē xué)*. Shanghai: Shanghai Science and Technology Publishing House, 1985: 298.

7. Peng Jian-Zhong and Yang Lian-Zhu, *Selected Case Studies from Master Zhao Shao-Qin (Zhào Shào-Qín lín zhèng yàn àn jīng xuǎn)*. Beijing: Learning Garden Publishing House, 1996: 40.

8. White Tiger Decoction *(bái hǔ tāng)* was discussed in Chapter 7.

9. Calm the Palace Pill with Cattle Gallstone *(ān gōng niú huáng wán)* was discussed in Chapter 7.

10. Regulate the Stomach and Order the Qi Decoction *(tiáo wèi chéng qì tāng)* was discussed in Chapter 7.

11. Purple Snow Special Pill *(zǐ xuě dān)* was discussed in Chapter 7.

12. Dong Jian-Hua et al., *Selected Case Studies from Famous Modern Chinese Doctors (Zhōng guó xiàn dài míng zhōng yī yī àn jīng huá)*. Beijing: Beijing Publishing House, 1990: 1841.

13. Great Treasure Special Pill *(zhì bǎo dān)* was discussed in Chapter 7.

14. Clear the Nutritive Level Decoction *(qīng yíng tāng)* was discussed in Chapter 7.

15. This is the immature leaves of Lophatheri Herba *(dàn zhú yè)*, which are difficult to find outside of East Asia. Substitute with Lophatheri Herba *(dàn zhú yè)*

16. Chongqing Traditional Chinese Medicine Research Institute, *Traditional Chinese Medicine and Acute Conditions Report*, vol. 8 *(Zhōng yī jí zhèng tōng xùn)*. Chongqing: Chonging Traditional Chinese Medicine Research Institute, 1985: 6.

17. Increase the Fluids and Order the Qi Decoction *(zēng yè chéng qì tāng)* was discussed in Chapter 8.

18. This is a type of "wood ear" fungus that is sweet and neutral and enters the Stomach and Large Intestine channels. It cools blood and stops bleeding, and is used for bloody stools, dysenteric disorder, abnormal menstrual bleeding, and hemorrhoids.

19. Peng Jian-Zhong, Yang Lian-Zhu. *Selected Case Studies from Zhao Shao-Qin (Zhào Shào-Qín lín zhèng yàn àn jīng xuǎn)*. Beijing: Learning Garden Publishing House, 1996: 11.

20. Modified Transform Maculas Decoction *(huà bān tāng)* was discussed in Chapter 8.

21. Dong Jian-Hua et al., *Selected Case Studies from Famous Modern Chinese Doctors*, 1304. This case was presented by Xu You-Ling.

22. Antelope Horn and Uncaria Decoction *(líng jiǎo gōu téng tāng)* was discussed in Chapter 8.

23. Calm the Palace Pill with Cattle Gallstone *(ān gōng niú huáng wán)* was discussed in Chapter 7.

24. This formula was first recorded in Li Chan, *Introduction to Medicine (Yī xué rù mén)*. Beijing: Chinese Medicine Publishing House, 1995: 633. It contains Aconiti Radix lateralis preparata *(zhì fù zǐ)* (1g), Gastrodiae Rhizoma *(tiān má)* (1g), Saposhnikoviae Radix *(fáng fēng)* (1g), Ziziphi spinosae Semen *(suān zǎo rén)* (1g), Cinnamomi Cortex *(ròu guì)* (2.3g), Saigae tataricae Cornu *(líng yáng jiǎo)* (2.3g), Glycyrrhizae Radix *(gān cǎo)* (1.5g), Notopterygii Rhizoma seu Radix *(qiāng huó)* (1.5g), and a small amount of Bambusae Succus *(zhú lì)*.

25. Dong Jian-Hua et al., *Selected Case Studies from Famous Modern Chinese Doctors*, 1193. This case was presented by Ni Xuan-Hua.

26. Ass-hide Gelatin and Scutellaria Decoction *(ē jiāo huáng qín tāng)* was discussed in Chapter 9.

27. He Lian-Chen. *Revised Classified Case Studies from Nationally Famous Doctors (Chóng dìng quán guó míng yī yàn àn lèi biān)*. Shanghai: Shanghai Science and Technology Publishing House, 1959: 195.

28. See Chapter 4 for a discussion of these ideas, which were developed by Wang Shi-Xiong.

29. Three-Nut Decoction *(sān rén tāng)* was discussed in Chapter 12.

30. This is one of the author's cases.

APPENDIX D

Pinyin-English Cross Reference of Formula Names

PINYIN	ENGLISH	PAGE
ān gōng niú huáng wán	Calm the Palace Pill with Cattle Gallstone	232
bái hǔ tāng	White Tiger Decoction	224
bái hǔ jiā cāng zhú tāng	White Tiger plus Atractylodes Decoction	395
bái hǔ jiā rén shēn tāng	White Tiger Decoction plus Ginseng	369
chāng pǔ yù jīn tāng	Acorus and Curcuma Decoction	444
cōng chǐ jié gěng tāng	Scallion, Prepared Soybean and Platycodon Decoction	255
dà dìng fēng zhū	Major Arrest Wind Pearl	296
dá yuán yǐn	Reach the Source Drink	426
dǎo chì chéng qì tāng	Guide Out the Red and Order the Qi Decoction	271
dǎo chì qīng xīn tāng	Guide Out the Red and Clear the Heart Decoction	476
dú shēn tāng	Unaccompanied Ginseng Decoction	452
èr jiǎ fù mài tāng	Two Shell Modified Decoction to Restore the Pulse	295
èr jiǎ jiǎn zhèng qì sǎn	Second Modification of Rectify the Qi Powder	432
fāng xiāng yǐn	Fragrant Drink	341
fú líng pí tāng	Poria Peel Decoction	433
gān lù xiāo dú dān	Sweet Dew Special Pill to Eliminate Toxin	445

525

PINYIN	ENGLISH	PAGE
wǔ yè lú gēn tāng	Five Leaves and Reed Decoction	449
wǔ zhī yǐn	Five Juice Drink	324
xī dì qīng luò yǐn	Rhinoceros and Rehmannia Drink to Clear the Collaterals	478
xī jiǎo dì huáng tāng	Rhinoceros Horn and Rehmannia Decoction	283
xiǎo chéng qì tāng	Minor Order the Qi Decoction	448
xiǎo xiàn xiōng jiā zhǐ shí tāng	Minor Sinking into the Chest Decoction plus Unripe Bitter Orange	216
xīn jiā huáng lóng tāng	Newly Augmented Yellow Dragon Decoction	268
xīn jiā xiāng rú yǐn	Newly Augmented Mosla Drink	387
xìng rén huá shí tāng	Apricot Kernel and Talcum Decoction	442
xìng sū sǎn	Apricot Kernel and Perilla Leaf Powder	316
xuān bái chéng qì tāng	Disseminate the White and Order the Qi Decoction	218
xuān bì tāng	Disband Painful Obstruction Decoction	441
xuān qīng dǎo zhuó tāng	Decoction to Disseminate the Clear and Guide out the Turbid	436
Xuē shì jiě biǎo shèn shī xiè rè fāng	Xue's Formula to Release the Exterior, Leach Out Dampness, and Drain Heat	418
Xuē shì xīn xiāng jiě biǎo fāng	Xue's Acrid and Aromatic Formula to Release the Exterior	418
yī jiā jiǎn zhèng qì sǎn	First Modification of Rectify the Qi Powder	431
yì yǐ zhú yè sǎn	Coix and Lophatherus Powder	439
yín qiào sǎn	Honeysuckle and Forsythia Powder	199
yù nǔ jiān	Jade Woman Decoction	275
Yú shì qīng xīn liáng gé sǎn	Yu's Clear the Heart and Cool the Diaphragm Powder	348
yù yào shi	Jade Key	347
zēng yè chéng qì tāng	Increase the Fluids and Order the Qi Decoction	264
zhēn wǔ tāng	True Warrior Decoction	452
zhì bǎo dān	Greatest Treasure Special Pill	233
zhǐ shí dǎo zhì tāng	Unripe Bitter Orange Decoction to Guide Out Stagnation	474
zhǐ shí dǎo zhì wán	Unripe Bitter Orange Pill to Guide Out Stagnation	438
zhì zǐ chǐ tāng	Gardenia and Prepared Soybean Decoction	214
zǐ xuě dān	Purple Snow Special Pill	234

Materia Medica
and Formula Index

529

—— O

Olibanum *(rŭ xiāng)*, 340, 434

Ophiopogonis Radix *(mài mén dōng)*, 107, 142, 145, 148, 150, 153, 154, 180, 184, 198, 201, 220, 221, 224, 227, 229, 236, 239, 240, 264, 265, 266, 267, 268, 269, 270, 272, 275, 280, 294, 295, 296, 297, 321, 322, 324, 345, 354, 370, 371, 373, 375, 376, 382, 384, 393, 469, 477, 512, 513, 514, 515, 519

Oranges, 324

Order Qi and Nourish the Nutritive Decoction *(chéng qì yăng yíng tāng)*,15

Oroxyli Semen *(mù hú dié)*, 206

Ostreae Concha *(mŭ lì)*, 296, 297, 376

—— P

Paeoniae Radix alba *(bái sháo)*, 144, 149, 223, 258, 259, 266, 267, 269, 270, 279, 280, 283, 284, 285, 286, 290, 291, 292, 293, 294, 295, 296, 297, 315, 325, 353, 354, 426, 427, 452, 514, 515, 517

Paeoniae Radix alba, dry-fried *(bái sháo)*, 382

Paeoniae Radix rubra *(chì sháo)*, 143, 149, 165, 170, 183, 202, 230, 258, 269, 272, 276, 277, 278, 282, 283, 286, 339, 349, 351, 353, 441, 469, 478, 516

Panacis quinquefolii Radix *(xī yáng shēn)*, 150, 154, 184, 221, 270, 293, 322, 354, 371, 376

Patriniae Herba *(bài jiàng cǎo)*, 219, 272, 340, 349, 352

Peach Kernel Decoction to Order the Qi *(táo rén chéng qì tāng)*, 163, 274, **285-87**, 302

Peach Pit Decoction to Order the Qi *(táo hé chéng qì tāng)*, 286

Pear juice, 15, 224

Pears, 148, 184, 315, 322, 324, 507

Perillae Caulis *(zĭ sū gěng)*, 168, 317, 447

Perillae Folium *(zĭ sū yè)*, 207, 316, 317, 318, 359, 429

Perillae Fructus *(zĭ sū zĭ)*, 211

Persicae Semen *(táo rén)*, 116, 149, 183, 201, 278, 286, 327, 328, 385, 478

Peucedani Radix *(qián hú)*, 204, 207, 316, 317, 318, 390

Phaseoli radiati Semen *(lǜ dòu)*, 320

Phaseoli Semen *(chì xiǎo dòu)*, 441

Phellodendri Cortex *(huáng bǎi)*, 142, 145, 154, 155, 165, 272, 279, 280, 340, 360

Pheretima *(dì lóng)*, 379, 444

Phragmitis Rhizoma *(lú gēn)*, 137n6, 145, 152, 156, 180, 197, 199, 200, 201, 205, 207, 208, 212, 214, 224, 263, 272, 322, 324, 346, 349, 351, 352, 353, 397, 437, 446, 447, 449, 450, 506, 507, 509, 510

Phragmitis Rhizomatis Succus *(lú gēn zhī)*, 107

Pinelliae massa fermentata *(bàn xià qū)*, 168

Pinelliae Rhizoma preparatum *(zhì bàn xià)*, 59, 158, 165, 171, 175, 206, 211, 216, 217, 317, 318, 360, 374, 391, 420, 421, 422, 423, 424, 425, 428, 429, 430, 431, 437, 440, 441, 442, 446, 447, 473, 476, 509, 522

Pini Semen *(sōng zĭ rén)*, 327, 328

Piperis longi Fructus *(bì bá)*, 434

Plantaginis Herba *(chē qián cǎo)*, 325, 397

Plantaginis Semen *(chē qián zĭ)*, 361

Platycladi Cacumen *(cè bǎi yè)*, 211, 393, 451

Platycladi Cacumen, charred *(cè bǎi tàn)*, 284

Platycladi Semen *(bǎi zĭ rén)*, 327, 328

Platycodi Radix *(jié gěng)*, 153, 154, 157, 158, 199, 200, 201, 204, 205, 207, 208, 212, 223, 231, 256, 277, 316, 317, 318, 319, 320, 326, 338, 339, 346, 348, 349, 360, 361, 415, 418, 419, 506, 509

Pogostemonis/Agastaches Folium *(huò xiāng yè)*, 418, 419, 425, 430, 431, 449, 450

Pogostemonis/Agastaches Herba *(huò xiāng)*, 85, 108, 155, 158, 159, 161, 168, 200, 223, 359, 360, 361, 370, 389, 391, 395, 397, 416, 418, 420, 421, 422, 423, 431, 432, 445, 446, 450, 469

Polygonati odorati Rhizoma *(yù zhú)*, 145, 150, 180, 221, 269, 270, 315, 471

Polygonatum Odoratum Decoction *(wei rui tang)*, 9

Polygoni cuspidati Rhizoma *(hŭ zhàng)*, 219

Polygoni multiflori Radix, fresh *(xiān hé shŏu wū)*, 329, 449

Polyporus *(zhū líng)*, 85, 179, 280, 361, 416, 420, 421, 422, 434, 436

Poria *(fú líng)*, 85, 158, 161, 280, 290, 291, 292, 298, 317, 318, 341, 342, 360, 361, 373, 374, 391, 420, 421, 429, 432, 436, 438, 439, 440, 452

Poria Peel Decoction *(fú líng pí tāng)*, 160, **433-34**, 454

General Index

541

—— X

—— Y